W9-BXG-100

NURSES AND THE LAW

A Guide to Principles and Applications

Second Edition

Nancy J. Brent, JD, MS, RN

Attorney at Law
Chicago, Illinois

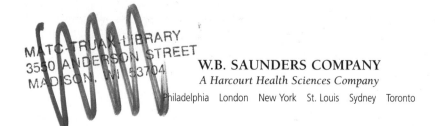

W.B. SAUNDERS COMPANY
A Harcourt Health Sciences Company
Philadelphia   London   New York   St. Louis   Sydney   Toronto

W.B. SAUNDERS COMPANY

A Harcourt Health Sciences Company

The Curtis Center
Independence Square West
Philadelphia, Pennsylvania 19106

Library of Congress Cataloging-in-Publication Data

Brent, Nancy J.
    Nurses and the law : a guide to principles and applications / Nancy J. Brent.—2nd ed.
      p.   cm.
    Includes index.
    ISBN 0-7216-9195-1
    1. Nursing—Law and legislation—United States. I. Title.

    KF2915.N8 B74 2001
    344.73'0414—dc21

                                00-049269

Vice President, Nursing Editorial Director: Sally Schrefer
Senior Editor: Michael S. Ledbetter
Senior Editorial Assistant: Avery C. Roberts
Production Manager: Donna L. Morrissey

NURSES AND THE LAW   ISBN 0-7216-9195-1

Printed in the United States of America

Last digit is the print number: 9   8   7   6   5   4   3   2   1

To my nephew,
Tristan Edward Weiss ("Teddy"),
who makes me laugh

About the Author

Nancy J. Brent received a Bachelor of Science degree with a major in nursing from Villa Maria College in Erie, Pennsylvania. Her Masters Degree in psychiatric–mental health nursing was obtained from the University of Connecticut in Storrs. After holding a number of clinical and teaching positions in nursing, Ms Brent attended Loyola University Chicago School of Law, graduating in 1981. Since 1986, Ms Brent has practiced law as a sole practitioner in Chicago, concentrating her practice in legal representation, consultation, and education for health care practitioners, health care delivery systems, and school of nursing faculty. She has published extensively in the area of law and nursing practice and has conducted many seminars across the country on law and health care delivery. The first edition of *Nurses and the Law* was named the *American Journal of Nursing* Book of the Year in Quality Improvement/Risk Management and in Nursing Administration. The text was also included in the 1998 Brandon Hill list as one for initial purchase in the area of law and nursing practice.

Contributors

MARGARET R. DOUGLAS, MS, RN
Associate Professor
Saint Xavier University School of Nursing
Director, Chicago Institute for Nursing Education
Chicago, Illinois
Ethics and Nursing Practice; Ethics Connections

MARY LINN GREEN, JD, MS, RN
Partner and Attorney at Law
Kostantacos, Reuterfors, McWilliams, Brandt & Green, PC
Rockford, Illinois
The Nurse in the Community

PAULA HENRY, JD, NP-C, BSN, RN
Attorney at Law
Lewis, D'Amato, Brisbois & Bisgard
Costa Mesa, California
The Nurse in Advanced Practice

Preface

The law and nursing practice continue to intertwine, indeed more deeply. Although some of the same legal issues that haunted nursing a short 4 years ago (e.g., unlicensed assistive personnel, work redesign [now often called "reengineering"], managed care) continue to do so now, new problems have developed. One such concern is of paramount importance, not only to nursing but also to consumers of health care around the world: the current nursing shortage. It is probably fair to say that this shortage has grown mainly out of the difficulties faced by nursing 4 years ago: managed care, declining student enrollments in baccalaureate nursing programs, the increased acuity of patients treated in hospitals, and the aging "baby boomer" population resulting in more and more retirements of nurses in the clinical, administrative, research, and academic areas.[1,2] Despite its origins, the shortage, already seen in the United States, Canada, England, the Philippines, Australia, and Western Europe, is ominous. Estimates indicate that in the year 2010, only 656,000 registered nurses with a baccalaureate will be available, whereas the need for the baccalaureate prepared registered nurses alone will be 1,385,000.[3]

The legal implications of such a shortage are numerous. Who, for example, will care for those acutely ill patients who need skilled care, whether on a "general" medical-surgical unit or in the ICU? What kind of care can be given if there are not adequate numbers of registered nurses and/or registered nurses skilled and experienced in the nursing care they provide? Will the standard of care currently required of the registered nurse by law change to a lesser standard? After all, if injury or death of patients occurs because of a number and experience shortage, should the registered nurse be held to a standard of care that may become impossible to meet? And who will educate the men and women who enter nursing education programs if "older" faculty retire and there is no one to replace them? The answers to these and many other questions are not easily found.

Mandatory nurse staffing ratios are a second legal implication that has come to the profession's and the public's attention in the last few years. California was the first state to pass such legislation,[4] but the true impact of this and other laws that may be passed mandating staff numbers is still to be determined. Proponents of such bills believe that requiring certain nursing staff numbers is at least a "start" in preserving the quality of patient care and in helping staff nurses achieve a better working environment.[5] Opponents, however, clearly argue that mandatory ratios are not the answer because any staffing number must also reflect other factors, including the nurse's education and experience, patients' acuity, and nursing administration resources available to the staff nurse while he or she is on duty.[6] Additionally, opponents argue that mandatory nursing staff ratios may indeed become more *maximum* indicators of staffing rather than *minimum* totals.[7] Regardless of the position taken on mandatory nurse staffing ratios, it is a moot issue if there are simply not enough registered or other nurses to fill the ratios adopted.

On the brighter side, many nurses who are still practicing are continuing to contribute to the nursing profession and the public's well-being through the establishment of their own businesses. These nurse entrepreneurs are involved in establishing free-standing clinics, establishing and running consultation businesses in such areas as patient classification systems and nursing informatics, and inventing health care products.[8] Entrepreneurship is not for everyone, however, nor is it something that is usually taught in nursing education programs. The legal implications of establishing and running a business are also numerous and include the organization structure of the business, professional and other liability insurance concerns, and employment considerations.

Although the legal issues intertwined with nursing practice that are mentioned here are by no means an exhaustive list, they illustrate the continued relationship that law and nursing experience. It is clear that the relationship between law and nursing will not end. If anything, it will become stronger and continue to change. In fact, a recent study of 634 nursing school administrators of National League for Nursing (NLN)–accredited nursing programs and their inclusion of legal aspects in nursing content in the programs revealed that legal issues in nursing practice is "emerging as essential content in nursing curricula."[9]

It is hoped the second edition of *Nurses and the Law* will help both students of nursing and practicing nurses achieve a better understanding of the long-standing role of law in nursing practice. As was done in the first edition, this edition identifies legal principles and applies them to nursing practice. A new feature in this text is the application of ethical principles to nursing practice. In addition to writing the excellent chapter Ethics and Nursing Practice (Chapter 3), Margaret Douglas has developed Ethics Connections to help the reader critically analyze ethical ideals and apply them to nursing practice.

The text has been organized in much the same manner as the first edition was organized. Part One consists of an overview of the law and of ethics as it applies to nursing practice generally. Part Two identifies fundamental legal and ethical concerns common to all areas of nursing practice. Part Three applies specific legal and ethical issues to identified roles in specific practice settings.

Readers saw the identification of legal principles at the beginning of each chapter as a helpful feature in the first edition. As a result, they are again listed at the beginning of each chapter. The use of actual court cases and examples of the application of legal principles from clinical practice were also identified as helpful features in the first edition, so they are also included in this edition. The added use of ethical principles and their discussion throughout the text will, I believe, enhance the reader's understanding of those principles and support the reader in comparing and contrasting the legal and ethical concerns inherent in nursing practice in today's world.

Tables are used liberally throughout the book to help the reader view material in a compact format. The Documentation Reminders provide a checklist approach to the reader for consideration when documenting patient care. Each chapter also ends with a list of topics for further inquiry. The topics lists have been used to provide additional study projects for nursing students, either as part of their initial course on nursing and the law or as a beginning point for more advanced scholarly inquiry.

Every attempt was made to ensure that the information in this book, both legal and ethical, is up-to-date, current, and accurate. Even so, the same caveat given in the first edition bears repeating in this edition. The law is not static; rather, it is ever changing. So, too, are the ethical issues confronting nursing practice in a state of constant flux. As a result, the reader must be certain to supplement the text with the latest information available on new court decisions, keep up with new legislation passed on both the state and federal level, and explore new areas of ethical concerns in nursing practice.

Change, it is said, is inevitable. This statement is certainly applicable to health care delivery and to nursing, especially today. Nursing cannot afford, then, to remain static. Rather, it must be pliable, clever, and proactive while still retaining what does not need to be changed. Critically analyzing the law and ethics and how each fits into their respective relationship with nursing will be one of the continuing challenges of each and every nurse and of the nursing profession generally.

Nancy J. Brent

REFERENCES

1. Sigma Theta Tau International Society of Nursing. *Facts About Nursing.* July 1999, 1–4. Available on the society's web page at http://www.nursingsociety.org/media/facts_nursingshortage.html. Accessed July 20, 1999.
2. Margaret M. Sloan, "Who Will Fill the Shoes of Aging Nurses?" 12(5) *Nursing Spectrum* (1999), 4–5; Margaret M. Sloan, "Aging Faculty Adds to RN Shortage," 12(5) *Nursing Spectrum* (1999), 6.
3. *Facts About Nursing, supra* note 1, at 2.
4. Leah Curtin, "Staffing: Kicking 'butt' California Style!" 2(1) *Curtin Calls . . .* (2000), 1–2.
5. *Id.*
6. American Nurses Association. *Principles on Nurse Staffing with Annotated Bibliography.* Washington, DC: Author, 1999.
7. Leah Curtin, *supra* note 4, at 2.
8. "The Entrepreneurs: Nurses Inspired with Ideas and Innovations," 25(2) *Reflections,* 1999 (entire edition dedicated to nurse entrepreneurs).
9. Mable Smith-Pittman, Joann Richardson, and Chouh-Jiaun Lin, "An Exploration of Content on Legal Aspects of Practice in Nursing Programs," 38(9) *Journal of Nursing Education,* 1999, 406.

Acknowledgments

It is amazing to me how many people it takes to write and produce a book. Even with my experience of knowing what is needed from the work on the first edition, I somehow erased that knowledge from my memory until I started working on this edition. Although the computer greatly aided me in doing most, if not all, of the research that took at least five people to do for the first edition, there was still a great deal of research needed. Checking for new case law, evaluating legal and nursing journal articles, identifying position statements, and finding informative web sites took a great deal of *my* time. I am thankful that I had such a great computer to work with and am thankful for the creative and accessible web sites with legal information available at the click of a mouse. I am also eternally grateful to my high school typing teacher who forced me to learn to type, using various threats that were probably legal at the time but which would not be acceptable today. I remember thinking of her class as an "easy class," a welcome relief from the academic courses I was taking. Little did I know how important her class would be as I went on to college, graduate school, law school, and undertook two editions of this text.

I also would like to thank my friends, family, and my nursing and law colleagues for their support during this edition's work. Many endured long silences from me and rescheduled lunch and visits as I slaved to finish the revisions. As was the case during the work on the first edition, many offered to help with proofreading, gathering references, or suggesting ideas.

I must also thank Linda Semenzin, my computer person, for her loyal and unwavering work on this edition. Her skill and expertise in doing all the revisions in an accurate and timely manner were invaluable. Although I would like to think the process this time around was a little easier because we had computer disks from the first edition to work with, the revision process was still tedious, detailed, and time consuming for her. Her contribution is even more amazing for two reasons. First, Linda began working full-time at a great job before we started on the revisions. So her work on the book had to take place during the evening after a long day at work and on weekends. Yet she did so without complaining and without missing deadlines we had to adhere to. Second, Linda continued working on the book even when hospitalized for a yet-to-be identified illness. When she called to tell me she was going to be hospitalized, one of her first concerns was the work still to be done on the book. I told her we would deal with that when she found out what she needed to do for herself. As it turned out, she was able to finish the work on the book with minimal delay. She is home, working, and feeling better too. She is truly amazing, and I am forever grateful to her.

My husband has also been patient and supportive during the work on this second edition. He still asked about the book's completion on a regular basis (like he did with the first edition), but the form of the question became, "Can we start living again soon?"

Thomas Eoyang, the editor of the first edition of the book, became the editor for this edition as well. I was grateful for his presence again this time around, since we work well together and have always been able to openly communicate our issues and concerns and above all get the "work" done. I was saddened when Thomas informed me near the completion of the revisions that he was leaving publishing to pursue other career opportunities. Selfishly, I wanted him to stay forever—or at least until I finished the book. But I am happy and excited for him as he explores new challenges in his life. I know, though, that I would not have attempted a second edition if he had not been the editor at the start of this project. His suggestions, support, and experience in the world of publishing were such assets for me. I will miss him in this role but look forward to what he decides to become in his next role. We will be keeping in touch.

Nancy J. Brent

Contents

PART ONE

Overview

The Government and the Law

1

KEY PRINCIPLES

- Constitution
- Bill of Rights
- Separation of Powers Doctrine
- Right
- Due Process of Law
- Equal Protection of the Law

The United States had its first constitution embodied in the Articles of Confederation, which was in effect from 1781 until 1789.[1] The Articles established a loose alliance of independent states with a central government. The powers of the government were limited, and there was no judiciary. Furthermore, the executive powers of the estab-lished system were weak at best.[2] As a result, Congress was given most of the power in the early system of government.

On March 4, 1789, the "new" federal Constitution, which had been formulated at the 1787 Constitutional Convention and eventually ratified by 11 states, became the second framework of the government. It was composed of a preamble stating its purpose, articles, and several amendments.[3] The articles governed such topics as (1) the legislative, executive, and judicial branches of the government; (2) the relationship of the states to each other and to the central government; and (3) ways in which the Constitution could be amended.[4]

Although the new Constitution was seen by many as an improvement over the Articles, for some it did not contain adequate protections for the continued sovereignty of the states and individual rights. Thus, specific amendments to the Constitution were proposed to "limit and qualify the powers of the government."[5] Those amendments, which were accepted by the states in 1792, became known as the Bill of Rights.

Despite the attempt to balance the powers of the federal government with those of individuals and states, the struggle did not end. Because the Constitution was established as the "supreme law of the land,"[6] the courts continued to further define and interpret the respective relationship between the federal government and the state governments and their citizens. Moreover, the Constitution itself continued to change. As of 1983, 26 amendments or articles to the federal Constitution had been ratified.[7]

Interestingly, before development of the federal Constitution, states tried to define their power by adopting their own constitutions. The definition of power by the states focused on several issues: their respective abilities to govern their particular state, limitations on the ability of the state government to usurp individual state citizens' rights, the interrelationship between the state governments, and where the federal government's power ends and a state's power is at least shared with the federal government or becomes supreme. Although each state eventually adopted its own constitution, these issues are still of concern today.

Clearly, the federal Constitution and state constitutions are ever-changing documents.

Clearly, the federal Constitution and state constitutions are ever-changing documents. Their applicability to all aspects of life, whether in the 1800s or the 21st century, is ever present, albeit in differing interpretations and applications of those charters. This chapter will present selected aspects of the U.S. Constitution and state constitutional principles as they apply to the nurse and health care delivery. The chapter illustrates the respective governments' abilities to directly or indirectly influence a nurse in his or her individual and professional life in two major areas: individual constitutional rights and the legislative process.

ESSENTIALS OF THE GOVERNMENT AND THE LAW

There is no question that the government influences a person's life, whether professional or private. What is unique about this influence is twofold. One distinctive aspect is the balancing of the state governments' power with federal governmental power. The second is the emphasis on the balancing of governmental power with the personal and collective liberties citizens possess.

The Constitution

A constitution is the primary law of a nation or state that establishes the character and organization of its government, limits and distributes power within the government, and establishes the extent and manner of the exercise of the government's power.[8]

Federal Constitution

The federal Constitution is composed of seven articles and 26 amendments, the first 10 of which have traditionally been called the Bill of Rights.[9] However, all 26 amendments focus on individual rights that are protected against governmental intrusion.[10]

The Constitution's purpose, included in its Preamble, is to "form a more perfect Union, establish justice, insure domestic tranquility, provide for the common defence, promote the general welfare, and secure the blessings of Liberty to ourselves and our Posterity."[11] The original seven articles are summarized in Table 1–1.

BILL OF RIGHTS. The American Bill of Rights (Table 1–2) is included in the U.S. Constitution and is composed of the first 10 amendments to the original articles. The first 10 amendments were ratified December 15, 1791, and the remaining amendments were enacted in the period from 1795 to 1971.

It is interesting to note that the Bill of Rights, and the subsequent amendments, have essentially remained unchanged since their adoption. This fact is particularly interesting since the Bill of Rights was passed when the Constitution was less than 5 years old.[12] Furthermore, only three amendments (XI, XIV, and XVI) were enacted to overturn Supreme Court decisions.[13] Thus, although the character of the Constitution and the Bill of Rights may change with court decisions interpreting the

TABLE 1-1

Articles of U.S. Constitution

ARTICLE	ESSENCE OF ARTICLE
I	Establishes legislative branch of government, Congress, with a Senate and House of Representatives; powers and limitations of Congress listed, including promoting the general welfare, regulating interstate commerce, and establishing courts inferior to the Supreme Court
II	Establishes executive power in the U.S. president; spells out how president is elected; makes president commander in chief of Army and Navy; allows president to recommend legislation; provides for State of the Union reports to Congress
III	Bases judicial power in one Supreme Court and inferior courts established by Congress; provides for Supreme Court to review "Article III" lower court decisions where jurisdiction exists (e.g., constitutional questions, laws of the United States, and treaties)
IV	"Full Faith and Credit" given by each state to other states' "Acts, Records and Judicial Proceedings"; citizens in each state granted "privileges and immunities" of citizens in all states; guarantees to all states a "Republican Form of Government"
V	Enumerates the manner in which amendments to the Constitution can occur
VI	Establishes the Constitution and the laws of the United States as the "supreme Law of the Land"; Congress is bound by oath to uphold Constitution; no "Religious Test" can be required as a qualification for any U.S. office or public trust
VII	Ratification of the Conventions of nine States required to "establish" Constitution

"black letter language" of this document, its basic framework continues to survive.

State Constitutions

State constitutions vary in their organization and content, so it is difficult to summarize their contents. However, in the Illinois Constitution, as an example, there are 14 articles covering such topics as a bill of rights—for example, freedom of speech, due process protections, and the rights of one accused of a crime (Article I), powers of the state (Article II), the respective branches of the government (Articles IV, V, VI), and the manner in which the state constitution can be revised (Article XIV). Clearly, a state constitution will include topics similar to those included in the federal Constitution. However, it is important to note that because the U.S. Constitution is the principal law, no state law (or court, for that matter) can reduce the guarantees afforded by the U.S. Constitution.

Separation of Powers of Government

The Separation of Powers Doctrine is an essential foundation of constitutional law and the respective organization of the United States and state governments. Basically it is the practice of dividing the powers of a government among its constituent parts to avoid a concentration of power in any one part, which could lead to abuse.[14] In the U.S. Constitution there are two parts to the doctrine:

a *functional* demarcation between the government and the governed and between the branches of the government (the legislative, executive, and judicial); and a *regional* distinction between federal and state governments.[15]

State constitutions also utilize the functional demarcation. The regional distinction is also incorporated within state constitutions; however, its character is composed of a delineation between the state and local governments.

> *. . . on both the federal and state levels, there is a tripartite system of government, each branch having its own distinct powers.*

Thus, on both the federal and state levels, there is a tripartite system of government, each branch having its own distinct powers. For example, the legislative division (Congress or a particular state legislature) passes laws. In contrast, the executive branch (the president or the governor) is charged with carrying out the laws enacted by the legislature. The judicial division is responsible for interpreting, construing, applying, enforcing, and administering the laws of the state or federal government.[16]

TABLE 1-2

Amendments to the U.S. Constitution

AMENDMENT	ESSENCE OF AMENDMENT
I	Congress cannot pass laws concerning (1) establishment of religion or its free exercise; (2) limits on freedom of speech, the press, or the right of peaceful assembly; and (3) the right to petition the government for redress of grievances
II	States cannot be limited in their ability to establish their own military to maintain security, nor can states limit the people in their right to keep and bear arms
III	In peacetime, no soldier can be housed in any private home without the owner's consent; in war, housing soldiers in private homes may occur, but only by law
IV	No unreasonable search or seizure of property or person can take place; a warrant can be issued only for probable cause, supported by an oath or affirmation, and must include a description of the place to be searched and the person and property to be seized
V	Prosecution of criminal offenses must be initiated with an indictment of a grand jury (except for U.S. or state armed forces); protection against being tried for the same offense twice (double jeopardy); no individual can be compelled to be a witness against himself in criminal case; no deprivation of life, liberty, or property without due process of law; no private property taken for public use without just compensation
VI	In criminal cases, accused has right to (1) speedy and public jury trial; (2) notice of nature and cause of accusation; (3) face witnesses against him; (4) use established procedures to require favorable witnesses to be present at trial; (5) an attorney
VII	In common lawsuits in which the amount in controversy is more than $20, trial by jury shall exist; when a jury renders its verdict, no fact shall be reexamined except pursuant to established common law rules
VIII	In criminal cases, no excessive bail or fines can be imposed, nor cruel and unusual punishment inflicted upon prisoners
IX	The constitutional rights shall not be used to deny or disparage others retained by the people
X	The powers not delegated to the United States by the Constitution or prohibited by it are retained by the respective states or by the people
XI	Limits the power of the federal courts to hear cases in law or equity in which one state sues another or in which the case involves citizens of any foreign state
XII	Enumerates procedures for the election of president and vice president; limitations on presidential terms and the succession of the president in event of death, resignation, or incapacitation
XIII	Abolishes slavery and involuntary servitude
XIV	Declares that persons born or naturalized in the United States and subject to its jurisdiction are U.S. citizens and citizens of the state where they live; prohibits a state from passing or enforcing any law that diminishes privileges or immunities of U.S. citizens; a state cannot deprive a person of life, liberty, or property without due process of law, or deny any person within its jurisdiction equal protection of the law; enumerates certain voting rights (male and over 21 years); grants Congress the power to pass legislation to enforce amendment
XV	Says that U.S. citizens' voting rights cannot be denied or limited by any state or the United States on account of race, color, or previous servitude
XVI	Establishes the ability of Congress to impose and collect taxes on income.
XVII	Provides for the direct election of U.S. senators
XVIII	Prohibited manufacture, sale or transportation, importation and exportation of intoxicating liquors in United States and all territories
XIX	Prohibits denial or limitation by any state or United States of voting rights on account of sex; grants Congress the power to pass legislation to enforce amendment
XX	See comment for Amendment XII
XXI	Repealed Amendment XVIII; transportation or importation of intoxicating liquors into a state in violation of state law prohibited
XXII	See comment for Amendment XII
XXIII	Grants District of Columbia residents the right to vote for president and vice president
XXIV	Eliminates poll tax in federal elections
XXV	See comment for Amendment XII
XXVI	Prohibits denial or limitation by a state or United States of voting rights on account of age for citizens 18 years of age and older

This organization serves as a system of checks and balances within the three components of a particular government to ensure a balance of power among the three. For example, when a decision is made by the U.S. Supreme Court (judicial branch) that interprets a particular federal law contrary to the intent of Congress (legislative branch) when that law was passed, Congress can, through its established processes, pass another amendment to the law in question that essentially nullifies the Supreme Court decision. Or, if the governor of a particular state vetoes a particular bill the state legislature has passed, it can attempt to override the veto in a special legislative session.

Some of the powers exclusively given to one branch of government may be exercised by another branch as well. For example, on the state level, the governor appoints heads of administrative agencies, such as the head of the department responsible for enforcing professional practice acts. In essence, the governor delegates to the appointed head the power to carry out the acts. Any delegated power cannot be exceeded, however. If that does occur, then there can be a challenge to the actions of the agency, person, or department that has allegedly exceeded the powers delegated to perform the responsibilities of the position.

Also, the president of the United States (executive branch) can issue executive orders or regulations (legislative function) that provide guidance for the implementation of, interpretation of, or credence given to a particular provision of the Constitution, a law, or a treaty.[17] The power to issue the orders or regulations, published in the *Federal Register* and codified in Title 3 of the *Code of Federal Regulations,* illustrates a *unique* variation of the executive branch's traditional power.

Individual Rights and Governmental Powers

A right is a power or privilege to which a person is entitled.[18] There are various rights, including moral, human, and legal ones. Each right possesses a different basis and character. Human rights, for example, are basic and fundamental ones that every individual should enjoy. They are expressed in many documents, including the United Nations Universal Declaration of Human Rights.

A right is a power or privilege to which a person is entitled.

Legal rights, in contrast, are those conveyed by constitution, statute, or common (case) law.[19] They include personal rights (e.g., personal liberty), civil rights (e.g., trial by jury and the equal protection of the laws), constitutional protections (e.g., freedom of speech and the press), and political rights (e.g., voting and citizenship).

Furthermore, a right may be absolute or conditional.[20] Thus, a nurse has the right to believe whatever he or she wants to. However, when that belief impinges on another person's rights, as when the belief is used in a discriminatory manner to withhold care from a particular group of patients, then the right of acting on that belief becomes conditional.

Rights may also be substantive or procedural. Substantive rights are the rights themselves, that is, the essence of the particular power or privilege. Procedural rights are those that govern the process and methods whereby governmental policies are carried out and actions occur. For example, a nurse's First Amendment right of free speech may be violated, which is a substantive violation. In addition, however, if the government did not use the required approach in limiting or restricting the speech (refusing to respond to the nurse's request for a rally permit, for example), then the nurse would be able to allege a procedural violation as well.

The individual rights guaranteed by the United States and the various state constitutions are numerous, complex, and ever changing. Although they will be discussed as they relate to the nurse as an individual and as a professional in various chapters throughout this book, a brief, general overview of selected rights follows. Such an approach will aid the reader in further developing knowledge about them when studying a particular right in subsequent chapters.

First Amendment Rights

First Amendment rights, such as freedom of religion, press, and speech, are self-explanatory. However, these individual rights can change their character in health care. For example, freedom of religion takes on a new meaning when an individual refuses treatment based on his or her religious beliefs. Moreover, the right becomes more complex when it is exercised by a parent on behalf of a minor child.

Likewise, when a nursing faculty member's ability to speak in class is limited in some way by a public institution, his or her First Amendment rights are potentially at risk. Similarly, if a public university limits a nursing student's ability to participate in a rally against restricting abortion rights, his or her right of association is threatened.

Fourth Amendment Rights

The freedom from unreasonable searches and seizures clearly includes protection from governmental invasion of one's home without justification and the rights of one accused of a crime when there is an attempt to use evidence at trial in violation of these rights. This amendment, and parallel state constitutional protections, also protect the nursing student in a public university who may be asked to provide a urine or blood sample for drug screening or a patient in a government hospital who is searched for drugs in its emergency room.

Fifth and Fourteenth Amendment Rights

The Fifth and the Fourteenth Amendments to the U.S. Constitution protect certain individual rights from being restricted by the federal and state governments, respectively. Both amendments state, among other things, that no federal or state government can deprive a person of "life, liberty, or property" without due process of law. Throughout the Bill of Rights' history, this language has been at the center of a multitude of lawsuits that have attempted not only to define what due process is, but also to delineate what life, liberty, and property include.

What is clear is that life, liberty, and property protected in these amendments have literal interpretations as well as more abstract meanings. For example, one accused of a crime is afforded many protections during the legal process so that his or her liberty and, possibly, life are not taken without due process. Furthermore, a person's real property (a house or parcel of land) cannot be taken by the government for a state road or federal highway without due process. These amendments protect more conceptual rights as well, such as a nursing license (property) or one's reputation and ability to be accepted into an academic program (liberty).

In addition, the Fourteenth Amendment's protections have been extended by various court decisions to other situations not specifically mentioned in the amendment's language. One such protection is the right of privacy. Thus the protection of privacy has been interpreted to mean that one has a right to refuse treatment, to have an abortion, and to decide whether or not to use birth control without undue governmental restriction.

> *Procedural due process . . . has been defined by the courts as what is fair under the circumstances.*

Although still far from clear, due process has generally been divided into two types: *procedural* and *substantive*. Procedural due process, like procedural rights, is composed of the methods used by the government in executing its policies. Thus, it has been defined by the courts as what is *fair* under the circumstances. To define each and every circumstance and each and every procedural protection that would be afforded in those circumstances would be difficult, however. Therefore, courts have customarily looked at the right that might be limited or eliminated by the particular government and then determined what process would be due to ensure fairness. Thus an individual charged with a crime would be afforded *more* due process protections than would an individual whose driver's license needed renewal.

Keep in mind that due process protections are mandated only when the federal or state government encroaches upon individual rights guaranteed by the two respective amendments. The requirement does not apply to private actions. When a state government is involved, the action is called "state action" or is referred to as being carried out "under color of state law."

Fourteenth Amendment's Equal Protection Clause

The Equal Protection Clause located in the Fourteenth Amendment to the U.S. Constitution prohibits state governments from making unreasonable classifications in their laws. The federal government is also prohibited from doing so by the Fifth Amendment's Due Process Clause.[21]

In essence, this mandate requires that all people similarly situated be treated the same under the law of the particular government. This mandate has also been tested in the courts throughout its history with varying results. The differences in court decisions can be attributed to many factors, including (1) the existence of a *reasonable,* as opposed to an *unreasonable,* classification being passed by a government; and (2) individuals challenging a particular law not being "similarly situated" to the group or class they were comparing themselves to.

If there is an equal protection challenge to a particular governmental classification, the court will evaluate the distinction by utilizing several tests. If, for example, the categorization creates a "suspect class" (based on race or national origin) or impacts a *fundamental* right, the "compelling interest" or "strict scrutiny" test will be applied. The category would be upheld under this test only if it promoted a compelling interest or purpose of the government.

A second test applied by the courts to evaluate governmentally based classes is the "rational basis" test. This test is used for laws relating to economics and social welfare issues. If the questioned law is "rationally related to a legitimate governmental interest" and not arbitrary, it can be upheld.

A third test relates to those classes that are not included in the first two categories. It has been called the "rationality plus" test, and is often used by the court when interpreting a classification impacting sensitive classes, such as those of gender. So long as there is a "fair and substantial" relationship to a government's purpose, the classification is often found to be constitutional.

An example of the equal protection concept would be found in the state's ability to regulate the practice of nursing. Classifications exist in nurse practice acts regulating who can obtain a professional or practical nursing license and who cannot. This is a legitimate exercise of the state's police power in regulating the practice of the nursing profession. If that regulation became discriminatory, however, it could be challenged.

For example, if a state did not allow males who met the requisite requirements to apply for a nursing license, a male could challenge the classification and the way in which it was administered in his situation as a violation of his equal protection rights. Most probably, the court would apply a "rationality plus" test, and unless the state could show that gender was related to a particular governmental purpose, the classification would be struck down as unconstitutional.

THE LEGISLATIVE PROCESS

Federal Legislative Body

The legislative body of the federal government is Congress, which is composed of the House of Representatives and the Senate. The Senate has 100 members and the House is composed of 435 members. Their composition and powers are spelled out in the U.S. Constitution. The primary function of Congress is to enact statutes by vote of the entire membership.[22]

State Legislative Bodies

State legislative bodies, called a legislature or assembly, are similarly organized as in the federal system, although variations exist according to the state's constitution. For example, the Illinois General Assembly is composed of a senate and a house of representatives, whereas Nebraska's legislature consists of one house called a senate. In New Hampshire the legislature is called the General Court.

How a Bill Becomes Law
Initiation of the Process

Laws arise when a need or change is identified by someone. The impetus to initiate the legislative process can come from individuals, professional or voluntary groups, the governor or president, or a legislator or assembly member. Once the idea concerning the proposed need or change is crystallized, the proposal is drafted into acceptable legislative form and language. Then a sponsor of the bill is obtained. In Congress, the sponsor must be a senator or a representative. The selection of a sponsor is critical to the success or defeat of the proposed bill, for the legislative sponsor's commitment to the proposal is vital if it is to survive the next step of the process.

Introduction of the Proposed Bill

Once drafted and prior to its introduction into the legislative body, a proposed bill is given a number. For example, if a bill is introduced on the federal level into the House of Representatives, it is given an H.R. designation and number (e.g., 1234). A proposed bill in the Senate is given an S. designation and number (1234). Proposed bills may also be the result of joint sponsorship from the two assemblies and would be denoted with an "H.J.Res." or "S.J.Res." title and number.

The impetus to initiate the legislative process can come from individuals, professional or voluntary groups, the governor or president, or a legislator or assembly member.

Assignment to Committee

Once introduced into the "chamber of origin," the bill is assigned to a committee or subcommittee of that chamber. The assignment depends on the subject matter of the proposed legislation. For example, in Congress, three sets of House and Senate committees authorize laws governing the Public Health Service, set limits on spending, and appropriate moneys yearly for the Service's programs.[23]

The work done while the bill is in committee is legion and extremely important. Generally several actions can be taken in reference to the proposal, including refusal to consider it; major or minor changes; and approval and return of the proposal to the chamber floor.[24] If the bill is not rejected immediately, the committee work then involves four major activities: (public) hearings; "markups" (changes made in the legislation); voting on the proposal by the committee; and reporting back to the legislative body (to apprise the members so they can cast their votes).[25]

Floor Action

The proposed bill is sent to the "originating chamber" by the committee, and the bill is debated, amended, and voted upon. If it is defeated, the proposed bill dies. If it is passed, it then goes to the other assembly, if one exists, and the entire process of committee work and floor action is repeated. Any differences in the proposed bill must be reconciled between the two chambers. If that does not occur, the proposed bill dies. If passed by the entire legislative body, the proposal is sent to the president or governor for consideration.

Action by the President or the Governor

The chief executive has two options when proposed legislation reaches his or her desk. It can be signed or not signed within the applicable time frame (for example, the president of the United States has 10 days, excluding Sunday, to act upon the proposal); in either case, the proposal becomes law. The proposal can also be vetoed. If vetoed, the proposal is usually sent back to the legislative body with the chief executive's rationale for the veto.

If it so chooses, the state or federal legislative branch can attempt to override the veto pursuant to the applicable constitution. For Congress, a two-thirds vote of each house will override the president's veto. For most state legislatures, a two-thirds or three-fifths majority of both houses is required.

Bill Becomes Law

Many bills contain provisions that specify when the bill will become law. The provision may indicate that the effective date is 1 year from ratification or that enactment is immediate, or it may delineate some other time frame. If a bill does not contain an effective date provision, in the federal system a bill becomes law on the date it is signed by the president or on the date the veto is overridden. State procedures for effective dates vary if the date is not specified in the bill.

Once passed into law, the bill is given a public law designation and number. For example, Congress's designations indicate the Congress that passed the bill and what number the bill was. Thus, Public Law 105-123 indicates that the 105th Congress passed the 123rd bill. Similar designations are given to state laws. For example, in Illinois, Act 91-20 indicates that the 91st General Assembly passed the 20th bill.

Implementation of the New Law

Once passed, the law must be carried out consistent with its stated purpose. A particular state or federal agency or agencies will have the responsibility to administer the act. This is most often done by passing rules and regulations consistent with the process established by state or federal law. This aspect of implementation is discussed at length in Chapter 8.

Budget/Revenue Concerns and the Legislative Process

The process of passing legislation in a state or the federal system is intricate. In addition to the logistics required to pass a particular bill into law, revenue is also needed to carry out the newly passed law. State legislatures have varying powers to pass their own budgets, with or without executive oversight from the governor in the state. In

Congress, appropriations bills originate in the House and must be passed by both chambers. Clearly, without revenues to carry out a particular piece of legislation, the newly passed law is truly a hollow victory.[26]

> *Clearly, without revenues to carry out a particular piece of legislation, the newly passed law is truly a hollow victory.*

SUMMARY OF PRINCIPLES AND APPLICATIONS

With all of its shortcomings, the U.S. Constitution has endured its initial test of time. It has existed essentially unchanged since its inception. Likewise, the individual rights protected by the framers of the federal Constitution continue to exist, albeit in differing and ever-changing ways. Whatever continues to occur with the various constitutions, the nurse must be constantly aware of how the state and federal charters affect his or her personal and professional life and the lives of patients. Thus the nurse needs to:

- Keep abreast of changes that occur in state and federal constitutions
- Identify constitutional concepts inherent in everyday life and professional practice
- Protect individual freedoms in all situations, but especially when delivering health care or teaching in any public institution
- Become involved in the legislative process by providing testimony at public hearings, writing legislators, participating in lobbying, and supporting bills that advance quality health care and individual rights
- Actively support candidates for political office at the state or federal level who further individual rights and professional goals
- Consult with an attorney when individual rights are threatened to obtain both substantive and procedural protections
- Exercise the right to vote

- Be active in state and national nursing organizations, including political action committees (PACs) that support individual and professional rights
- Never take individual freedoms or the U.S. systems of government for granted

TOPICS FOR FURTHER INQUIRY

1. During a given period, identify constitutional rights that are present during the care of patients. Analyze how each right was protected or violated. Suggest ways in which the patients' rights could have been better protected.

2. Write a position paper on a patient right that conflicts with your belief(s) about that particular right. Identify the basis for your beliefs and suggest ways in which you can resolve the conflict between your beliefs and the patient's.

3. Track a bill affecting health care from its inception in the legislative process until its completion, on either the state or federal level. Evaluate nursing's participation, if any, in the process. Analyze how the bill would impact upon nursing practice if it became law. Suggest how nursing's involvement in the legislative process might have changed the process or the actual bill itself.

4. Interview a state or federal representative to determine his or her priority concerning a topic related to nursing practice. Identify the elected official's understanding of nursing practice and the profession. Discuss how many times nurses have contacted the representative concerning legislation affecting health care and the profession. Suggest ways in which communication between the representative and nurses could be improved.

REFERENCES

1. Ralph Chandler, Richard Enslen, and Peter Renstrom. *Constitutional Law Deskbook: Individual Rights*. 2nd Edition. Rochester, New York: Lawyers Cooperative Publishing, 1993, 2 (with Cumulative Supplement issued May 1999).
2. *Id.* at 2–3.
3. *Id.* at 14.
4. *Id.* at 14.
5. John Neary, "Roots and Radicals," *Life* (Fall 1991), Bicentennial Issue: The Bill of Rights, 43, *quoting* James Madison.
6. See, generally, *Marbury v. Madison*, 1 Cranch 137 (1803).
7. Chandler, Enslen, and Renstrom, *supra* note 1, at 14.
8. Henry Campbell Black. *Black's Law Dictionary*. 7th Edition. St. Paul, Minn.: West Group, 1999, 306–307.
9. Chandler, Enslen, and Renstrom, *supra* note 1, at 5.

10. *Id.* See also Neil Cogan, Editor. *The Complete Bill of Rights: The Drafts, Debates, Sources & Origins.* New York: Oxford University Press, 1997.

11. U.S.C.A. Const. Preamble.

12. Ronald Rotunda, "Celebrating the Bicentennial of the Bill of Rights," 79 *Illinois Bar Journal* (December 1991), 610.

13. *Id.*

14. Chandler, Enslen, and Renstrom, *supra* note 1, at 60–64.

15. *Id.*

16. Black, *supra* note 8, at 850.

17. *Id.* at 591.

18. Chandler, Enslen, and Renstrom, *supra* note 1, at 691.

19. *Id.*

20. *Id.*

21. *Id.* at 308.

22. Richard Abood and David Brushwood. *Pharmacy Practice and the Law.* 2nd Edition. Gaithersburg, Md.: Apsen Publishers, Inc., 1997, 13. More information on the Senate and House of Representatives can be found on their respective websites: http://www.senate.gov/ and http://www.house.gov/.

23. John Iglehart, "Politics and Public Health," in *Health Policy and Nursing: Crisis and Reform in the U.S. Health Care Delivery System.* Charleene Harrington and Carroll Estes, Editors. Sudbury, Mass.: Jones and Bartlett Publishers, 1997, 493.

24. Abood and Brushwood, *supra* note 22, at 13.

25. *Id.*

26. See generally *Health Policy and Nursing: Crisis and Reform in the U.S. Health Care Delivery System, supra* note 23.

The Nurse and the Judicial System

2

The public views the judicial system and the law with many emotions: awe, confusion, mistrust, fear, and anxiety, to name a few. These emotions are probably the result of many factors, including prior experience with a particular aspect of the law or legal system or, alternatively, no exposure to the workings of the law.

Regardless of the basis of the emotions felt by the public, the law and the legal system are more intimately involved in each person's life, directly or indirectly, than is acknowledged. The law provides society with a set of rules to live by and highlights one's rights as well as responsibilities.[1] Thus, whether driving a car, starting a business, or practicing one's profession, the law and the judicial system are central to those activities. In fact, Lawrence Friedman, a well-known author on the historical development of American law, has described law "as a mirror held up against life."[2]

The American judicial system had its roots, as did much of the development of American law, in the English system.[3] Its character and structure have undergone immense changes from their early beginnings, including division of the system into civil and criminal courts, a separate system for federal and state courts, and development of special courts, such as juvenile and equity courts.

Despite its many changes, the roles of the judicial system have remained constant: dispute resolution, behavior modification, allocation of gains and losses, and policy making.

Despite its many changes, the roles of the judicial system have remained constant: dispute reso-lution, behavior modification, allocation of gains and losses, and policy making.[4] How those roles are carried out, and the ultimate decisions that are reached, do fluctuate by necessity, however, because the law—and its judicial system—reflect society's wishes and needs.[5]

This chapter will present an overview of the American judiciary, with particular emphasis on the civil trial system and its applicability to the nurse. Although some of the same information presented here is relevant to the criminal justice system, the latter is a distinct system with a distinct set of procedural, and other, rules.

THE JUDICIAL SYSTEM OR JUDICIARY

The judiciary is the branch of the government that interprets, construes, and applies the law.[6] It is composed of many parts and subparts or branches, including the state judicial system, the federal judicial system, respective trial and appellate courts, civil courts, criminal courts, and special courts.

The judiciary carries out its responsibilities with the help of prior decisions, federal and state statutes and their concomitant legislative history, and the federal and state constitutions. The various sources of law used by the judicial system are listed in Table 2–1.

There are also specific rules of procedure, both civil and criminal, both federal and state, that guide the courts and the various parties to a suit in relation to their conduct while a case is pending before the court.

Federal Judicial System

The federal system's basis for existence is Article III, Section 1, of the U.S. Constitution, which enables the U.S. judicial power to "vest in one Supreme Court, and in such inferior courts as the Congress may from time to time ordain and establish."[7] The federal system is composed of the federal district courts (the trial courts), the federal courts of appeals, and the Supreme Court. In addition, there are several special courts in the federal system that are analogous to the trial and appellate courts, but which hear specific types of cases, such as tax or military matters. Figure 2–1 depicts the organization of the federal courts.

TABLE 2–1

Sources of Law

SOURCE	COMMENT
1. Federal Constitution	Balances powers of government and protects individual rights; includes Bill of Rights (first 10 amendments) and remaining amendments
2. Respective state constitutions	Balances powers of government and protects individual rights; may vary in terms of additional rights granted by each state over rights granted by federal Constitution
3. Statutes	Laws passed by Congress (federal), state, or local legislative bodies
4. Administrative law, rules, and decisions	Decided by agencies delegated this power by the respective legislative body
5. Common law	"Judge-made" or "court-made" decisions; based on precedent, custom, usage, and tradition; also called case law
6. Other	Executive orders from the president or the governor; treaties; principles of equity

Data from: Nancy J. Brent, "Legal Implications in Nursing," in *Foundations of Nursing Practice: A Nursing Process Approach.* Julia Leahy and Patricia Kizilay, Editors. Philadelphia, Penn.: W. B. Saunders Company, 1998, 62–63.

> *There are 94 geographic federal district courts, or trial courts, with at least one in every judicial district.*

There are 94 geographic federal district courts, or trial courts, with at least one in every judicial district. Most often, a judge, with or without a jury, hears cases in the district courts, although some of the trial courts use magistrates. A federal magistrate may try certain civil and misdemeanor criminal cases or may be given responsibilities such as pretrial hearings.[8] A decision by a federal district trial court is binding only on that district.

The actual trial process in a federal district court is the same as in a state trial court and is discussed in the section Essentials of the Civil Trial Process.

There are 13 U.S. Courts of Appeals. The 11 geographic circuits are composed of varying numbers of states, as is illustrated in Figure 2–2. The District of Columbia constitutes the 12th circuit. The 13th appeals court is the Court of Appeals for the Federal Circuit located in Washington, D.C.

The appellate courts sit in review of cases appealed from the federal trial courts. The court's role is to ensure that the law was applied correctly by the trial court. Usually the cases are decided by a panel of three judges, although on special cases, the entire court can decide to review a case

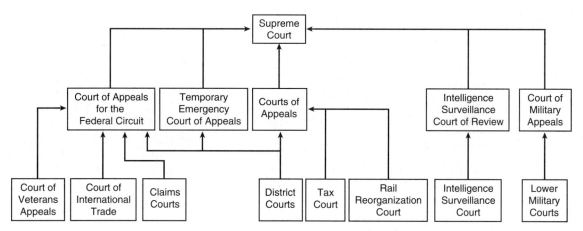

FIGURE 2–1. Organization chart of the federal court system. (From: Lawrence Baum. *American Courts: Process and Policy.* 4th Edition. Copyright © 1998 by Houghton Mifflin Company. Adapted with permission.)

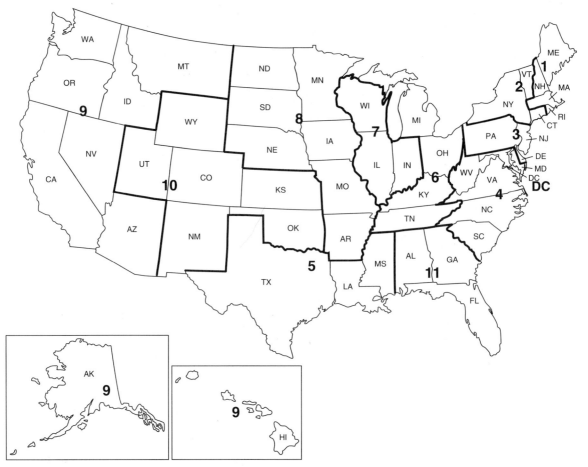

FIGURE 2–2. The federal judicial circuits. (From: Lawrence Baum. *American Courts: Process and Policy.* 4th Edition. Copyright © 1998 by Houghton Mifflin Company. Adapted with permission.)

en banc (full bench). The number of appellate judges in each district varies from 4 to 28.[9]

A decision by a particular appellate court is not binding on any other judicial circuit, except for a decision by the Court of Appeals for the Federal Circuit, which, as shown in Figure 2–1, reviews cases from *all* 12 circuits. Thus, only those states included in the particular circuit would be required to comply with a decision by its appellate court. If a decision that binds all states is sought, an appeal to the U.S. Supreme Court must occur.

The U.S. Supreme Court is the "supreme court of the land" and is therefore the final court to which a case can be appealed.

The U.S. Supreme Court is the "supreme court of the land" and is therefore the final court to which a case can be appealed. The Court is composed of nine justices. Most often, all of the justices participate in a decision (*en banc*). However, at least four justices must agree to grant review of a case brought before it by a *writ of certiorari.*[10]

One exception to the Court's full membership participating in a case is when a particular justice, in his or her role as a *circuit justice,* hears a special case from the circuit assigned to him or her when the Court itself has other matters pending before it. A common example of a special case that utilizes one justice to make a decision is a request for a stay of execution in criminal cases.

Like the appeals courts, the Supreme Court sits in review of cases from the lower federal and state courts.

It is important to note that federal judges and Supreme Court justices are nominated by the president of the United States and confirmed by the Senate. This is in contrast to judges in the state system who are most often elected to their position.

State Judicial System

Because each state has its own judicial system, the state system has been described as fragmented and varied.[11] In addition, the District of Columbia and the territories of the United States also have their respective courts comparable to the state system. Because each state has the power to organize its own judicial system, each is unique, and no one system is representative of all of the others. Even so, there are some similarities that can be summarized.

> *. . . the state [judicial] system has been described as fragmented and varied.*

To begin with, the general framework of a state court system is identical to that of the federal system in that there are trial courts, appellate courts, and a state supreme court. However, the specifics of each state system may vary. For example, some states possess one level of trial court, as represented in Figure 2–3 (Illinois state court system), while others have major and minor trial courts, meaning that they are divided in terms of the seri-

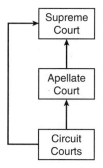

FIGURE 2–3. Organization chart of the Illinois court system. (From: Lawrence Baum. *American Courts: Process and Policy*. 4th Edition. Copyright © 1998 by Houghton Mifflin Company. Adapted with permission.)

ousness of the cases each division hears. If the latter structure exists, the major courts may function as appellate courts in reviewing some cases decided in the minor courts.[12]

Furthermore, some states have divided their trial courts into ones of general or limited jurisdiction. Illinois, for example, has given its trial courts general jurisdiction to hear all matters, despite the fact that the trial courts do have divisions, such as the traffic and the municipal courts.

The names of the state trial courts also vary. They may be called district courts, courts of common pleas, or circuit courts. In systems with limited jurisdiction, minor courts may be known as magistrate courts, justice of the peace courts, or juvenile courts.

State trial courts, or those considered "major" courts, can conduct jury trials (with a judge presiding) and bench trials (in which the judge acts as the jury). "Minor" courts and those with limited jurisdiction usually do not conduct jury trials.[13]

State appellate courts can be organized in either a one-tier or two-tier system.[14] Furthermore, some states divide their appeals courts into ones for criminal cases and ones for civil cases. How the appeals courts hear their respective cases also varies; some use a panel of judges while others require the entire court to review an appealed case. Regardless of their structure, the appeals courts' jurisdiction is "mandatory"; that is, the court must hear each case appealed to it because of the fundamental doctrine in the judicial system that parties are entitled to one appeal.[15]

A state supreme court is the final court of appeal in the state system.[16] As such, its decision is binding only on the state in which it sits. The number of judges sitting on a state supreme court varies between five and nine.[17] How many state supreme court judges are needed to decide a case also varies from state to state. The jurisdiction of the court is generally discretionary, especially when lower appellate courts exist in the state system. As a result, the judges have the ability to decide which cases they will hear and which they will not decide. However, some cases must be heard by the state supreme court, including trial decisions from criminal courts that impose a life sentence or the death penalty.

Jurisdiction

Jurisdiction is the authority by which a court recognizes and decides cases.[18] The rules governing jurisdiction are set by respective state and federal constitutions and statutes, spelling out what kinds of cases a particular court can hear and which court is the correct forum for a particular case.[19] Jurisdiction can be defined as applied to one particular court (e.g., an Illinois criminal court) or the particular court system as a whole, such as the federal judicial system, including its organizational structure.[20]

Jurisdiction is the authority by which a court recognizes and decides cases.

The concept of jurisdiction is complex and varied, especially because of the two separate and distinct judiciaries in the United States, the state and federal systems. Even so, by analyzing each of these systems, certain common themes emerge. In doing so, it is helpful to think of jurisdiction both in terms of the two systems and in terms of a whole that incorporates both the essence and structure of the particular system.

Subject Matter Jurisdiction

Subject matter jurisdiction of the federal judicial system is predicated on the Constitution and various federal statutes. Thus a federal court hears criminal and civil cases such as those involving issues in which (1) the federal government is a party (federal party jurisdiction); (2) two or more states are parties (diversity jurisdiction); and (3) a challenge under federal law is raised (federal question jurisdiction).[21]

Subject matter jurisdiction in the state court system is defined by the state constitution and statutes and includes such issues as family matters, criminal matters, and the amount of money that is sought in the lawsuit.

Personal Jurisdiction

Personal jurisdiction in both the federal and state court systems is defined as the power of the court over the individual and is contrasted with *in rem* jurisdiction, meaning the court's power over one's property.[22] Depending on the nature of the suit—against the person, against a person's property, or both—the correct jurisdiction must be established for the court to render a judgment against the party or the party's property. Thus, for

example, a suit in federal court in Ohio could not be sustained if that court had no power over a nurse defendant located in Wyoming whose conduct was the subject of the suit.

Structural Jurisdiction

The structural jurisdiction of both the federal and state court systems is both vertical and horizontal.[23] In both systems the vertically organized courts are specified as either trial courts or appellate courts. The higher-level courts function as courts of review or appeal from the courts below.[24] Similarly, the horizontally organized courts, usually at the trial court level, possess specific jurisdiction to hear certain types of cases, such as domestic relations and probate (wills, guardianship) matters. Structural jurisdiction can be easily visualized by referring to Figures 2–1 and 2–2.

Venue

A particular concept related to the horizontal jurisdiction of a court system is that of venue. Although it is sometimes incorrectly referred to as jurisdiction, it involves the place or geographic area where a court with jurisdiction can hear and determine a case.[25] For example, depending on the particular state rules, if a nurse employee decides to sue her employer alleging a breach of an employment contract, the nurse must do so in the state court located where the case arose, where the nurse resides, or where the employer conducts business.

Legal Precedent

The American system of determining legal rights and responsibilities is based on prior case decisions, rulings, rationale, and custom. Thus, when a case, legal issue, or motion comes before the court, the judge must make a determination in *that* situation by reviewing prior case decisions and their rationale and applying those prior decisions to the case before the court. Generally the prior rulings are followed by the court. If either party is unhappy with reliance on the prior law, he or she can appeal the decision, particularly if it is believed there is a chance to "make new law" or challenge prior decisions because of some unique aspect of the case.

Stare decisis

In contrast to legal precedent, *stare decisis* ("to stand by cases decided") refers to the court following its own principles of law and those of inferior courts as applied to a particular set of facts.[26] Clearly, unless there is a superior court ruling or holding overturning decisions of the lower court, this doctrine binds the court hearing a particular case to apply the same ruling as has been reached before, so long as the facts of the current case fit within the principle of law decided earlier. Parties to the suit can always challenge a ruling based on *stare decisis* by appealing the decision to a higher court.

. . . stare decisis ("to stand by cases decided") refers to the court following its own principles of law and those of inferior courts as applied to a particular set of facts.

Res judicata

Res judicata stands for the principle that once a final decision in a case has been determined by a court having jurisdiction, it is binding on all of the parties and is therefore an absolute bar to any further legal action that involves the same claim, demand, or cause of action.[27] Thus, if a nurse is a defendant in a professional negligence claim and there is a final decision by a jury in his or her favor, the plaintiff in that case cannot file another case alleging the same causes of action against him or her for the same injury.

ESSENTIALS OF THE CIVIL TRIAL PROCESS

Despite the many variations among state court systems in organizational structure, there are certain common phases and steps in the trial process in most state court systems. These phases and steps are helpful in many ways. Most important, they provide an organized and fair process for the resolution of the controversy that is the basis of the suit. Thus, one can determine how a case proceeds to trial and where in the judicial system a particular case may be (where it is pending) once it is filed.

Initiation of a Civil Suit
Evaluating Possibility for Suit and Drafting Complaint

When an individual believes he or she has suffered a loss or injury because of someone else,

whether the loss is bodily injury or property damage, the person will consult with an attorney concerning the possibility of filing a suit to compensate for the loss or injury. When the wrong suffered is allegedly the result of a health care professional's negligence, the attorney who is consulted will review the medical record. If the potential cause of action (the grounds that serve as the basis for the suit) is based on another legal theory, such as a breach of contract, the attorney will review any documents that would support the individual's theory. In addition, the attorney will carefully interview the individual for additional information concerning the alleged wrong.

If the attorney determines that a suit can be initiated on behalf of the client, then a complaint is drafted and its accuracy is confirmed by the client. A complaint is one type of pleading. Pleadings are the formal, written allegations by parties in a case about their respective claims and defenses.[28] The state or federal rules of civil procedure—the procedures, methods, and practices to which attorneys and the court must adhere in civil cases—define, among other things, types of pleadings and their content. Several pleadings are generally utilized in civil cases. They are listed in Table 2–2.

The client who initiates the suit becomes the *plaintiff* (or *petitioner*) in the suit and those who are sued are the *defendants* (or *respondents*).

The complaint specifies with particularity the alleged wrongs of the defendants in paragraphs called *counts*. There may be one or several counts against a defendant or defendants. Figure 2–4 contains a portion of a sample complaint.

The plaintiff or petitioner who decides to bring the suit may also need to *verify* the complaint; that is, swear and sign under oath that it is accurate and truthful. If a complaint is verified, usually all other pleadings filed in the case must also be verified.

The attorney must also prepare a *summons*. A summons is the official notification to the defendant that a suit has been filed against him or her. The summons states that the defendant is required to file his or her appearance, either himself or herself or through an attorney, and answer the complaint by a certain date. The summons must be attached to the complaint so that the defendant is apprised of the nature of the suit against him

<table>
<tr><td colspan="2" align="center">**TABLE 2-2**</td></tr>
</table>

Common Pleadings in Civil Cases

NAME	PURPOSE
Complaint	Initiation of case; must clearly inform defendant of allegations against him or her and relief requested; that plaintiff is entitled to relief; and that court has jurisdiction
Answer	Defendant's written assertion either denying plaintiff's allegations in the complaint or admitting them but then setting forth defenses against them
Counterclaim	Defendant's allegations of his or her own causes of action against the plaintiff in the same case to defeat plaintiff's case; used by a defendant with a denial of the allegations in the complaint
Reply	Plaintiff's response to defendant's counterclaim; can also be used after a motion is filed in a case (see Table 2-3) or at any other time the court orders either party to file one
Cross-claim	Allegations of co-parties—either co-plaintiffs or co-defendants—against each other that are germane to the case and may avoid liability for that party
Third-Party Complaint	Defendant's complaint to bring third party (not originally sued by plaintiff) into suit because third party may be liable for plaintiff's injury

Data from: Henry Campbell Black. *Black's Law Dictionary*. 7th Edition. St. Paul, Minn.: West Group, 1999.

or her. A portion of a sample summons is contained in Figure 2–5.

A summons is the official notification to the defendant that a suit has been filed against him or her.

Filing the Suit

Once the evaluation and pleadings are complete, the suit must be filed with the court. The summons and complaint is taken to the clerk of the court's office where it is given a number that is required to be on all pleadings. For example, the case number often begins with the year the case is filed, followed by a designation as to the court division it is filed in, and is completed with the consecutive number of that particular case. Therefore, if a case were filed in the law division of a particular state court in the year 1999, it would have a number similar to 99 L 12345. The next case filed after it would have the number 99 L 12346.

The filed summons and complaint must then be *personally served* (delivered) to all of the defendants named in the suit. Service of the summons and complaint can take place in several ways, based on the state or federal civil practice rules, including by mail or by a sheriff or other agent delivering them to the defendant (or his or her agent) in the defendant's home or workplace. The defendant will not know about the case, or be required to respond to it, until receipt of the copy of the complaint and summons. The *service of process* formally begins the jurisdiction of the court over the defendant and the subject matter of the case.

It is important to remember that the case must be filed with the court within the applicable statute of limitations. A state or federal statute of limitations, along with the statute of repose included in the statute of limitations, specifies the time frames within which a case must be filed. For civil cases, the time limitations vary because of the nature of the suit and the various time frames adopted by the state or federal legislatures respectively in their civil practice rules and procedures. For example, an action alleging defamation must usually be brought within 1 year from the time the defamation occurred, whereas a suit alleging professional negligence generally has a 2-year statutory limitation.

Filing of Appearance and Answer by Defendant

Once the defendant is properly served, a certain number of days—usually 30—is granted within which to respond to the complaint. The defendant's attorney will file an appearance with the court within the time frame so that the court has a record that the defendant is represented and has complied with the summons. A copy is also sent to the plaintiff's attorney.

In addition, if no objections are raised by written motion as to the court's personal jurisdiction over the defendant or the subject matter, an answer to the allegations in the complaint is prepared,

IN THE CIRCUIT COURT OF COOK COUNTY
COUNTY DEPARTMENT-LAW DIVISION

Mary Jones,
          Plaintiff
 	
     v.
 	
ABC Hospital, Fred Free, M.D.,
and Susan Nega, R.N., M.S., individually
and as an employee of ABC Hospital,
          Defendants
	)
	)
	)
	)
	) 92 L 1234
	)
	)
	)
	)
	)
	)
	)

COMPLAINT AT LAW

COUNT I

Now comes the Plaintiff, MARY JONES, by and through her attorney, SUSAN SMITH, and by way of her Complaint At Law against the Defendant, ABC HOSPITAL (hereinafter referred to as HOSPITAL), an Illinois not-for-profit corporation, alleges as follows:

1. On January 15, 1999, and for some time prior thereto, HOSPITAL operated a medical facility located in Chicago, Cook County, Illinois, for the care and treatment of patients.

2. On January 15, 1999, and for some time prior thereto, HOSPITAL undertook the care and treatment of the Plaintiff, MARY JONES.

3. Specifically, Plaintiff, MARY JONES came to HOSPITAL'S EMERGENCY ROOM on or about January 15, 1999, complaining of severe chest pain at about 10:45 a.m. . . . .

COUNT II

Now comes the Plaintiff, MARY JONES, by and through her attorney, SUSAN SMITH, and by way of her Complaint At Law against the Defendant, FRED FREE, M.D., alleges as follows:

1. On January 15, 1999, and for some time prior thereto, FRED FREE, M.D., was a licensed physician in the State of Illinois, having received his license in Illinois in 1980.

2. On January 15, 1999, and for some time prior thereto, FRED FREE, M.D., was employed by HOSPITAL as an Emergency Room physician. . . . .

COUNT III

Now comes the Plaintiff, MARY JONES, by and through her attorney, SUSAN SMITH, and by way of her Complaint At Law against the Defendant, SUSAN NEGA, R.N., M.S., alleges as follows. . . . .

1. On January 15, 1999, and for some time prior thereto, SUSAN NEGA, R.N., M.S., was a licensed professional registered nurse in the State of Illinois, having received that license in 1982.

2. On January 15, 1999, and for some time prior thereto, SUSAN NEGA, R.N., M.S., was employed by HOSPITAL as an emergency room nurse. . . . .

WHEREFORE, Plaintiff, MARY JONES, prays this honorable Court enter judgment in her favor against the Defendant, SUSAN NEGA, in the amount in excess of $50,000.00.

_____
Susan Smith, Attorney
for Plaintiff, Mary Jones

FIGURE 2–4. Portion of sample complaint.

2120 - Served	2121 - Served
2220 - Not Served	2221 - Not Served
2320 - Served By Mail	2321 - Served By Mail
2420 - Served By Publication	2421 - Served By Publication
SUMMONS	**ALIAS - SUMMONS**

(Rev. 9/3/99) CCG 0001

IN THE CIRCUIT COURT OF COOK COUNTY, ILLINOIS
COUNTY DEPARTMENT, _____ DIVISION

(Name all parties)

No. _____

v.

SUMMONS

To each defendant:

YOU ARE SUMMONED and required to file an answer to the complaint in this case, a copy of which is hereto attached, or otherwise file your appearance, and pay the required fee, in the office of the Clerk of this Court at the following location:

❑   Richard J. Daley Center, 50 W. Washington, Room _____, Chicago, Illinois 60602

❑   **District 2 - Skokie**   ❑   **District 3 - Rolling Meadows**   ❑   **District 4 - Maywood**
    5600 Old Orchard Rd.   2121 Euclid   1500 Maybrook Ave.
    Skokie, IL 60077   Rolling Meadows, IL 60008   Maywood, IL 60153

❑   **District 5 - Bridgeview**   ❑   **District 6 - Markham**
    10220 S. 76th Ave.   16501 S. Kedzie Pkwy.
    Bridgeview, IL 60455   Markham, IL 60426

You must file within 30 days after service of this summons, not counting the day of service.
IF YOU FAIL TO DO SO, A JUDGMENT BY DEFAULT MAY BE ENTERED AGAINST YOU FOR THE RELIEF REQUESTED IN THE COMPLAINT.

To the officer:

This summons must be returned by the officer or other person to whom it was given for service, with endorsement of service and fees, if any, immediately after service. If service cannot be made, this summons shall be returned so endorsed. This summons may not be served later than 30 days after its date.

Atty. No.: _____

Name: _____

Atty. for: _____

Address: _____

City/State/Zip: _____

Telephone: _____

WITNESS, _____, _____

_____
Clerk of Court

Date of service: _____, _____
(To be inserted by officer on copy left with defendant or other person)

Service by Facsimile Transmission will be accepted at: _____
(Area Code)   (Facsimile Telephone Number)

AURELIA PUCINSKI, CLERK OF THE CIRCUIT COURT OF COOK COUNTY, ILLINOIS

FIGURE 2–5. Sample summons. (From: Cook County Circuit Court Form CCG 0001 [9-3-99]. Used with permission of Aurelia Pucinski, Clerk of the Circuit Court of Cook County, Illinois.)

based on the defendant's discussions with his or her attorney. The answer is filed with the court and a copy is sent to the attorney for the plaintiff.

In addition to preparing an answer to the complaint, the attorney may determine that a counter-claim or a cross-claim is indicated (see Table 2–2). Either of those options would be filed with the answer.

It is important for the nurse to keep in mind that once served, he or she should not discuss anything about the case with anyone other than the attorney representing the nurse. The nurse sued for alleged professional negligence may use the attorney who works for the health care facility where the nurse is employed if, for example, the nurse is covered under the employer's professional liability insurance policy. Or the attorney may be one retained personally by the nurse if, for example, the nurse has purchased his or her own professional liability insurance.

A portion of a sample answer to the complaint in Figure 2–4 is illustrated in Figure 2–6.

Pretrial Phase

Period of Discovery

Once the court obtains jurisdiction over the party or parties to a suit, the next step in the trial process is called the *period of discovery*. It is a time during which all the parties to a suit are given the opportunity to obtain information about the issues contained in the suit from the other parties, witnesses, or other sources. It also ensures a fair and equitable manner by which the parties obtain relevant information concerning the suit to avoid surprise concerning evidence should the case go to trial. It may also help settle a case prior to trial if adequate evidence indicates that a settlement might be an equitable way to resolve the allegations in the suit.

Any of the parties in the suit have access to the same discovery methods. The more common ones will be addressed.

WRITTEN INTERROGATORIES. *Interrogatories* are questions directed at one party concerning information needed by another party, who files them with the court and sends copies to all the other parties. The party to whom the questions are addressed must answer the questions in writing and under oath. The answers are also filed with the court and copies sent to all parties.

The questions request information needed by the party who filed them. For example, in a professional negligence case against a nurse, the plaintiff might ask for information concerning the nurse's education, certifications, any involvement as a defendant in other professional negligence suits, and places of employment since graduation from his or her nursing program.

DEPOSITION. A *deposition* is a procedure whereby a party in the case or a witness gives his or her statement concerning the case under oath with all parties and their attorneys present. To request the deposition of a party to the case, one serves notice to the party's attorney. If, however, a nonparty's deposition is requested, the court issues a *subpoena*. The subpoena is used to ensure the presence of the person who is not named in the suit but whose testimony as a witness in a particular case is needed.

A deposition is a procedure whereby a party in the case or a witness gives his or her statement concerning the case under oath with all parties and their attorneys present.

If the subpoena is a *subpoena duces tecum,* the person is required to appear and bring to the deposition (or trial) any documents specified in the subpoena that are in his or her possession.

The format in a deposition is a question and answer one; that is, the attorney who is taking the statement questions the deponent (the one giving the testimony) and the deponent answers. A court reporter transcribes everything said during the deposition and reproduces the transcript of the deposition for use by the attorneys.

During the deposition, the other attorneys are given the chance to cross-examine the person giving the statement. In addition, throughout the deposition, objections to questions, answers, and other issues may be raised by any of the attorneys.

Depositions are an important method of discovery for several reasons. Because the testimony is given under oath, any later deviation from the statement during trial can be used to impeach (question the credibility of) the deponent. Second,

IN THE CIRCUIT COURT OF COOK COUNTY
COUNTY DEPARTMENT-LAW DIVISION

Mary Jones, 　　　　Plaintiff	)))	
v.	)))	92 L 1234
ABC Hospital, Fred Free, M.D., and Susan Nega, R.N., M.S., individually and as an employee of ABC Hospital, 　　　　Defendants	))))))	

ANSWER TO COMPLAINT AT LAW

Now comes the Defendant, SUSAN NEGA, R.N., M.S., by and through her attorney, NANCY J. BRENT, and by way of Answer to the Plaintiff's Complaint At Law, states:

COUNT I

Defendant, SUSAN NEGA, R.N., M.S., makes no response to Count I as Count I is not directed against her.

COUNT II

Defendant, SUSAN NEGA, R.N., M.S., makes no response to Count II as Count II is not directed against her.

COUNT III

1. Defendant admits the allegations in Paragraph 1 of Count III.
2. Defendant admits the allegations in Paragraph 2 of Count III.
3. Defendant . . . .

WHEREFORE, Defendant, SUSAN NEGA, R.N., M.S., denies that the Plaintiff is entitled to the relief prayed for or any relief whatsoever, and prays this honorable Court enter judgment in her favor and against the Plaintiff.

—————————————————
Nancy J. Brent, Attorney
for Defendant, Susan Nega, R.N., M.S.

FIGURE 2–6. Portion of sample answer.

depositions provide the opportunity to "discover" the deponent; that is, to see how the deponent appears; how he or she responds to the questions asked; how credible he or she is; and other issues critical to the success or failure of the testimony at trial. A deposition can also help obtain more information concerning the case: who might be potential additional witnesses (and defendants), whether settling the case may be more appropriate than proceeding to trial, and who might have been incorrectly included as a defendant.

Depositions can be taken as evidence depositions. If this is specified when the notice of the deposition is sent to all the attorneys involved, the statement will be introduced into evidence at the trial upon a motion by the attorney who asked that it be taken. Evidence depositions are used when there is a concern that a particular deponent may not be available at trial because of age, illness, or recently establishing residence in another state or country.

REQUEST TO PRODUCE CERTAIN DOCUMENTS. A Request to Produce Certain Documents is used during the discovery phase to obtain materials and information from parties that are essential to the case. Most often, the request will be filed prior to a deposition so that the materials and information can be utilized during the deposition.

A request would be used, for example, when a nurse sues an employer alleging wrongful discharge. The nurse files the request seeking copies of any and all material in his or her personnel file.

REQUEST TO ADMIT FACTS. This type of discovery tool is used to ask that one of the parties admit or deny certain facts that are at issue in the case. The party to whom the request is directed must file a response within a certain time frame and admit or deny what is asked in the request. Most civil practice rules state that if the request is not responded to, the facts contained in the request are admitted.

Like the Request to Produce Certain Documents, this tool is helpful in resolving many of the facts concerning the case as early as possible. Or, if facts are denied, it serves to crystallize the contested issues early in the pretrial process.

COURT MOTIONS AND ORDERS. During the discovery phase, attorneys for all of the parties will seek orders from the court if it is determined that, for example, a party is not cooperating with the discovery process, if there are objections to the types

or number of questions in the written interrogatories or deposition, or if a request for documents is unduly burdensome or irrelevant to the case. In addition, the court can dismiss a defendant from the suit during this phase if the results of discovery show that the particular defendant did not contribute to the injury or damages sustained by the plaintiff. A particular defendant might also ask for a judgment in his or her favor at this time, again because there was no liability for the alleged damages.

All of these requests are made through motions, in which the parties in a case, through their respective attorneys, ask that the court rule on a particular matter or order a party to do something or refrain from certain conduct. Most often they are written documents and are presented to the court after written notice has been given to all parties in the suit. Motions can, however, be oral, and these occur most often during a trial or hearing as legal issues and questions are raised for resolution by the court. Moreover, motions can take place *after* a trial; for example, when a party asks the court to order a new trial.

Some of the more common motions in civil cases are presented in Table 2–3.

TABLE 2–3

Common Motions in Civil Cases

NAME	PURPOSE
Motion to Quash service of summons	Seeks to render void the service of the summons and complaint on a party; if granted, requires another try at service because court does not have power over party unless properly served
Motion to Dismiss	Usually made before hearing or trial, it attacks the suit by alleging insufficient legal basis to sustain suit
Motion for Summary Judgment	Asks court to dismiss case because there is no contest about the facts in the case and party making the motion is entitled to ruling in his or her favor as a matter of law
Ex parte motion	Meaning "one side only"; may be used in rare circumstances in which giving notice to the other party may not be possible or helpful; is often used when one party seeks an injunction or restraining order against another
Discovery motions	Used during the discovery phase of a case when the parties are experiencing difficulties with each other in obtaining requested material or taking a deposition, for example; may also be used when unique discovery is needed or is not consistent with civil practice rules
Motion to Strike	Requests that biased, immaterial, or harmful information included in a pleading or in oral testimony be removed from the pleading or record and disregarded
Motion for Directed Verdict	Requested by either party during trial, asks that a verdict in one's favor be granted because the party with the burden of proof did not meet that burden
Motion for Judgment Notwithstanding the Verdict	Requested by either party after judge or jury reaches decision, asks that despite decision, movant is entitled to judgment in his or her favor
Motion for Mistrial	Requested by either party before the jury's verdict or judge's decision, it seeks an order to render the trial void; can be due to a highly prejudicial remark or error; judge can also declare mistrial if jury cannot make decision; a retrial must occur if mistrial granted

Data from: Henry Campbell Black. *Black's Law Dictionary.* 7th Edition. St. Paul, Minn.: West Group, 1999.

Pretrial Conference

The pretrial conference is the final step in the pretrial phase and is attended by the attorneys, the judge, and, if they wish to be present, the parties to the case. Its purpose is to clarify and fairly resolve any pending issues in the controversy prior to trial. In addition, if possible, there is always the attempt to settle the case rather than have it proceed to trial. A settlement is not an admission of liability or fault; in fact, if a case is settled, any and all documents surrounding the settlement clearly state that the defendant admits no liability.

If a settlement is reached, the cause of action cannot be brought again against any of the defendants who participated in the settlement. It may be, however, that not all defendants settle with the plaintiff. If that occurs, the case would proceed to trial against any remaining defendants in the suit.

Factors that are evaluated in determining whether to settle a suit include the expense, both personal and financial, of continuing to trial; the credibility and strength of the evidence obtained during the discovery phase; and the uncertainty of what the jury's verdict will be at trial.

Trial Phase

Assignment of Case to Judge and Selection of Jury

When a case comes up on the trial calendar, it is immediately assigned to a trial judge. The trial judge is usually *not* the same judge who presided over the pretrial motions, period of discovery, and pretrial conference. If one of the parties has asked for a jury trial, the judge's role during the trial is that of "referee"; that is, he or she interprets the law as it pertains to the case before the trial court. The jury, after ruling on the facts of the case, renders a verdict.

If, on the other hand, there is no demand for a jury, then the judge also determines the facts at issue and renders a verdict. Jury trials are much more common than bench trials, however, and the selection of a jury usually follows the assignment of the trial judge.

Jury selection, the *voir dire,* is conducted by either the trial judge or the attorneys, depending on the state or federal civil practice requirements. In either case, questions are asked of the panel of potential jurors about matters relevant to the trial.

Potential jurors may be dismissed (excused from jury duty) *for cause* (where prejudice or bias is found, for example) or *without cause* (peremptory challenges). Depending on the state or federal rules, each attorney in the case has a certain number of peremptory challenges.

The number of jurors needed in a civil trial varies. In federal courts and some state courts 12 jurors are required. Other state courts require only 6 jurors.[29]

Opening Statements

After the jury is selected, the trial begins with opening statements by all of the attorneys. The opening statement informs the jury of what that particular party intends to prove during the trial and what evidence will be used to do so. Most often, the plaintiff's attorney is the one who is the first to give his or her opening statement because the plaintiff has the burden of proving the case. The *burden of proof* means the obligation to affirmatively convince the judge or jury that the allegations contained in the complaint forming the basis of the suit are true. The burden is different, depending on the type of suit. For example, in a civil suit, the plaintiff must usually prove his or her case "by a preponderance of the evidence," whereas in a criminal case, the state must prove a criminal defendant guilty "beyond a reasonable doubt."

> The burden of proof *[for the plaintiff]* means the obligation to affirmatively convince the judge or jury that the allegations contained in the complaint forming the basis of the suit are true.

Testimony of Parties and Witnesses

PLAINTIFF. The plaintiff is the first to present his or her case. Specifically, the plaintiff and any other witnesses are called individually to give their testimony under oath under the direct examination of the plaintiff's attorney. Witnesses that corroborate (strengthen or support) the plaintiff's testimony are usually called *occurrence witnesses.*

However, other witnesses may be called, including an *expert witness.*

After each witness has testified under direct examination, the attorneys representing the defendants or other parties in the suit cross-examine the witness, each taking his or her turn individually. The purpose of cross-examination is to discount or render unimportant the witness's testimony in the eyes of the jury. After cross-examination, the attorney who originally called the witness, or the attorney for any other party, can ask additional questions to rebut (refute) the testimony.

Once the plaintiff's attorney has called all witnesses, the attorney rests the case. The defendant's attorney then has a turn at presenting the case to the jury.

DEFENDANT. Before beginning to call witnesses, the defendant's attorney will attempt to dispose of the case in his or her client's favor by asking the judge to grant a directed verdict (see Table 2–3) because the plaintiff did not meet the burden of proof. If the judge grants the motion, the case is dismissed. Most often, however, the judge does not grant such a motion, and the defendant begins to present his or her case.

The attorney for the defendant then calls the defendant and witnesses to testify. As before, once each witness has testified, cross-examination takes place, and there is an opportunity to present rebuttal testimony. The defendant's attorney rests the case once all the testimony and evidence has been presented to the court.

The defendant's attorney may again request that the court enter a directed verdict for his or her client. The plaintiff's attorney can also make the same request. If granted, the case is dismissed. If not, the next step in the trial process takes place.

Closing Arguments and Jury Instruction

Each side presents closing arguments, with the plaintiff doing so first. After all closing arguments have taken place, the judge then instructs the jury on the applicable law, how they are to determine money damages, and the burden of proof applicable to the hearing. In the federal judicial system and many state systems, the judge's instructions to the jury consist of suggestions from the attorneys in the case. In other states, model or pattern jury instructions must be used, or substantially followed, by the judge.

The jury then retires to deliberate its verdict.

The Jury's Verdict

During its deliberations, the jury is sequestered (isolated from the public). Depending on the cause of action, or what the attorneys stipulated (agreed to), a unanimous verdict or a majority verdict may be required. If no decision can be reached, a "hung jury" occurs, and a new trial would need to take place. If a decision is reached, however, and there are no challenges to that decision (e.g., for tampering with the jury), then the jury announces its decision in open court and the judge enters a judgment and dismisses the jury.

Appeals Phase

If either party or parties are unsatisfied with the verdict, an appeal can be taken to the next highest court in the state or federal system. The party bringing the appeal is the *appellant,* and the one against whom the appeal is taken is the *appellee.* The appellant must file the notice of appeal in the manner and within the time specified in the applicable civil practice rules. Most often, appellants are required to file their notice within 30 days from the verdict.

The party bringing the appeal is the appellant, *and the one against whom the appeal is taken is the* appellee.

Depending on the subject matter of the case and the appeal, the appellate court may be *mandated* to review the case, or the review may be *discretionary.* A discretionary review is often sought through a petition asking the court to review the case. When the court grants such a request, it issues a *writ of certiorari.*

If the appellate court decides to review a decision of a lower court, it does so based upon the record in that hearing or trial, briefs, and other documents submitted by the appellant and appellee, and in some states, oral arguments by the attorneys. Once a decision is made, it is binding on the parties unless the next level of appeal is taken.

Appeals courts have the power to affirm lower court decisions (in which case the lower court ruling is final); to overturn the decision (in which case the lower court must render a verdict consistent with the higher court's decision); or to reverse, modify, or vacate a decision (in which instance the case is remanded [sent back] to the lower court for additional consideration).[30]

Ensuring Compliance with the Final Outcome

Once all appeals have been taken, the outcome of the litigation must be complied with by the losing party or parties. Thus, if the case involved the professional negligence of a nurse and the judgment against the nurse was upheld, then the nurse must pay whatever monetary amount of damages he or she was found responsible for. If, in contrast, the nurse was a plaintiff who sued a former employer for wrongful discharge, and the court decision included reinstatement to his or her position, that reinstatement would have to occur without delay.

If a defendant refuses to comply with the outcome of the case, it is necessary to ensure it through various legal procedures. For example, if damages are not paid as ordered by the court, then an *execution of judgment* to enforce payment is filed. Or, an *injunction* may be sought to require a party to follow the judgment of the court or jury.

Role of the Nurse in the Trial Process

Obviously the nurse may be involved in the trial process in any of the roles discussed. The nurse may be a plaintiff in a suit if he or she, for example, sues an employer for wrongful discharge or defamation. However, the nurse's role as a defendant is perhaps the most familiar role, particularly in relation to professional negligence suits. The nurse may also be involved in the trial process as an *occurrence witness*; that is, someone who will be able to support or refute allegations against another nurse colleague or other party. Last, and by no means least, the nurse may be an expert witness (either the plaintiff's or the defendant's expert) in a professional negligence suit against a nurse.

ALTERNATIVES TO THE CIVIL TRIAL PROCESS

Factors such as financial cost, length of time, and the adversarial nature of the litigation process fueled dissatisfaction with the trial process as a means of settling controversies between litigants. Although alternatives to litigation (called alterna-

tive dispute resolution or ADR) existed in the United States since before the Declaration of Independence and the Constitution,[31] they were not utilized extensively by society as a whole (business and labor sectors being an exception).[32] Alternative dispute resolution did not become "officially institutionalized" in the United States until 1922.[33] Even so, as court dockets became increasingly backlogged, attempts to find alternatives to "traditional litigation" became necessary.[34]

Alternative dispute resolution (ADR). . . include(s) but is not limited to mediation, arbitration, conciliation, and screening panels.

Efforts to establish and/or use alternatives to litigation have resulted in several options in place of the trial process. They include but are not limited to mediation, arbitration, conciliation, and screening panels. These ADR methods are used regularly today and are an effective means of deciding all kinds of disputes. Furthermore, court-mandated arbitration exists in all 50 states.[35]

In addition to ADR methods discussed thus far, others have been established by state and federal laws for particular situations. In relation to health care, for example, on the federal level the Federal Mediation and Conciliation Services (FMCS) has the power to conduct mandatory mediation of contract negotiation disputes when difficulties exist among employers, employees, and a union under the National Labor Relations Act (NLRA). In addition, some states have passed legislation providing for arbitration when a disagreement arises between a patient and a health care provider and the parties have a written agreement to submit the disagreement to binding arbitration.[36]

Although the purpose of each ADR method is to avoid litigation, the procedures vary. A comparison of the more common options is important for the reader to understand their commonalities and differences. It is important to keep in mind, however, that the methods may be combined or blended to form "hybrid" alternatives in a particular situation or state.

Mediation

Mediation is usually an informal process in which the parties in dispute will attempt to voluntarily resolve their differences by utilizing a private mediator or mediation service. They hope the process ends with an agreement concerning the disputed issues.

Mediation may also occur, however, as part of the litigation process and is then termed court-annexed mediation. For example, in some state courts, parties contemplating divorce when children are involved are required to see a mediator to attempt to resolve such matters as child custody and support. In court-required mediation, the mediator cannot make a decision concerning the issues discussed in mediation. Rather, he or she aids the parties to reach agreement concerning the issues under consideration so that they do not have to be litigated. A final report concerning the mediation, whether successful or unsuccessful, is usually filed with the court.

Mediation may also be ordered by the court when a motion is presented to the judge during a pending lawsuit. For example, if a nurse has filed for divorce and custody issues are not being easily resolved, the nurse's attorney may file a motion asking that the parties submit to mediation.

Arbitration

Arbitration is defined as a more formal process in which a dispute is submitted to a third neutral party, or a panel of arbitrators, to hear arguments, review evidence, and render a decision.[37] In some arbitration agreements, the decision rendered—the award—is given the same weight as a court decision; that is, it is *binding*. If so, it is final, and the parties must abide by the decision.

Arbitration is defined as a more formal process in which a dispute is submitted to a third neutral party, or a panel of arbitrators, to hear arguments, review evidence, and render a decision.

Arbitration may be voluntary and done by a private organization and result in a binding resolution. This often occurs, for example, in grievance procedures established by employers for employees who want to challenge a disciplinary action. Binding arbitration is usually the last step of the procedure. Most often, the procedure clearly spells out the process for the selection of the arbitrator, who is required to pay for it, and how the decision of the arbitrator will be treated. Binding arbitration is also included in many union contracts whereby the union agrees to submit any union member-employee's work-related problems to an arbitrator rather than go through the nonunion employee's grievance procedure.

Arbitration may also be required before litigating the issues in court, but the decision of the arbitrator is nonbinding. With this approach, arbitration is similar to mediation.

A third approach to arbitration is court-annexed arbitration. Court-annexed arbitration is governed by a state mandatory arbitration act that includes the procedures and process of arbitration, including the types of cases that will be heard (for example, civil cases), any jurisdictional amounts required (for example, cases asking for compensation between \$2,500 and \$15,000), and qualifications for arbitrators. Usually, court-annexed arbitration is not binding, and a losing party may reject the arbitrator's decision within the time specified in the particular arbitration act and then move for a *de novo* trial (starting anew).[38]

When arbitration does not involve court-annexed arbitration, arbitrators are often selected by the parties from a list of qualified arbitrators compiled by the Board of the American Arbitration Association. Or, for state and federal organizations that require arbitration, such as the railroad and airline industries, the National Mediation Board was established to promote and select arbitrators for contract disputes in those industries.[39]

Conciliation

The purpose of conciliation is to improve communications and decrease tensions between the parties to a dispute. A third neutral party attempts to do so by interpreting issues, providing any technical assistance that may be needed, and suggesting solutions.[40] The process may be informal or formal. Conciliation is often a part of the mediation or arbitration process.

SUMMARY OF PRINCIPLES AND APPLICATIONS

The civil judicial system, both federal and state, can be confusing for the nurse because it is complex and foreign. In addition, alternative dispute resolutions provide options that may prove more beneficial in terms of time and cost but add to the general confusion about resolving disputes. The nurse can attempt to resolve uncertainty about the civil judicial system by

- Becoming familiar with his or her state civil judicial system

- Comparing the state judicial system with the federal court system

- Comparing and contrasting the state civil justice system with its criminal justice system

- Serving as a juror when summoned to do so in his or her state

- Obtaining legal representation when contemplating the filing of a civil suit, when served with a summons and complaint as a named defendant, or when subpoenaed to testify at a deposition or at trial

- Cooperating with legal counsel when involved in a civil suit, regardless of the role

- Investigating alternative dispute resolution methods and, if possible and beneficial, incorporating them into any employment agreement, employee handbook, or other legal document governing the relationship between the parties

- Becoming involved in efforts to improve the civil judicial system, whether state or federal

TOPICS FOR FURTHER INQUIRY

1. Review at least three employee handbooks from health care delivery systems and analyze the type(s) of alternative dispute resolution methods they use for employee grievance resolution.

2. Analyze the types of cases and the awards given to plaintiffs in cases in which a nurse is a named defendant, during a 2- or 3-month period, in the state and federal courts in your state.

3. Attend a nursing negligence trial, identify the role(s) of any nurse in the trial, and evaluate his or her effectiveness in that role.

4. Do a comparative study of the number of civil cases involving nurses and civil cases involving at least three other health care providers.

REFERENCES

1. Henry Campbell Black. *Black's Law Dictionary*. 7th Edition. St. Paul, Minn.: West Group, 1999, 889.
2. Lawrence Friedman. *A History of American Law*. New York: Simon & Schuster, 1985, 695.
3. *Id.* at 19.
4. Lawrence Baum. *American Courts: Process and Policy*. 4th Edition. Boston: Houghton Mifflin Company, 1998, 7–9.
5. Friedman, *supra* note 2, at 695.
6. Black, *supra* note 1, at 850.
7. U.S.C.A. Const. Article III, Section 1.
8. Baum, *supra* note 4, at 31.
9. Henry Abraham. *The Judicial Process: An Introductory Analysis of the Courts of the United States, England, and France*. 7th Edition. New York: Oxford University Press, 1998, 181.
10. *Id.* at 195.
11. Baum, *supra* note 4, at 42–43.
12. *Id.* at 44–45.
13. *Id.* at 5–6.
14. *Id.* at 46–47.
15. *Id.*
16. Abraham, *supra* note 9, at 157.
17. Baum, *supra* note 4, at 47.
18. Black, *supra* note 1, at 855.
19. Baum, *supra* note 4, at 22.
20. *Id.*
21. Ralph Chandler, Richard Enslen, and Peter Renstrom. *Constitutional Law Deskbook: Individual Rights*. 2nd Edition. Rochester, New York: Lawyers Cooperative Publishing, 1993, 673–674 (with May 1999 Cumulative Supplement).
22. Black, *supra* note 1, at 857.
23. Baum, *supra* note 4, at 24.
24. *Id.*
25. Black, *supra* note 1, at 1553–1554.
26. *Id.* at 1414.
27. *Id.* at 905.
28. *Id.* at 1173.
29. Abraham, *supra* note 9, at 121.
30. Baum, *supra* note 4, at 269–270.
31. Bette J. Roth, Randall Wulff, and Charles Cooper. "Introduction," in *The Alternative Dispute Resolution Practice Guide*. St. Paul, Minn.: West Group, 1998, Chapter 1:1, 1–2.
32. *Id.* at 1–3.
33. *Id.*
34. *Id.*
35. *Id.* at Appendix 2.
36. See, for example, 710 ILCS 15/1 *et seq.* (1976).
37. Baum, *supra* note 4, at 234.
38. Roth, Wulff, and Cooper, *supra* note 31, Chapter 22:1, 22:2, 22:3.
39. James Hunt and Patricia Strongin. *The Law of the Workplace: Rights of Employers and Employee*. 3rd Edition. Washington, D.C.: Bureau of National Affairs, 1994, 170.
40. See generally, Roth, Wulff, and Cooper, *supra* note 3.

Ethics and Nursing Practice

3

Margaret R. Douglas, MS, RN

KEY PRINCIPLES

- Relationships between Ethics and Law
- Conflicts between Ethics and Law
- Bioethics
- Ethical Theories
- Moral Principles
- Moral Reasoning
- Ethics of Care
- Covenantal Relationships

Nurses face increasingly complex ethical concerns as changes in economics, technology, law, and morality interact within the context of human health. Once viewed primarily as a human service, health care has become a profitable business. Corporate values and practices interact and sometimes conflict with the values and practices of health care professionals, including nurses. Health care resources are finite. Financial benefits and burdens, once dismissed lightly, have become important considerations in health policy and clinical decision making. In addition, beliefs about the nature and development of human life and health care are being challenged as never before. On the one hand, genetic and technological innovations produce possibilities for creating and controlling new life. On the other hand, values about sanctity and quality of life compete with one another at the end of life. Nurses collaborate in providing technologically superior care to some persons, while they seek to limit the intrusions of technology into the lives of others. There is a "digital divide" in which people who have access to electronic information technology can be informed about state-of-the-art treatments for disease conditions, while those without such access continue to depend upon the treatment recommendations of their health care providers. Nurses work to improve basic primary health care services in communities that are struggling with poverty and its correlates—violence and inadequate housing, sanitation, nutrition, education, and access to health care. Paradoxically, nurses in the United States are practicing in what is simultaneously among the best and the worst of health care systems in the industrialized world.

> *. . . nurses in the United States are practicing in what is simultaneously among the best and the worst of health care systems in the industrialized world.*

It is not surprising, therefore, that ethics is central to nursing knowledge and practice. McAlpine[1] asserts that interest in ethics has grown from "cottage to growth industry status." Morally responsible individual and institutional comportment requires reasoning that is grounded not only in ethical theories and moral principles but also in moral reasoning, caring, and evolving conceptions of organizational or institutional ethics. This chapter presents an overview of the relationships between ethics and law, ethical theories, moral principles, moral reasoning, nursing ethics as the ethic of care, and a model for ethical decision making. Contemporary ethical issues related to advanced nursing practice, genetics, managed care, and institutional ethics are included.

BIOETHICS, NURSING ETHICS, AND BIOMEDICAL ETHICS

What is nursing ethics, and how is it similar to and different from biomedical ethics and law? Ethics, or moral philosophy, is concerned with the systematic study of morality—standards of moral conduct and moral judgment. Morality addresses traditions of belief about right and wrong human conduct.[2] Not all values or customs governing human conduct are moral values. Some customs or values may refer to other matters, such as economics, etiquette, esthetics, or culture. To differentiate morality from other norms of human conduct, Beauchamp[3] identified four properties that frequently are present in moral judgments. A judgment generally is considered to be a moral judgment if it has overriding social importance, prescribes a general course of action, is universalizable, and/or pertains to the general welfare of a social group.

Normative ethics refers to application of ethical theories, moral principles, and/or rules to specific situations or acts. Bioethics is the application of ethical theories and moral principles to life and to work. Nursing ethics, biomedical ethics, and ethics of other health care disciplines such as medical social work are dimensions of bioethics (see Figure 3–1).

RELATIONSHIPS AMONG ETHICS, LAW, AND NURSING PRACTICE

In a culturally pluralistic nation such as the United States, the dominant pattern of ethical norms is not easy to discern, let alone legislate. Given the changes that occur in all three areas—ethics, law, and nursing—it is not surprising that the relationships among the three sometimes are dissonant. Law, ethics, and nursing all are altered as society, conceptions of the moral good, and health care change. For example, rapid technologi-

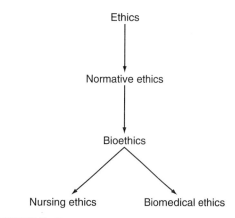

FIGURE 3–1. Nursing ethics as a component of normative ethics. From: D. M. Goldstein, "Scope Note 19: Nursing Ethics: A Selected Bibliography, 1987 to Present, 2(2) *Kennedy Institute of Ethics Journal* (1992), 177–192.

cal advances require that we address new legislation, nursing practice, and ways of balancing the burdens and benefits of technology. Exponential changes in information technology, such as increased use of the Internet by health care consumers, have influenced ethics, law, and nursing practice in the emerging field of "telehealth." In genetics research and practice, technological advances have been so rapid that the U.S. Human Genome Project[4] is expected to be completed in 2003, two years ahead of schedule. Furthermore, this project has allocated a percentage of its total budget to attend to the ethical, legal, and social issues that may be consequences of the project. This allocation is an unprecedented acknowledgment that "science tells us what is possible, but it does not tell us what is right."[5]

Recent changes in health care law include, but are not limited to, legislation concerning use of fetal tissue, assisted suicide, health care rationing, advanced practice nursing, and institutional staffing patterns and practices. Recent changes in health care ethics include expanding from a focus on individual morality to organizational or institutional ethics that includes greater attention to fiduciary morality. As more nurses are prepared in advanced practice roles, nursing practice is becoming more autonomous and collaborative. The *Code for Nurses with Interpretive Statements*[6] is being revised to explicitly address nurses' accountability to clients rather than to physicians and employers. The basic tenets of this code have not changed since 1973, although the *Interpretive Statements*

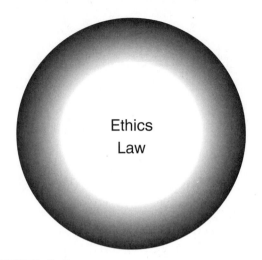

FIGURE 3–2. Coextensive relationship between ethics and law.

were revised in 1985. In a parallel way, nursing ethics itself is moving away from a reliance upon moral principles to a process of critical, reflective thinking that includes contextual, relational reasoning that frequently is referred to as an "ethic of care."

Thus, the relationships between law and ethics are complex and dynamic. Law and ethics serve to inform one another in a relationship that occasionally is cohesive but frequently is characterized by tension. There is, however, a pattern to the relationships that characterizes both the interrelationships and the way that the relationships change.

In an effort to clarify the interrelationships of ethics and law, Diane Kjervik,[7] a nurse-attorney, analyzed writings in both law and ethics to identify patterns of connection between the two. She concluded that there were at least three possible views: (1) *coextensive,* (2) *separate,* and (3) *partially overlapping.*

Patterns of Relationships between Law and Ethics

Coextensive Relationships

In the coextensive relationship (Figure 3–2), "law and ethics share the same scope in terms of matters considered."[8] In a pluralistic society such as the contemporary United States, the coextensive view more frequently represents the ideal than does the actual relationship between ethics and law. In the coextensive relationship, law and ethics may inform one another in at least two ways. When there is genuine, principled disagreement about

what is "good" or "just," law may help to inform ethics. Conversely, values may need to be negotiated through persuasion so that an overriding moral value may be discerned. In this latter situation, ethics would inform law. The Patient Self-Determination Act[9] is a close, although not perfect, example of coextensive relationships. In the Patient Self-Determination Act, the moral principle of respect for autonomy is affirmed through legislation requiring health care entities and providers receiving Medicare and Medicaid funds to ask persons if they have an advance directive, and if not, if they wish to execute an advance directive to express their treatment preferences in certain situations.

Separate Relationships

A separate relationship between law and ethics that Kjervik[10] identified is illustrated in Figure 3–3.

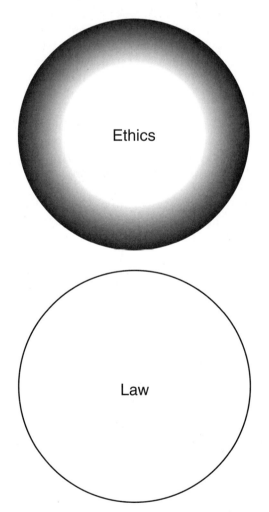

FIGURE 3–3. Separate relationship between ethics and law.

In the separate relationship, law and ethics are discrete and independent of one another. Each is concerned with "entirely distinct matters." If law and ethics were considered to be mutually exclusive, then one would not appeal to law for resolution of ethical issues. Furthermore, when existing legislation clearly conflicts with morality, one may argue that civil disobedience is morally required. The current effort to legislate a bill of rights for clients of managed care organizations illustrates a relationship between ethics and law.

Partially Overlapping Relationships

A partially overlapping relationship between law and ethics is the third possible relationship described by Kjervik.[11] Partially overlapping relationships are represented in either of two ways, depending upon the context. One form of the relationship may be illustrated by two interlocking circles (Figure 3–4), the second form by a circle within a larger circle (Figure 3–5). Of the two possibilities, Kjervik prefers the latter when the larger circle represents ethical matters and the smaller circle represents legal circumstances. The idea that law is embedded within ethics is consistent with the observation that some ethical issues extend beyond the boundaries of law.

Societal pluralism is another factor in determining the relationships between ethics and law in any given situation. In a pluralistic society, the prevailing moral values may be diverse and conflicting, thus making it difficult to discern whose values are being represented in any given legislation. The long-standing conflict between "pro-choice" and "pro-life" constituencies in the United

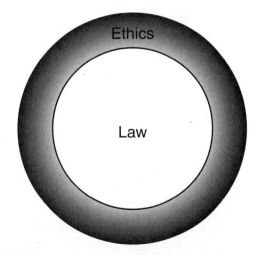

FIGURE 3–5. Partially overlapping relationship between ethics and law.

States highlights the difficulties of attempting to enact legislation that is in harmony with the dominant values of a pluralistic society. In another example, the Patient Self-Determination Act is based upon respect for autonomy as a dominant value in the United States. Cross-culturally, however, interdependence and community may be of greater value to some people than a given individual's autonomy. Among many indigenous people throughout the world, decisions are made within the context of the family and/or the community.

Time is another consideration in the relationship among law, ethics, and values. In the case of some civil rights, nearly a century passed before legislation was enacted that reflected the changing national moral values. That century was punctu-

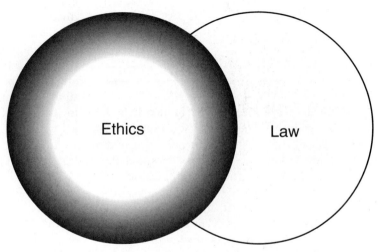

FIGURE 3–4. Partially overlapping relationship between ethics and law.

ated by warfare, other forms of violence, and civil disobedience.

Law, Ethics, and Complexity

In another view of the relationships between law and ethics, Schneider[12] asserts that law provides a "systematically disciplined," albeit inept, language for thinking about ethics as well as a tool through which to achieve action. Schneider claims that bioethics is a political movement as well as an academic discipline. The language of bioethics is broader in scope than the language of law. To illustrate the difference between the language of law and the language of bioethics, Schneider[13] contrasts the moral principle of autonomy with the legal concept of rights. Although bioethics can describe a principle of autonomy in such a way as to encompass its full meaning, the legal language of rights is more limited in scope. Law is an agency of social regulation and therefore must find authority in legal precedent of the past, while recognizing that it is setting legal precedent for the future.

The cases of *Roe v. Wade*[14] and *Cruzan*[15] illustrate the deliberative support of existing rights without establishing new rights. In *Cruzan,* the U.S. Supreme Court was asked to declare a constitutional right to die. Schneider contends that the Supreme Court might have supported a constitutional right to die had it not been for the right to abortion that was established by *Roe v. Wade,* a decision that has been contested for two decades.

. . . the language of law is designed to fulfill its task of social regulation, not to address the full and complex scope of morality . . .

Although "privacy" rights were at stake in both cases, the majority of the Court did not find a constitutional "right to die" in *Cruzan.* Citing Oliver Wendell Holmes,[16] Schneider shows that the language of law is designed to fulfill its task of social regulation, not to address the full and complex scope of morality. Further, there is danger in thinking that the languages of law and of bioethics are the same. "Nothing but confusion of thought

can result from assuming that the rights of man in a moral sense are equally rights in the sense of the Constitution and the law."[17] Bioethicists who refer to the law as the moral minimum[18] also address the usefulness of law in social regulation and its limitation in the complex, dynamic discourse of bioethics.

Although Kjervik's and Schneider's models may account for some of the relationships between ethics and law, the full array of influences on both law and ethics is extremely complex. For example, values help to inform both law and ethics in intricate patterns of relationships. The values that interact with law and ethics include, but are not limited to, cultural, spiritual, religious, and economic values. When economic resources are or are purported to be scarce, the relationship of economic values to law and morality becomes more critical than in times when resources are abundant. Managed care illustrates the connection of economic values with law and ethics. The current controversies and issues surrounding access to health care and managed care highlight the interaction of economics with law and ethics. Law, ethics, and other values may interrelate in many ways, including the possibilities of coextension, separation, and overlapping described by Kjervik.

Conflicts between Law and Ethics

Conflicts between legal and moral rights are common. Moral rights frequently are considered to exist independently of and form a basis for justifying or criticizing legal rights. Rights are the mirror images of duties or obligations. In their text *Principles of Biomedical Ethics,* Beauchamp and Childress define rights as "justified claims that individuals can make upon others or upon society."[19] For each duty, there is a corresponding right. Moral rights are claims that are grounded in moral principles and/or rules. Legal rights are claims that are based upon legal principles and rules. Discussions of rights to health care, for example, may focus on health care as a moral right or as a legal right.

In addition to being categorized as moral or legal, rights also can be considered either *positive* or *negative*. A positive right is a claim that requires that some action be taken in behalf of individuals with justifiable claims. The right to information about health care treatment options is an example of a positive right that obligates health professionals to provide patients with the material necessary to make informed choices about treatment. In the United States, Congress generally is concerned with legal rights. The United Nations, on the other hand, focuses on human rights, moral rights that are intended to correct deficiencies in legal rights in various nations.

The right to health care is an example of a conflict between legal and moral conceptions of rights. Individuals whose liberty interests have been curtailed, perhaps by imprisonment or institutionalization for mental illness, do have a positive legal right to health care. Others do not. Arguments supporting health care as a positive right sometimes contend that health care is a public good analogous to education and police or fire protection. Such arguments generally have not prevailed. In fact, according to Powers,[20] opponents of health care as a positive right have countered with the argument that state and local governments have no constitutional obligation to provide any "substantive services within their borders." The failure of the Clinton administration to create universal access to health care in the United States exemplifies the conflict between moral and legal rights.

Court decisions in the United States have tended to support negative rights with no corresponding entitlements. Negative rights require others to refrain from acting. The right to refuse treatment and the right to die are examples of negative rights that obligate professionals not to intervene. For example, in abortion decisions in the early 1980s, courts held that even though women had a fundamental right to abortion without governmental interference, there was no corresponding obligation of the federal government to pay for the abortion procedures, except to save the mother's life or in cases of rape or incest.[21]

Ethical-Legal Influences on Nursing Practice

The dialogue between case law and case analysis in ethics has helped to clarify the position of nursing and other disciplines regarding a number of issues, especially those concerned with refusal of life-sustaining (or life-prolonging) measures. In less than 50 years, industrialized societies have needed to modify the goal of prolonging life through curative treatments for terminal or incapacitating diseases and/or injuries. As life-sustaining and/or prolonging technology has de-

veloped, questions of balancing the benefits and burdens of duration of life with those of quality of life have arisen. The availability of technological cures that both enhance and devastate human life is relatively recent and requires an interdisciplinary dialogue to address in a responsible, compassionate way. Lawson[22] concludes that "whatever it is that we should value in life, it should not be made a function of what medical science renders possible."

The Patient Self-Determination Act[23] and state advance directive and health care surrogacy legislation are examples of how the moral principles, such as respect for autonomy, are supported by laws that affirm individuals' positive right to have information about treatment options and to express those choices in advance directives, such as living wills or durable powers of attorney. In the Patient Self-Determination Act, there is a corollary obligation of institutions and other health care providers to provide clients with information about their rights regarding treatment alternatives and the right to refuse treatment. The political, economic, ethical, and legal positions represented in the Patient Self-Determination Act emerged, in part, from the widely publicized *Cruzan*[24] case and the earlier *Quinlan*[25] case. Cases such as that of Helga Wanglie[26] and the Lakeberg conjoined twins[27] may help to clarify the boundaries between required and optional treatment and care. Whatever the structures of the relationships among ethics, law, and nursing practice, the processes are fluid and dynamic.

As legislation and morality change, nursing's positions on related issues change as well. Florence Nightingale, in *Suggestions for Thought,* wrote, "Ideas make progress. And the meanings attached to words which express these ideas cannot, therefore, remain the same."[28] Changing meanings of nurses' social responsibilities, rights, and moral codes are reflected in professional documents such as the *Code for Nurses with Interpretive Statements*[29] and *Nursing's Social Policy Statement.*[30] Changes in meaning and practice also are illustrated in position statements crafted by professional nursing organizations, such as the American Nurses Association (ANA), the National League for Nursing (NLN), and the American Association of Colleges of Nursing (AACN). Both the ANA and NLN have published position statements on assisted suicide, for example. Such codes, policies, and position statements are central to professional practice.

Managed Care and Ethics

The margins of practice are blurring still further as the dialogue extends to both extremes of treatment—from the need to cease futile treatment to the obligation to assist clients to obtain essential treatment that might not be approved by their health care carrier. Nurses have an advocacy role in helping people to secure the nature and quality of care that is essential to life and health. This advocacy role is becoming critically important in this managed care environment. Managed care is associated with the current trend toward institutional ethics. Managed care emphasizes aggregate rather than individual health and favors beneficence over autonomy.

Managed care is a contemporary, economically driven model of health care delivery that poses special concerns for ethics, law, and nursing practice. Some advocates of managed care argue that it provides opportunities as well. Acknowledging that managed care "has introduced conflicts of interest in health care," Koloroutis and Thorstenson[31] identified an ethics framework for organizational change within a context of managed care. The framework is intended to guide decision making at both clinical and institutional levels. Development of the framework was guided by three assumptions: stewardship of scarce resources; the centrality of caring, healing, and compassion; and the provision of physician and patient incentives to provide and receive appropriate care.

also varies. Generally, they are interdisciplinary and include health care professionals and community representatives. Typically, committees have representation from nursing, spiritual care, medical social work, law, medicine, hospital administration, and the community served by the institution. Some hospitals or medical centers have separate nursing ethics committees.

Early committees usually were prognosis committees. Subsequently, the committees expanded their functions to provide ad hoc and retrospective case consultation, including ethics rounds, in hospitals and medical centers. In the next stage of development, ethics committees provided ethics education programs and developed policies concerned with common ethical issues and concerns. Educational and policy-development initiatives addressed but were not limited to responses to health care legislation and regulation, such as the Patient Self-Determination Act and Joint Commission on the Accreditation of Healthcare Organizations (JCAHO)[33] criteria regarding patient rights. JCAHO requires that hospitals have processes to ensure a "patient's right to considerate care that preserves dignity and respects cultural, psychosocial, and spiritual values." In this era of managed care, ethics committees are again in transition, moving beyond concern for individual moral comportment to addressing organizational ethics, including moral fiduciary accountability, in a more systematic way.

Whatever the structures of the relationship among ethics, law, and nursing practice, the processes are fluid and dynamic.

Ethics committees are again in transition, moving beyond concern for individual moral comportment to addressing organizational ethics.

The Development of Ethics Committees

From their beginning as a consequence of the *Quinlan*[32] case, ethics committees have undergone several functional and structural transitions. Generally, these changes have occurred gradually, and the functions of each developmental stage have been retained in subsequent stages. Some functions are retained by the full committee. Others, such as case consultation and ethics rounds, may be delegated. The structure of ethics committees

Perhaps ethics committees will be transformed into what Christopher[34] refers to as "integrated ethics programs." Integrated ethics programs would extend into all areas of policy development and organizational structure, not only those that ordinarily are regarded as ethics related. Lawson[35] suggests that this transition would require that ethicists have a much broader knowledge of business and economics than they currently have. In addition, key decision makers would need to be educated and become involved as "ethics advocates." In managed care organizations, ethics committee members may be called upon to consider a wide range of issues about the allocation and distribution of resources, including whether an institution should reduce its marketing budget in order to provide more charitable care. Some aspects of labor relations issues also may be addressed by ethics committees or their counterparts in managed care organizations.

The present shift to institutional ethics in this era of managed care is complex and challenging. In this emerging ethics committee model, collaboration between bioethicists and institutional economists may be required to create models of institutional ethics that are just. Few bioethicists currently are prepared by either education, experience, or philosophical stance to create a model that addresses all facets of institutional ethics. Institutional economists, too, are limited. Generally, they have backgrounds in business ethics, not bioethics. Although there are some bioethicists who also are grounded in economics and some economists with strong backgrounds in bioethics, they are in the minority.

ETHICAL THEORIES, MORAL PRINCIPLES, AND MORAL REASONING

In recent decades, nursing ethics has been influenced by philosophy, theology, and psychology, as well as nursing praxis. A variety of ethical theories and moral principles from philosophical and theological ethics have offered a way of thinking about the moral life and ethical decision making in health care and nursing. Although each category of theories and principles is useful in informing ethical decision making in nursing, all are limited in addressing the universe of ethical issues encountered in contemporary practice. This is particularly the case in this technological information age and managed care environment in which moral and economic values coexist, not always peacefully. Although bioethicists disagree about the extent to which applying ethical theories and moral principles is useful in practice, an overview of philosophical ethics is offered for consideration as general guides for ethical judgments.[36]

Ethical Theories

Three categories of philosophical ethical theories—virtue, consequentialist, and deontologi-

cal—historically have served as a foundation for ethics in health care and nursing. Table 3–1 lists selected ethical theories and their relationship to nursing ethics.

Contractarian and rights-based theories sometimes are considered to be separate ethical theories. They will be considered here to be types of deontological theories. *Contractarian ethical theory* has some features in common with the Anglo-American legal system. In contract theory, the rules of ethics are a product of negotiated consensus. Contracts can be either formal or informal, individual or societal. Valid contracts hold that each party to the contract has duties to other parties.

Moral Principles

Moral principles serve as a foundation for reflection on moral conduct and general guides for ethical decision making in nursing. Although less abstract and more context specific than ethical theories, moral principles are at a higher level of abstraction than are rules or specific actions. For example, rules about informed consent are based on the moral principle of respect for autonomy.

What are the key moral principles and how many are there? Moral philosophers disagree about the number of key moral principles. Some moral philosophers like Beauchamp and Childress[37] argue that there are four moral principles. Others, such as Veatch,[38] identify six or more. The four principles of respect for autonomy, nonmaleficence, beneficence, and justice proposed by Beauchamp and Childress will be accepted for purposes of discussion in this chapter. Other moral principles that are generally included in discussions of ethics in nursing include fidelity or promise-keeping, veracity or truth-telling, confidentiality, and privacy. These additional principles will be considered to be rules that are grounded in the four moral principles, especially in respect for autonomy.

The principles do not have an inherent rank order. Until recently, however, there has been a high value for autonomy in the U.S. In institutional ethics, however, there is a trend toward focusing on beneficence (the good for society as a whole). In the current ANA *Code for Nurses with Interpretive Statements*,[39] there is no consensus about the rank ordering of moral principles. However, in the proposed revision, autonomy is regarded highly. Eth-

TABLE 3–1

Selected Ethical Theories and Their Relationship to Nursing

ETHICAL THEORY	PHILOSOPHER/ETHICIST	CENTRAL THESIS	RELEVANCE TO NURSING
Consequentialist (Teleological or Utilitarianism)	Jeremy Bentham John Stuart Mill	Outcome-oriented (from *telos* "end")— The principle of social utility, the greatest good or least harm for the greatest number	The principle of utility undergirds much of clinical nursing practice, social policy, and quantitative nursing research. Nursing process is goal-directed and outcome-oriented, as are critical pathways and Diagnostic Related Groups (DRGs)
Deontological	Immanuel Kant	Process-oriented (from *deon* "rule")— The rightness or wrongness of an act is determined by its inherent moral significance, not outcome	The *Code for Nurses: With Interpretive Statements* has a strong deontological focus. In early stages of nurse-patient relationships, standards of practice, institutional policies, etc. help to establish parameters of appropriate moral conduct
Virtue	Aristotle Alasdair MacIntyre	Person-oriented—Addresses moral life and values. Moral goodness or badness is discussed in terms of the moral value attached to the character trait or virtue	Historically, virtue theory was the basis for nursing's emphasis on the moral character of the nurse

Data from: J. Bentham. *An Introduction to the Principles of Morals and Legislation.* New York: Hafner, 1948; J. S. Mill. *Utilitarianism.* G. Sher, Editor. Indianapolis: Hackett Publishing Company, 1979; I. Kant. *Grounding for the Metaphysics of Morals.* J. Ellington, Trans. Indianapolis: Hackett Publishing Company, 1981; ANA. *Code for Nurses: With Interpretive Statements.* Kansas City, Mo.: Author, 1985; Aristotle. *Nichomachean Ethics,* Book 2, A. E. Wardman Trans., in R. Bambrough. *The Philosophy of Aristotle.* New York: Mentor Books, 1966; A. MacIntyre. *After Virtue.* Notre Dame, Ind.: University of Notre Dame Press, 1981.

icists frequently disagree about the overriding moral principles that inform decisions in specific cases. The four moral principles relevant to nursing are defined in Table 3–2.

The Moral Principle of Respect for Autonomy

Respect for autonomy generally refers to individual freedom of choice or liberty interests. However, autonomy is not an "all-or-nothing" phenomenon. There are gradations of autonomy.[40–43] Threats to autonomy arise from several sources, including uncertainty about how to interpret and respect autonomy. Autonomy is threatened in two major ways: interfering too much (excessive control) and not interfering enough (neglect). There is a fine line between respect for autonomy and abandonment, particularly in care of uninsured, underinsured, chronically ill, mentally ill, physically disabled, adolescent, and elderly patients. Respect for autonomy is also threatened when the exercise of one person's autonomy rights interferes with another person's freedom of choice and ac-

tion. This situation frequently occurs when ill persons are cared for at home by a family caregiver.

Much of the work on autonomy has been done in acute care settings. With managed care, prospective payment systems, and early hospital discharge, the ethics of community, home, and long-term care need to be addressed more adequately than in the past. The predominant North American value for keeping patients out of nursing homes has the potential for threatening the autonomy of at least three categories of individuals: patients, their family caregivers, and their formal caregivers.

INFORMED CONSENT. As is the case with autonomy in general, processes and practices that are associated with autonomy also are changing. For example, the processes of giving informed consent in clinical practice and research are being challenged. With the current focus on communitarian ethics, ethical dimensions of informed consent are in transition. In clinical ethics, informed consent was once considered to be primarily or solely the right of the individual or surrogate decision maker. Currently, informed consent is beginning to be

TABLE 3-2	

Definitions of Moral Principles Relevant to Nursing

MORAL PRINCIPLE	DEFINITION
Respect for Autonomy	Self-determination. Recognizes the right of persons to choose their actions freely without being constrained by the will or governance of others. Generally refers to individual freedom of choice or liberty interests. Three conditions of autonomous action are (1) intentionality, (2) understanding, (3) absence of controlling influences
Nonmaleficence	Doing no harm. Generally considered to be the first principle of human interaction (sometimes incorporated into the principle of beneficence)
Beneficence	Preventing harm, removing harm, and doing good
Justice	Fairness; giving to each his or her due (claim or entitlement)

Data from: T. L. Beauchamp and J. F. Childress. *Principles of Biomedical Ethics.* 4th Edition. New York: Oxford University Press, 1994.

examined from the perspective of family.[44] This shift in considering informed consent as a process rather than an event acknowledges that individuals' values change over time. When their values are stable, individuals can decide about important life events in a way that is congruent with their values. If, however, a person's beliefs and moral ideals are in transition, consent becomes an interpretive process that is made in collaboration with others, such as family. This communal approach to informed consent assumes that "values do not simply emanate from some ineffable core within us but take shape through interaction with our environment."[45] Legal aspects of informed consent are discussed in Chapter 12.

The Moral Principle of Nonmaleficence

The principle of nonmaleficence holds that one should do no harm. Discerning what is harmful is one of the most difficult problems in clinical practice. Although it is relatively easy to understand that some actions in and of themselves will be harmful to human life and/or health, it is harder to determine when an action that is intended to be helpful actually harms. It is even more difficult to discern when intentionally or unintentionally refraining from action harms or risks harm to another. Few treatments are entirely beneficial and without risk of harm.

PAIN MANAGEMENT. The dilemma of pain management in terminally ill clients illustrates the principle of nonmaleficence in both acting and refraining from acting.[46] As disease progresses and death becomes imminent, persons may experience excruciating pain, pain that is managed by increasingly large and potentially lethal doses of medication.[47-49] Nurses who struggle with the clinical judgment of whether and when to administer such treatments must consider the issue of harm, the standard of due care, and the ANA's *Code for Nurses with Interpretive Statements.* Nurses have developed great skill in helping clients to manage their pain.

Pro bono or volunteer work is a professional obligation of beneficence. For example, some nurses and other health care professionals volunteer several hours per month at storefront clinics for homeless persons.

The Moral Principle of Beneficence

Some ethicists consider that the principle of beneficence incorporates nonmaleficence. Beneficence, as explicated by Beauchamp and Childress,[50] entails the obligations to (1) prevent harm, (2) remove harm, and (3) do good. The idea of balancing risks, harms, benefits, and effectiveness is grounded in the principle of beneficence. Although there is general agreement that beneficence involves personal, professional, and societal obligations, there is disagreement about the strength and boundaries of those obligations. *Pro bono* or volunteer work is a professional obligation of beneficence. For example, some nurses and other health care professionals volunteer several hours per month at storefront clinics for homeless persons.

INSTITUTIONAL ETHICS AND MANAGED CARE. In the evolving communitarian ethics and in managed care systems, there is a trend away from focusing on individual autonomy toward greater emphasis on beneficence.[51] This view of beneficence encompasses the good not only of the individual but of the institution and society as a whole. The movement away from individualistic ethics toward institutional ethics favors beneficence as a dominant moral principle.

RESEARCH: PROTECTION OF HUMAN SUBJECTS. Beneficence also figures prominently in the ethics of research. From a research perspective, consent to participate in research studies also encompasses moral principles besides beneficence, including nonmaleficence, respect for autonomy, and justice. Ethical guidelines for the conduct of research and protection of human subjects originated with the *Nuremberg Code,* in response to the atrocities committed in the name of experimentation in World War II concentration camps. Subsequent guidelines include the international *Declaration of Helsinki* and the *Belmont Report.*[52] These documents were used by the U.S. National Commission for the Protection of Human Subjects of Biomedical and Behavioral Research to develop the 1978 national policies for the protection of human subjects. The ANA *Guidelines for Nurses in Clinical and Other Research*[53] also reflect the principles presented in the *Belmont Report.*

Institutional review boards (IRBs) have developed protocols for the protection of human subjects that comply with the national guidelines. In recent years, however, there has been a dramatic increase in the amount of research that needs to be reviewed and monitored, without a corresponding increase in the human and material resources allocated to IRB offices and staff. With the increased workload, insufficient institutional resources, and changes in research methodologies, some IRBs have been reported for failure to follow the rules for research review processes. Charges of scientific misconduct also have been made.[54-57] The National Institutes of Health (NIH) Office for Protection from Research Risks (OPRR) placed a moratorium on clinical research, including nursing research, in several prestigious medical centers. This recognition of lapses in the protection of human subjects of research has led to productive national problem-solving and educational forums for IRB members and staff. The ethical dimensions of research will be much more carefully attended to in the future than they have been in the recent past, both nationally and internationally. Nurses who conduct or participate in clinical research must continue to be mindful and vigilant in the protection of human subjects in research. Like physicians, nurses who are both researchers and clinicians must be aware of how their dual roles may be perceived by patients who also are research subjects.

The Moral Principle of Justice

Justice refers to fairness or to receiving one's due. One type, distributive justice, is concerned with the allocation and distribution of scarce benefits when there is competition for them. Theories of distributive justice typically address one or all of the following considerations about the distribution of benefits and burdens to each person: (1) an equal share, (2) according to individual need, (3) according to individual effort, and (4) according to societal contribution.

The language of justice frequently is used to discuss issues and policies concerning the allocation and distribution of scarce resources, including health care resources.[58-61] Table 3–3 lists several concepts of justice and their impact upon health care allocation.

Rawls's *A Theory of Justice*[62] is an example of a conception of justice that sometimes is used to guide actual or proposed social policy development. The recent and continuing issue of transforming the current health care system in the United States emerges, in part, from a question whether there is a moral right to access to health care goods and services. If so, then the question of how those goods and services can be fairly distributed among the population becomes a central concern. Claims that some managed care organizations are unjust arise from the view that those who are most vulnerable have the least access to care; thus they bear a greater burden than those who can afford to pay for health care.

In addressing the need for health care reform, May[63] appeals to a reaffirmation of

> our foundations as a people. Our founders assumed that if a nation could create a common good, it should make that good common. We can now deliver health care to all our people, and this good will help secure and enhance the life, liberty, and welfare that is our nation's promise to its citizens. It is time to reconfirm that promise to one another. Such a renewal of

TABLE 3–3

Conceptions of Distributive Justice That Inform Health Care Allocation

CONCEPTION	PHILOSOPHER	MAJOR IDEAS	HEALTH POLICY IMPLICATIONS
Egalitarian	Aristotle	Equality in all respects of condition being considered (i.e., health care)	One-tier system. No one would be entitled to more or fewer benefits than anyone else in society.
Libertarian	John Stuart Mill	Individual liberty should not be restricted on any grounds except that of harm to others (Mill)	Two-tier system. Minimal health care benefits would be provided for those who have no resources to purchase more extensive goods and services. Goods and services beyond the minimum would depend upon one's ability to pay.
	Robert Nozick	The minimal state is the most extensive state that can be justified (Nozick)	
Decent minimum	John Rawls	Fairness: (1) Each person is to have an equal right to the most extensive basic liberty compatible with a similar liberty for others. (2) Social and economic inequalities are to be arranged so that they are both (a) reasonably expected to be to everyone's advantage, and (b) open to all	A system that would define a standard of minimally decent health care that no one would fall below. Everyone would be able to compete for access to goods and services beyond the decent minimum.

Data from: Aristotle, *Nichomachean Ethics,* Book 2, A. E. Wardman, Trans., in R. Bambrough, *The Philosophy of Aristotle.* New York: Mentor Books, 1966; J. S. Mill, *Utilitarianism.* G. Sher, Editor. Indianapolis: Hackett Publishing Company, 1979. (Original work published 1861); R. Nozick. *Anarchy, State, and Utopia.* New York: Basic Books; J. Rawls. *A Theory of Justice.* Cambridge, Mass: Harvard University Press, Belnap Press, 1971.

a covenant seems difficult, coming as it does, so late in the day and with well-established interests already in the field. It will surely require a broad appeal to self-interest. But it will also need to appeal to . . . those angels that Tocqueville must have discerned when he wrote that a "covenant exists . . . between all citizens of a democracy when they all feel themselves subject to the same weakness and the same dangers; their interests as well as their compassion makes it a rule with them to lend one another assistance when required."

JOHN RAWLS ON JUSTICE, INSTITUTIONS, AND LAW

Justice is the first virtue of social institutions as truth is of systems of thought. A theory, however elegant and economical, must be revised if it is untrue; likewise, laws and institutions, no matter how efficient and well-arranged, must be reformed or abolished if they are unjust.[1]

[1] J. Rawls. *A Theory of Social Justice.* Cambridge, Mass.: Belnap Press of Harvard University Press, 1971, 3.

Moral Reasoning

Moral reasoning is the psychological interpretive process that helps to connect one's moral values with one's ethical choices. Through moral reasoning, one examines the salient features in an ethical situation and makes a judgment or chooses a course of action that is, presumably, congruent with one's moral beliefs and values. Moral values are not static, but change as persons mature. Theorists of moral reasoning are attempting to discern the developmental patterns of moral values. Such developmental conceptions of moral reasoning include those of Piaget,[64] Kohlberg,[65, 66] Gilligan,[67, 68] and Rest.[69] Piaget was among the first psychologists to propose a developmental approach to the study of human values.

Kohlberg extended Piaget's work and proposed a linear, hierarchical model of three sequential levels, each of which contained two stages. In the first and lowest level, *preconventional morality,* moral behavior is grounded in external rules about right and wrong. In the second level, *conventional morality,* moral conduct is based on a sense of order and human relationships. In the third and highest level, *principled morality,* behavior is governed by a sense of social responsibility and justice.

A PHYSICIAN SPEAKS OF SOCIAL JUSTICE

The United States "is, first, a country morally imperiled, and those of us who care for patients cannot but do so in bad faith. This country and South Africa stand alone among industrial powers in having no national system of health care. Here, we have elected the commercialization of medicine rather than its socialization. The only aspect of our health policy which resembles a system is the systematic exclusion of millions. It is the fittest who benefit, not the frail, and not the vulnerable."[1]

---

[1] D. McGuire, "Forward: Medicine: a Bedside View," Editor. in *The Crisis in Health Care: Ethical Issues*. N. McKenzie, New York: Meridian, 1990, 11–18.

Based on extensive comparative studies using Kohlberg's interviews and the *Defining Issues Test* (DIT), Rest[70] and colleagues suggested that moral development is more complex than Piaget and Kohlberg had proposed. Rest proposed a model of moral action stating that four types of psychological processes are required for a person to take moral action: (1) moral sensitivity, (2) moral reasoning, (3) moral commitment, and (4) moral action.

Gilligan,[71] a moral psychologist, has discerned two moral orientations in human development. She argues that two moral visions—one of justice and one of care—recur in human experience. The *justice orientation* focuses on oppression and inequality and values reciprocity and equal respect. The *care orientation* focuses on detachment or abandonment and values attention and response to need. Although both men and women evidence both justice and care concerns as they discuss moral issues, women tend to adopt a care perspective and men, a justice orientation.

Although both men and women evidence both justice and care concerns as they discuss moral issues, women tend to adopt a care perspective and men, a justice orientation.

Gilligan and her colleagues are discerning a different moral developmental pattern, one that reflects a high value for the contextual relevance of a situation. Gilligan's work, with its emphasis on human relationships and caring, resonates with nursing's contemporary focus on the ethics of care. Although several models of moral development have been explored in nursing,[72] no one model of moral reasoning has adequately explained the complexities of ethical decision making in the nursing profession. In addressing Gilligan's studies, Ray commented that Gilligan's work "reinforces the complexity of the ethical caring perspective."[73]

No one model of moral reasoning has adequately explained the complexities of ethical decision making in the nursing profession.

There is agreement among moral developmental theorists, however, that moral reasoning is linked to ethical decision making. One's pattern of moral reasoning may help to determine the pattern of principles or values that is associated with ethical decision making.

NURSING ETHICS AS THE ETHICS OF CARE

Nursing ethics, although long embedded within the context of bioethics and biomedical ethics, is emerging as a distinct type of normative ethics, an ethics of care.[74] Definitions of caring vary so widely that a substantive discussion about what caring means is beyond the scope of this chapter. Nevertheless, common themes in the caring literature suggest that caring is concerned with reciprocal human connections and relationships,[75–77] preserving personhood in a world of objectivity,[78] and alleviating vulnerability.[79] The status of caring as a moral standard is still in a fluid, evolutionary state. Caring is argued to be a virtue, an imperative,[80] or a moral ideal.[81, 82] Despite such ambiguity, caring is considered to be an emerging foundation for ethics in nursing.[83–85]

As nursing matures as a discipline and as the solutions of science simultaneously resolve and create health care problems, the need for an ethic of relationship that cherishes all persons has seldom been greater. The work of Carol Gilligan[86] and nurse philosophers and theorists such as Patricia Benner,[87] Barbara Carper,[88] Sally Gadow,[89] Madeleine Leininger,[90] Margaret Newman,[91] and Jean Watson[92, 93] explores how an ethic of care may serve to create moral community as nurses and others affirm the value of relationship in health care. Watson proposes that "an ethic of care has a distinct moral position: caring is attending and relating to a person in such a way that the person is protected from being reduced to the moral status of objects."[94] Nursing ethics as the ethic of care is grounded in the human-to-human relationships that are referred to as the nurse-patient/client relationship.

Covenantal Relationships

A covenantal relationship model of nurse-patient relationships is consistent with nursing ethics as an ethic of care.[95, 96] A variety of models of physician-patient relationship have been examined for their relevance to nurse-patient relationships.[97–100] Covenantal relationships are characterized by (1) mutual exchange of gifts, (2) entrustment, and (3) endurance.[101] Patients give at least two kinds of gifts to nurses—the individual gift of participation and presence in the relationship and the social gift of support for education and regulation of professional practice. Nurses give patients the gift of competent, caring practice that is consistent with professional standards and statutory regulations.

Although patients and nurses are strangers when they first meet, they trust each other to fulfill the expectations that they have of each other. In most instances, nurses expect that patients will be open and honest in the information they share about their own health and experiences of illness. Patients expect that nurses will be competent to practice according to legal and professional standards. In addition, nurses expect that patients will engage in the health practices or treatments that are negotiated through the nursing process. Patients, in turn, expect that the nurse will provide care as long as it is needed. Covenantal relationships are not static. According to Beauchamp,[102] they are a process of mutual discovery of those health practices that are *negotiated* within the context of ongoing developing relationship. Furthermore, the *mutuality of perspectives* is *constantly evolving* and must be reevaluated as goals emerge that were not clearly seen before. Finally, and perhaps most importantly, each person is changed in the relationship. Table 3–4 illustrates the characteristics of covenantal nurse-patient relationships.

Covenantal Relationships and Conflict

Covenantal relationships are not idyllic connections in which everything always goes smoothly. The assumption that nurses will not abandon patients is being challenged as nursing practice is influenced by unevenly distributed financial resources. Societal patterns of drug use and violence against strangers limits patients' willingness to be open and honest in entrusting their

---

	TABLE 3–4	

Characteristics of Covenantal Nurse-Patient Relationships

CHARACTERISTICS OF COVENANTAL RELATIONSHIPS	NURSES	PATIENTS
Exchange of gifts	Professional practice: competence in nursing knowledge and skills; commitment to attending and practicing according to legal and professional standards	Enabling privilege of professional practice: willingness to participate in nurse-patient relationship and societal support of health care and educational institutions and regulation of practice
Entrustment	Willingness to enter as strangers into a continuing relationship	Willingness to entrust life and health to professional strangers
Endurance	Commitment to "walk with" patient through experiences of wellness and illness; promise not to abandon	Commitment to follow through with recommended treatments or to be open with nurse about decision to refuse treatments

Data from: J. L. Allen. *Love and Conflict.* Lanham, Md.: University Press of America, 1995.

well-being to strangers. Furthermore, some believe covenantal relationships contain seeds of conflict. External threats to covenantal relationships between physicians and clients have been addressed by May.[63] He specifically cites managed care and assisted suicide as threats to the physician's covenant. Both managed care and assisted suicide are concerns for nurses, as well. The ANA has issued statements opposing assisted suicide.[104, 105]

Allen,[106] in his book *Love and Conflict,* proposes two categories of covenants: inclusive and special. Inclusive covenants are open to all persons by virtue of their being human. Inclusive covenants are concerned with basic human rights and obligations. Special covenants are open only to those persons who meet specific criteria for membership. Examples of special covenants include marriage, family, and professional covenants. Parents, for example, have obligations for the health and safety of their own children that exceed the obligations they have for the children of strangers. People have a wide variety of covenantal relationships all at once. For instance, nurses are members of inclusive covenants that connect them with all other humans. In addition, they are in special covenantal relationships with their families, their employers, and their professional organizations.

Conflict occurs when the needs or obligations of some covenants are at odds with the needs or obligations of other covenants. When conflicts occur between two or more special covenants, creativity and negotiation skills can be used to preserve the integrity of the relationships. For example, nurses who are single mothers frequently experience such conflict when they are scheduled to work at the same time that one of their children is ill. Another family member, friend, or neighbor may care for the child, or another nurse may be willing to work an extra shift or work on a day off.

When conflicts occur between inclusive covenants and special covenants, however, Allen argues that the commitment to the inclusive covenant should take precedence over the commitment to the special covenants. For example, a nurse who witnesses the abuse of an elderly person is morally obligated to intervene to protect the person's safety and well-being even if a colleague or employer demands that the nurse overlook the situation. "Whistleblowing" often occurs in situations in which nurses recognize that a person's human rights or welfare are violated. This is an example of choosing to support the inclusive covenant of human rights rather than the special covenant of employer-employee relationships.

Although it is emerging as a distinctive branch of bioethics and is clearly differentiated from biomedical ethics, nursing ethics, as the ethic of care, values ethical theories and moral principles as reference points and guides with which to appraise specific actions and arrive at moral choices together with patients. The technological maze of possibilities for treatment and the managed care environment create new challenges for everyone involved. Ethicists, lawyers, legislators, and health care professionals are struggling with the uncertainties about what is beneficial, burdensome, efficient, affordable, and compassionate. Earlier ways of examining ethical issues in health care, although necessary as reference points, are not sufficient to address the contextual complexities of health care possibilities and problems. Therefore, ethical theories and moral principles are necessary but not sufficient foundations for the moral life in nursing. Such theories and principles offer structure and clarity to the covenantal dialogue. Together with a covenantal nurse-patient relationship, examination of relevant ethical theories and moral principles can help more fully to inform the moral life of nursing practice and the institutions with which nurses are associated.

Earlier ways of examining ethical issues in health care, although necessary as reference points, are not sufficient to address the contextual complexities of health care possibilities and problems.

NARRATIVE AS A WAY OF REVEALING MORAL COMPORTMENT

Narrative discourse or story is at the heart of the ethics of care and of covenantal relationships. Narrative is a way of revealing community beliefs and values, of understanding which moral principles are operating and in what context. Benjamin commented that "narrative achieves an amplitude that information lacks."[107] Such narratives can appear in many forms as prose, as poetry, and as other media. Diekelmann,[108] for example, has found that through the sharing of stories in clinical and educational settings, nurses are coming to a greater trust in their own clinical judgment and are valuing collaboration with colleagues and patients. Gadow[109] asserts that in nursing, story is truth.

The communal moral conversation will be fuller and richer if it acknowledges all who comprise the moral community, especially clients. Narrative and theoretical work, together, offer a fuller understanding of nursing ethics than is possible with either approach alone. In addressing the need to value both theoretical or propositional and narrative types of discourse, Carson[110] remarked that in bioethics, propositional discourse is useful in selecting relevant ideas and arguing their merit, but narrative offers a way of synthesizing sense and reason. Bioethical rationality, he continues, has lost sight of the importance of imagination, which is composed of the emotions and the intellect. Narrative can help all who participate in ethical decision making to find moral peace, if not moral certainty.

In ordinary moments of their everyday professional lives, nurses are privileged to participate in extraordinary moments in the lives of others. Yet, much of what is most important to nurses in their practice is private. Nursing practice must become more visible if the full scope of nurses' work is to be valued in this era of managed care. In a discussion of caring and gender-sensitive ethics, Bowden contends that nursing and the recipients of nursing care have been disproportionately affected when institutional costs are cut. "Although historically the major part of hospital incomes has derived from selling nursing services—especially in the early part of the century when medicine had few services to offer—invisibility in billing and on the governing boards of hospitals has made nursing care the obvious source of cost control . . . nursing care has always been severely and disproportionately constrained by health care budgets."[111] One way that nurses have begun to make their practice more visible, and therefore more powerful, is through the use of narrative, or story.

Narrative discourse or story is at the heart of the ethics of care and of covenantal relationships. Narrative is a way of revealing community beliefs and values, of understanding which moral principles are operating and in what context.

ETHICAL DECISION MAKING: A PROCESS AND A MODEL

Theories and moral principles serve as a reference point in the contextual, relational dimensions of nurse-patient covenants. From the perspective of truth as found in narrative, linear models of ethical decision making have limits. Frequently what seems like an ethical conflict really is lack of information or understanding about the facts of the situation. Like the Sufi legend of the blind men describing an elephant, each person may possess different data and/or interpret the same data differently. A process of ethical decision making that is grounded in an ethic of care and in covenantal relationships is contextual and communal. The kinds of questions asked and the alternatives proposed reflect an assumption that humans live in communities, not in isolation. Whenever possible, all persons who are involved in the decision are part of the process. The options proposed are not usually standard choices, but are creative alternatives that are unique to the persons and the communities involved. Some of the key questions are shown in Table 3–5.

A process of ethical decision making that is grounded in an ethic of care and in covenantal relationships is contextual and communal. The kinds of questions asked and the alternatives proposed reflect an assumption that humans live in communities, not in isolation.

TABLE 3–5

Considerations Relevant to Ethical Decision Making

1. The facts:

What are the facts of the situation? All too frequently, what appears to be an ethical issue is really misunderstanding of the information available, lack of information, lack of access to the information, and/or inadequate communication about the situation.

What are the cognitive, emotional, spiritual, cultural, ethical, legal, and other decisional influences relevant to interpretation of the facts?

2. The persons:

Who is/are/should be involved in the situation?

What are their beliefs, values, knowledge, and decisional capacity with respect to the situation?

3. The institutions:

What institutions are involved in the situation (consider many levels from family to national/international institutions).

What norms, values, policies, regulations, laws, and economic considerations are relevant?

4. The relationships:

What covenantal relationships have bearing on the situation? Of these, which are inclusive; which are special?

Which of these relationships are in harmony; which are in conflict?

5. The issue(s):

What is a clear, concise, communal statement of the issue(s) in the situation?

Which of the issues are ethical? (Which are emotional, economic, legal, spiritual, cultural, etc?)

6. The options:

What are the alternative courses of action? (Generate as many as possible. Try not to fall into the either/or trap; think of creative possibilities.)

What are the consequences of each alternative?

What are the benefits of each option?

Who benefits?

What are the burdens?

Who bears the burdens?

For which option(s) do the benefits most outweigh the burdens (or which options are least burdensome) and for whom: the client, the community, both client and community?

7. The choice(s):

Who should decide?

What should be decided?

Who should communicate the decision?

Who should carry out the chosen action(s)?

8. The evaluation:
Formative (Process):

Are the actions as beneficial as anticipated?

Are the burdens as onerous as anticipated?

Are the actual benefits greater than the actual burdens (or is this actually the least burdensome alternative?)

If not, what alternative courses of actions are available/preferable?

Summative (Outcome):

Was the intended benefit achieved? Were the anticipated burdens present?

What can we learn from this situation that will help to inform our future decision making, communication patterns, policies, and/or practices?

A STORY OF SUFFERING?

Bernard Gert, a philosopher and member of an ethics committee, shares a story about how he helped to identify the intent of a son's and daughter's request to continue to give morphine to their father, who was unconscious and dying from cancer:

"We started talking about the likelihood of their father actually suffering any pain or discomfort. The son was prepared to believe that their father was not suffering at all, but the daughter thought there was some slight possibility that he was suffering. However, when I pointed out to her that there was absolutely no change in his behavior before and after the morphine had been stopped, she admitted that this was correct. Eventually it became clear to all of us that the primary reason for their wanting morphine was to hasten death, that pain relief provided a rationalization for their insisting on the administration of morphine, but that neither of them had any firm conviction that their father was suffering."[1]

[1]B. Gert, "A Philosophical Consultation," in *Ethics at the Bedside*. C. M. Culver. Hanover, N.H.: University Press of New England, 1990, 29–39.

IMPLICATIONS FOR NURSING PRACTICE

Morally responsible nursing practice requires that nurses know and examine their own values as well as the codified and emerging values of the discipline. Although it is important for nurses to be aware of the dramatic dilemmas that frequently accompany crises at the beginning and end of life, they also must be sensitive to the more subtle ethical issues that are part of their history and are encountered every day. For example, changing staffing patterns in hospitals frequently raise issues of safety and effectiveness of nursing care. Error in medicine, nursing, and health care is a grave, international concern that is being addressed collaboratively by professional organizations. Several states have crafted safe staffing legislation as a response to the unsafe conditions created by inadequate staffing and mandatory overtime.

The use of a model of ethical decision making that is consistent with their values and beliefs will help nurses to thoroughly and systematically review the complex aspects of ethical situations in clinical practice. Nurses must develop the habit of thinking systematically and regularly about the ethical dimensions of their practice not only at the level of nurse-patient relationships but at a broader institutional level as well. They must be visible and vocal when policies and practices related to moral situations are discussed or developed. For example, nursing should have representation on institutional ethics committees and be involved in developing and/or revising policies related to ethical concerns such as advance directives (e.g., under what circumstances they are or are not honored). Nurses should know the forum for discussing ethical issues in their institutions and be aware of when and how to seek consultation from ethics committees or ethics consultants. They should develop comfort in discussing ethical issues with their patients and the patients' families. All nurses, especially those who are self-employed or employed in areas where there are no ethics committees, should cultivate a moral community, a safe haven for the discussion of the ethical issues they encounter in practice.

TOPICS FOR FURTHER INQUIRY

Until recently, research in nursing practice and nursing ethics has tended to focus on the characteristics of nurses and their moral reasoning processes and patterns with respect to their ethical decision making. As the context and communal nature of ethics in nursing and other health care professions is emerging as an important dimension of nursing ethics, research should focus on questions that address but are not limited to the following.

1. Phenomenological inquiry, including the lived experiences of communal moral relationships and/or decision making

2. Phenomenological and descriptive inquiry regarding moral and ethical issues in managed care, case management, and critical paths—for example, to what extent, if at all, is the quality of nursing care (with respect to professional norms and standards such as ANA *Standards of Nursing Practice,* state nurse practice acts, and professional credentialing criteria) altered for clients in managed care systems as compared with fee-for-service and/or other reimbursement/delivery models and questions regarding delegation to technicians, and the like

3. Phenomenological and descriptive studies of ethical considerations, issues, values, and the like in advanced nursing practice roles, such as clinical nurse specialists,

nurse practitioners, nurse anesthetists, and nurse-midwives

4. Phenomenological and descriptive studies of interdisciplinary patterns of the moral professional life and decision making

5. Phenomenological, descriptive, explanatory, predictive, and intervention studies to understand, describe, predict, and rectify such social justice concerns as restricted access to health care goods and services because of poverty and its consequences

6. Educational and evaluative research concerned with empowering students of nursing to act in accordance with their moral choices and to have a voice in interdisciplinary and community groups

7. Educational and evaluation research oriented toward heightening awareness of advance directives, consequences of managed care, and the like among well persons, so that individuals, families, and communities are not confronted with the need to make critical health care decisions during times of crisis when they are most vulnerable

8. Replication of the fine array of existing studies in nursing so that the emerging knowledge in nursing ethics can be verified and used in practice

REFERENCES

1. Heather McAlpine. "Critical Reflections about Professional Ethical Stances: Have We Lost Sight of the Major Objectives?" 35 *Journal of Nursing Education* (1996), 119–126.

2. Thomas L. Beauchamp and James F. Childress. *Principles of Biomedical Ethics*. 4th Edition. New York: Oxford University Press, 1994.

3. Thomas Beauchamp. *Philosophical Ethics: An Introduction to Moral Philosophy*. New York: McGraw-Hill Book Company, 1982.

4. See, generally, *Ethical, Legal, and Social Issues (ELSI) of the Human Genome Project,* located on the *Human Genome Project Information* Web site at http://www.ornl.gov. hgmis/resource/elsi/html, February 20, 1998.

5. Catherine L. Lawson. "The Second Stage of Bioethics and Institutionalist Economics." 32(4) *Journal of Economic Issues,* 1998, 985–988.

6. American Nurses Association. *Code for Nurses with Interpretive Statements.* Kansas City, Mo.: Author, 1985.

7. Diane Kjervik, "Legal and Ethical Issues: The Connection between Law and Ethics," 6 *Journal of Professional Nursing* (1990), 138, 185.

8. *Id.*

9. Omnibus Budget Reconciliation Act (OBRA). (Pub. L. No. 101-158, Sections 4205–5207; Sections 4751–4752), 1990. (Patient Self-Determination Act passed November 6, 1990).

10. Kjervik, *supra* note 7.

11. Kjervik, *supra* note 7.

12. C. E. Schneider, "Bioethics in the Language of the Law," *Hastings Center Report* (July-August 1994), 16–22.

13. *Id.*

14. *Roe v. Wade,* 410 U.S. 113 (1973).

15. *Cruzan v. Director, Missouri Department of Health,* 497 U.S. 261 (1990).

16. O. W. Holmes, "The Path of the Law," in O. W. Holmes, *Collected Legal Papers.* New York: Harcourt, Brace, 1920, 170.

17. *Id.*

18. E. Pellegrino, "Withholding Treatment, Surrogate Decisions and Rationing: Some Selected Aspects," in *Health Care Law and Ethics.* R. Southby and J. Hirsh, Editors. Washington, D.C.: George Washington University, 1989, 151–172.

19. Beauchamp and Childress, *supra* note 2.

20. M. Powers. *Legal Rights to Health Care.* Paper presented at the Advanced Bioethics Course II: Ethics and Health Care Allocation. Kennedy Institute of Ethics, Washington, D.C., March 1990.

21. *Id.*

22. Lawson, *supra* note 5.

23. OBRA, *supra* note 9.

24. *Cruzan, supra* note 15.

25. 70 N.J. 10 (1976), 355 A.2d 647 (1976).

26. *In re the Conservatorship of Wanglie,* No. PX-91-283 (Minn. Dist. Ct. Hennepin Co. July 1991).

27. D. C. Thomasma, J. Muraskas, and P. A. Marshall, "The Ethics of Caring for Conjoined Twins: The Lakeberg Twins," 26 *Hastings Center Report* (July/August 1996), 4–12.

28. M.D. Calabria and J. A. Macrae. Editors. *Suggestions for Thought by Florence Nightingale: Selections and Commentaries.* Philadelphia: University of Pennsylvania Press, 1994, 15.

29. ANA, *supra* note 6.

30. American Nurses Association. *Nursing's Social Policy Statement.* Washington, D. C.: Author, 1995.

31. M. Koloroutis and T. Thorstenson, "An Ethics Framework for Organizational Change," 3 *Nursing Administration Quarterly* (1999).

32. *Quinlin, supra* note 25.

33. C. Krozek and A. Scroggins, "Patient Rights . . . Amended to Comply with 1999 JCAHO Standards." *CINAHL Information Systems* (Glendale, Cal.), http://ovid1.aiss.uic.edu/ibis/ovidweb/ov...3&totalCit=127& D=nursing&S=AIP PPPOPFCIHJM, November 15, 1999.

34. M. J. Christopher, "Integrated Ethics Programs: A New Mission for Ethics Committees," 10 *Bioethics Forum* (Fall 1994), 19–21.

35. Lawson, *supra* note 5.

36. Beauchamp and Childress, *supra* note 2.

37. *Id.*

38. R. Veatch. *A Theory of Medical Ethics.* New York: Basic Books, 1981.

39. ANA, *supra* note 6.

40. G. Agich, "Reassessing Autonomy in Long-term Care," 20(2) *Hastings Center Report* (March-April 1990), 12–17.

41. B. Collopy, N. Dubler, and C. Zuckerman, "The Ethics of Home Care: Autonomy and Accommodation," 20(2) *Hastings Center Report* (March-April 1990), S1–S16.

42. B. Collopy, P. Boyle, and B. Jennings, "New Directions in Nursing Home Ethics," 21(2) *Hastings Center Report* (March-April 1991), S1–S15.

43. B. Collopy, "Autonomy in Long Term Care: Some Crucial Distinctions," 28(3) *Gerontologist* (1988), 10–17.

44. *Id.*

45. M. G. Kuczewski, "Reconceiving the Family: The Process of Consent in Medical Decisionmaking," 26 *Hastings Center Report* (March-April 1996), 30–37.

46. *Id.*

47. M. Makielski and C. Broom, "Administering Pain Medications for a Terminal Patient. (Case study and commentary)." 11(3) *Dimensions of Critical Care Nursing* (1992), 157–161.

48. M. E. Greipp, "Undermedication for Pain: An Ethical Model," 15(1) *Advances in Nursing Science* (1992), 44–53.

49. L. A. Copp, "An Ethical Responsibility for Pain Management," 18(1) *Journal of Advanced Nursing* (1993), 1–3.

50. Beauchamp and Childress, *supra* note 2.

51. J. W. Glaser. *Three Realms of Ethics: Individual, Institutional, Societal-Theoretical Model and Case Studies.* Kansas City, Mo.: Sheed and Ward, 1994.

52. U.S. National Commission for the Protection of Human Subjects of Biomedical and Behavioral Research. *The Belmont Report: Ethical Principles and Guidelines for the Protection of Human Subjects of Research.* DHEW Publication No. (OS) 78-0012. Washington, D.C.: U.S. Government Printing Office, 1978.

53. American Nurses Association. *Human Rights Guidelines for Nurses in Clinical and Other Research.* Kansas City, Mo.: Author, 1985.

54. V. Foubister, "More Centers Cited for Ethics Lapses in Research," 42(41) *American Medical News* (1999).

55. R. H. Nicholson, "Unity in Diversity," 29(2) *Hastings Center Report* (January-February 1999).

56. J. Palca, "Institutional Review Boards: A Net Too Thin," 26(3) *Hastings Center Report* (1996).

57. D. F. Phillips, "IRBs Search for Answers and Support During a Time of Institutional Change," (institutional review boards) (Medical News & Perspectives), 283(6) *JAMA* (2000), 729.

58. Aristotle. *Nichomachean Ethics,* Book 2, A. E. Wardman, Trans., in R. Bambrough, *The Philosophy of Aristotle.* New York: Mentor Books, 1966.

59. J. S. Mill. *Utilitarianism.* G. Sher, Editor. Indianapolis: Hackett Publishing Company, 1979. (Original work published 1861.)

60. R. Nozick. *Anarchy, State, and Utopia.* New York: Basic Books, 1974.

61. J. Rawls. *A Theory of Justice.* Cambridge, Mass.: Harvard University Press, Belnap Press, 1971.

62. *Id.*

63. W. F. May. *Testing the Medical Covenant: Active Euthanasia and Health Care Reform.* Grand Rapids, Mich.: Wm. B. Eerdmans Publishing Co., 1996.

64. J. Piaget. *The Moral Judgment of the Child.* New York: Free Press, 1965.

65. L. Kohlberg. *The Psychology of Moral Development: Essays on Moral Development, 1.* San Francisco: Harper Row, 1981.

66. L. Kohlberg. *The Psychology of Moral Development: Essays on Moral Development, 2.* San Francisco: Harper Row, 1984.

67. C. Gilligan. *In a Different Voice: Psychological Theory and Women's Development.* Cambridge, Mass.: Harvard University Press, 1982.

68. C. Gilligan, J. V. Ward, and J. McL. Taylor. Editors. *Mapping the Moral Domain: A Contribution of Women's Thinking to Psychological Theory and Education.* Cambridge, Mass.: Harvard University Press, 1988.

69. J. Rest. *Development in Judging Moral Issues.* Minneapolis: University of Minnesota Press, 1979.

70. *Id.*

71. Gilligan, *supra* notes 67 and 68.

72. S. Ketefian and I. Ormond. *Moral Reasoning and Ethical Practice in Nursing: An Integrative Review* (National League for Nursing Pub. No. 15-2250). New York: National League for Nursing, 1988.

73. M. Ray, "Communal Moral Experience as the Starting Point for Research in Health Care Ethics," 42(3) *Nursing Outlook* (1994), 104–109.

74. D. M. Goldstein, "Scope Note 19: Nursing Ethics: A Selected Bibliography, 1987 to Present," 2(2) *Kennedy Institute of Ethics Journal* (1992), 177–192.

75. N. Noddings, "In Defense of Caring," 3(1) *Journal of Clinical Ethics* (1992), 15–18.

76. N. Noddings. *Caring: A Feminine Approach to Ethics and Moral Education.* Berkeley: University of California Press, 1984.

77. M. S. Katz, N. Noddings, and K. A. Strike. Editors. *Justice and Caring: The Search for the Common Ground.* New York: Teachers College Press, Columbia University, 1999.

78. J. Watson. *Human Science and Human Care.* Norwalk, Conn.: Appleton-Century-Crofts, 1985.

79. S. Gadow, "Nurses and Patient, the Caring Relationship," in *Caring, Curing, and Coping.* A. H. Bishop and J. R. Scudder, Editors. Tuscaloosa, Ala.: University of Alabama Press, 1985, 31–43.

80. M. A. Newman. *Health as Expanding Consciousness.* 2nd Edition. New York: National League for Nursing Press, 1994.

81. J. K. Brody, "Virtue Ethics, Caring, and Nursing," 2 *Scholarly Inquiry for Nursing Practice* (1988), 87–96. Also see S. T. Fry, "Response to 'Virtue Ethics, Caring, and Nursing'." 2 *Scholarly Inquiry for Nursing Practice* (1988), 97–101.

82. J. Watson, "Introduction: An Ethic of Caring/Curing/Nursing qua Nursing," in *The Ethics of Care and the Ethics of Cure: Synthesis in Chronicity.* J. Watson and M. Ray, Editors. New York: National League for Nursing, 1988.

83. E. H. Condon, "Nursing and the Caring Metaphor: Gender and Political Influences on an Ethics of Care," 40(1) *Nursing Outlook* (1991), 1–19.

84. P. Benner. *From Novice to Expert: Excellence and Power in Clinical Nursing Practice.* Menlo Park, Cal.: Addison-Wesley, 1984.

85. P. Benner and J. Wrubel. *The Primacy of Caring: Stress and Coping in Health and Illness.* Menlo Park, Cal.: Addison-Wesley, 1989.

86. Gilligan, *supra* note 67 and 68.

87. Benner, *supra* note 84 and 85.

88. B. Carper, "The Ethics of Caring," 3(3) *Advances in Nursing Science* (1979), 11–19.

89. S. Gadow, "Clinical Subjectivity: Advocacy with Silent Patients. Ethics, Part I: Issues in Nursing," 24 *Nursing Clinics of North America* (February 1989), 535–541.

90. M. M. Leininger, Editor. *Ethical and Moral Dimensions of Care.* Detroit: Wayne State University Press, 1990.

91. Newman, *supra* note 80.

92. Watson, *supra* note 78.

93. Jean Watson. *Nursing: Human Science and Human Care: A Theory of Nursing.* New York: National League for Nursing, 1988. (Publication Number 15-2236).

94. *Id.*

95. M. C. Cooper, "Covenantal Relationships: Grounding for the Nursing Ethic," 10(4) *Advances in Nursing Science* (1988), 48–59.

96. M. Douglas and N. Brent, "Substance Abuse and the Nurse Manager: Ethical and Legal Issues," 2(1) *Seminars for Nurse Managers* (1994), 16–26.

97. J. C. Tronto, "An Ethic of Care," 22(3) *Generations* (Fall 1998), 15–20.

98. May, *supra* note 63.

99. W. May. *The Physician's Covenant.* Philadelphia: Westminster Press, 1983.

100. E. D. Pellegrino and D. C. Thomasma. *A Philosophical Basis of Medical Practice: Toward a Philosophy and Ethic of the Healing Professions.* New York: Oxford University Press, 1981.

101. J. Allen. *Love & Conflict.* Lanham, Md.: University Press of America, 1995.

102. Beauchamp, *supra* note 3.

103. May, *supra* note 63.

104. Anonymous, "ANA Weighs in on Supreme Court Case on Assisted Suicide," 67(1) *Massachusetts Nurse* (1997), 2.

105. American Nurses Association, "American Nurses Association Position Statement: Assisted Suicide . . . Effective Date: December 8, 1994," 14(7) *Maryland Nurse* (1995), 3–4.

106. Allen, *supra* note 101.

107. W. Benjamin. *Illuminations.* New York: Schocken Books, 1968, 89.

108. N. Diekelmann, "Behavioral Pedagogy: A Heideggerian Hermeneutical Analysis of the Lived-Experiences of Students and Teachers in Nursing," 32(6) *Journal of Nursing Education* (1993), 245–250.

109. S. Gadow, "Advocacy Nursing and New Meanings of Aging," 14 *Nursing Clinics of North America* (1979), 81–91.

110. R. A. Carson, "Spirit, Emotion, and Meaning: The Many Voices of Bioethics." *Hastings Center Report* (May-June 1994), 23–24.

111. P. Bowden. *Caring: Gender-Sensitive Ethics.* London: Routledge, 1997.

Concepts of Negligence, Professional Negligence, and Liability

4

KEY PRINCIPLES

- Tort
- Negligence/Professional Negligence
- Personal Liability
- Vicarious Liability
- *Respondeat superior*
- Corporate/Institutional Theory of Liability
- *Res ipsa loquitur*
- Expert Witness
- Statute of Limitations
- Immunity from Suit

Negligence is a fairly familiar term to most individuals, whether they be professional nurses or laypeople. However, a clear understanding of what constitutes negligence and professional negligence or malpractice is elusive for many of those same individuals. Indeed, it has been only since the early part of the 19th century that the law has held negligence to be a distinct basis of liability, separate from other types of tort actions.[1] Since this separation, however, negligence has emerged as the "dominant cause of action for accidental injury in this nation today."[2]

This chapter will present the theory of negligence, professional negligence, and liability when negligence is found to be present. Information will focus on the elements, standards of care, and defenses to a cause of action in negligence. In addition, special considerations in this area of the law will be discussed, including product liability law and wrongful death actions.

ESSENTIALS OF NEGLIGENCE AND PROFESSIONAL NEGLIGENCE LAW

Definitions

Tort Law

Tort law includes negligence and professional negligence. The word *tort* is derived from the Latin word "tortous." In the French language, a tort is a civil wrong, other than breach of contract, for which the law will provide a remedy by allowing the injured person to seek damages.[3] The definition describes the conduct that is the basis of a tort: conduct that is "twisted," "crooked," "not straight."[4] The law of torts seeks to protect others from unreasonable and foreseeable risks of harm by enforcing duties established by law that individuals have to each other. It does so by allowing compensation (money) to the victim of the injury "at the expense of the wrongdoer."[5]

A tort is a civil wrong, other than breach of contract, for which the law will provide a remedy by allowing the injured person to seek damages.

Negligence

Negligence is defined as "conduct which falls below the standard established by law for the protection of others against unreasonable risk of harm."[6] The unreasonable risk of harm in negligence includes the concept of foreseeability. That is, the harm that occurred could be anticipated by the defendant at the time of injury because a reasonable likelihood existed that it could take place.[7] The conduct in question is measured by an objective standard of "due care" in the circumstances and has come to be known as "the ordinary, reasonable, and prudent" person standard (of care). In other words, when negligence is alleged, the conduct complained of is compared with what the ordinary, reasonable, and prudent person would have done in the same or similar circumstances. If the conduct being analyzed is in conformity with this objective gauge, then the individual is not negligent. If, however, the jury determines that the behavior was not consistent with this standard, then a verdict is returned against the person, finding that he or she was negligent.

In every negligence action, four essential elements must be proven for a cause of action in tort to be successful:

1. A duty must exist between the injured party and the person who allegedly caused the injury;
2. A breach of the duty must occur;
3. The breach of duty must be the proximate (legal) cause of the injury (including the element that the defendant's conduct was the "cause-in-fact" of the injury); and
4. Damages or injuries or both, which are recognized and compensable by law, must be experienced by the injured party.[8]

In instances in which the defendant's or defendants' conduct was "evil," "outrageous," or intentional, damages may consist not only of compensatory payment but also of "punitive" or "exemplary" damages. The latter serve as a deterrent, at least in theory, to warn others in society that such conduct will not be tolerated.

Negligent conduct can occur when acts of commission or omission take place. For example, negligent conduct can be alleged when an individual does something in a negligent manner or does something that an ordinary, reasonable, and prudent person *would not* do. This type of conduct is negligence by commission. In contrast, negligence by omission takes place when one fails to do something when a duty exists to do so. For example, a driver who fails to stop at a stop sign (duty exists) and runs into another car traveling through the intersection most probably would be found negligent. By not stopping at the sign, he or she could be found just as negligent as the driver who *does* stop, but who does not look carefully before proceeding into the intersection and hits the car.

It is important to be clear about the fact that in negligence the individual does not *intend* or *want* to bring about the injury or injuries that result from his or her behavior. Rather, the essence of the law of negligence is that the individual, knowing there is a risk of those results, has a duty to "anticipate them and guard against them."[9]

Nonprofessional negligence claims include suits filed for property damage (an improperly built garage, for example, which collapses on the car parked in it), personal injury (the improperly built garage collapses onto an individual in the garage at the time), or both. Most of the personal injury cases filed, however, result from injuries sustained in motor vehicle accidents.[10]

Professional Negligence

Professional negligence (or professional malpractice as it may also be called) involves the conduct of professionals (e.g., nurses, physicians, dentists, and lawyers) that falls below a professional standard of due care. Professionals possess knowledge, skill, and expertise upon which laypeople rely. Therefore, the law requires that their conduct conform with the applicable standard of care for that professional group. The applicable standard includes a "standard minimum of special knowledge and ability."[11]

Professional negligence . . . involves the conduct of professionals (e.g., nurses, physicians, dentists, and lawyers) that falls below a professional standard of due care.

Thus, when the professional nurse's conduct is alleged to be negligent and a patient is injured, the nurse's conduct should be compared with that of other ordinary, reasonable, and prudent professional nurses in the same or similar circumstances. Furthermore, for professionals generally, the standard of due care is framed in relation to what the reasonably well qualified professional(s) in the same or similar locality would do.

The latter standard, known as the locality rule, has been utilized less and less in recent years. Initially, the rule was used to avoid liability in smaller hospitals and health care centers that did not have the ability to "keep up" with large urban health care facilities and providers. Today, however, with the development of advanced methods of communication and information exchange, the availability and use of new technologies, and national licensing examinations, among other factors, the "locality rule" has outlived its initial purpose. Even so, some jurisdictions still use the locality standard or some remnant of it.

In either event, the standard is established by an expert witness who testifies at the trial. An expert witness is an individual who, by training, education, and/or experience, is qualified by the court as able to assist the jury in understanding subjects not within the knowledge of the average layperson.[12] Many states have specific statutory provisions in their civil practice rules concerning who can function as an expert witness. In professional negligence suits, an expert witness is generally required because the jury's knowledge about health care and health care professionals is limited. Thus, the expert witness must testify to the standard of care and give an opinion whether it was met in a case before the court.

The expert witness may come from another jurisdiction than the nurse defendant, or may be from the nurse's own state. He or she will be required to testify in accordance with whatever rule—local or national—is used in that state to establish the standard of care.

Liability

The word *liability* is often defined in many diverse ways. When the word is used liberally, however, it means responsibility for a possible or actual loss, penalty, evil, expense, or burden for which law or justice requires the individual to do something for, pay, or otherwise compensate the victim.[13]

For example, the rule of personal liability holds everyone responsible for his or her own behavior, including negligent behavior. This rule makes it difficult, if not impossible, to shift total liability to another person or entity.

. . . the rule of personal liability holds everyone responsible for his or her own behavior, including negligent behavior.

Vicarious liability, also called imputed liability or imputed negligence, refers to the responsibility one is found to have for the actions of other individuals because a special relationship exists between those individuals.[14] A common example of such a special relationship is that of employers and employees (master/servant). The basis of this theory is that when employees are hired to carry out the business of the employer, they may cause injuries. When this happens, the employer is in a better position to bear the financial cost of injuries to consumers than is the injured party.[15] Furthermore, if the employer may also be held responsible for employees' negligent acts, it is an incentive to the employer to hire, orient, and carefully supervise employees to reduce, insofar as it is possible, the employer's liability under this doctrine.[16]

Respondeat Superior

Respondeat superior is a Latin term meaning "let the master speak" and is based on vicarious liability. It requires that, for the employer (master) to be vicariously liable for the negligent acts of employees (or its agents), the act must have occurred during the employment relationship *and* have been part of the employee's job responsibilities (that is, within the employee's scope of employment). Thus, if a nurse who is an employee of a particular hospital is providing care within the scope of his or her job responsibilities (e.g., giving an injection) and an injury takes place, the injured patient alleging negligence can sue the nurse *and/or* the hospital under this theory of liability.

There are two unique applications of the *respondeat superior* doctrine. One is called the borrowed servant doctrine and the other is titled the captain of the ship rule. Traditionally, both have been applied to the operating suite, but with the many changes in health care delivery today, their applicability to *any* service in the hospital is possible. What each doctrine does, briefly put, is to shift the employer-employee relationship from the hospital *to* another health care provider or entity vis-á-vis the nurse.

With the borrowed servant approach, the employer of the staff nurse in the operating suite is the physician, not the hospital. For the doctrine to apply, however, the staff nurse must technically become the physician or surgeon's "temporary employee"—that is, working under the direct control and supervision of that individual—during the operation. The individual who becomes the temporary employer must be in a position to exert specific control over the staff nurse in relation to the *specific* conduct that caused the injury. If this can be shown, then the hospital may be absolved of any vicarious liability for the staff employee for the injury, and the physician, surgeon, or other health care provider can be found liable for his or her temporary employee's acts.

It is important to note that this doctrine does not normally apply in most health care delivery situations where the staff nurse carries out orders of a physician or other health care provider. Likewise, when a nursing supervisor directs a nurse to perform certain functions, the nurse does not become the borrowed servant of that nurse supervisor. Rather, the doctrine arises in unique situations in which the nurse is clearly under the management of the surgeon. For example, if the surgeon utilizes his or her own nurse when performing surgery, or when an operating team utilizes its own nursing staff to assist during surgical procedures, this doctrine would most probably apply.

The captain of the ship rule is similar to the borrowed servant doctrine in that it holds the chief surgeon to be the one who controls, and is thus responsible for, all individuals in the operating room. Thus, the employees of the operating suite become his or her temporary employees, and any injury during the course of that relationship becomes the vicarious responsibility of the chief surgeon.[17] It is important to note that neither doctrine has been widely embraced for various reasons, including the recent acknowledgment of nursing practice as an independent and accountable profession, regardless of the speciality area.

For example, in a 1997 case, *Starcher v. Byrne*,[18] the Mississippi Supreme Court held that neither the captain of the ship rule nor the borrowed servant doctrine applied in the case against a surgeon and a certified registered nurse anesthetist (CRNA) working with him. During the surgery to correct a ventral hernia, the CRNA administered the anesthesia because her employer, Dr. Coursey, could not do so. The patient suffered a bronchospasm. The patient's heart stopped and CPR was instituted. The patient suffered brain damage and sued the surgeon, alleging that he was responsible for the CRNA's negligent administration of anesthesia. The Mississippi Supreme Court held that, among other things, the CRNA was not the employee of Dr. Byrne, but was the employee of Dr. Coursey, who was not present during the procedure. Moreover, if the CRNA believed the orders of Dr. Byrne, the surgeon, were incorrect, she was under no obligation to obey them. Last, since the CRNA was

not negligent (according to the findings of the trial court), neither doctrine could apply in this case.

Although the case does not specifically utilize the doctrines by name, Key Case 4–3, discussed later in this chapter, illustrates the difficulty in identifying exactly *who* is a nurse's employer, especially in some of the newer practice arrangements. Nurses who are employed by nurse agencies or registries, or employed by a specific surgical group or other practice group, may face the legal question of who employs the nurse when a suit is filed.

Corporate or Institutional Theory of Liability

In *Darling v. Charleston Community Memorial Hospital*,[19] the Illinois Supreme Court formulated this theory concerning the liability of health care delivery systems. In essence, the theory states that the health care delivery system—whether a hospital or an ambulatory care center, for example—can be sued when it (allegedly) breaches any of its direct duties to its patients. Although many duties have been specified in numerous court cases across the country, some of the direct duties that health care delivery systems have to health care consumers include (1) maintaining the facilities to avoid unreasonable and foreseeable risks of harm (this includes not only the physical plant of the entity but also safe equipment for patient care); (2) providing competent, qualified, trained, and licensed health care providers, including medical staff; (3) properly orienting and supervising staff; and (4) adopting and enforcing adequate institutional policies, procedures, rules, and bylaws.[20]

Because a health care delivery system is managed by its board of directors, chief executive officer (CEO), and his or her administrator(s), the standard of (due) care when determining if the health care delivery system was negligent is measured by what other ordinary, reasonable, and prudent boards, CEOs, or administrators would have done in the same or similar circumstance(s).

Immunity from Suit

If applicable, immunity from suit exempts an individual or entity from liability in certain situations. At one time, the doctrines of charitable and sovereign immunity protected charitable (nonprofit) hospitals and governmental health care delivery systems from suit. Currently, however, only seven states apply the charitable immunity doctrine to health care.[21]

The sovereign immunity doctrine has also been somewhat eroded on both the state and federal levels. Thus, when allowed under either state or federal law(s), governmentally sponsored health care delivery systems can be sued pursuant to those laws.[22]

It is important to note that immunity provisions in a state statute do not prevent a suit from being filed against a person who is immune. Rather, they provide the basis for dismissal of the suit against that defendant, if found by the court to apply. Also, immunity is never absolute. If, for example, an individual's alleged negligent conduct is determined to be willful, wanton, gross, or reckless, then immunity from suit would not apply.

Statute of Limitations

Whether passed by a state or federal legislature, a statute of limitations establishes the time periods within which a claim may be filed or within which certain rights can be enforced.[23] For negligence and professional negligence claims, that time period is a specified period (2 years, for example) from the date of the injury, or if the jurisdiction has adopted the discovery rule, a specified period from the discovery of the injury by the plaintiff, or from the time at which, using reasonable diligence, the plaintiff should have discovered the injury.[24]

. . . a statute of limitations establishes the time periods within which a claim may be filed or within which certain rights can be enforced.

Exceptions to these general statutory limitations are often placed on filing a suit. For example, a minor (as defined by state law) may be provided with a longer time within which to file a suit.

A statute of repose is often incorporated into a statute of limitations. This statutory language places an outermost limit on the time frame(s) within which a suit can be filed. The purpose of the statute of repose is to provide some mitigation of the hardship that is placed on defendants exposed to potential suits for negligent conduct under the "discovery rule."[25] Its application is often narrowly applied in certain cases, such as construction cases.

Res Ipsa Loquitur

Meaning, literally, "the thing speaks for itself," *res ipsa loquitur* is a rule of evidence that allows for an inference of negligence on the part of the defendant because of the circumstances surrounding the injury. The inference is not automatic, however. It occurs because the plaintiff offers circumstantial evidence that allows the inference to be made. That evidence must consist of proof that (1) the injury normally does not occur in the absence of negligence; (2) the defendant(s) had exclusive control over the object that caused the injury; and (3) the injury cannot have occurred as a result of any voluntary action on the part of the injured party.[26]

Practically, what this rule does for the plaintiff depends on the jurisdiction. In some, it affects the strength of the inference that can be drawn by the jury concerning the injury. It allows the case to continue because the evidence concerning the injury, although inferred, is enough for the jury to make its decision. In others, it shifts the burden of proof to the defendant, requiring him or her to introduce evidence to rebut the inference of negligence.[27]

Examples of professional malpractice cases in which this doctrine was allowed by the court include (1) foreign bodies (sponges, surgical instruments) left in a patient after surgery[28]; (2) a (wrongful) pregnancy after bilateral tubal ligation[29]; and (3) footdrop immediately after a nurse administered an injection to an infant.[30]

It is important to note that the doctrine can also be applied to multiple defendants. In the landmark case *Ybarra v. Spangard,*[31] the operating room team refused to discuss what had taken place during an appendectomy that resulted in permanent injury to a patient's right arm. The team believed if they did not testify concerning what had occurred, the injured plaintiff would lose his suit because he could not prove who had exclusive control over him. The California Supreme Court held, however, that the team's silence would not deter a verdict in favor of the injured party. It decided in favor of the plaintiff. The court reasoned that a different decision would result in injured patients being unable to win a suit when health care providers simply decided not to disclose the facts of the incident.

PROFESSIONAL NEGLIGENCE CLAIMS AGAINST NURSES

Professional negligence claims against health care providers, including nurses, are based almost exclusively on *personal* injury. According to a recent research study analyzing *nursing* negligence in hospitals,[32] examples of personal injury allegations against nurses include death, fracture, dislocation, neurovascular/peripheral nerve damage, and a retained sponge or other object.

Furthermore, the types of personal injuries that occur when nurses provide patient care result from varied negligent conduct on the part of the nurse. Five common types of conduct alleged against nurses in lawsuits include inadequate assessment, inadequate communication, medication administration error, poor documentation, and failure to follow established policy.[33] Some common allegations against nurses and case examples are listed in Table 4–1.

Regardless of the type of conduct that ultimately is determined to be negligent, however, the case alleging negligence must prove, to the court's satisfaction, the necessary components of the case. Simply put, the plaintiff must plead and prove his

TABLE 4–1

Common Allegations of Negligent Conduct Against Nurses

CONDUCT	CASE EXAMPLES
Medication errors (wrong dose, wrong route, wrong patient)	*Fleming v. Baptist General Convention*[34]
Improper monitoring or assessment	*Adams v. Cooper Hospital*[35]
Improper use of equipment	*Dent v. Memorial Hospital of Adel*[36]
Failure to communicate patient condition to M.D. or others	*Karney v. Arnot-Ogden Memorial Hospital*[37]
Failure to follow physician order(s)	*District of Columbia v. Perez*[38]
Failure to follow hospital or other delivery system policies and procedures	*Helman v. Sacred Heart Hospital*[39]
Failure to provide proper patient care or to deliver patient care properly	*Montgomery Health Care v. Ballard*[40]

or her case, which includes meeting the burden of proof by affirmatively proving the facts in dispute.

Cases against nurses are no different. How the interplay of the essentials of professional negligence takes place in the courtroom is illustrated by analyzing several cases involving nurses.

KEY CASE 4–1   Fraijo v. Hartland Hospital et al. (1979)[41]

FACTS: Annette Boyd, 39 years old, married and the mother of three children from prior marriages, was not feeling well because of an asthmatic condition. She had sought medical help at an ER a number of times for her distress, and she was told to contact her regular physician about this but did not do so. On June 13, 1979, Ms. Boyd went to the ER of Hartland Hospital, where she was seen by one of the ER physicians. The doctor thought that she was in "moderate respiratory distress" but believed that she should be hospitalized because of the prior recent attacks. After standard treatment in the ER and the proper authorizations for admission were obtained, Ms. Boyd was admitted to a ward in the hospital.

The "backup" physician assigned to Ms. Boyd initiated a plan of care, including laboratory work, consultation with an asthma specialist, and the medications Demerol and Phenergan PRN for pain. In addition, he testified at the trial that he also ordered Solu-Cortef again (because it had not yet been given) and blood gas studies when he visited Ms. Boyd at about 10:15 P.M. According to the doctor, the

Key case continued on following page

KEY CASE 4–1

Fraijo v. Hartland Hospital et al. (1979)[41] *Continued*

patient was still dyspneic but "was not in peril." The RN assigned to care for Ms. Boyd testified at the trial that she saw no physician visit the patient between 10:00 and 11:00 P.M. but called the doctor shortly after 10:00 P.M. to inform him that Ms. Boyd's pulse and respiration were increased. He then ordered the Solu-Cortef and asked the nurse to call him later concerning the patient's condition.

Despite the provision of the care ordered, Ms. Boyd's condition continued to worsen (increased pulse, respiration, and increased blood pressure). In addition, she began to experience chest pain. The medication nurse administered the Demerol.

Shortly after the Demerol was administered IM, Ms. Boyd became cyanotic, and the nurse called for inhalation therapy. Ms. Boyd convulsed and stopped breathing. A "Code Blue" was called, but despite efforts to save her from cardiopulmonary arrest, Ms. Boyd was declared dead at 12:15 A.M.

No autopsy was done. There was an investigation by the coroner's office, which concluded that death was caused by "heart and lung failure." The husband and other surviving family members filed a wrongful death suit against the hospital, the physicians, and the medication nurse alleging malpractice.

Plaintiff's experts testify that medical care was "substandard," and caused death

TRIAL COURT DECISION: At trial, the primary issue was the cause of Ms. Boyd's death. The plaintiffs' theory was that Ms. Boyd's care had been negligent from the beginning of her treatment. The expert witness also testified that the care given by the physicians was "too little, too late," and the Demerol, as the final example of "substandard medical practice," caused the patient's death. The defendants' two expert witnesses, both physicians, testified as to other theories concerning the death, stating that the medical care was "adequate"; that the death was probably caused by a pulmonary embolism, myocardial infarction, or spontaneous pneumothorax; and that the Demerol administered IM could not have acted within 5 minutes to cause the convulsion and apnea.

Defendant's expert witnesses testify as to different causes of death

Physician expert witness gives opinion about nursing care

One physician expert witness also testified about the medication nurse giving the Demerol. He believed her actions to be within the standard of care for a nurse in that situation.

The jury returned a verdict in favor of all of the defendants. The plaintiffs asked for a new trial, but that motion was denied by the court. They then appealed the judgment on the basis that the trial court made "serious errors" in the jury instructions. Specifically, they alleged that the instructions concerning the nurse's judgment when administering medications were not correct. They also alleged "serious errors" in an evidentiary ruling.

APPEALS COURT DECISION: The appellate court affirmed the trial court's decision. It held that the "serious errors" in the jury instructions, which involved the medication nurse's duty of care, did not exist because the instructions were modified to reflect the current practice of nursing, in which a nurse does make "independent" decisions concerning the care given a patient, including the administration of medications. Also, the court opined that a nurse's conduct is tested "with reference to other *nurses*, just as is the case with doctors."

Standard of care for professional nurse is to compare nurse's conduct with that of other nurses

The evidentiary issue concerned the court's refusal to admit the drug manufacturer's insert on Demerol as evidence during the testimony of one of the nurses, but later allowing it when one of the medical experts was testifying. The court held that the proper foundation had not been laid during the nurse's testimony.

Judge has discretion to select jury instructions about cause of death

Last, the appellate court held that the judge's choice of instructions given to the jury concerning the cause of Ms. Boyd's death (proximate cause vs. legal cause instructions) was within the discretion of the trial judge.

ANALYSIS: This case illustrates how important the standard of care is in a professional negligence case. Clearly the plaintiffs had hoped that by challenging what the court sanctioned as the *professional* standard for a nurse (comparing her conduct with that of other *nurses* in the same or similar situation) would bring them a new trial. The court's support of the expanded role of the nurse in its opinion, and specifically in relation to making judgments about medication administration, is also important. What is problematic about the case, however, is the use of a *physician,* as opposed to a nurse, as an expert witness concerning *nursing* roles. This case was decided before another California case, *Fein v. Permanente Medical Group,*[42] in which the California Supreme Court held that the standard of care for the professional nurse is that of another professional nurse, not a physician. With this decision firmly in place, it is doubtful that a California court today would allow a physician to be used as an expert witness to establish the standard of care for a professional nurse. Even so, more recent decisions by other state courts have allowed a physician to be used as an expert witness to establish the standard of care for a professional nurse.[43] Generally, however, a nurse is not able to testify as an expert witness to establish the standard of care for a physician.[44]

FACTS: After Victor Mather's birth, his condition deteriorated rapidly, and he developed breathing problems. One of the nurses in the delivery room began suctioning the baby and administered oxygen. The baby stopped breathing. The physician inserted an endotracheal tube and attempted to suction the infant through the tube, but the nurse could not supply the doctor with the correct tubing to fit the endotracheal tube. The tube was removed, oxygen administered, and a second endotracheal tube inserted. Next, the doctor asked for an Ambu bag. The only one available had a mask attached to it, which could not be used with an endotracheal tube. Neither the doctor nor the nurse could remove the mask. The baby's condition continued to worsen. The doctor blew air into his lungs until appropriate equipment arrived. The infant survived, but suffered many injuries, including cerebral palsy.

Key case continued on following page

*Nurse testifies to her conduct
during incident*

The parents filed a suit against the hospital and the doctor, alleging professional negligence. The allegations against the hospital were based on the delivery room nurse's conduct, specifically that she failed to supply the delivery room with necessary equipment and supplies and that she could not operate the equipment needed in the situation.

TRIAL COURT DECISION: The trial court jury returned a verdict against the hospital and found the physician not negligent. It did so based on the nurse's own testimony at trial. She testified that (1) it was her responsibility to equip the delivery room and know how to use the equipment there; (2) she failed to remove the mask, although she did not know why she failed to do so; (3) it was her responsibility to restock the supplies in the delivery room but she did not restock the suction tubes because she assumed she would not need them; (4) prior to the incident, she had not been working for 9 weeks; and (5) she had never assisted in a delivery room where an Ambu bag was used.

*Experts testify that hospital
breached its standard of care*

*Doctor testifies nurse's conduct
led to infant's injuries*

Two experts, one for the plaintiff and one for the physician, also testified. Both concluded that failure to have proper equipment available and train employees in its use is a breach of the hospital's standard of care.

The doctor's testimony also supported the fact that the nurse's conduct led to the injuries sustained by the infant.

The hospital appealed the $9 million verdict to the Connecticut Supreme Court.

*Supreme Court affirms sufficient
evidence for verdict against
hospital*

CONNECTICUT SUPREME COURT DECISION: The Connecticut Supreme Court upheld the trial court's verdict as well as the amount of the jury's award. It clearly stated that sufficient evidence existed in the transcript of the trial to support the breach of the standard of care by the hospital.

Furthermore, it held, there was sufficient evidence to link the cerebral palsy to the oxygen deprivation.

ANALYSIS: This case is interesting because it illustrates two important concepts: The first is that of corporate or institutional liability. Clearly, the hospital had duties of care to its patients. When the delivery room nurse's conduct was analyzed, the hospital's breach of its duties was clear. The trial court heard much testimony that indicated that if the hospital had provided an update or "refresher" orientation to the nurse regarding her responsibilities and the use of equipment in her position, the injuries that were sustained by the infant may have been avoided.

If this case were brought today, the delivery room nurse would also be sued as an individual defendant under the theory of personal liability. A plaintiff's attorney will plead as many causes of action as he or she in good faith can plead. Therefore, the nurse employee must be clear about the fact that he or she is responsible for his or her own conduct. This, of course, includes continuing education updates and reorientation to equipment and responsibilities. However, an employer may also be named in a suit and liability assessed against it when it breaches one of its duties of care to the patient.

Hansen v. Caring Professionals, Inc.[46]

FACTS: Adriana Hansen was admitted to Mt. Sinai Hospital Medical Center for surgery. The surgery went well. But while she was recovering from surgery, a central venous catheter (CVC) attached to her jugular vein became disconnected when one of the nurses providing care to Ms. Hansen placed her in a sitting position on the bed. According to the allegations in the case, the disconnected CVC allowed air to enter the patient's blood stream and an air embolus moved to her brain, resulting in severe brain damage and total disability. Ms. Hansen's husband and guardian sued Caring Professionals, Inc., the agency which "employed" the nurse, alleging that one of the nurses providing care to Ms. Hansen was referred to Mt. Sinai by Caring Professionals, that the nurse worked at Mt. Sinai on a temporary basis, that as a result of the nurse's negligent conduct, Ms. Hansen was injured, and that the nurse was the agent and employee of both Mt. Sinai and Caring Professionals.

Referring agency brought into suit under vicarious agency theory

TRIAL COURT DECISION: Caring Professionals moved for a summary judgment, claiming that as a matter of law, it could not be vicariously liable for the negligent act(s) of the nurse because the nurse was not an agent or employee of Caring Professionals. Ms. Hansen responded to the motion for summary judgment by citing the *Illinois Nurse Agency Licensing Act,* which defined the relationship between nurse agencies and the nurses it referred as that of employer-employee. Even if the Act did not apply, Hansen argued that the summary judgment should not be granted because there existed a material issue of fact that should be decided by a trial. The trial court granted a summary judgment to Caring Professionals. Ms. Hansen appealed the decision.

Trial court grants summary judgment to Caring Professionals holding that it was not the employer of the nurse, nor was the nurse an agent of Caring Professionals

APPEALS COURT DECISION: The 1st District Appellate Court, without dissent, upheld the trial court's decision. The court opined that Caring Professionals was a referring agency only and was not in the business of treating patients. It further explained the concept of master-servant within the context of the employment relationship as defined by Illinois law. For a master-servant relationship to exist, the right of control, which includes the power to discharge an employee, must be present. The control must be over the manner and method in which work is to be done. Caring Professionals did not have the power to direct or control the nurse's work while she was at Mt. Sinai. To hold Caring Professionals accountable for conduct it cannot direct, control, or oversee would be contrary to the notions of fairness, according to the court.

Appeals Court upholds trial court's ruling

ANALYSIS: This case is an important one in health care delivery today, for traditional employer-employee relationships do not always exist. The use of nurse agencies is not new. This decision clearly supports a clear principle: Simply referring potential health care provider names to health care delivery system employers, who control the manner, time, place, and scope of the work, will not invoke the vicarious liability doctrine. Professional nurses who obtain positions in an arrangement similar to the one involved in this case will need to be certain that they understand the legal ramifications. Whether the nurse is considered an employee has little impact on his or her *individual* liability.

Key case continued on following page

KEY CASE 4–3	Hansen v. Caring Professionals, Inc.[46] *Continued*

The *Hansen* case does *not* deal with nurse registry situations in which the nurse is clearly an employee of that agency and the latter has much more control over the nurse in relation to performance, type of compensation arrangement, and the termination of employment. In such a situation, the agency would most probably be considered the employer. However, with unique and innovative employment agencies continuing to proliferate, their legal status, and that of the nurse obtaining work through them, will continue to be tested in the courts when patient injuries occur.

Undoubtedly, the few cases discussed do not illustrate each and every possible type of professional negligence case a nurse may be involved in. In fact, that would be difficult, at best, to do, for negligence *and* professional negligence cannot fit into any specific formula or rule.[47] Rather, it is "relative to the need and occasion."[48] Despite the impracticality of analyzing a myriad of cases concerning professional negligence, one thing is certain: The nurse must be ever vigilant in maintaining standards of care and providing patient care consistent with those standards. The specific standard of care will depend, again, on the circumstances and the area of nursing practice.

> *. . . The nurse must be ever vigilant in maintaining standards of care and providing patient care consistent with those standards.*

DEFENSES AGAINST NEGLIGENCE AND PROFESSIONAL NEGLIGENCE ACTIONS

Whenever an individual is sued, it is important for that person to defend himself or herself—that is, to attempt to establish that, by law or by fact, the plaintiff should not be awarded that which he or she seeks.[49] In defending oneself against allegations of negligence and professional negligence, there are several defenses that, if successful, would result in a verdict for the defendant(s) and against the plaintiff. It is important to note, however, that although it is not a guarantee, the *best* defense against inclusion in a lawsuit is to practice nonnegligently. Adherence to a risk-management approach when delivering patient care is also essential.

Failure of Plaintiff to Prove Essential Elements

One vital defense against allegations of any negligent conduct is the inability of the injured party to prove all of the elements of the cause of action—duty, breach of duty, proximate cause, and injuries/damages. Although this defense does not prohibit the case from being filed, it would prohibit a verdict against the defendant or nurse defendant.

Failure of Plaintiff to Prove Defendant(s) Acted Unreasonably

If the plaintiff cannot prove that the defendant acted unreasonably in the situation, then the plaintiff would be unable to have a verdict returned in his or her favor. Negligent behavior requires that the defendant place the injured party in danger of a "recognized" risk and then conduct himself or herself "unreasonably." Again, there are no guidelines or rules to follow concerning what conduct would satisfy these definitions. Rather, a risk-benefit form of analysis is used that takes into consideration, among other things, (1) the probability and extent of harm, (2) the social interest the actor is seeking to advance, and (3) what alternative actions are open to the actor.[50]

For example, when a nurse notifies all necessary staff who must be informed when a patient's condition worsens and initiates any and all actions needed to protect the patient from any further deterioration in condition, the nurse's conduct would be seen as reasonable. Thus, the nurse would not be found to be professionally negligent, even if injury or harm resulted to the patient.

Assumption of Risk by Plaintiff

Assumption of risk is an affirmative defense (meaning that the defendant(s) must plead it as a defense in the answer to the complaint). It simply states that the defendant should not be held responsible for an injury the plaintiff received if the plaintiff (1) had knowledge of the facts that constituted the dangerous condition, (2) knew it was dangerous, (3) recognized the nature and extent of the danger, and (4) voluntarily chose to assume the danger.[51] The defendant(s) must prove all elements of the defense for it to be successful.

In nonprofessional negligence situations, this defense might be pleaded when, for example, someone is injured at a golf course by an uncontrolled golf ball or when a car accident occurs and the injured party was driving the car with faulty brakes for some time before the accident. In professional negligence actions, this defense may be used when the patient has been informed of specific, unavoidable results of a particular course of treatment but elects the treatment nonetheless.

However, under this defense, an individual *never* assumes the risk of negligent treatment.[52] Thus, injury to a patient's arm resulting from negligent administration of a chemotherapy agent by a nurse, rather than due to the propensities of the toxin itself (which had been discussed with the patient as an adverse result), would not fall under this defense.

At one time, the successful utilization of the assumption of risk defense barred any liability on the defendant's part. However, with the advent of the comparative negligence doctrine (see discussion below), the total prohibition against liability is being reevaluated.[53] Currently, courts apply the defense differently with comparative negligence, some using it as a total bar to liability if the assumption of risk was "express," and others not using it as a bar when the defendant's negligence

forced the plaintiff into a situation in which he "reasonably" assumed the risk.[54]

Plaintiff Filed Suit After the Statute of Limitations Has Run

This defense, if successful, requires a case filed after the required time to be dismissed, usually with prejudice, meaning that it cannot be filed

---

again. Sometimes, however, by the time a layperson becomes aware that an injury suffered may be due to negligence of a health care provider, the period within which a person must file the case has already passed. Thus, the law allows extensions of time to file cases for those individuals who find themselves in certain situations.

One such situation occurs when, for example, there has been an attempt by the health care provider or health care delivery system to conceal or act fraudulently with regard to an injury. When such behavior on the part of the defendant can be proven, courts have consistently held either that the defense is barred (cannot be used) or that the statute of limitations was tolled (stopped running) during the period of concealment or fraud. In either case, the court allows the case to proceed, despite the fact that the statute of limitations has actually passed.[55]

Another circumstance in which the statute of limitations defense may arise is when the plaintiff attempts to characterize a malpractice case as something else, for example, a breach of contract action. Because a contract action has a longer statute of limitations (5 years as opposed to 2 years, for example), the plaintiff may try to file the action long after the malpractice statute of limitations has run. The longer filing period for such actions is one reason that health care professionals, including nurses, and health care delivery systems are cautioned *not* to guarantee (specific) results in health care. Among other problems, it raises the possibility of a valid allegation that a contract was entered into. If this is proven, the longer filing period might then apply.[56]

Defendant's Immunity from Suit

Immunity from suit can occur in certain situations, as when the local, state, or federal legislature passes laws that protect entities from liability under certain circumstances. Thus, a nurse working for a county hospital and the county hospital (as the employer) who were sued for alleged negligence may be able to successfully obtain a dismissal of the suit if they had immunity for the alleged conduct.

Despite the gradual erosion of the doctrines of sovereign and charitable immunity, one possible area of immunity that exists for health care providers, including nurses, is the state's Good Samaritan act or sections of specific practice acts (e.g., the

state's nurse practice act). This law provides immunity from suit for acts or omissions when the nurse provides care to an individual in an accident, in an emergency, or under other specified conditions. Most often, the care must be provided under certain circumstances: for example, without compensation, with no prior knowledge of the injury, and in good faith. Thus, a suit against the nurse would not be sustained for any injuries unless the nurse's conduct was willfully or wantonly negligent (that is, intentional or with reckless disregard for the safety of another).[57] Similarly, some states allow immunity to the nurse who volunteers services at certain functions, such as a health fair or religious camp.[58]

. . . one . . . area of immunity that exists for health care providers, including nurses, is the state's Good Samaritan acts or sections of specific practice acts . . .

It is important to note that the immunity provided by Good Samaritan acts, in whatever form, was not traditionally applied to emergency room care by physician or nurse staff, or in any other emergency situation in a health care delivery setting in which staff provided care to patients. However, several state courts have begun to apply this doctrine to such situations, albeit under varying circumstances. Illinois and California are two states that have applied Good Samaritan immunity to physicians when they provided emergency care to hospital patients who were not under their personal care.[59]

Plaintiff's Contributory Negligence

This defense, one of the most common utilized against negligence allegations,[60] states that the plaintiff's conduct contributed to the injuries he or she sustained and that the conduct was below the standard that the plaintiff was to uphold for his or her own protection.[61] If the plaintiff is negligent, in most states he or she *cannot* recover any damages from the defendant. Rather than support the defendant's lack of negligence, this defense sees both parties as being "at fault," but because plaintiff did not act with reasonable care, he or she is barred from being enriched from it.[62]

This defense can be very successful in both negligence and professional negligence actions. For example, if a pedestrian is hit by the driver of a car and sues, and the defendant driver proves that the pedestrian had crossed the street against a no-walk sign, thus "contributing" to his or her injury, the driver can obtain a verdict in his or her own favor. Likewise, if a home health care nurse provides instructions concerning medications and diet and a patient is injured, he or she may sue the nurse under a negligent teaching theory. So long as the nurse can prove that it was not his or her instructions, but rather the patient's failure to follow the regimen presented, that caused the patient's injuries, a verdict would be returned in the nurse's favor as well.

Because of the obvious harshness of this defense—the plaintiff recovers nothing even though suffering injury—many states have modified the defense to that of comparative negligence.

Plaintiff's Comparative Negligence

Rather than operate as an absolute bar to a plaintiff's recovery of damages for injuries sustained, comparative negligence allows for "comparing" the negligence of the plaintiff *and* the defendant, and any damages awarded to the plaintiff are adjusted accordingly. Thus the plaintiff does recover for his or her injuries but only to the extent that he or she was not negligent. Three versions of comparative negligence exist: pure, modified (50%), and slight-gross.[63]

In a pure comparative negligence jurisdiction, the damages awarded to the plaintiff would be reduced by the respective negligence of the plaintiff and defendant. Thus, if a jury returned a $50,000 verdict against a nurse because his or her home care instructions to the plaintiff were negligent, but the plaintiff's failure to follow them were determined to be 20% of the reason for his injury, the verdict would be reduced by that 20%. The nurse's verdict amount, then, would be $40,000, a reduction of $10,000.

In a modified or 50% jurisdiction, the same example would result in reduction of the amount awarded to the plaintiff by whatever percentage his or her own conduct contributed to the injuries, so long as the negligence was less than the established "threshold" limit—usually 50%. If, however, the plaintiff's negligence exceeds that limit, then the plaintiff recovers nothing. Thus, if a patient's actions were found to be 35% responsible for the injuries and the defendant's conduct 65% responsible, the plaintiff could recover from the defendant because his or her negligence was under the threshold 50% "fault" limit. Even so, he or she could recover only 35% of the verdict amount. Using the above example, that would be $17,500.00.

The third version, slight-gross, allows recovery for the plaintiff only if his or her negligence is "slight" in comparison with the defendant's "gross" negligence. Reduction in the verdict based on the proportion of total negligence attributed to the plaintiff then occurs, as has already been illustrated.[64]

SPECIAL CONSIDERATIONS

Survival Actions

Historically, when a plaintiff or defendant died before completion of a suit based on a tort, the action died along with the person. Today, however, through survival statutes, a personal injury action can continue after the death of either party.[65] State survival statutes vary greatly, but they generally provide a "transfer" of the case to the personal representative, who can continue with a suit and recover the same damages the decedent would have been entitled to at his or her death.[66] Most survival statutes allow the cause of action to continue, whether or not death was due to the defendant's tort. Some, however, do not allow the action to continue if the cause of death was the defendant's tortious conduct. Rather, a "new" claim must be initiated on behalf of the beneficiaries under the wrongful death statute.[67]

Likewise, federal survival laws include protections for civil rights violations, for federal employees, and perhaps even for those discriminated against in employment, especially when economic injury is alleged.[68]

Many states exclude certain torts, such as defamation, and specific damages, such as punitive or exemplary, from surviving the death of either party.

Wrongful Death Actions

As was the case historically with survival actions, the common law did not allow a deceased's heirs or dependents to sue, in their own behalf, for their loss due to the death of the family member. However, with the passage in England of the Fatal Accidents Act in 1846, English and American law, both in every state and at the federal level, provided statutory remedies for the wrongful death of a family member.[69] Generally speaking, the various statutes allow the action to be filed when death occurs as a result of negligent and intentional torts, under a strict liability theory, and, in some instances, for a breach of contract and a breach of warranty.[70]

Which family members are able to bring a wrongful death action are specified in each statute, usually by group. Thus, a spouse or children are examples of family members who can recover economic losses they might have reasonably expected to receive had the family member not died (e.g., the value of the decedent's companionship).[71]

Wrongful Pregnancy Actions

In a wrongful pregnancy suit, the plaintiff seeks damages for the emotional, physical, and economic injuries allegedly sustained because the physician negligently performed a procedure that was to prevent further childbearing.[72] The injury sued for is the birth of a healthy child who was not planned for.[73]

Wrongful pregnancy actions can be based on negligence (e.g., an improperly performed sterilization or abortion), on a lack of informed consent (e.g., the physician failed to inform the plaintiff fully of all risks concerning possible pregnancy *despite* the procedure), or on a breach of warranty action (the physician *guaranteed* that no pregnancy would occur after the procedure, for example).[74] Damages that can be awarded include the costs associated with the pregnancy and delivery, the costs of any medical complications due to the pregnancy, and, in some instances, the costs of raising and educating the child.[75]

Wrongful Birth Actions

This tort is based on the idea that the *parents* of an expected child born with congenital anomalies should be compensated for the birth of the child because the physician failed (1) to inform them of the risk(s) of giving birth to a deformed child or (2) to advise them to undergo diagnostic tests that would have discovered the fetus's condition.

In either case, the parents were not able to make a choice whether to forgo pregnancy altogether or, alternatively, to terminate the pregnancy once the defects were discovered.[76]

Damages recoverable under this cause of action generally include the costs determined to be necessary to care for the child as a result of his or her impairment. Many states do not allow the plaintiff to recover damages for his or her own emotional anguish in witnessing the child's birth or because he or she will experience suffering because the child is suffering.[77]

Although traditionally this cause of action has been filed against obstetricians, nurse-midwives may face inclusion in such suits if they fail to advise patients concerning genetic counseling and diagnostic testing. Nurse-midwives will need to ensure that an accurate and complete family history is taken when a new case is initiated. Referral of the client to the appropriate health care provider for counseling and testing is essential. Because nurse-midwives limit their practice to normal deliveries, the client should be referred to a physician if a complicated pregnancy is anticipated. This is also important to avoid inclusion in wrongful life suits.

Wrongful Life Actions

Wrongful life actions are brought by the parents of a child with congenital anomalies on behalf of the child who has been born with those deformities. Essentially, the gist of the action is based on the position that the child should never have been born at all, and thus the court must compensate the child for that harm. Because of the difficulty in measuring that "harm," as well as the philosophical difficulties in supporting a position that an individual should never have been born, most jurisdictions deny recovery to a child for general suffering in being born in a defective condition.[78]

Product Liability Actions

Product liability is an area of tort law that deals with the liability of a manufacturer, seller, and others in the "chain of distribution" who supply goods or products to the public when an injury occurs due to "defects" in those products.[79] The rationale for the development of a product liability law was to protect the public by requiring that a manufacturer and/or seller of goods introduced into the marketplace ("stream of commerce") bear the cost of any injury that might be sustained by the user of the product (or a bystander).

Several legal theories have developed under product liability, and the injured party, including a patient who alleges injury due to a product used in his or her care (medicine or patient care equipment, for example) can sue by alleging negligence, breach of an express or implied warranty, or strict liability in tort. Because negligence law (or the law of negligence) has been developed at length in this chapter, utilizing this theory in a product liability action will not be discussed, other than to remind the reader that all of the essential elements of a cause of action in negligence must also be pled in a products liability case based on it. The two other theories, warranty and strict liability, will be briefly addressed.

Warranty

Most goods/products are covered by a state's Uniform Commercial Code (UCC), which covers, among other things, express or implied warranties for goods/products manufactured, sold, and distributed. An express warranty is one that is given orally or in writing concerning a characteristic of the good/product, while an implied warranty is one that exists because of the operation of the law.[80] Under the UCC, there are two particular warranties important in relation to health care goods/products—the warranty of fitness and the warranty of merchantability.[81] Both are implied warranties.

The implied warranty of fitness states that the product sold is "fit" for its intended use, that the buyer (a hospital, for example) is relying on the skill of the seller to select and furnish the suitable good/product, and that the seller, retailer, or manufacturer knows any particular purpose of the item.[82] The implied warranty of merchantability maintains that the item purchased is adequately contained, packaged, and labeled; conforms to the promises or assertions on the container or label; is fit for the "ordinary purpose" the good/product is used for; and would successfully pass inspection by those in the "trade."[83]

When a patient is injured allegedly because of a product used in his or her care (a Stryker frame, for example), he or she may initially be unsure who is ultimately responsible for the injury: the manufacturer or seller of the product, because of a breach of the implied warranty of fitness or merchantability, or the hospital, for its failure to maintain the equipment properly or to adequately train staff to use the equipment. As a result, the patient will most probably include the manufacturer or seller in a products liability count in the suit. Moreover, although the hospital would be included in the malpractice suit under a liability theory other than product liability, it will need to provide testimony regarding the conditions discussed above concerning the implied warranty of fitness it relied on when it purchased the equipment.

It is important to note that some warranties may be disclaimed in certain situations. If allowed and properly worded, a disclaimer may defeat an individual's action against the manufacturer or others in the "chain of distribution."

Strict Liability

Strict liability in tort for products means that the manufacturer and others will be held liable for an injury without regard to the fault or intent of those individuals to harm or injure another. Although this is a sweeping liability theory, the injured person—the patient—must plead and prove all of the following: (1) the product was defective; (2) the defect existed at the time the product left the possession of the defendant(s) (e.g., the manufacturer or seller); (3) the product was unreasonably dangerous (e.g., defectively designed or manufactured, or bearing a defective warning); (4) injuries were sustained by the individual; and (5) the defect was the legal cause of injury to the plaintiff.[84]

If the defendant(s) can prove that a product alleged to be defective was "unavoidably unsafe" (that it could not be made "safe" for its ordinary and intended use), then no liability would be present under the strict liability theory. An example of such a product is a vaccine that may be needed to immunize the public, but which poses the inherent risk of the recipients' contracting the disease. Historically, the polio vaccine was one such product.[85]

Because nursing care is often delivered with equipment—monitors, surgical instruments, and syringes, for example—and most often with medications, product liability has more applicability to nursing than might initially be thought.

Because nursing care is often delivered with equipment—monitors, surgical instruments, and syringes, for example—and most often with medications, product liability has more applicability to nursing than might be initially thought. Because the provision of nursing care is usually considered a service and not the provision of a product, most nurses would not be involved in a strict liability suit as a defendant. However, implications do exist for both the nurse and the employer whenever a patient injury occurs with the use of a product. They are summarized in Table 4–2.

In addition to the implications noted in Table 4–2, it is important for the nurse to keep in mind that liability under a professional negligence theory may exist for the nurse who utilizes equipment that is faulty or is used incorrectly. Thus, when equipment is not working properly, the nurse must inform those who are to be notified of the malfunction so the problem can be corrected immediately. Furthermore, adequate training on new equipment is essential so that no unreasonable and foreseeable injury is experienced by a patient because of the nurse's lack of expertise with that equipment.

TABLE 4–2

Implications for Nurses Utilizing Products in the Provision of Patient Care

- Consider membership on policy and procedure committees to ensure clear policies concerning product identification, evaluation, and repair
- Learn policies and procedures concerning actions to be taken when an injury or death occurs with equipment, including but not limited to whom to contact and preservation of the product
- Store medications, tubing, and other patient care equipment according to manufacturer's directions
- Administer medications, ointments, and other drugs according to manufacturer's instructions
- Adequate in-service and orientation to new patient care equipment
- If involved in purchasing equipment and other patient care products, obtain representations by company in writing
- Conduct a thorough assessment of the patient with regard to drug allergies and any previous problems when patient care equipment was used
- If a patient experiences a reaction to a particular medication, stop its use and notify the physician
- Document all instances of patient injury accurately and completely in the patient's record and other required forms

Data from: Nancy J. Brent, "Assessing, Evaluating and Selecting Patient Care Products," 9(2) *Home Healthcare Nurse* (March/April 1991), 9–10; Patricia Kingsley and Dick Sawyer, "Making Medical Devices Safer," 12(21) *Nursing Spectrum* (1999), 10–11.

Safe Medical Devices Act (SMDA)

The SMDA, effective November 28, 1991,[86] requires hospitals, nursing homes, and other medical "device-user facilities" to report a serious injury, illness, or death that "reasonably suggests" it took place because of the use of a medical device. The report is to be made to the Food and Drug Administration within 10 working days of awareness of the incident, and, if the identity of the manufacturer is known, to the manufacturer of the device.

All medical products except those absorbed into the body are included in the Act's definition of "medical device." Thus, when a serious injury, illness, or death occurs with the use of a monitor, syringe, or other patient care product, the institution must report (1) its name; (2) the name, serial number, and model number of the medical device, if known; (3) the name and address of the manufacturer of the device; and (4) a brief description of the event.[87]

Although the duty to report is clearly the *institution's,* the nurse providing care with any medical device covered under the act should (1) follow agency policies when an injury, illness, or death occurs and a medical device is believed to be involved in some way; (2) document the incident accurately and completely in the medical record, incident report, and agency reporting forms; (3) discontinue the use of the medical device (and replace it immediately with another); and (4) record the ID number of patient equipment in the medical record and/or other forms on a regular basis.[88]

ALTERNATIVE MEDICINE/NURSING

In recent years, alternative medicine (also called complementary, integrative, or unconventional medicine) has been gaining in popularity. Defined as "medical interventions not taught widely in U.S. medical schools or generally available at U.S. hospitals,"[89] such treatments are the focus of research, articles, and commentaries.[90] Although there is no one list of what therapies are included in the alternative health care group, some examples include massage therapy, touch therapy, homeopathy, acupuncture, and hypnosis.[91] In 1990 alone, chiropractors, naturopaths, and other alternative medicine practitioners received 425 million visits costing patients $10.3 billion in out-of-pocket costs.[92] Most often, patients utilizing alternative health care are self-referred.[93]

Western medicine has always been skeptical of alternative therapies. In addition to a concern about whether the complementary practices will indeed help the patient, traditional health care practitioners are also concerned about their legal liability should a patient allege a poor outcome after being referred to the alternative practitioner by his or her health care provider.

A recent study evaluating insurance claims for chiropractors, massage therapists, and acupuncturists from 1990 to 1996 shows, however, that the concern for legal liability may not be as real as it might seem. In fact, the data studied indicated that claims against these practitioners occurred less frequently than claims against physicians during the same time period.[94] In addition, the injuries sustained by those who consulted alternative health practitioners were less severe than those suffered by patients when seeing traditional physicians.[95]

Even so, as in any situation where a health care provider, including a nurse and especially an advanced practice nurse, has a duty to prevent a foreseeable and unreasonable risk of harm to a patient, certain factors must be considered when providing care in a complementary therapy or when referring a patient to an alternative medicine practitioner.

To begin with, it is imperative that the nurse know as much as possible about the practitioner and the type of therapy he or she offers. Contacting the practitioner about his or her services is essential. Participating in educational offerings and reading about the complementary treatment modality[96] can also help the nurse evaluate whether this type of treatment might be beneficial to the patient.

A second concern for the nurse is whether an alternative health care practitioner is regulated in his or her state. Does the state require a certificate

---

ETHICS CONNECTION 4–2

More and more health care consumers choose nonallopathic healing practices (alternative medicine) as supplements or alternatives to their usual medical treatment (allopathic medicine). This increased variety of health treatments has implications for ethics. There are ethical issues concerning but not limited to disclosure, competence, and reimbursement. From the perspective of covenantal nurse-patient relationships, discussed at length in Chapter 3, disclosure is a moral obligation of both consumers and health care professionals. On one hand, consumers who seek allopathic treatments frequently also use alternative methods but do not disclose their alternative healing practices to their nurses or physicians. This can lead to serious consequences, especially drug interactions or overdoses. This is especially a problem if the client is using nonformulary products, such as herbal preparations. On the other hand, consumers are now expecting that health care professionals will inform them about nonallopathic treatments. The father of a 6-year-old who died from a rare, highly malignant brain tumor raised the question of whether physicians are obliged to tell patients about "an alternative remedy—even if it's unproven and most physicians are skeptical about the inventor's claim of incredible success."[1]

In order to provide consumers with alternative treatments, nurses and other health professionals must understand the treatments and know which treatments are safe and effective and which are not. If nurses choose to practice nonallopathic healing, they must be competent to do so. Credentialing and certification for holistic health practitioners currently is not well regulated. Ethical practice, therefore, requires that nurses who choose to incorporate nonallopathic treatments into their practice be prepared in the most rigorous educational programs available. For example, many nurses have chosen to complete educational programs in massage therapy before they include massage as one of their treatment practices. The National League for Nursing has produced educational materials about selected practices, such as Therapeutic Touch. Several schools of nursing in the United States offer masters or doctoral programs in holistic health or healing, and the number of complementary healing or holistic health nursing texts and reference books has increased in recent years.

Reimbursement for nonallopathic services is an ethical issue with the moral principle of distributive justice. Few third-party payers reimburse for nonallopathic treatments such as aromatherapy, music therapy, and the like. Consumers who prefer to use nonallopathic remedies generally pay for such services "out of pocket."

[1]Sarah Scott, "Father Sues Doctor over Right to be Told of Alternative Therapy for Child's Brain Tumor," 171(3) *Western Journal of Medicine* (1999), 208.

to practice acupuncture, for example? Or is a license issued only after the successful completion of a nationally recognized examination?

If a nurse decides he or she would like to practice nursing within a complementary nursing model, the nurse must be certain that the practice does not conflict with the definition of *nursing* in the state nurse practice act. Can the alternative method of health care be seen as an extension of his or her nursing practice? Or, could it be seen as the practice of some other type of health care profession? For example, if massage therapy requires a license in the state where the nurse practices, the nurse would probably be on safer regulatory ground to also obtain a license as a massage therapist before initiating massage therapy in his or her practice.

Another concern for those who practice alternative therapies is which standard of care would be applied to the practitioner if a professional negligence suit were filed.[97] The reader will recall that the standard of care discussed earlier in the chapter is what other ordinary, reasonable, and prudent professional nurses would do in the same or similar circumstances. If alternative health care is not "mainstream," if there are few nurses who practice complementary health care, how will the standard be established?

This and other issues (e.g., third-party reimbursement, informed consent) concerning the practice of alternative health care and referral to its practitioners will surely be answered in the years ahead, not only by professional associations, health care practitioners, and the public, but also by the courts, regulatory bodies, and statutory law.

SUMMARY OF PRINCIPLES AND APPLICATIONS

The law of negligence and professional negligence is complex and vast. The basic concepts and principles presented in this chapter are a framework that will be discussed in most of the other chapters in the book, especially in the following two chapters and those in Part Three. In those chapters, the principles and concepts will be applied to the many roles and specialty areas of nursing practice. However, certain guidelines are important to review here:

- Negligence and professional negligence are examples of torts

- The essential elements of a cause of action in negligence are duty, breach of duty, proximate cause, and damages

- When professional negligence is alleged against a nurse, the nurse's conduct will be compared with that of other ordinary, reasonable, and prudent *nurses* in the same or similar circumstances in the same or similar community

- The use of an expert witness to establish the standard of care is essential in professional negligence cases

- Although the concept of personal liability is important for the nurse to be aware of, also important is the potential liability of the employer under two theories, the corporate theory and *respondeat superior*

- There are many defenses against allegations of negligence and professional negligence, including assumption of risk, untimely filing of the case, and immunity from suit

- Tort causes of action that may also result in nurses being named as defendants include wrongful birth and wrongful life actions

- Survival actions allow a case to continue against a health care provider after the death of the plaintiff

- Although product liability cases may not include nurses as defendants unless they are involved in the "chain of distribution," providing patient care with any product—medications, monitors, or surgical tape—has clear implications for the nurse

- The *Safe Medical Devices Act* requires certain health care delivery systems to report to the Food and Drug Administration serious injury, illness, or death that may have resulted from the use of a medical device

- Alternative health care options require the nurse to be ever vigilant about new and different legal and ethical issues in this emerging area of health and nursing care

TOPICS FOR FURTHER INQUIRY

1. Do a paper comparing and contrasting two different types of alternative health care treatment modalities. Identify the ways in which nursing's role might change in the two modalities and analyze any concerns for increased legal liabilities for nurses practicing in them.

2. Do a statistical analysis of the types of cases in which nurses are named as defendants and compare them with cases involving another professional group pro-

viding direct patient care. Discuss the differences and similarities, if any.

3. Develop interview questions, and then interview nurses to evaluate their understanding of professional negligence.

4. Interview jurors who have served in a nursing malpractice case. Identify the issues that were important to them in deciding on a verdict in the case, such as the credibility of the expert witnesses, the injury involved, the length of time the nurse practiced, and the demeanor of the nurse defendant during his or her testimony.

REFERENCES

1. W. Page Keeton, General Editor. *Prosser and Keeton on The Law of Torts*. 5th Edition. St. Paul, Minn.: West Publishing Company, 1984 (with 1988 pocket parts), 160–161.
2. *Id.* at 161.
3. Henry Campbell Black. *Black's Law Dictionary*. 7th Edition. St. Paul, Minn.: West Group, 1999, 1496.
4. Keeton, *supra* note 1, at 2.
5. *Id.* at 7.
6. *Restatement (Second) of Torts,* Section 282 (1972) (with updated pocket parts).
7. Keeton, *supra* note 1, at 170, *citing Stewart v. Jefferson Plywood Co.,* 469 P.2d 783, 786 (1970).
8. Keeton, *supra* note 1, at 164.
9. Keeton, *supra* note 1, at 169.
10. Lawrence Baum. *American Courts: Process and Policy.* 4th Edition. Boston: Houghton Mifflin Company, 1998, 242.
11. Keeton, *supra* note 1, at 185; See also American Nurses Association. *Legal Aspects of Standards and Guidelines for Clinical Nursing Practice.* Washington, D.C.: Author, 1998.
12. Black, *supra* note 3, at 600.
13. Black, *supra* note 3, at 925.
14. Keeton, *supra* note 1, at 499.
15. *Id.* at 500.
16. *Id.*
17. Theodore LeBlang, Eugene Basanta, Robert Kane, and others, "Malpractice Law," in *The Law of Medical Practice in Illinois.* Volume I. 2nd Edition. St. Paul, Minn.: West Group, 1996, 789–790 (with December 1998 Cumulative Supplement).
18. 687 So. 2d (1997)
19. 211 N.E.2d 253 (1965), *cert. denied,* 383 U.S. 946 (1966).
20. Christopher Kerns, Carol Gerner, and Ciara Ryan, Editors. *Health Care Liability Deskbook.* 4th Edition. St. Paul, Minn.: West Group, 1998, 1:9, 1-19–1-22; George Pozgar, *Legal Aspects of Health Care Administration.* 7th Edition. Gaithersburg, Md.: Aspen Publishers, Inc., 1999, 165–181.
21. Some states that adhere to some form of charitable immunity doctrine are Arkansas, Maryland, Ohio, and Rhode Island. Kerns, Gerner, and Ryan, *supra* note 20, at 1–27.
22. The federal government has consented to be sued in certain situations under the *Federal Tort Claims Act* of 1946, originally enacted and found at 60 Stat. 843. State governmental consent for suit varies from state to state.
23. Black, *supra* note 3, at 1422–1423.
24. Keeton, *supra* note 1, at 166.
25. *Id.* at 167–168.
26. Keeton, *supra* note 1, at 244.
27. *Id.* at 257–259.
28. *Fieux v. Cardiovascular & Thoracic Clinic,* 978 P.2d 429 (Oregon 1999).
29. *Clay v. Brodsky,* 499 N.E.2d 68 (1986).
30. *Edgar County Bank and Trust v. Paris Hospital,* 312 N.E.2d 259 (1974).
31. 154 P.2d 687 (Cal. 1945).
32. Janet Pitts Beckman. *Nursing Negligence: Analyzing Malpractice in the Hospital Setting.* Thousand Oaks, Cal.: Sage Publications, 1996.
33. *Id.;* Marianne Demilliano, "8 Common Charting Mistakes to Avoid," *NSO Risk Advisor,* 1992, 3–6.
34. 742 P.2d 1987 (Okla. 1987).
35. 684 A.2d 506 (N.J. 1996).
36. 509 S.E.2d 908 (Ga. 1998).
37. 674 N.Y.S.2d 449 (N.Y. 1998).
38. 694 A.2d 882 (D.C. 1997).
39. 381 P.2d 605 (Wash. 1963).
40. 144 So. 2d 249 (La. Ct. App. 1962).
41. 160 Cal. Rptr. 246 (1979).
42. 211 Cal. Rptr. 368 (Cal. 1985), *appeal dismissed,* 474 U.S. 892 (1985).
43. See, for example, *McMillan v. Durant,* 439 S.E.2d 829 (S.C. 1993).
44. See, for example, *Arlington Memorial Hospital Foundation v. Baird,* 991 S.W.2d 918 (Tex. 1999). However, in *Carolan v. Hill,* 553 N.W.2d 882 (Iowa 1996), a certified registered nurse anesthetist (CRNA) was permitted to testify as an expert witness against a physician who was not an anesthesiologist but who administered anesthesia to a patient. Because of the improper positioning of the patient's arm during surgery, he suffered ulnar nerve injury to his left arm. The CRNA's expert testimony was allowed because of the CRNA's expertise which related directly to the precise issue in the case.
45. 540 A.2d 666 (Conn. 1988).
46. 676 N.E.2d 1349 (Ill. 1997).
47. Keeton, *supra* note 1, at 173.
48. *Id.*
49. Black, *supra* note 3, at 430.
50. Keeton, *supra* note 1, at 169–173.
51. Black, *supra* note 3, at 121.
52. See generally, Keeton, *supra* note 1, at 480–498.
53. Keeton, *supra* note 1, at 496.
54. *Id.* at 495–498.
55. See, for example, *Mueller v. Thaut,* 430 N.W.2d 884 (Neb. 1988), in which the physician who negligently delivered the Muellers' child told the parents that their daughter's death was due to her "severe deformity." When the parents obtained the death certificate to file a life insurance claim and discovered the true cause of death was "traumatic injury" sustained at birth, they filed a wrongful death action against Dr. Thaut. He attempted to raise the statute of limitations as a defense, but the court held that his misrepresentation of the true cause of the child's death delayed the filing of the suit, and the parents were allowed to go forward with their cause of action.
56. See, for example, *Stanley v. Chastek,* 180 N.E.2d 512 (Ill. App. 2nd Dist. 1985); *Doerr v. Villate,* 220 N.E.2d 767 (Ill.

App. 2nd Dist. 1966); *Murray v. University of Pennsylvania Hospital,* 490 A.2d 839 (Pa. 1985). Approximately 26 states clearly permit a medical malpractice suit to allege a breach of contract theory, in addition to alleging professional negligence. Kerns, Gerner and Ryan, *supra* note 20, at 1:15–1-18.

57. Black, *supra* note 3, at 1057.

58. See, for example, 745 ILCS 49 *et seq.* (1997) (Good Samaritan Act).

59. See *McKenna v. Cedars of Lebanon Hospital,* 93 Cal. App. 3d 282, 155 Cal. Rptr. 631 (1979); *Burciaga v. St. John's Hospital,* 187 Cal. App. 3d 710, 232 Cal. Rptr. 75 (1986); *Johnson v. Mitaviuw,* 531 N.E.2d 970 (Ill. App. 1st Dist.) (1988), *cert. denied.,* 125 Ill. 2d 566 (1989).

60. Keeton, *supra* note 1, at 451.

61. Pozgar, *supra* note 20, at 137.

62. *Id.*

63. Keeton, *supra* note 1, at 74.

64. *Id.* at 474.

65. *Id.* at 942.

66. *Id.* at 943.

67. *Id.*

68. *Id.* at 944.

69. *Id.* at 945.

70. *Id.* at 946–947.

71. Kerns, Gerner, and Ryan, *supra* note 20, at 1:5, 1-18.

72. *Id.* at 2:5, 2-8-2-11.

73. *Id.*

74. *Id.*

75. *Id.*

76. Keeton, *supra* note 1, at 370.

77. LeBlang et al., *supra* note 17, Vol. 2, 556.

78. Keeton, *supra* note 1, at 371. The case that brought wrongful life actions to the nation's attention was *Gleitman v. Cosgrove,* 227 A.2d 689 (1967).

79. Keeton, *supra* note 1, at 677.

80. Black, *supra* note 3, at 1582.

81. Uniform Commercial Code, Section 2-314 (1995).

82. *Id.*

83. *Id.*

84. *Restatement (Second) of Torts,* Section 402A (1965); Keeton, *supra* note 1, at 692–702.

85. *Restatement (Second) of Torts, Id.,* Comment K.

86. Pub. L. No. 101–629, 104 Stat. 4511 (November 28, 1990).

87. *Id.* at Section 8, Stat. 4511–4512.

88. Nancy J. Brent, "High Tech Care and Medical Devices: The Safe Medical Devices Act of 1990," 10(3) *Home Healthcare Nurse* (May/June 1992), 11–12; Jeanne Beers Blumenthal and E. Jean Hayes, "Home Health Care Nursing: Liability and Risk Management For 'Informed Consent' and the Safe Medical Devices Act Duties," 28(5) *Journal of Health and Hospital Law* (September/October 1995), 289–290.

89. David Studdert, David Eisenberg, Frances Miller and others, "Medical Malpractice Implications of Alternative Medicine," 280(18) *JAMA* (November 11, 1998), 1610.

90. See generally, Michael Cohen. *Complementary & Alternative Medicine: Legal Boundaries and Regulatory Perspectives.* Baltimore: Johns Hopkins University Press, 1998.

91. *Id.* at xii.

92. Studdert, et al., *supra* note 89, at 1610.

93. David Eisenberg and others, "'Unconventional' Medicine in the United States: Prevalence, Costs, and Patterns of Use," 328(4) *New England Journal of Medicine* (1993), 246–252.

94. Studdert, et al., *supra* note 89, at 1610.

95. *Id.*

96. See, for example, Rena J. Gordon, Barbara C. Nienstedt, and Wilbert Gelser, Editors. *Alternative Therapies: Expanding Options in Health Care.* New York: Springer Publishing Company, 1998.

97. For an interesting case focusing on the applicable standard of care for a licensed physician whose homeopathic remedies resulted in a license revocation by the North Carolina Board of Medicine, see *In Re Guess,* 393 S.E.2d 833 (N.C. 1990).

Professional Negligence: Prevention and Defense

5

Chapter 4 presented general concepts of negligence and liability. This chapter will focus on guidelines to aid the nurse in avoiding, insofar as humanly possible, unnecessary inclusion in lawsuits alleging professional negligence. It is important to keep in mind, however, that because professional negligence does not require the intent to be negligent—that is, the intent to expose another to an unreasonable and foreseeable risk of harm—there is no absolute way to avoid being named in such a lawsuit. Therefore, the information presented in this chapter consists only of suggestions that *might* preclude allegations of professional negligence against the nurse.

The guidelines presented—adequate orientation, adherence to job descriptions, and proper documentation in the patient's medical record, for example—are familiar to nurses in almost any health care delivery system and in whatever role they undertake in them. Even so, they bear highlighting within a preventive focus aimed at raising one's awareness of professional negligence.

In addition to discussion of guidelines, the defense of a lawsuit alleging professional negligence will also be examined.

PREVENTION

Adherence to Legal Standard of Care

It is important to keep in mind that the law *does not* require the nurse to protect against every possible harm to the patient. Rather, the law requires the nurse to carry out care in accordance with what other reasonably prudent nurses would do in the same or similar circumstances. Thus, the nurse's provision of high-quality care consistent with established nursing standards of care and standards of professional performance is vital if the nurse is to meet the legal standard of care when negligence is alleged.[1]

> *. . . the law requires the nurse to carry out care in accordance with what other reasonably prudent nurses would do in the same or similar circumstances.*

Adhering to established standards of care requires that the nurse be knowledgeable about them. Attending continuing education courses that focus on established or new standards; continually evaluating skills through regular skills-testing courses (whether employer sponsored or through other programs); and updating one's information concerning new developments in patient care are pivotal. These can be accomplished by reading journal articles and professional organization publications (American Nurses Association, National Association of Critical Care Nurses, and the Association of Women's Health, Obstetric and Neonatal Nurses, for example) and attending conferences sponsored by the professional groups.

Certification

Obtaining postbasic program certification in the nurse's area of practice is another way of providing quality care to patients. Certification recognizes that the individual nurse possesses either (1) a basic level of knowledge in the specialty beyond that of entry level into practice or (2) an advanced level of practice which indicates entry-level competence in that advanced practice (e.g., nurse-midwifery).[2]

The first type of certification—by a professional nursing certification board or organization—is the most universal. Whatever organization certifies the nurse (there are more than 30 nursing organizations with certification programs, including the American Board for Occupational Health Nurses, Inc., the American Nurses Credentialing Center, and the American Academy of Nurse Practitioners), the nurse must meet rigorous prerequisites to sit for the certification examination. The certification examination tests performance-based criteria in the area of specialty practice. Reexamination or continuing education is usually required to maintain certification, which is an additional way the provision of quality care to patients is maintained.

Although certification is often a voluntary means of credentialing, in many states it is required for a nurse to obtain a license for advanced practice as a nurse practitioner, a nurse-midwife, a nurse anesthetist, or a clinical nurse specialist. When certification and education are required by a state for licensure, the regulatory agency in the state sets the minimum legal requirements to obtain licensure and practice in that state.

A third type of certification—institutional—is done by academic entities. It acknowledges that the nurse has met the requirements of the particular program of study in the specialty area. For example, many colleges and universities offer a post-master's certificate program in gerontologic or trauma nursing.

Despite the nursing profession's support of certification, the certification organizations vary widely in terms of prerequisites (e.g., should a bachelor of science degree be required for any certification program?), the procedures, and when and how evaluation of continued competency (recertification) occurs.[3] In addition, although there is a need for empirical data linking certification to improved patient outcomes, no organized solution to conducting necessary research and reporting results currently exists.[4]

Because certification is an essential component of professional practice, nursing certification boards and organizations will need to continue to collaborate in order to clearly define the professional and legal parameters of certification.

Orientation to Job/Position

Adequate orientation to a new patient care job may be an important aspect in avoiding unnecessary inclusion in a professional negligence lawsuit. This is particularly so with a new graduate nurse or when the new position is one in which the nurse has had no previous experience. It may be, for example, that a nurse with inpatient medical surgical nursing experience has been hired as a home health care nurse. Despite possessing excellent medical surgical nursing skills, the nurse's use of these skills is very different in the home setting. Health care delivery systems should require that all nurse employees successfully complete an orientation program before being assigned to provide care. In addition, the use of preceptors to work with the new employee for a specified period after orientation is helpful. The nurse can be given time to achieve a level of comfort in the new setting or position before working more independently with patients.

Once adequately oriented, the nurse will need to provide care consistent with patient care policies and procedures. If the nurse needs additional familiarization, he or she should voice that need. Furthermore, periodic evaluations of performance (performance appraisals) are important to substantiate quality care and identify areas in which improvement in patient care may be needed.[5]

ETHICS CONNECTION 5–1

Currently, there is an acute nursing shortage, including a shortage of nurse educators. This shortage contributes to a dual problem of adequately preparing nursing students for professional practice and of providing orientation and continuing education so that professional nurses can function safely and effectively in their jobs. As the nursing workforce decreases, economic demands require staff nurses to care for more patients in less time than ever before. At a time when more is demanded of staff nurses, less on-the-job orientation is provided for them. This imbalance between the productivity expected of nurses and the institutional support to assure safe, effective practice raises serious ethical concerns. See Chapter 3 regarding covenantal relationships and the moral principle of nonmaleficence.

In addition, the reduced length of stay for patients in acute care institutions has increased the need for nurses who are qualified to work in community settings. This shift of many nurses from hospitals and medical centers to community-based practice contributes to the cost of orientation for acute care institutions. In the past, nurses who sought community-based positions were expected to have at least a year of practice experience in acute care settings. Thus, hospitals and medical centers bore the burden of orienting nurses who then sought positions outside the hospitals. Hospital nursing administrators argue that this practice places an unfair burden on the educational resources of hospitals and medical centers. They are orienting nurses who then leave the hospital to work elsewhere. Viewing this practice as an issue of social justice, acute care institutions are calling for other community agencies to share the cost of orienting nursing staff.

Job Descriptions

Whenever a nurse seeks a position, he or she should ask for and carefully review its job description. Job descriptions can provide a wealth of information to the nurse, for among other things they include the qualifications necessary to perform the job and define patient care responsibilities. The nurse employee who believes the job requirements are beyond his or her level of experience should reject the position or, at a minimum, should ask for additional orientation and supervision to fulfill the position responsibilities.

The acceptance of a position requires the nurse to perform his or her role's responsibilities within the confines of its description. If there is an injury and professional negligence is alleged, the job description and other patient care documents, like policies and procedures and orientation information, may be introduced into evidence at trial to support conformity—or lack of conformity—with them.[6]

Conformity with a job description is important not only from a liability perspective, but also because of the position the nurse employee may be placed in vis-á-vis the employer. Not adhering to a job description, or performing a task that the nurse was not proficient in pursuant to the institution's internal monitoring system, can result in a theoretical, if not actual, adversarial posture between the employer and the nurse employee. Such a stance may prove quite beneficial to the plaintiff during the course of the trial, especially if the nurse and employer attempt to shift the "blame" for the injury to each other on the basis of the adopted policies, job descriptions, or skills proficiency evaluation.

Patient Care Policies and Procedures

Well-developed policies and procedures can be of great help in the provision of nonnegligent care. Because they are based on current, accepted practice, adherence to them may help the nurse avoid omissions in patient care that might result in injury to a patient. Their development is influenced by many factors, including accreditation standards, court decisions, patient care rights, and state and federal legislation. Health care delivery system policies and procedures are concerned with, among other things, promoting quality care, delineating lines of authority and communication, and meeting accreditation requirements. As a result, they should be updated on a regular basis.[7]

Well-developed policies and procedures can be of great help in the provision of nonnegligent care.

Although policies and procedures are used in conjunction with each other and are related, they have separate definitions. A policy is a guideline that has been formulated by administrative authority and directs action to some purpose.[8] A policy does not eliminate the need for individual judgment and decision making, nor does it negate the nurse's accountability for decision making.[9]

A procedure, in contrast, is a detailed, step-by-step description of what is required for a particular situation; for example, in giving patient care, under what circumstances notification to administration must occur, and to whom a situation is to be reported. Procedures cannot be blindly followed by the nurse employee, however; individual decision making and accountability still exist for the nurse employee.

Once oriented to the policies and procedures for the health care delivery system, the nurse needs to familiarize himself or herself with them and utilize them in the provision of patient care. Should changes be necessary because a procedure is out of date or inconsistent with the nurse's scope of practice, the nurse should discuss this with the policy and procedure committee within the institution. In addition, membership on the committee is a responsibility of the nurse employee and nursing administration.

When deviation from established policies and procedures occurs, liability may result for the institution and its nursing staff.

Accreditation, Licensing, and Other Standards

Knowing and adhering to accreditation, licensing, and other standards can help to reduce lawsuits by providing care consistent with those standards. Health care delivery systems are highly regulated by federal, state, and sometimes local laws. In addition, many private agencies also affect those systems.

State Regulatory Laws

State laws such as a hospital licensing act and a home health care agency act grant a state administrative agency the power to adopt standards the entity must meet, grant licenses to conforming institutions, and enforce compliance with the laws and regulations promulgated by the agency.[10] Compliance with the act not only provides continued licensure, it also can provide guidelines for patient care, especially as to staffing requirements, qualifications, eligibility for staff membership, and other aspects of patient care delivery.

If compliance does not occur, and a patient is injured, he or she will attempt to prove that the noncompliance was the cause of the injury. As a result of the *Darling v. Charleston Community Hospital* case discussed in Chapter 4, applicable licensing standards can be utilized in a trial to support this allegation.

Accreditation Standards

Like licensing standards, accreditation standards for all types of health care delivery systems can provide precepts to adhere to when providing care. Accreditation is given by private organizations, such as the Joint Commission on the Accreditation of Healthcare Organizations (JCAHO) and the American Osteopathic Association (for osteopathic hospitals). Adherence to their standards is not legally mandated, as is the case with licensing requirements. However, submitting to the voluntary accreditation process speaks to the intent of the health care delivery system to provide quality care to patients.

Furthermore, as with licensing standards, accreditation standards provide guidelines in the provision of acceptable care. They too can be utilized in a trial to prove conformity—or lack of conformity—with them when a patient injury occurs. For example, in a 1990 Illinois appellate case, *Roberts v. Sisters of Saint Francis,*[11] the appellate court discussed the use of Joint Commission standards in relation to the case generally and to their use in the jury instructions against the physician named in that case. The court clearly stated that the commission's standards could be used if they had been dealt with properly at the trial level.

Federal Regulatory Laws

Perhaps the best-known federal law regulating health care delivery—and thus establishing patient care guidelines—is Medicare. Its "Conditions of Participation for Hospitals" (and for other health care delivery settings)[12] set patient care guidelines that, if adhered to, can be helpful in proving the provision of acceptable, nonnegligent care.

Continuing Education

Keeping abreast of the newest developments in patient care issues is another essential element in staying out of a professional negligence suit. Participating in seminars and classes on the clinical care of patients, scope of practice issues, patient rights, and patient relations can be helpful in focusing the nurse's awareness on the issues and providing him or her with the updated skills to provide patient care safely and effectively. This is particularly so when clinical classes require an evaluation of the skills acquired during the course or workshop.

Keeping abreast of the newest developments in patient care issues is another essential element in staying out of a professional negligence suit.

Also important to include in continuing education programs is information on risk management and the fundamentals of liability law.

Open Lines of Communication

It may seem simplistic to think that open lines of communication can guard against a lawsuit alleging professional negligence. However, effective communication is "the foundation for delivery of competent nursing care."[13] Thus, the nurse must ensure open and ongoing lines of communication with other staff nurse colleagues, nursing management, hospital administration, risk management, physicians, and other health team members. If changes in a patient's condition are quickly communicated and intervention occurs, if a problem concerning disagreement with patient care is appropriately shared and resolved within the health care delivery system hierarchy, or if needed changes in patient care procedures are brought to the appropriate staff committee for needed revi-

---

ETHICS CONNECTION 5–2

The ethical issue of commercial support of continuing education confronts nurses, physicians, and other health professionals. The costs of providing continuing education have escalated while institutional support for such programs has diminished. Consequently, commercial funding of continuing education programs by pharmaceutical and other health care product companies has grown, together with the possibility of moral conflict of interest. Professional organizations such as the American Nurses Association (ANA) have issued position statements about commercial support for continuing education.[1] Ethics committees in hospitals and medical centers have begun to recommend policies and practices about vendor funding of continuing education. These guidelines and policies are aimed at protecting the mission of the health care or educational institution by prohibiting the commercial sponsor from planning the program, disclosing the commercial sponsors, and restricting product promotion during the continuing education program.

---

[1]American Nurses Association. *Position Statements: Guideline for Commercial Support for Continuing Nursing Education.* Washington, D.C.: Author, 1997.

---

sions, patient injury may be avoided. In fact, in a study of 747 malpractice cases involving nurses from 1988 to 1993, "communication negligence" was responsible for 203 (27.17%) of the adverse events (injuries or death) experienced by patients.[14]

Open and ongoing lines of communication with the patient and his or her family are also essential. This includes, of course, providing information to the patient and the family, informing them of changes in care, and keeping them abreast of hospital policy and procedures generally. It also includes more subtle ingredients, however, that lie at the heart of treating individuals with dignity and respect. Thus, establishing rapport, practicing "active listening," acknowledging feelings, and responding to the concerns of the patient or the family are essential.

Although it is difficult to say with certainty that being treated in a humane and caring manner will always avoid a lawsuit, especially when a "bad medical outcome" occurs, studies indicate that one factor patients use to evaluate medical care is their level of satisfaction with the care. Researchers in

one study focusing on obstetricians concluded that even if a patient does not file a suit, physicians who have been involved in one or more lawsuits are the objects of more patient complaints concerning their unsatisfactory communication skills.[15] In another study of 160 adults who watched a videotape of physicians communicating medical outcomes (e.g., "positive result," "poor result") and a relationship to possible physician fault for those outcomes, results indicated that good communication skills (e.g., a caring attitude) might decrease the risk that the adult would file a suit, even if the physician was at fault for the bad outcome.[16] Moreover, according to one commentator, today's consumers of health care do not tolerate a "patronizing relationship" with health care providers.[17] Rather, they want providers who will listen to their concerns, respect their wishes, and accommodate their needs.[18]

Documentation of Patient Care

The medical record is an essential and necessary part of patient care. The medical record is to be a complete and accurate account of the patient's care while receiving treatment in the health care delivery system. Its contents are regulated by many sources, including licensing, accrediting, and professional organization (for example, the American Nurses Association) standards, case law, and state practice acts. Common requirements from those sources include the medical history, physical examination results, reports of laboratory and other diagnostic tests, nursing assessments and care provided, informed consent for procedures, and the documentation of any patient and/or family teaching done.[19]

The uses of the medical record are as varied as the sources that affect its contents. Within the health care delivery system, the record is used to communicate between and among staff, departments, and health care providers concerning the patient and his or her care. It is also used by the system's risk management department and utilization management and quality management committees to evaluate patient care and its need and to determine where improvements should occur.

Outside the health care delivery system itself, the medical record is used by third-party payers, private and governmental, including Medicare and Medicaid, to ensure that they are paying for actual services provided; by researchers in health care;

and for initial and continuing accreditation or licensing grants by health care administrative agencies.

The patient's medical record is also used in legal proceedings, whether by administrative agencies required to enforce social benefit programs such as worker's compensation laws, by the state's attorney or other prosecutorial body to enforce criminal laws, or by a civil court to determine the extent of the injured person's injuries in a car accident or due to alleged negligence on the part of a health care provider.

The medical record is also used in litigation in which professional negligence is alleged (and is the first piece of potential evidence that is extensively evaluated by the plaintiff's attorney when consulted by an injured patient concerning a suit). Therefore, it must be viewed as a viable way by which to defend against allegations of professional negligence. If the medical record is complete and accurate and reflects the documentation of high-quality, nonnegligent care, it can be the nurse's "best defense" against allegations of negligence. If, however, the documentation is incomplete, contains gaps, is not consistently done pursuant to policies, and is inaccurate, then the record can, and will, be used to support the allegations of negligence in the patient's complaint. Thus, adhering to guidelines for proper documentation is essential.

The following guidelines are general ones for the nurse to keep in mind when documenting in the medical record. They are not meant to be all inclusive. Therefore, the nurse should consult other available guidelines, such as accreditation standards. In addition, review of Parts Two and Three for specific DOCUMENTATION REMINDERS pertinent to those areas of practice is also recommended. Guidelines for computer documentation of patient care will be discussed separately.

Documentation Guidelines

1. Write legibly.
2. Use black, permanent ink for entries. Do not use colored pens, pencils, or felt-tip pens.
3. Date and time all entries.
4. Every entry must be accounted for; that is, the nurse must sign his or her name and list credentials and other required data for every entry reflecting patient care. No nurse should document in the medical record for another person, unless that practice is "standard" practice, as in emer-gency room nursing. Even so, when documenting for another, the nurse "scribe" must accurately reflect who is providing care and who is documenting the care. Under no circumstances, however, should the nurse sign another nurse's name in any portion of the record.

5. No blank spaces should be left in any area of the documentation. If space is left on a line after the entry is complete, the nurse should draw a line through the space to the end of the page. If larger areas are available on form sheets (e.g., comments section or other section) and are not used, a line should be drawn diagonally through them so it is clear that documentation in the section was not overlooked. Documenting something like N/A (for not applicable or not assessed), if documentation policies allow for this, is also acceptable.

6. There should be no erasures, obliterations, or "whiting out" on any portion of the medical record. If an error in the record must be corrected, it should be done by drawing one line through the error, initialing and dating the line, and continuing the documentation of the correct information on the next available space or line.[20]

7. Factual entries are essential. The medical record is no place for opinions, assumptions, or meaningless words or statements ("Had a good day"). Rather, the entry should be factual, complete, and accurate, containing observations, clinical signs and symptoms, patient quotes (if applicable), interventions, and patient reactions.

Factual entries are essential. The medical record is no place for opinions, assumptions, or meaningless words or statements ("Had a good day").

---

8. The use of correct spelling, punctuation marks, and grammar is important.

9. Every medical record page should reflect the patient's correct name and other identifying information.

10. Abbreviations used in the medical record must be confined to ones adopted by the health care delivery system only, and used according to

the meanings assigned them. If there is no adopted policy concerning abbreviations, then the nurse should not use them, but write out all words instead. Also, the nurse should not use his or her own abbreviations, however clever and time saving they may be. Last, adopted abbreviations should be used consistently throughout the institution; for example, it would not be acceptable to use *pp* as "post partum" on the labor and delivery service but use it for "pedal pulse" in other areas of the hospital.

11. Documentation in the record should occur as soon as possible after the care is given. Entries should never be made before a procedure or medication is given.

12. When a physician, supervisor, or others (including other staff nurses) must be contacted concerning a patient's condition, that information should be entered in the record in a factual and accurate manner and include the manner of communication, the names of those contacted, what was discussed, and what response took place as a result of the contact. Any new orders must be documented according to policy, along with the care provided, the patient's response to the newly ordered care, and any other necessary information. An incident or occurrence report may also need to be filled out.[21]

13. Any order, narcotics count, narrative entry, or other documentation should not be countersigned unless the countersigner can attest to the accuracy of the information and that he or she has personal knowledge of it. If a nurse cannot speak to both of those issues, it is best to qualify the countersignature in some way; for example, documenting that the nurse has only reviewed the entry and signed it.

14. When an unusual incident occurs, such as a fall or other type of patient injury, in addition to documenting the information on an occurrence or incident report, the situation must also be documented in the patient's medical record. The filing of an incident report *does not* take the place of documenting the information in the record.

15. Whenever a patient leaves the nurse's care (for diagnostic work, for example) or the nurse leaves the patient (when a home health care nurse leaves the home after provision of care), an entry in the medical record should reflect the time, the condition of the patient upon leaving, and any other information the reader of the entry should be aware of.

16. A patient transfer requires that information concerning the transfer be documented in the record, including the date and time of transfer, patient condition when transferred, who (if anyone) accompanied the patient, who provided the transfer, where and to whom the patient was transferred, and manner of transfer (for example, wheelchair or ambulance).

17. Consent for, or refusal of, treatment must be documented in the record, either by written consent or refusal forms or by the physician documenting this information in his or her progress notes. If the nurse is involved in a consent or refusal situation, the incident should be documented in his or her nursing notes.

18. Patient and/or family teaching, as well as discharge planning, must also be documented in the medical record. The use of teaching forms for the purpose of documenting the teaching that took place is an acceptable way of doing so, as long as the forms can withstand legal challenges to their completeness, accuracy, and the patient's ability to understand them. Likewise, discharge planning must be complete, specific to the needs of the patient and the family, and communicated to the patient and others who may be involved in his or her care.

19. The existence and disposition of any personal belongings of the patient—dentures, glasses, jewelry, and money, for example—need to be recorded. If, for example, the patient's glasses are placed in the bedside stand, or given to the family to take home, there must be factual documentation in the record.

20. Patient responses to medications, treatments, patient teaching, and any other interventions by the nursing staff should be documented. It *is* important to intervene with a patient care problem. It is equally important, however, to assess and document the patient's response to the care provided.

21. Agency or institution policies should be reviewed regularly and adhered to when documenting in the patient's record.

22. When it is necessary to add omitted information to an already existing entry, policies and procedures should be consulted and followed. Most often, the addition of information is coded on the next available line or space as a "late entry" or "addition to nursing note of _____ ," the date and time of the information that is being

added is documented, and the additional information is then placed in the record.

Computer Documentation Guidelines

Computers in health care have become commonplace to health care providers. Computers are in use in many health care delivery systems across the United States, albeit in varying degrees. The variety is based mainly on the regulation of computers in health care by state regulatory agencies, such as the hospital licensing board. For example, some states may authorize health care institutions to utilize electronic documentation only for medical test results or nursing entries, while others have allowed electronic documentation for the entire patient care record.

The ability to capture, store, retrieve, and transmit data about a patient's health care is indeed remarkable. When the nurse uses a computer rather than handwritten entries to provide information concerning patient care, however, additional legal concerns exist. Clearly, policies and procedures must address those concerns, including confidentiality and privacy of patient data in the computer; access to the patient data stored in the computer system; authentication of entries in the patient's computer record; ongoing review procedures for evaluation of the completeness, accuracy, and timeliness of record entries; and error correction.[22]

Electronic documentation guidelines include:

1. The nurse must protect the user identification code, name, and/or password given for documentation. They should not be given to anyone else for his or her "temporary" use or for another to document for the nurse who has been assigned those access identifiers.

2. The nurse should access information and document only where and how authorized to do so. For example, the nurse's attempt to obtain information concerning a unit or patient without authorization would be a clear breach of confidentiality and privacy (e.g., substance abuse or mental health care).

3. The nurse should not ignore any "expert reminders" that show up for a particular patient. For example, if the nurse did not code information correctly, or if important data were overlooked, the computer would alert the nurse to those omissions.

4. Late entries and error corrections will be handled differently than under a narrative format. The nurse will need to be clear about the procedure for adding information into the system *after* exiting a particular patient's file or the program itself.

5. Utilization of the correct user identification code of the nurse *and* the correct patient code (for the patient record itself) is essential.

6. Printouts of patient information must be handled correctly and pursuant to the institution's policy. At a minimum, the printout should be shredded, or patient identification information should be removed before the printout is disposed of if no shredding occurs.

7. Keeping current when changes in the documentation format occur will be important.[23] The staff education department can help with this by providing in-services to nursing staff when new formats are adopted.

DEFENSE

The defense of a case is the defendant's answer or response to a claim or suit. It sets forth the reasons why the defendant is not liable and why the relief requested should not be granted.[24] The defense of a case includes, but is not limited to, the filing of an answer; raising specific, affirmative defenses against the allegations; obtaining evidence to support one's position; and identifying the best strategic overall approach to the case.

The defense of any case alleging professional negligence against the nurse also involves proving to a judge (bench trial) or jury (jury trial), through the use of established rules of evidence and court procedures, that the relief requested by the plaintiff should not be granted. Several specific topics pertaining to the defense of professional negligence suits will be highlighted here. The reader is also encouraged to review Chapter 2 for further elaboration of the civil judicial system generally, especially in relation to the defense of any civil suit.

Selecting an Attorney

If the nurse's attorney is provided under the contract of insurance, the selection of the attorney remains with the insurer. If the nurse is not comfortable with the attorney assigned, or if, on the other hand, the nurse is not covered by a professional liability policy for whatever reason and must select an attorney for representation, Appendix A should be reviewed to aid the nurse in resolving his or her concerns surrounding the selection of an attorney.

Selecting an Expert Witness

The use of an expert witness in a professional negligence case is necessary in most jurisdictions. Thus, selecting the appropriate person who can best educate the jury concerning the nurse's conduct in the particular case and the applicable standard is important.

The selection of an expert witness can occur in various ways. First and foremost, it is important to retain a nurse expert who has had experience in testifying in that role. Those individuals can sometimes be identified through state nursing associations or through the national nurse attorney association (The American Association of Nurse Attorneys). In addition, local attorneys and nurse attorneys are good resources for information concerning nurse expert witnesses.

Second, the nurse expert witness must possess the credentials necessary to qualify as an expert witness in the particular state. In addition, appropriate credentialing can be helpful in avoiding a successful attempt by opposing counsel to question the nurse expert's credentials during cross-examination. Credentials would include educational preparation, experience, publications, and honors received by the nurse expert witness.

Third, the nurse expert witness must be able to testify accurately and with confidence. Guidelines for nurse expert testimony are discussed below.

Preparation for Trial

A civil suit has many phases, the last of which chronologically is the actual trial itself. Prior to trial, the discovery period is an active and intense time during which facts and information about the case are obtained from all the parties involved to assist in preparation for trial.[25] Guidelines for one specific tool used during the discovery phase, the deposition, and actual trial testimony will be briefly discussed.

A deposition is a pretrial discovery method whereby the statement of a party or witness is taken under oath.

A deposition is a pretrial discovery method whereby the statement of a party or witness is taken under oath. The deponent (person giving the deposition) may be asked questions by all attorneys for the named parties (plaintiff[s] and defendant[s]). If the deposition is a *discovery* deposition, it usually cannot be introduced into evidence at trial. It can, however, be used to impeach the deponent at trial if his or her testimony varies from the deposition testimony. In contrast, if the deposition is an *evidence* deposition, it can be introduced into evidence at the trial (thus eliminating the need for the witness to be present at trial). Evidence depositions are often used for parties or witnesses who may not be able to attend the trial for many reasons, including living in another state or terminal illness.

In contrast, testifying at the trial is the process of providing evidence, through one's statement under oath, for the purpose of establishing or proving a fact or facts in a judicial inquiry.[26]

The following suggestions are not meant to be all-inclusive or absolute. Rather, they provide ways in which a suit against the nurse can be better defended. As a general rule, these guidelines are important to consider whether giving a deposition or testifying at trial.

As a Named Party or Witness

1. Always be prepared to testify. This includes a thorough review of the situation that gave rise to the suit and all documentation concerning the incident (e.g., the medical record). Talk with your attorney about what can be expected at the deposition or at trial.

2. Testifying truthfully is essential. Falsified or otherwise untrue testimony can create more problems than it solves in the defense of a case. In addition, perjury is a crime under federal and most state laws.

3. The nurse must be open and honest with his or her attorney. Although doing so may be "embarrassing" or uncomfortable for the nurse, the attorney must not be shielded from information

that compromises his or her ability to defend the case to the fullest extent possible. This is particularly important if the nurse does not share information with his or her counsel and the attorney for the other party does discover it and uses it during the deposition or at trial. This situation could result in compromising the credibility of the nurse.

4. The nurse should dress conservatively and professionally when giving testimony. Because impressions will be important, whether during a deposition or at trial, the nurse's appearance is important. During the deposition, the others present want to "discover" how the deponent (the person providing the testimony) looks and responds during the deposition *in addition to* hearing the actual testimony. Many times, cases are settled, or a decision made to go to trial, based on a witness's or party's demeanor during a deposition. At trial, how the jury perceive an individual and the testimony given can influence their ultimate decision.

5. Controlling one's anger, anxiety, and frustration is important. During the deposition and trial, opposing counsel may attempt to reduce the credibility of the nurse's testimony. Many times that attempt includes trying to manipulate the witness (being hostile, then nice); intentionally misstating prior testimony; appearing surprised at anything that is said; using hypothetical situations quite different from the incident that formed the basis of the suit; and questioning professional competence. Ignoring these and other tactics, and answering as confidently, normally, and nondefensively as possible, will weaken, if not totally destroy, these maneuvers.

Furthermore, questions involving a hypothetical situation should probably be objected to by the nurse's attorney as irrelevant to the nurse's testimony. Although hypothetical situations are used by the expert witness in many states, their use with named parties or occurrence witnesses is questionable. If the nurse, however, is asked to respond to a hypothetical situation, he or she should do so only after differentiating it from the case before the court.

6. The nurse should answer only those questions asked of him or her. Many times, nurses involved in the legal system try to cooperate so fully that they do the work for the opposing side. It is the lawyer's responsibility and obligation to elicit testimony; make him or her do that job.

7. Waiting until the entire question is asked before answering is vital. Again, in an attempt to appear cooperative, or because of anxiety, the nurse involved in testifying may begin an answer before the question is clear. Doing so may volunteer information not asked, and once they hear it, those attending the deposition or the trial jury will find it difficult to "disregard" the statement.

8. Waiting a few seconds before answering *after* the question is asked is also helpful, for it gives the nurse's attorney the opportunity to object to the question asked. Once an answer is given, an objection can still be made. However, as is true with an answer given before the question is completed, the jury may find it difficult to disregard the answer despite instructions by the judge to do so. Furthermore, only if an objection to a question is sustained is the answer stricken from the record.

9. The nurse should not guess at any answers. If the nurse does not know an answer, does not remember something, or cannot estimate about a particular issue, he or she should say so. The attorney for the nurse can deal with these inabilities through various trial techniques. Also, if those techniques are not helpful to the nurse in providing the requested testimony, then it is best not to try to answer a question under oath when one is not as reasonably certain as can be about that answer.

10. Testifying as clearly as possible is important. Overusing "medicalese" can be problematic, although there must be a balance between using "appropriate" medical terms and descriptions and using it to excess. This is particularly important at trial, for the jury must be convinced that the nurse knows what he or she is testifying to—is a competent and nonnegligent professional, in other words—but the jury cannot be "lost" in the process.

11. Although the nurse may want to appear friendly during the trial, it is important that the nurse defendant or witness *not* talk with the jury in any manner during the trial. Attempting to do so may lead to a mistrial being granted by the judge or charges of jury tampering being alleged against the nurse.

12. The nurse must be careful not to personalize anything about the suit. Although the nurse's conduct is in question if named as a defendant in the suit, the tendency to see oneself as a "bad nurse" or "doing something wrong" is a common, but not helpful, reaction.[27]

13. The nurse must rely on the advice his or her attorney provides. The defense of any lawsuit,

including a professional negligence suit, is complicated, diverse, and foreign to most nurses. Although the advice the attorney provides may not seem "correct," the attorney is the one with the most knowledge in the situation concerning the law and its application. If the nurse simply cannot follow the attorney's advice and direction, however, he or she should discuss this with the attorney. It may be that another attorney will need to be assigned to the case, or perhaps the "differences" can be worked out when information and rationale are provided. In any event, the nurse must be clear about the fact that the attorney is *his or her advocate*. Advocacy depends on a relationship of mutual trust and honesty and open lines of communication.

Although the nurse may want to appear friendly during the trial, it is important that the nurse defendant or witness not talk with the jury in any manner during the trial.

As an Expert Witness

In addition to the suggestions given for the nurse defendant or witness, the nurse who functions as an expert witness has additional concerns in relation to his or her testimony and its impact on the defense of the case. The following general guidelines are also important during a deposition or trial in which the expert witness is testifying.

1. The nurse expert witness must testify accurately and completely as to his or her qualifications. A thorough review of education, positions held, publications, and honors is vital, along with applicable dates.
2. Preparation is essential. Many sources of information must be reviewed to provide an opinion, because the expert usually does not possess direct, actual knowledge concerning the case. Those sources include the medical record, nursing tests and articles, the state nurse practice act, national standards applicable to the case, the agency or institution policy and procedure manual, and depositions.

3. The nurse expert witness will need to be familiar with the law of the state where he or she will be testifying as it relates to the form the opinion will take. In some states the expert witness is asked directly to give his or her opinion after a review of the medical record and the testimony at trial. Other states present a hypothetical situation based on the case, and the expert witness is then asked to give an opinion based on the theoretical circumstance. In either case the nurse must testify honestly concerning whether or not the standard of care for the nurse in the case was maintained or breached.
4. The role of the expert witness is to educate the jury to the standard of care. Thus, his or her testimony must be clear, concise, and complete. This requires judicious use of medicalese so that the jurors can understand the testimony.

The role of the expert witness is to educate the jury to the standard of care.

Ramifications for Other Liability

The defense of any case, including the defense of a professional negligence case, must take into account the potential for other liability. Thus, the attorney who represents a nurse in a professional negligence suit must analyze the conduct that formed the basis of the suit to determine if criminal liability or disciplinary action is possible. If so, the professional negligence suit must be defended with those other possible legal actions in mind. Initial consultation with attorneys who concentrate their respective practices in those areas is well advised so that the strategies of the suits can be planned. The nurse may need to raise this concern with his or her attorney at the beginning of the defense of the negligence suit so that additional problems can be planned for if further legal action is taken against the nurse.

INSURANCE ISSUES

Self-Insurance

Most nurses named in lawsuits are covered by some form of professional liability insurance.

The insurance coverage may exist under the employer's self-insurance plan. With this type of self-insurance, the insurance statement/contract is drafted by the employer and establishes conditions under which the self-insurance applies (e.g., coverage and loss).[28] The institution's self-insurance may be in the form of a self-insurance fund, channeling (where attending physicians are voluntarily included in the insurance program or trust), a trust fund, or disbursement from operating funds.[29] Self-insurance is seen as beneficial for several reasons, including the fact that the institution controls the claims and claims process, self-insurance is less expensive than purchasing liability insurance from an insurer, and it provides a sense of cohesion among the staff when a suit is filed.[30]

Professional Liability Insurance Policy

A professional liability insurance policy is a contract whereby an insurer agrees to enter into a policy of insurance with the insured (e.g., the hospital or the nurse) to provide coverage for delineated professional activities. If the hospital and/or nurse is found to be liable for the plaintiff's injuries or damages due to conduct covered under the insurance contract, the insurer (the insurance company) will pay that amount on behalf of the insured. Liability insurance contracts commonly include professional negligence (or malpractice), errors, omissions, and/or mistakes in rendering nursing services as covered events.

The nurse may carry his or her own professional liability insurance or may rely on coverage under the institutional liability policy. The latter will cover the nurse only when functioning as an employee and working within the scope of his or her employment. Regardless of whether the nurse purchases his or her own professional liability insurance or relies on the employer's, the nurse should evaluate certain factors concerning the insurance policy, and these factors are summarized in Table 5–1.

Applicable Professional Liability Insurance

If the nurse named in a lawsuit is covered under a policy of professional liability insurance, the policy will usually stipulate that an attorney be employed by the insurer to represent the insured.

Although the insurer may have the obligation to provide counsel, if the nurse is not satisfied with the selection of the attorney, he or she should make that dissatisfaction known to the insurer. Furthermore, if the nurse's concerns are not heeded by the insurer, the nurse may retain private counsel at his or her own cost to obtain effective representation. In such a situation, the insurance attorney would most probably withdraw from representing the nurse, and there may be another suit filed concerning the insurance contract and the potential breach of the insurer to provide competent counsel.

> *If the nurse named in a lawsuit is covered under a policy of professional liability insurance, the policy will usually stipulate that an attorney be employed by the insurer to represent the insured.*

The insurance policy provisions will also specify whether it is the "primary insurance," provides "secondary" coverage, or is an "excess" policy. Generally speaking, if only one policy is carried by the nurse, it will be the primary insurance policy. If, however, the nurse is covered by two professional liability insurance policies—one purchased by the employer and one purchased by the nurse personally, for example—one may become the secondary policy based on the language of the respective policies. If, in contrast, the nurse's employer is self-insured and the nurse is covered in that manner, his or her own commercial policy would most probably become the primary coverage and the employer's self-insurance would be utilized as an excess fund.[31]

It is difficult to predict with certainty how coverage questions would be resolved, for each situation must be analyzed in view of the specific language of the policy and applicable state laws.[32] Thus, if named in a suit, the nurse should obtain as much information as possible concerning the coverage issue and, if needed, obtain an independent, objective opinion as to his or her rights and responsibilities in the situation.

TABLE 5–1

Factors to Evaluate with Professional Liability Insurance Policies

TYPE OF POLICY—CLAIMS MADE (covers a claim only if injury occurs and claim filed while the policy is in effect) or OCCURRENCE (covers a claim regardless of when filed so long as the incident arose while the policy was in effect); if policy CLAIMS MADE, tail coverage needed to cover claim made after policy no longer in effect.

AMOUNT OF COVERAGE—Adequate coverage important. Based on type of practice, cost of coverage, any ceilings (caps) on the amount injured parties can recover for, and own assets that need protecting. Insurer will pay only for damages as specified in the insurance contract. Dollar limits are usually expressed as $A/$B; *A* represents the amount paid per claim and *B* the aggregate amount paid under the policy in a given year.

INSURED'S OBLIGATIONS UNDER POLICY—Full and honest disclosure concerning type of nursing practice and responsibilities; cooperating with the insurer in defending any suit; notifying the insurer if named in a suit, if a patient is injured as a result of care rendered, or if a suit is threatened against the nurse.

INSURER'S OBLIGATIONS UNDER POLICY—A general duty to defend any and all allegations against the insured that are covered by the policy; pay for any and all expenses to do so (unless limited by the terms of the policy); provide effective legal representation (if included in policy); and notify the insured within specified time frames if the insurance policy is going to be canceled.

EXCLUSIONS IN THE POLICY—Generally, no coverage for intentional torts, criminal charges, exceeding the scope of one's practice as defined by state nurse practice acts, or punitive damages.

INDEMNIFICATION AND CONTRIBUTION CLAUSES—Clauses in the contract of insurance covering the right of one of the parties to seek reimbursement for any costs and damages paid on behalf of the other party, and the right of the insurer to share a payment proportionally in accordance with the policy limits when more than one policy covers the loss. Although separate and distinct clauses, both are important to the insured and should be carefully reviewed. Depending on how they are written in the policy, the nurse may seek recovery from the insurance company for some or all monies paid personally to defend against a suit under the indemnification language. Or, with a contribution clause, if two liability insurance policies cover the same event, the two insurance companies will be determining each's respective "contribution" to any judgment entered against the nurse.

"OTHER INSURANCE" CLAUSE—A clause describing which policy of insurance will control if more than one exists. Terms such as *primary, excess,* and *secondary* will usually be present. Other clauses that control the contribution of the policy, once its role is established, are *excess* (no payment will occur until all other sources of coverage are expended); *pro rata* (sharing of the loss according to the contract); and *escape* (no coverage or payment if other insurance coverage exists). In addition, the insurance policy may have language in it allowing the company to settle a case without the consent of the insured (nurse). Although this is often a troubling requirement for the nurse defendant, it is important to remember that its inclusion in a policy is based not on the merits of the case but on financial considerations of continuing a suit. In other words, if it is more beneficial for the insurance company to "cut its losses" and end the suit rather than proceed further, it will do so.

Data from: The American Association of Nurse Attorneys. *Demonstrating Financial Responsibility for Nursing Practice.* Pensacola, Fla.: Author, 1989; George D. Pozgar. *Legal Aspects of Health Care Administration.* 7th Edition. Gaithersburg, Md.: Aspen Publishers, Inc., 1999, 425–438; Vickey Masta-Cornic, "A Basic Insurance Primer," in *The Risk Manager's Desk Reference.* 2nd Edition. Barbara Youngberg, Editor. Gaithersburg, Md.: Aspen Publishers, Inc., 1999, 202–214.

SUMMARY OF PRINCIPLES AND APPLICATIONS

The defense of a professional negligence suit requires a great deal of time, effort, and strategy. Perhaps the best defense, however, is to avoid being included in such a suit. Although this is easier said than done, and although there is no absolute way to avoid being named in a suit that alleges professional negligence, the nurse can avoid unnecessary inclusion in such a suit by:

- Practicing nursing in accordance with licensing standards, professional standards, well-developed policies and procedures of the health care system, and accreditation standards

- Asking for orientation to a new position

- Reviewing the job description of the position

- Documenting care in accordance with accreditation and licensing standards, agency policy, and applicable national standards of documentation of nursing care

- Maintaining open lines of communication with fellow health care workers and patients and their families

- Maintaining and updating credentials and certification for areas of nursing practice, including specialty areas of practice

- Keeping current on nursing practices, procedures, and other developments in the delivery of nursing care

- Carefully evaluating professional liability insurance coverage, including whether to purchase one's own policy, what type of policy is being purchased, and what the nurse's obligations are under the policy

- Practicing within the scope of nursing practice, including any specialty area of nursing

When inclusion in a suit does occur, the nurse can help in his or her own defense by:

- Cooperating fully with his or her attorney
- Testifying in a competent and professional manner
- Utilizing expert witness testimony by a nurse to establish the standard of care
- Remaining confident of his or her professional abilities despite inclusion in a suit

TOPICS FOR FURTHER INQUIRY

1. Critically evaluate at least three different professional liability insurance policies. Look for similarities and differences in terms of coverage amounts, definitions of nursing in the policy, and exclusions and costs, as well as other provisions. Decide which policy provides the best protection for the nurse.

2. Interview a nurse who has been named in a suit and has had to go through at least a portion of the trial process. Ascertain the nurse's perception of her attorney's role during the deposition or trial testimony. Have the nurse identify ways in which he or she believed the attorney's role could have been different or more helpful.

3. Locate and interview several nurses who function as nurse experts in your area of nursing specialty. Compare and contrast each nurse expert's experience as a part of the litigation team.

4. Analyze several documentation policies from health care facilities for how, if at all, the policies protect the nurse in documenting from a "defense" position. Identify ways in which the policies could be improved.

REFERENCES

1. American Nurses Association. *Legal Aspects of Standards and Guidelines for Clinical Nursing Practice.* Washington, D.C.: Author, 1998, 3.
2. ONCC Research Committee and Executive Staff, "Report of a State-of-the-Knowledge Conference on U.S. Nursing Certification," 31(1) *Image Journal of Nursing Scholarship* (1999), 52–53.
3. *Id.*
4. *Id.*
5. Fay Rozovsky. *Liability and Risk Management in Home Health Care.* Gaithersburg, Md.: Aspen Publishers, Inc., 1998, 12:6–12:7.
6. *Darling v. Charleston Community Hospital,* 211 N.E.2d 253 (1965), *cert. denied,* 383 U.S. 946 (1966).
7. Barbara Stevens Barnum and Karlene M. Kerfoot. *The Nurse as Executive.* 4th Edition. Gaithersburg, Md.: Aspen Publishers, Inc., 1995, 131.
8. *Id.*
9. See, for example, *Convalescent Services, Inc. v. Schultz,* 921 S.W.2d 731 (Texas 1996).
10. Theodore LeBlang, W. Eugene Basanta, Robert John Kane, and others. *The Law of Medical Practice in Illinois.* Volume 1. 2nd Edition. St. Paul, Minn.: West Group, 516–523 (with 1998 pocket part supplement).
11. 556 N.E.2d 662 (1st District 1990). See also *Advincala v. United Blood Services,* 678 N.E.2d 1009 (1996).
12. 42 U.S.C.A. Section 1395x(e)(1994); 42 C.F.R. Part 482 (1998 revisions).
13. Janet Pitts Beckmann. *Nursing Negligence: Analyzing Malpractice in the Hospital Setting.* Thousand Oaks, Cal.: Sage Publications, 1996, 268.
14. *Id.* at 36.
15. G. Hickson, E. Clayton, S. Entman, and others, "Obstetricians' Prior Malpractice Experience and Patients' Satisfaction with Care," 272(20) *JAMA* (November 1994), 1583–1587.
16. Gregory Lester and Susan Smith, "Listening and Talking to Patients: A Remedy for Malpractice Suits?" 158 *West. J. Med.* (1993), 268–272; See also Ann Scott Blouin and Nancy J. Brent, "Creating Value for Patients: A Legal Perspective," 28(6) *JONA* (June 1998), 7–9.
17. Mark Smith, "Growth of Managed Care," 2(4) *Front & Center* (Summer 1998), 3.
18. *Id.*
19. William H. Roach, Jr. and the Aspen Health Law and Compliance Center. *Medical Records and the Law.* 3rd Edition. Gaithersburg, Md: Aspen Publishers, Inc., 1998, 28–43.
20. *Id.* at 59–61.
21. See generally Beckman, *supra* note 13, at 258–261, 268–269.
22. Elizabeth C. Mueth, "Computer-Based Patient Records," in *Nursing Documentation: Legal Focus Across Practice Settings.* Sue E. Miner. Thousand Oaks, Cal.: Sage Publications, 1999, 29–39; Roach and the Aspen Center, *supra* note 19, at 290–309.
23. Close monitoring will be needed for the changes proposed in the way health care systems develop health information systems and electronically transmit specified health information as proposed under the Health Insurance Portability and Accountability Act, signed into law on August 21, 1996. For an excellent overview of the proposed rules, see Adele A. Waller, "Preparing for the Complexities of Administrative Simplification Under HIPAA," in *1999 Health Law Handbook.* Alice G. Gosfield, Editor. St. Paul, Minn.: West Group, 677–727.
24. Henry Campbell Black, Black's Law Dictionary. 7th Edition. St. Paul, Minn.: West Group, 1999, 430.
25. *Id.* at 478.
26. *Id.* at 1485.

27. Being sued is also described by many nurses as one of the most traumatic experiences a nurse can have. Linda Shinn, "What to Do If You Are Sued," in *Take Control: A Guide to Risk Management*. Linda Shinn, Editor. Chicago, Ill.: Kirke-Van Orsdel, Inc. and Chicago Insurance Company, 1998, VII-1–VII-14.

28. Vickey Masta-Gornic. "A Basic Insurance Primer," in *The Risk Manager's Desk Reference*. 2nd Edition. Barbara Youngberg, Editor. Gaithersburg, Md.: Aspen Publishers, Inc., 1999, 208.

29. *Id.* at 208–211.

30. *Id.*

31. The American Association of Nurse Attorneys, Inc. *Demonstrating Financial Responsibility for Nursing Practice*. Pensacola, Fla.: Author, 1989, 4.

32. A recent case dealing with insurance coverage, nursing liability, and whether a nurse should carry personal professional liability insurance is *Patient's Compensation Fund v. Lutheran Hospital*, 588 N.W.2d 888 (Wis. 1999).

The Nurse and Quality Patient Care

6

- Quality Management
- Utilization Management
- Risk Management
- Peer Review

The provision of quality patient care is of constant concern and a goal of most health care delivery systems and health care providers, especially in view of the legal obligation of both to provide reasonable, nonnegligent care. That concern and goal can be thwarted, however, when additional factors exert equally compelling influences on their achievement. Such factors include economic concerns over the ever-rising costs of health care; the proliferation of third-party payers in health care; increased regulation of health care delivery by state and federal governments, including the establishment of the federal Agency for Health Care Policy and Research in 1989 (recently renamed the Agency for Health Research and Quality); the current worldwide nursing shortage, both in terms of numbers of nurses and nurses with needed specialties, skills, and experience; rising competition among health care systems; the use of practice policies; and the increasingly sophisticated health care consumers who demand quality care.

It is clear that these factors have created a focus on cost containment, and that focus has affected the provision of quality patient care. Two authors have clearly identified the pivotal issue in cost containment and its effect upon quality patient care. In the past, incentives in health care focused on doing more rather than less because payment was based on the services provided.[1] Today, however, incentives are reversed so that doing the minimum is becoming the norm.[2] Indeed, a minimalistic approach has raised the concern, ignored by society and the legal system, as to what role "undue economic influence" may have on physician/health care provider–assisted suicide.[3] Because patients are so powerless in a minimalistic health care system, another author suggests they need to be enabled. One way that can occur is through the use of the class action suit as a way of empowering consumers of health care and, at the same time, possibly improving health care quality, costs, and access.[4] Also, the ever-present question of the allocation of scarce resources has not been dissipated by cost containment.[5] If anything, the competition for limited resources has become more acute.

Although there may be general agreement that economic and other constraints may adversely affect patient care, there is little agreement on what quality patient care is. It has been defined as including clinical underpinnings but also economic, social, political, and cultural elements.[6] Others have defined it in terms of "process measures of health plans"; that is, for example, rates of immunizations. Quality patient care has also been analyzed according to data used to measure performance. Performance measures can include clinical data, financial data, and indexes of patients' satisfaction with care.[7] Whatever definition of quality patient care is used, there is no question that an internal peer review process that audits the quality of patient care is essential.[8] Indeed, without a well-developed program of analyzing and evaluating patient care provided within a health care delivery institution or system and the risks associated with the delivery of that care, the institution or system faces certain failure.

This chapter will explore the quality assurance mechanisms and risk management tools used in health care delivery.

ESSENTIALS OF MONITORING AND EVALUATING PATIENT CARE

Historical Overview

The mechanisms for evaluating patient care and avoiding risk have undergone many changes throughout the years, oftentimes reflecting concomitant changes in society. Nursing quality management most probably began with Florence Nightingale, who evaluated care given soldiers in the Crimean War in a systematic manner.[9] Quality management, utilization management, and risk management programs generally began as a response to the establishment of the Joint Commission on the Accreditation of Healthcare Organizations (JCAHO) in 1953 (then JCAH) and its subsequent standards for accreditation.[10] The federal government, through its Medicare and Medicaid programs, also enhanced the development of quality assurance programs.

*Nursing quality management
most probably began
with Florence Nightingale . . .*

With the advent of continuous quality improvement and total quality management programs in the 1980s, the focus on customer-driven improvement of patient care became more important than conformity with JCAHO standards.[11] This focus was soon replaced with an emphasis on evaluating outcomes, severity of illness measurements, and patient satisfaction, among other indicators.[12] Likewise, an increased concern for cost containment saw the establishment of case management programs.

Risk management's growth in health care was initially concerned with covering the financial loss from patient injuries, mainly through the purchase of professional liability insurance.[13] Since then, however, its focus has expanded to include many more responsibilities, not the least of which is evaluating and maintaining quality care to patients.

Definitions of Monitoring and Evaluating Patient Care

Quality Management

Quality management (QM) was once known as quality assurance. Today, however, QM has become varied and is known by many names in health care organizations (e.g., "clinical process improvement," "clinical resource management").[14] Regardless of its name, QM focuses upon the evaluation of the quality of patient care.[15] It is also concerned with the "business needs" of the organization, such as managed care contracting, case management, and organization reengineering.[16]

Recently, there has been a trend toward including in QM the functions of continuous quality improvement (CQI) and total quality management (TQM). TQM is defined as a group of quality improvement approaches that focus on "customer satisfaction" and the improvement of existing structures and processes.[17] Integrating TQM into QM is seen by many as being cost effective and reducing the duplication of evaluating and improving quality in the health care organization.[18]

Likewise, CQI involves improving performance at every "functional level of an organization's operation."[19] As a result, combining CQI into QM is an easy fit.

Although QM can be viewed as a process in and of itself, it can also be viewed as an integral part of other quality assurance programs—utilization management, risk management, and peer review. Indeed, many health care organizations are integrating quality management, utilization management, and risk management activities and operational improvements into one department.[20]

Utilization Management

Utilization management (UM) is a process to evaluate whether, based on preestablished standards, services provided to patients were medically necessary.[21] Recently, case management has become an integral part of UM.[22] The review process in UM can occur before services begin, concurrently (while the patient is still receiving services), or retroactively (after the termination of services). The process may be done by the health care organization itself, or the organization may use an outside UM firm. In addition, the federal and state governments through their Medicare and Medicaid programs and private insurance companies also do UM. Regardless of when UM is done, it is helpful in many ways. First, it can reduce costs. Second, it can help sustain quality patient care by attempting to maintain a high level of care even in an alternative setting or at a "lower level" of care.[23]

*Utilization management . . . can
reduce costs and . . . can help
sustain quality patient care . . .*

Despite the promises UM and other quality assurance procedures hold for sustaining quality health care, there are continuing concerns that these activities are seen more as "cost containment" methods than "quality control" procedures.[24]

Risk Management

Risk management (RM) is the systematic internal process of a health care delivery system aimed at reducing preventable injuries and accidents and reducing financial loss for the health care entity.[25] This is accomplished by reducing risks to the entity through "risk identification, risk analysis, risk treatment, and risk evaluation."[26]

Risk identification uses, among other methods, occurrence or incident reports, which identify concurrent risks as well as anticipate the risks associated with the provision of services.[27] Risk analysis evaluates identified risks in terms of the priority for addressing them. Risk evaluation looks at the "likely frequency of occurrence and severity of outcomes."[28]

Risk treatment includes controlling risks/losses and risk financing in three ways: risk elimination, risk prevention, and risk reduction.[29] Risk financing occurs through the purchase of liability insurance or through the establishment of a self-insurance program.

Risk management's concern of reducing the financial losses to the organization clearly expands to losses other than those that might occur in delivering patient care. For example, risk management is also concerned with employee issues (resolving grievances in a fair and expeditious manner) and avoiding injuries to employees and visitors that might occur on its premises.

Risk management must work hand in hand with QM and UM, whether or not the three quality assurance functions are integrated in a particular health care organization. All three processes share common concerns even if from different perspectives.[30] In fact, standards of one accrediting body, the Joint Commission on the Accreditation of Healthcare Organizations, link the three quality assurance functions.[31] Information from risk management activities that may be helpful in improving the quality of patient care must also be accessible to the other components of the quality assessment process.[32]

Peer Review

Another component of monitoring and evaluating patient care, peer review (PR) is carried out by the entity's practicing health care providers, including nurses. The purpose of peer review is to examine the quality of care provided by the health care provider group (physicians or nurses, for example) and the group's adherence to established standards of practice. Individual practitioner performance is also assessed.[33]

Peer review may result in an individual health care provider's clinical practice being terminated or limited in some way (for example, placing the individual on a probationary status). In addition, peer review may result in the individual practitioner being reported to the National Practitioner Data Bank (NPDB) and other banks, such as the National Council of State Boards of Nursing Data Bank (NDB).

Peer review decisions may also result in liability for the facility's peer review committee. As a result, many states have provided immunity from civil suit for individuals participating in peer review activities as part of an institution's established process of internal quality control, improving patient care, and reducing patient morbidity or mortality. The immunity often extends to individuals in various health care delivery systems, such as hospitals and long-term care facilities. These state immunity protections are often found in the statutes governing the establishment, licensure, and operation of the health care delivery system, such as the hospital licensing act and the home health care licensing act.

In addition to the state protections afforded peer review and the evaluative procedures for improvement of patient care generally, the National Practitioner Data Bank also offers immunity from suit for health care delivery systems that participate in its procedures.

Peer review can also occur outside the health care delivery system's established procedures. One way this occurs is through peer review organizations (PROs). PROs review services provided to Medicare and Medicaid recipients covered by health maintenance organizations to determine if care was reasonable, medically necessary, and in conformity with national standards of care, among other things. Peer review activities are carried out by the Health Care Financing Administration (HCFA).

Recently, the focus of PROs has changed toward patterns and outcomes of care and toward the promotion of quality improvement strategies.[34] As a result, PROs are now called Quality Improvement Organizations (QIOs).[35]

The Process of Monitoring and Evaluating Care

How a health care delivery entity decides to organize its quality assessment responsibilities varies. Whatever the decision, health care entities usually identify a "global method" that is to be used by all staff.[36] In addition, the health care entity uses a variety of tools and techniques to reach its goals, including flowcharts, benchmarking (the use of internal and external measures of "best performance" to set goals and improve the service under evaluation), and cause-and-effect diagrams.[37]

The internal process established must also take into account the many external aspects of monitoring and evaluating care discussed in other chapters in this book, including licensing, accreditation, and credentialing.

If the overall process of monitoring and evaluating care is to be successful, information flow among and between QM, UM, RM, and PR is essential. Information is gathered through many sources, including audit reports, research findings, patient complaints and satisfaction surveys, and length-of-stay data. Another source of helpful information for the organization's efforts to monitor and evaluate care is the use of incident or occurrence screening and reporting.

If the overall process of monitoring and evaluating care is to be successful, information flow among and between QM, UM, RM, and PR is essential.

Incident or Occurrence Screening and Reporting

Incident or occurrence screening is a systematic institution-wide process for identifying adverse patient care situations. Depending on how the institution organizes its quality assurance functions, the incident or occurrence report may go to the risk coordinator, a risk management committee, or the risk management department. In the screening process, the medical record is reviewed, either concurrent with the patient's stay or after discharge. The purpose is to "prevent" a patient care problem (if the patient is still being cared for) or prepare for the possibility of a suit (if the patient has been discharged).

Systematic screening is done regularly by utilizing a developed form with certain criteria listed for review. When a specific criterion is met, or a deviation from the criteria is discovered in the

record, it is then referred to a second phase of screening.

During the second phase, assessment and appropriate interventions are discussed. If the screening is a retrospective review, the information is categorized and used to initiate changes prospectively. In contrast, if the screening is concurrent, changes may be implemented in the care of that patient immediately to avoid or at least lessen a further untoward result.

In contrast to the screening process, incident or occurrence reporting is the way in which individual staff members communicate information concerning an adverse patient care situation to risk management utilizing the health care delivery system's policies and procedures for occurrence reporting. The incident or occurrence form is a formal document. It requests that staff supply certain objective information concerning the incident so that appropriate screening can take place and necessary interventions can be instituted, if possible.

Although the forms vary greatly in format, size, shape, and comprehensiveness, they most often include information concerning the patient, a factual description of the incident, any injuries sustained, and the outcome of the situation.[38] Figure 6–1 shows a conventional incident form.

With the increasing use of computers in health care, the sample conventional form may be replaced with a form that can be easily converted to use in the institution's computerized system.[39]

For a comprehensive risk management program to work, especially in relation to risk screening and reporting, the health care delivery system staff should be encouraged to use the reports without fear of retribution, loss of job, or other negative results. Only when staff, risk management, quality management, utilization management, and peer review work closely together in an atmosphere of trust and cooperation can patient care monitoring and evaluation work successfully.

Standards in Quality Management, Utilization Management, Peer Review, and Risk Management

Most health care delivery systems will utilize accreditation standards developed by private accrediting bodies such as the Joint Commission or other applicable entity in monitoring and evaluating patient care. Although an institution may de-

---

INCIDENT REPORT

Name of person

Mary J. Smith

Address

27 Morrison Street, Philadelphia, PA

Date of report	Date of incident	Time of incident	If ED patient, give unit number:
1/9/99	*1/9/99*	*8:30 a.m.*	

LOCATION OF INCIDENT
- ☐ patient room
- ☑ patient bathroom
- ☐ OR
- ☐ ED
- ☐ hospital grounds
- ☐ nurses' station
- ☐ other _____

IDENTIFICATION
- ☑ inpatient
- ☐ ED patient
- ☐ outpatient
- ☐ employee
- ☐ volunteer
- ☐ visitor
- ☐ other _____

Admitting diagnosis of patient

Diabetes mellitus

CONDITION BEFORE INCIDENT
Level of consciousness (previous 4 hours)
- ☑ alert
- ☐ confused, disoriented
- ☐ uncooperative
- ☐ sedated (drug:_____)
- ☐ unconscious

Ambulation
- ☑ OOB
- ☐ OOB with assistance
- ☐ bed rest with BRP
- ☐ complete bed rest
- ☐ not specified
- ☐ other (specify) _____
_____

Side rails
- ☐ up
- ☑ partially up
- ☐ down

Restraints
Present ☐ yes ☑ no
Ordered ☐ yes ☑ no

Call system within reach
- ☑ yes
- ☐ no

Bed height
- ☐ high
- ☑ low

NATURE OF INCIDENT
Fall
- ☐ while ambulatory
- ☐ while sitting
  - ☐ chair ☐ commode
- ☐ from bed
- ☐ off table, stretcher, or equipment
- ☑ found on floor
- ☐ other _____

Medication
- ☐ error in patient identification
- ☐ incorrect drug
- ☐ incorrect dosage
- ☐ incorrect route
- ☐ timing
- ☐ duplication
- ☐ omission
- ☐ incorrect I.V. solution hung
- ☐ incorrect I.V. rate
- ☐ other _____

Surgical
- ☐ consent problem
- ☐ incorrect sponge and instrument count
- ☐ foreign object left in patient
- ☐ other _____

FIGURE 6–1. Sample incident report (first page). (Used with permission from *Better Documentation/Clinical Skillbuilders*, 1992 © Springhouse Corporation.)

---

velop its own unique standards, it is hoped that working with a private accrediting entity's standards encourages compliance that leads to accreditation. Furthermore, because accrediting standards are often utilized by state licensing entities and in suits alleging negligence to establish standards of care, adherence to them can aid the health care delivery system in those situations as well.

Other standards that are used in quality management, utilization management, and peer review include Medicare and Medicaid (including the Health Care Financing Administration) guidelines and promulgated rules and regulations.

Guidelines in risk management are varied because of the unique nature of risk management and the possibility for diversity in its organization, scope, and functions within a health care delivery system or network. Even so, some standards do exist, and accreditation entity standards are one example.

NATURE OF INCIDENT *(continued)*

Equipment
Type _____
Control and serial number _____

_____

☐ malfunction
☐ shock
☐ burn
☐ other _____

Date of last maintenance _____
BioMed notified ☐ yes ☐ no
Risk Management notified ☐ yes ☐ no

Personal property
☐ damaged
☐ lost
☐ other _____

Describe items.

Miscellaneous
☐ patient refuses treatment
☐ needle stick
☐ injuries in treatment
☐ infection
☐ discharge against medical advice
☐ struck by door
☐ other _____

Describe the incident.
Pt. found sitting on floor in bathroom.
Pt. states she slipped.

Witnesses: ☐ yes ☑ no
If yes, note names, addresses, and phone numbers, and indicate if they're employees, visitors, etc.
1. _____   2. _____

DISPOSITION
Seen by
☑ attending doctor
☐ ED doctor

Treatment
☐ not indicated
☐ treatment given
☐ treatment refused
☑ X-ray ordered
☐ admitted to hospital
☐ follow-up care indicated

Examination findings:
Tender ⓛ shoulder
Doctor's signature:
John Moyer, MD

Notification
(include your name, the date, and the time)
Attending doctor notified
☑ yes   ☐ no
Jane Kelly, RN 1/9/99 8:45 a.m.
Supervisor notified
☑ yes   ☐ no
Jane Kelly, RN 1/9/99 8:47 a.m.
Noted in chart
☑ yes   ☐ no
Jane Kelly, RN 1/9/99 8:49 a.m.
Sick call request completed
☐ yes   ☑ no

Patient or family notified
☐ yes   ☑ no

☑ Documented in progress notes

FIGURE 6–1 *Continued. Sample incident report (second page). (Used with permission from Better Documentation/Clinical Skillbuilders, 1992 © Springhouse Corporation.) Illustration continued on following page*

Other standards for risk management come from standard forms used in occurrence screening developed by, as examples, the American Hospital Association and the Chicago Hospital Risk Pooling Programs. Also, through professional associations such as the American Society for Hospital Risk Managers (ASHRM) and the Risk Management Foundation, standards concerning education, credentialing, and the practice of risk managers have been established.

Recent Developments in Quality Assessment

Because lower costs, higher quality, and improved access to health care are vital to ensure the survival of a health care entity,[40] there has been increasing emphasis on merging quality assessment functions with "reengineering" and "process redesign." Quality management by any name is described as a "quick fix."[41] Reengineering, in contrast, is seen as a revolutionary and fundamental redesign of an entity's business processes to

GENERAL DATA
Attending doctor _John W. Moyer, MD_

Room number _439_   Bed number _1_   Shift ☑1 ☐2 ☐3

Additional details of incident

Pt. stated that she slipped on floor when getting out of the shower and hit her Ⓛ arm on the door. Pt. complaining of pain in Ⓛ shoulder. Pt. escorted back to bed. BP 124/80, P 84. Dr. Moyer notified @ 8:45 a.m.

Signature _Jane Kelley_   Title _RN_   Date _1/9/99_

Director's summary (detail follow-up to above incident and action taken)

Signature _____   Title _____   Date _____

FIGURE 6–1 *Continued.* Sample incident report (third page). (Used with permission from *Better Documentation/Clinical Skillbuilders*, 1992 © Springhouse Corporation.)

achieve improvements in "critical measures such as cost, quality, service, and speed."[42] Process redesign seeks to combine the two approaches by developing an organization's infrastructure to support any changes implemented.[43]

It is not yet certain how the wedding of quality management functions with the models of organizational change will affect the provision of quality patient care on a long-term basis. Even so, it is a marriage that is firmly established in health care today. Its impact can also be seen in texts in nursing practice and nursing management wherein nursing students and practicing nurses alike orient themselves—and their practice—to this phenomenon. Even so, the questions of how quality in health care can truly be ensured continue.[44]

IMPLICATIONS FOR NURSING

Because the provision of quality patient care is a fundamental part of nursing practice, nursing must be consistently and actively involved in monitoring and evaluating patient care. Clearly, nurse executives, whether the chief nurse executive or those holding other positions in upper nursing management, should be vigorously involved in quality assessment in the health care delivery system. Likewise, nurse managers, as well as staff nurses, need to be involved as quality management, utilization management, or risk management committee members if the organization uses a committee approach to monitoring and evaluating patient care. In addition, it is essential to participate in nursing audits, either as an auditor or one being audited, and to conduct or participate in research that may ultimately improve patient care.

Participation in peer review activities not only is a way of contributing to the monitoring and evaluation of patient care but also meets the need of the profession to monitor itself. Thus, when a nurse evaluates another nurse's performance within the context of their particular institution, he or she is also contributing to overall regulation and improvement of the profession.

A nurse can contribute to quality management by being active on other committees as well. Membership on the forms committee, policy and procedure committee, and staff development committee, for example, directly influences the provision of quality patient care. If membership is not possible, each staff nurse can augment a committee's work by sharing concerns and making suggestions to a member of the committee.

Nursing must also ensure that patient care is documented in accordance with institution or agency policy and with guidelines for good documentation. Because the medical record is a common component in both quality appraisal and risk management, it is vital to the overall success of both programs.

Likewise, the use of incident or occurrence reports must be stressed as a necessary component of the process of improving patient care. In addition, the guidelines for documentation in the patient's record should be followed for documenting on the incident form as well.

The nurse must also be knowledgeable about his or her responsibilities for reporting within the health care entity any quality management events that are monitored by outside agencies. For example, in 1998 the Joint Commission on Accreditation of Healthcare Organizations has initiated a new Sentinel Event Policy. It strongly recommends that health care organizations, among other things, self-report to the commission any "sentinel events"—those needing immediate investigation and response, such as a death, serious physical or psychological injury, or the risk of these situations.[45] Examples include medication errors, patient suicide, and surgical procedures done on the wrong site. Although it is not the nurse's responsibility to personally report these events to the commission, it is the nurse's obligation to follow established institutional policies to ensure that those in the organization who must be notified are informed. Thus, compliance with the commission's policy is possible, and necessary changes in patient care can be identified and initiated by the health care entity to rectify the original problem.

It is also important that the nurse feel comfortable in informally discussing potential patient care problems with fellow staff nurses, nurse managers, and committee members. Because risk prevention is one of the elements of patient care evaluation, identifying a particular concern about patient care that has not yet become a problem is a valuable way to improve patient care and serve the institution's goals of quality management as well.

The ability to share concerns with one another not only is important to quality appraisal and risk management but also is essential in weathering the storms of change essential in "reengineering" and "process redesign" as it affects QM, UM, RM, and PR efforts. Nursing must support each member's effort to provide quality patient care during organizational change. Moreover, the need to provide quality care must be a constant concern despite the restructuring that continues around the nurse who is providing care to patients. The changes that occur cannot alter the nurse's overriding duty to provide care that is nonnegligent and consistent with quality standards of care.

Other factors can decrease poor patient care and reduce risks to patients, nursing staff, and the employer. They include the establishment and use of a good orientation program for new staff, continual in-service programs for staff, support for attendance at continuing education programs, and establishment and updating of job descriptions.

SPECIAL CONSIDERATIONS

The Health Care Quality Improvement Act of 1986

The Health Care Quality Improvement Act (HCQIA) is a federal law passed by Congress in response to the increasing occurrence of malpractice in the United States and society's concern about the quality of health care.[46] The law's three stated purposes are to (1) improve the overall quality of health care, (2) limit the ability of incompetent physicians to move from state to state without disclosure or discovery of past performance, and (3) encourage and protect good-faith involvement by physicians in peer review activities.[47]

To carry out its purposes, the Act established the National Practitioner Data Bank as a national information system. Health care delivery systems, state medical and other boards, professional societies, and insurance companies are required to report certain activities and query the bank under certain situations.

The National Practitioner Data Bank is overseen by the U.S. Department of Health and Human Services. Information that must be reported to the bank by certain entities or groups includes:

1. any payment by a medical malpractice insurer (meaning an insurance company, self-insurance program(s), or self-insured individual practitioners, "or otherwise") on behalf of all licensed health care providers resulting from a written claim or judgment
2. any disciplinary action taken by any state licensing board
3. any disciplinary action taken by a state licensing board or agency against other health care providers, including nurses, under the Medicare and Medicaid Patient Protection Act of 1987[48] for clinical incompetence or professional misconduct
4. disciplinary actions for incompetence or unprofessional conduct by hospitals, group medical practices, and health maintenance organizations that adversely affect clinical privileges of physicians and dentists (if the action denies, limits, revokes, or suspends privileges for 30 days or more)
5. actions by a professional society for incompetence or unprofessional conduct that adversely affects membership in that society[49]

Hospitals are required to request information from the NPDB in two instances. One is when a health care practitioner (including, for example, a nurse-anesthetist or nurse-midwife) applies for clinical or medical staff membership. The second situation is on the 2-year anniversary of the grant-ing of privileges or membership, and then every 2 years thereafter.

Penalties for noncompliance with the Act exist. For example, failure of an insurance company to report a payment on behalf of a licensed health care provider can result in a $10,000 penalty.[50]

Certain benefits for compliance with the Act are also included. For example, a hospital, its agents and employees, and peer review committee members who make a report consistent with the act and "in good faith" are immune from civil suit for damages and antitrust liability as a result of the professional review process.[51]

The National Council of State Boards of Nursing Data Bank

The National Council of State Boards of Nursing Data Bank (NDB) was established as a voluntary reporting system for member state boards of nursing to convey data concerning disciplinary actions taken against nurses by the particular state board. Information that may be reported to the National Council of State Boards of Nursing Data Bank includes the nurse's name and other biographical information, action taken, and the type of violation (such as unprofessional conduct or incompetency). The bank notifies all state board members and the certification body of nurse anesthetists of any information it receives. The branches of the military and the U.S. Public Health Service may query the bank for information. Currently, no health care delivery systems have access to, or input into, the bank.[52]

Liability Concerns
Negligence/Professional Negligence

Whenever monitoring or evaluation of patient care is undertaken, there is always concern that the institution and individuals involved may be found liable if the process is done negligently. The potential liability exists because of established legal principles of *respondeat superior,* the *corporate theory of liability,* and other laws, including case law (specifically, the *Darling* case), discussed in Chapter 4.

Whenever monitoring or evaluation of patient care is undertaken, there is always concern that the institution and individuals involved may be found liable if the process is done negligently.

Because potential liability might discourage health care providers and health care systems from participating in patient care monitoring and evaluation, whether in the form of quality management, utilization management, or risk management, many states have passed statutes that provide civil immunity for those activities. Some states do not provide civil immunity for quality assessment responsibilities if the conduct questioned is willful or wanton. It is also important to note, however, that the immunity from suit applies only to conduct involved in the process and procedures of quality assessment. If the health care delivery system, or one of its employees, is negligent in the *treatment* of a patient, then no immunity exists for that alleged conduct.

Actions Involving Clinical Privileges

Peer review activities are protected from suit under the Health Care Quality Improvement Act for covered institutions, the peer review committee, any member of the committee, or anyone assisting with the peer review process. However, the immunity provisions apply only in certain conditions set forth in the Act. They include "adequate" due process protections for the health care provider under review (e.g., notice of rights, hearing within 30 days); "reasonable" efforts to obtain the facts concerning the conduct under review; the review is believed to be in the interest of quality care; a person giving any information to the committee concerning the competence or professional conduct of a person must do so truthfully; and the review is believed warranted by the actual facts of the situation.[53] In addition, adherence to reporting mandates and query schedules and truth in providing information to the peer review body are required.

In addition to the Health Care Quality Improvement Act, some states have passed laws protecting health care entities other than hospitals for their peer review processes. In Illinois, for example, the Long-Term Care Peer Review and Quality Assessment and Assurance Protection Act[54] specifically precludes liability for civil damages as a result of conduct during peer review or quality assessment and assurance activities, unless the person or committee is involved in willful or wanton misconduct.

Defamation

A health care provider's concern that his or her reputation may be damaged during any process of monitoring and evaluating patient care is understandable. The law of defamation protects certain individuals or groups with a qualified privilege to speak what might otherwise be defamatory to protect the free flow of information necessary as part of that individual's official duties. Thus, unless the qualified privilege is abused, information given and exchanged during the quality assessment process would be protected from suit.

In addition, the courts have generally held that any exchange of information during quality assessment activities by the health care entity and its committees is not a publication to "a third party" for the purposes of defamation. So long as the information is exchanged within the entity, the communication is characterized as only the corporation talking to itself.[55]

Even if the aforementioned two protections did not apply in a particular situation, the general immunity provisions of the HCQIA and state statutes for the improvement of patient care activities would protect the free exchange of information concerning a specific health care provider so long as the protections were not abused.

Confidentiality of Quality Management, Utilization Management, Risk Management Reports, Data, Committee Meeting Minutes, and Other Information

The free exchange of information concerning quality assessment procedures also requires that the information reviewed, received, and generated remain confidential, that is, not subject to release to those outside the process. Although there is some controversy surrounding the availability of information to outsiders, the general rule is that material generated pursuant to quality assessment is confidential and can be disclosed only under limited circumstances.

The HCQIA, for example, severely restricts access to the data bank to ensure the information in it is used solely for the improvement of patient care. Thus, access to data reported to the bank is limited to, for example, the individual health care provider who has been reported to the bank; hospitals that query concerning an individual on staff or one applying for clinical privileges; state regulatory agencies responsible for licensing health care providers; and attorneys filing malpractice claims. In fact, only an "edited version" of all data bank information is available to the public for research and other public-use purposes. It excludes specific names of patients, physicians, and other health care practitioners reported.[56] Other information, such as the type of entity filing the report and the dollar amount and date of any payments made upon settlement or judgment, is included in the data.[57]

Information in the possession of peer review organizations is also confidential, with a specific limitation on the release of the information concerning a particular patient or health care provider to the public.

State laws vary concerning the confidentiality of information received during patient care assessment and evaluation, but many states do provide statutory protection from disclosure as previously discussed. Additionally, some states, like Illinois, have enacted state statutes that protect all quality assessment data, including incident or occurrence reports, by prohibiting their release, discoverability, and introduction into evidence in any trial, administrative hearing, or judicial proceeding.[58]

It may seem clear that quality assessment materials are confidential. In reality, however, the interplay of the various state and federal laws, and the continued debate over whether the materials should be confidential, result in many cases being filed to test the ability of "outsiders" to obtain that information.

Moreover, other changes are taking place concerning the confidentiality of this kind of information. With the vast amount of information available on the "information superhighway," once inaccessible information can now be obtained by anyone with a computer. For example, the Health Care Financing Administration (HCFA) has its Nursing Home Data Base available on the Medicare Web site.[59] It provides "understandable information about every nursing home in the United States." It does so by providing summary information about a nursing home's last state inspection.

Antitrust Concerns

One of the unique concerns in quality assessment is the impact peer review may have on competition in health care. If the process impedes or eliminates the ability of health care providers to gain access to clinical privileges in health care delivery systems, or to maintain those privileges, then those health care providers may be unfairly kept from providing their services. Furthermore, consumers would be unable to choose treatment from these health care providers. Because this issue most often arises when the health care provider does not obtain privileges in a particular system, the law has seen fit to protect health care entities

---

ETHICS CONNECTION 6–1

In 1995, the Joint Commission for Accreditation of Healthcare Organizations required that health care institutions address "organizational ethics." Prior to that time, ethics in nursing tended to focus on individual rather than institutional ethics. Ethicists struggle to define and describe organizational ethics and to show the differences between institutional and interpersonal ethics. Identifying the limits and boundaries of organizational ethics is complex and challenging. This task is especially difficult because, although an organization has moral values that guide its practices, "individuals bear the responsibility"[1] of organizational ethics.

In 1998, in an effort to show how complex organizational ethics is, the Park Ridge Center used selections from a *New Yorker* article[2] about Michael Swango, "the poison doctor." The Swango case is discussed[3] and followed by responses from an ethicist,[4] a hospital administrator,[5] and an educator.[6] The conflict between an individual's and an organizations' rights to privacy and the obligations to disclose information that bears on patient safety are evident in the Swango case. Refer to Chapter 3 for further discussion of organizational ethics.

[1]Van Rensselaer Potter, "Individuals Bear Responsibility," 12(2) *Bioethics Forum* (Summer 1996), 27–28.
[2]James B. Stewart, "Professional Courtesy," *New Yorker* (November 24, 1997).
[3]Phillip Boyle, "The Poison Doctor Tests the Limits of 'Professional Courtesy,'" 1(3) *The Park Ridge Center Bulletin* (February/March 1998), 6–8.
[4]Phillip Boyle, "Organizational Teflon: Making Sure the Case Doesn't Stick," 1(3) *The Park Ridge Center Bulletin* (February/March 1998), 8–9.
[5]Ralph Muller, "A Hospital Administration Responds: Yes, Swango Could Go Undetected," 1(3) *The Park Ridge Center Bulletin* (February/March 1998), 9–10.
[6]Jean Lang. "Swango: The View from the Couch," 1(3) *The Park Ridge Center Bulletin* (February/March 1998), 10.

and those involved in peer review from antitrust challenges in certain situations.

One of the unique concerns in quality assessment is the impact peer review may have on competition in health care.

The Health Care Quality Improvement Act includes immunity for alleged antitrust violations, so long as the professional review activities comply with the act. Thus, if an action is taken in furtherance of professional review, based on the health care provider's "competence or professional conduct," and is consistent with the requirements discussed earlier, then no antitrust violations would be likely.[60]

The Health Care Quality Improvement Act notwithstanding, federal antitrust law also exempts certain peer review activities from its mandates. One such exemption is that of state action—when the review action can be attributed to the action of the state rather than to a private organization. This exemption or defense applies to a health care organization that is a "sovereign branch" of state government (e.g., the state university hospital) or a private facility whose challenged conduct is without question adopted by the state as state policy and supervised by the state itself.[61] Several court decisions have held that a private hospital's actions were not immune from the antitrust law because the peer review actions were not supervised by the state.[62] Thus, courts will no doubt continue to carefully scrutinize cases alleging a violation of federal antitrust laws when the defense is that a particular peer review process is exempt from those federal antitrust laws under this exemption.

Managed Care

Managed care has been defined in many ways. One definition sees it as "a continuum of plans that focus on utilization and price of service, with the goal of reducing health care costs and maximizing value to both patient and payor."[63] Regardless of the specific definition, it is, in reality, simply another name for cost control and access control in health care.

Although this chapter has discussed various immunities for activities that might directly or indirectly be characterized as cost control measures, certain actions and their subsequent impact on patient care are evaluated by the courts. Specifically, when compliance with limitations imposed by third-party payers on a health care delivery system or health care provider results in injury or death to the patient, courts are imposing liability for those limitations.

Managed care organizations—a health maintenance organization (HMO), a preferred provider organization (PPO), or a management service organization (MSO), to name a few—face liability concerns in many areas. Some include denial of treatment,[64] improper credentialing of health care providers, and utilization management services.[65]

Two early cases involving utilization management activities bear mentioning. In the first case, *Wickline v. State of California,*[66] the California appellate court reversed a trial court decision in favor of Mrs. Wickline and against Medi-Cal, a state medical assistance program. After Medi-Cal denied a request for further hospital days following several surgical procedures for circulatory problems, the physician did not appeal that decision and discharged Mrs. Wickline. She developed additional problems at home, was readmitted to the hospital, and underwent two amputations on the affected leg—first below the knee and subsequently above the knee.

The appeals court clearly stated that "while a third party payor may be held legally accountable for medically inappropriate decisions, in this case plaintiff's treating physicians were ultimately responsible for the decision to release her,"[67] especially when none of the physicians challenged the decision to discharge the patient.

Wilson v. Blue Cross of Southern California[68] reached a different result, even though it was decided in the same California appellate district and division as *Wickline.* The case involved a *private* health insurance company and its utilization review organization. The company denied additional days (only 10 days were allowed pursuant to the contract of insurance for psychiatric illness) for a psychiatric hospitalization for a severely emotionally ill young man, Harold Wilson, Jr. No appeal procedures for the denial existed, and the Wilsons had no money of their own to pay for additional hospitalization. The treating psychiatrist's evaluation indicated that 3 to 4 additional *weeks* of inpatient care were needed. Harold Wilson was discharged on March 11 and committed suicide on March 31.

In her suit against Blue Cross, the utilization review company, and others, Harold Wilson's mother was defeated at the trial level by a summary judgment motion. On appeal, the appellate court reversed the decision and remanded the case to the trial court. The court stated that the case should go to trial against the utilization review company to determine its liability for "tortious interference with the contract of insurance between the decedent (Wilson) . . . and Blue Cross and its role in causing the wrongful death of the decedent."[69] Additionally, the court held that the *Wickline* decision was not controlling in this case because of the many differences in the two cases. It also opined that language in *Wickline* concerning the liability of the physician was "overly broad" *dicta* (nonbinding language in a court opinion).

At the trial, the jury decided in favor of the private health insurance company but held that the insurance company wrongfully withheld benefits. In addition, the jury held that the insurance company did not deal with the insured "fairly" and "in good faith" because the insured's contract of insurance did not provide for utilization review "in the first place."[70] Even so, the jury did not award damages to the Wilson family because Mrs. Wilson failed to prove the insurance company acted with malice.[71]

These two cases provide basic guidelines for health care delivery systems and health care practitioners, including nurses, who may be involved in managed care decisions. Those guidelines include the following:

1. Liability may be present for managed care decisions that result in injury or death to a health care consumer.
2. Complete documentation is necessary concerning a patient's progress, or lack of progress, so that a managed care organization has all the information it needs to make a well-founded decision.
3. If the nurse is a reviewer, he or she will need to seek out as much information as possible concerning the patient to make a well-reasoned decision.[72]
4. The physician involved in a denial of additional days should vigorously exercise any established appeal procedures.

5. Nurses functioning as utilization management employees should be licensed and be competent in utilization review principles.
6. Each and every health care delivery system must regulate and oversee any outside managed care program, whether public or private.[73]

Clinical Practice Guidelines

Clinical practice guidelines, also called "practice policies," "clinical pathways," and "practice parameters," among other titles, are well entrenched in health care delivery today. They are seen as a tool to improve quality care, ensure the appropriate use of health care resources, and aid in the cost-effectiveness of health care.[74] Clinical practice guidelines were initially developed as a response to the establishment in 1972 of the professional standards review organization (PSRO) program, which focused on the evaluation and review of care provided to Medicare and Medicaid recipients.[75]

Clinical practice guidelines are defined as "systematically developed statements to assist practitioner and patient decisions about appropriate health care for specific clinical circumstances."[76] In nursing, they have been used to improve the time within which patients receive chemotherapy after admission to the health care facility, to adjust rest periods for patients after returning to the unit after physical therapy, and to decrease the readmission rate for neuroscience patients and patients with hip fractures.[77]

Although well entrenched in various forms in health care delivery, practice parameters are controversial. Some of the concerns surrounding their use include (1) whether they may increase liability for health care providers, (2) how and when variations in the recommended pathway or guideline should occur, and (3) the use of the guidelines for reimbursement purposes.[78]

Clinical practice guidelines are generally a good risk management tool. Even so, they must be developed carefully and with input from those health care providers who are expected to follow them. The guidelines should also be as comprehensive and specific as possible, based on current practice, and utilize relevant research findings and "appropriate clinical expertise" in the development process.[79]

The nurse working with practice guidelines should be involved in their development. In addition, it is important to remember that they must be updated on a regular basis. Moreover, the nurse providing care pursuant to practice guidelines must not blindly follow them. Rather, the guidelines are "flexible," allowing individualized application based on the specific needs and status of the patient.[80]

Corporate Compliance Programs

Due to the spiraling costs of health care resulting from unidentified health care fraud and abuse, in 1997 the federal government took proactive steps to curb, insofar as possible, additional instances of undetected fraud and abuse. Under various programs, including Operation Restore Trust (ORT), and the passage of the Health Care Insurance Portability and Accountability Act,[81] hospitals, home health care agencies, and other health care delivery institutions initiated corporate compliance programs. "Voluntary" in nature, the programs were developed under the guidance of the Office of the Inspector General (OIG) of the Department of Health and Human Services. The guidelines require that an oversight compliance program is to, among other things, reduce the likelihood of violations of federal laws pertaining to fraud and abuse, educate employees about health care fraud and abuse, establish a confidential "hotline" to allow employees to report questionable activities without fear of retaliation, and use mechanisms such as audits to monitor compliance with the established program.[82]

Compliance programs will be helped tremendously in their efforts to reduce fraud and abuse in health care by the Healthcare Integrity and Protection Data Bank (HIPDB). Effective October 1, 1999, the HIPDB collects data and centralizes information on "final adverse actions" taken against health care providers, suppliers, and practitioners across the United States.[83] Federal and state agencies and health care plans are required to report instances of health care–related criminal convictions and exclusions of health care practitioners, providers, and suppliers from participation in state and federal health care programs, among other events.[84] The reported information can be used by licensing boards, law enforcement agencies, and other "eligible users" when investigating instances of fraud and abuse. The reporting of incidents and querying the HIPDB is done on the World Wide Web at http://www.npdb-hipdb.com.[85]

Corporate compliance policies and procedures are an excellent quality management tool, in addition to being a vehicle to reduce illegality in the delivery of health care.[86] The nurse can contribute to the success of a corporate compliance program in many ways. The first is to know the established policies and procedures and strictly follow them. Second, accurate and complete documentation of all patient care given is also essential. Third, a nurse who suspects that illegal activity may be going on in the facility in which he or she works (e.g., billing for a home health care nurse when a home health aide visits) should report it consistent with established procedures. A fourth way in which a nurse can contribute to the facility's overall compliance program is to act as the corporate compliance officer. A person with a nursing degree and extensive clinical experience who also possesses good communication skills, utilizes critical thinking, and understands the law, among other characteristics, is an excellent candidate for this role.[87]

The Administration of Medications

There is no question that the administration of medications is one of the high-risk areas in nursing practice. When an error occurs, devastating results, including death, are possible. Studies have indicated that there are many reasons for an "adverse medication event," including fatigue,[88] failures in communication,[89] errors in transcription,[90] and failure to comply with facility policies.[91] Poor labeling and packaging of medications is also cited as a major factor that contributes to medication errors.[92] Despite the number of medication errors suspected (1.6% to 38%) for all medications administered, it is believed that only 25% of errors are reported.[93]

The avoidance of medication errors, then, is of primary concern to the nurse and the health care entity that want to ensure quality patient care. Table 6–1 lists some innovative guidelines for avoiding medication errors.

In addition to following the guidelines listed in Table 6–1, the nurse can also help avoid medication errors and thereby contribute to quality patient care by following well-established principles of medication administration. They include complying with the five "rights" of medication administration (right patient, right route, right dose, right

---

ETHICS CONNECTION 6-2

In corporate compliance programs, the institutional mission and the ethical concerns of employees meet. The following situation is an example of how a nurse identifies a corporate compliance concern about the potential for an improper referral.[1]

> Regina is a clinical nurse specialist at Charity who often works with Dr. Stone, a gastroenterologist who admits many patients to "Sweet Charity." She has noticed that when patients need gastrointestinal (GI) lab testing, Dr. Stone often refers them to a particular non-Charity facility even though Charity has its own well-run GI lab. Then she hears through the grapevine that Dr. Stone is a part owner of the other facility. She suspects a legal or ethical problem and wonders whether she should tell anyone in authority of her concerns.[2]

Whether or not the referrals to the GI lab violate the Ethics in Patient Referrals Act ("Stark" legislation), Regina has identified a pattern of referrals that morally risks the appearance of a conflict of interest.

---

[1]David E. Guinn and David B. McCurdy, "Corporate Compliance and Integrity Programs: The Uneasy Alliance between Law and Ethics," 31 *Insight* (Spring 1999), 2–10.
[2]*Id.* at 3.

time, right medication); focusing on the responsibility of medication administration and avoiding all distractions; seeking clarification and information from appropriate health team members (e.g., pharmacy and physician ordering medication) when uncertain or unsure about a medication order; and refusing to work extra shifts when fatigued or stressed.

Managed Care and Patient Well-Being

Separate from the liability and quality management concerns of health care practitioners surrounding managed care discussed in this chapter is the growing concern about its effect upon patient well-being.[94] In fact, a 1999 survey of 768 nurses and 1,053 physicians reveals that this concern has become a reality.[95] The nurses surveyed indicated a number of troublesome findings. Initially, about half of the nurses (48%) said that within the last 2 years a health plan decision resulted in a decline in health for their patients.[96] Moreover, the nurses in the study indicated that the primary negative effect of managed care was the "decreasing quality of care,"[97] despite its positive effect on preventive care, practice guidelines, and disease management. The "decreasing quality of care" identified by the nurses in the study included inadequate staffing

---

TABLE 6-1

Avoiding Adverse Medication Events

GUIDELINE	NURSING ACTION
Properly labeled stored drugs	Contact pharmacy when medication not labeled correctly; withhold administering medication until labeling issue clarified.
Medication room "user-friendly"	Provide input into design of medication room, if possible; suggest ways to improve already existing medication room (e.g., noise level, lighting, distractions); arrange stored medications to help nurse in preparing and administering meds (e.g., signs, markers, adherence to state/federal agency rules for storage)
Competence with medication administration equipment	Use only after orientation to equipment and demonstrated competence is achieved; ask for regular updates on use of equipment; seek in-service orientation for any new equipment
Read medication label three times	Read label before pouring medication, immediately before administering medication, and when placing medication "container" back in storage
Established procedures for administration of investigational medications	Follow institutional procedures; "double-check" high-dosage investigational drugs; participate in review of and approval of protocols.

Data from: J. Duncan Moore, "Accident Insurance: Dana-Farber Seeks Foolproof Ways to Stop Medical Errors," *Modern Healthcare* (1997), 44–45; Susan Grant, "Viewpoint: Who's to Blame for Tragic Error?" 99(9) *AJN* (1999), 9; Janet Pitts Beckmann. *Nursing Negligence: Analyzing Malpractice in the Hospital Setting.* Thousand Oaks, Cal.: Sage Publishers, Inc., 1996; National Coordinating Council for Medication Error Reporting and Prevention, "Recommendations for Avoiding Error-Prone Aspects of Dispensing Medications," May 19, 1999, and "Recommendations to Reduce Errors Related to Administration of Drugs," June 29, 1999, located at http://www.nccmerp.org/, accessed April 13, 1999.

ETHICS CONNECTION 6–3

Medication errors are a clear example of violation of the moral principle of nonmaleficence, the avoidance of harm. What is less clear, however, is the major source of medication errors. Both the American Nurses Association (ANA)[1] and the Institute of Medicine (IOM)[2] agree that most medication errors occur because of failures in the health care system rather than individual errors. After reviewing two highly publicized situations regarding nurses' medication errors, the ANA argued that the health care systems, rather than the individual nurses, were at fault. One situation was the involvement of 13 nurses in the 1994 Dana-Farber Institute chemotherapy overdose. The second was the indictment of three Colorado nurses on criminal charges following an infant's death from medication. The fine line between individual and institutional responsibility for safe, effective medication administration may become clearer as ethicists better understand organizational ethics.

Inadequate and/or inappropriate institutional staffing patterns undoubtedly contribute to medication and other errors that compromise patient safety. Nurses in several states are working to reduce such errors by improving staffing patterns. Sometimes, employers try to discourage nurses from publicly discussing patient safety issues that may result from unsafe staffing. For example, when an Oregon nurse testified about a life-threatening patient emergency that resulted from understaffing, the hospital's human resources department informed her that she should "deal with concerns about quality of patient care internally rather than making them public."[3] The ANA action report, "Shared Accountability in Today's Work Environment,"[4] recommends strategies to address concerns about patient safety, including (1) "educating policy-makers and the public on the effects of downsizing, restructuring, and reorganizing that lead to breakdowns in safety and quality"; (2) "work with other health care organizations to identify and correct systems errors that lead to patient injuries"; and (3) "support the role of the professional nurse in correcting systems errors through quality improvement initiatives and protect the nurse."

---

[1]Mary Foley, "News Release: Testimony of the American Nurses Association Before the Subcommittee on Labor, Health and Human Services, Education and Related Agencies Committee on Appropriations, United States Senate, on patient safety and medical errors," (December 13, 1999). http://www.ana.org/gova/federal/legis/testimon/1999/iom.htm

[2]Institute of Medicine. To Err Is Human: Building a Safer Health System. Washington, D.C.: National Academy Press, 2000.

[3]S. King, "Hospital Nurse Staffing—The Public's Interest," 64(3) *Oregon Nurse* (September 1999).

[4]House of Delegates, American Nurses Association. "Shared Accountability in Today's Work Environment," American Nurses Association (1998).

(69%), decline in a patient's health on a weekly or monthly basis (63%), and patient inability to obtain needed prescription medications.[98]

It is too early to say with certainty if the concerns expressed by the sample in this study will continue to exist. Additionally, more surveys of this kind are necessary to clarify the nursing profession's concerns about managed care and its effects on patient well-being. Even so, the nurse cannot ignore the findings of this study. The findings need to be proactively incorporated into the health care entity's plan to achieve quality patient care. The nurse can do so by voicing concerns

ETHICS CONNECTION 6–4

In managed care, ethics and economics meet. This encounter may be smooth or rocky, depending in part upon how effectively consumer's rights are protected within the managed care system. State and national professional nursing organizations have drafted guidelines to help nurses better understand how to maintain morally responsible practice in a managed care environment.[1] For example, the Massachusetts Nurses Association (MNA) has published guidelines for nurses' practice in managed care that are linked to the American Nurses Association (ANA) *Code for Nurses with Interpretive Statements.*[2] Mary Silva, a nurse ethicist, has provided an annotated bibliography that addresses specific ethical concerns and guidelines related to managed care.[3] See Chapter 3 for further discussion of ethical issues in managed care.

---

[1]"Ethical Guidelines for Nurses in Managed Care, Market-Driven Environment," 67(7) *Massachusetts Nurse* (August 1997), 11.

[2]American Nurses Association. *Code for Nurses with Interpretive Statements.* Kansas City, MO: Author, 1985.

[3]Mary Cipriano Silva, "Ethics and Managed Care: A Selected Annotated Bibliography," 18(2) *Plastic Surgical Nursing* (1998), 105–107.

about short-staffing to nursing administration, identifying declines in patient health and reporting those concerns to the physician and to appropriate departments or committees within the organization (e.g., quality management and risk management), and continuing to be a patient advocate.

In fact, patient advocacy may well be one of the best approaches to ensure quality patient care. The survey found that among doctors who intervened on behalf of their patients to obtain needed care, 42% indicated that the case was resolved in the patient's favor, 22% stated the case was resolved in the plan's favor, while 21% reported the outcome a compromise.[99] A small victory, perhaps, but a victory nonetheless in the overall battle to achieve quality patient care.

SUMMARY OF PRINCIPLES AND APPLICATIONS

The importance of monitoring and evaluating patient care will not diminish. In fact, as health care resources continue to shrink, access to health care becomes even more restricted, cost control remains ever present, and the many other legal and ethical issues surrounding quality care persist, its importance will continue to be emphasized.[100] Perhaps the following statement best describes the need for enduring scrutiny:

> We have granted the health professions access to the most secret and sensitive places in ourselves and entrusted to them matters that touch on our well-being, happiness and survival. In return, we have expected the professions to govern themselves so strictly that we need have no fear of exploitation or incompetence. The object of quality assessment is to determine how successful they have been in doing so; and the purpose of quality monitoring is to exercise constant surveillance so that departure from standards can be detected early and corrected.[101]

The nurse, then, must meet his or her responsibilities to ensure that quality assurance activities are successful by doing the following:

- Actively participating in quality management, utilization management, peer review, and risk management programs in the health care delivery system
- Understanding the different roles of quality management, utilization management, peer review, and risk

management, but also appreciating the uncommon interdependence of one with the others

- Accepting responsibility to become skilled in quality assessment through continuing education courses, academic courses, and other methods of learning
- Adhering to the mandates of state and federal law concerning confidentiality, immunity, and good-faith reviews as a committee member involved in quality assessment
- Working with risk management to ensure, insofar as possible, risk identification and risk avoidance of patient care problems
- Remembering that the ethical ramifications of quality management activities are important
- Carefully analyzing the patient care situation to provide the best-reasoned decision possible under the circumstances when reviewing patient care situations for continued coverage as a third-party utilization review employee
- As a staff nurse, aiding risk management with its responsibilities by not documenting in the patient care record that an occurrence or incident report was filled out and by forwarding the report to designated personnel as indicated in the entity's policies
- As a nurse manager, providing leadership in the quality assessment and evaluation process

TOPICS FOR FURTHER INQUIRY

1. Develop a questionnaire for staff nurses in the health care facility where you work concerning nurses' attitudes surrounding occurrence reports. Evaluate their opinions about the purpose of the reports, how many times they have filled one out pursuant to policy, any retaliation issues they fear as a result of their use of the reports, and other issues. Compare and contrast the results among the respondents and suggest ways for the facility to improve its occurrence reporting system.

2. Identify cases in your state that have been filed alleging a cause of action against a managed care organization. Determine what causes of action are the most predominant. Suggest ways in which such liability may be avoided in the future through the development of policies and procedures in a particular facility or type of facility (e.g., home health care agency, ambulatory clinic).

3. Interview nurses in your health care facility who have taken active roles in the facility's quality assessment programs. Obtain information from the nurses as to how they functioned in their roles. How was their input used in comparison to others? What did the nurses see as their roles? Were they as active as they could have been with their responsibilities? Compare and contrast the results among the interviewees and suggest ways for the facility to improve the participation of nurses in the quality assessment program.

4. Write an in-depth paper on clinical practice guidelines and their use in nursing. Include their strengths and weaknesses in everyday practice. Identify ways in which a specific practice guideline discussed in the paper could be improved, and analyze the reasons for the changes from clinical, legal, and ethical perspectives.

REFERENCES

1. Joanne Comi McKloskey and Helen Kennedy Grace, "Preserving Quality in an Era of Cost Containment," in *Current Issues in Nursing.* 5th Edition. Joanne Comi McCloskey and Helen Kennedy Grace, Editors. St. Louis, Mo.: Mosby, 1997, 288.

2. *Id.*

3. Fred Garzino, "Undue Economic Influence on Physician-Assisted Suicide," 1(3) *DePaul Journal of Health Care Law* (Spring 1997), 537–578.

4. Kathy L. Cerminara, "The Class Action Suit as a Method of Patient Empowerment in the Managed Care Setting," 24(1) *American Journal of Law & Medicine* (1998), 7–58.

5. See, for example, Sarah T. Fry, "The Ethics of Health Care Reform: Should Rationing Strategies Target the Elderly?" in McCloskey and Grace, *supra* note 1, 626–631.

6. John D. Blum, "Achieving Quality in Managed Care: The Role of the Law," in *Achieving Quality in Managed Care: The Role of the Law.* Chicago, Ill.: Health Law Section of the American Bar Association (1997), 1.

7. Arnold Epstein, "Performance Reports on Quality-Prototypes, Problems, and Prospects," in *Health Policy and Nursing: Crisis and Reform in the U.S. Health Care Delivery System.* 2nd Edition. Charlene Harrington and Carrol Estes, Editors. Boston, Mass.: Jones and Bartlett, 1997, 243–245.

8. Fred LeMire and John Hesse, "Managed Care Contracting," in *The Risk Manager's Desk Reference.* 2nd Edition. Barbara Youngberg, Editor. Gaithersburg, Md.: Aspen Publishers, Inc. (1998), 483.

9. See, generally, Florence Nightingale. *Notes on Nursing: What It Is and What It Is Not.* New York: Dover Publications, Inc., 1969.

10. Barbara J. Youngberg and Diane Weber, "Integrating Risk Management, Utilization Management, and Quality Management: Maximizing Benefit Through Integration," in Youngberg, *supra* note 8, at 27.

11. *Id.* at 29.

12. *Id.*

13. *Id.* at 28.

14. Youngberg and Weber, *supra* note 10, at 29.

15. *Id.*

16. *Id.*

17. Bette Keeling, Sherry Baker, Linda Thompson, and others, "Process Redesign: Beyond TQM and Reengineering," in *Process Centered Health Care Organizations.* Suzanne P. Smith and Dominick L. Flarey, Editors. Gaithersburg, Md.: Aspen Publishers, Inc., 1999, 95; Fay A. Rozovsky. *Liability and Risk Management in Home Health Care.* Gaithersburg, Md.: Aspen Publishers, Inc., 1998, 10:2.

18. Youngberg and Weber, *supra* note 10, at 29.

19. George D. Pozgar, "Tort Reform and Reducing the Risks of Malpractice," in *Legal Aspects of Health Care Administration.* 7th Edition. Gaithersburg, Md.: Aspen Publishers, Inc., 1999, 524.

20. Youngberg and Weber, *supra* note 10.

21. Youngberg and Weber, *supra* note 10, at 29.

22. George D. Pozgar, "Managed Care and Organizational Restructuring," in *Legal Aspects of Health Care Administration, supra* note 19, at 485.

23. *Id.*

24. See, generally, Claire M. Fagin and Suzanne Gordon, "Conclusion: What Can We Do To Protect Quality Care?" in *Abandonment of the Patient: The Impact of Profit-Driven Health Care on the Public.* Allen D. Baer, Claire Fagin, and Suzanne Gordon, Editors. New York: Springer Publishing Company, 1996, 101–110.

25. George D. Pozgar, *supra* note 19, at 485.

26. Rozovsky, *supra* note 17, at 10:4–10:6.

27. *Id.* at 10:8.

28. *Id.* at 10:5.

29. *Id.* at 10:6.

30. Youngberg and Weber, *supra* note 10, at 30–31.

31. Joint Commission on Accreditation of Healthcare Organizations. *Comprehensive Accreditation Manual for Hospitals.* Oak Brook Terrace, Ill.: Author, 1994.

32. Youngberg and Weber, *supra* note 10, at 30, 39–40.

33. Christopher Kerns, Carol J. Gerner, and Ciara Ryan. *Health Care Liability Handbook.* 4th Edition. St. Paul, Minn.: West Group, 1998, 14:1–14:2.

34. Beth C. Weitzman, "Improving Quality of Care," in *Health Care Delivery in the United States.* 6th Edition. Anthony Kovner and Steve Jonas, Editors. New York: Springer Publishing Company, 1999, 392.

35. *Id.*

36. Diane Weber, "Incorporating Quality Improvement Strategies and Benchmarking into Risk Management," in Youngberg, *supra* note 8, at 47.

37. *Id.* at 47–55.

38. See, generally, "Discovery and Admissability of Medical Records," in *Medical Records and the Law.* William H. Roach, Jr. and the Aspen Health Law Center. 3rd Edition. Gaithersburg, Md.: Aspen Publishers, Inc., 1998, 255–257.

39. See, generally, "Computerized Medical Records," in Roach and Aspen, *supra* note 38, at 290–327.

40. Keeling et al., *supra* note 17, at 95.

41. *Id.* at 98.

42. *Id.* at 96.

43. *Id.* at 97.

44. See, generally, McKloskey and Grace, *supra* note 1; Fagin and Gordon, *supra* note 24.

45. *Sentinel Event Policy and Procedures,* located on the *American Society for Healthcare Risk Management* Web site at http://www.ashrm.org/sentinelpp.htm, accessed November 10, 1998. See also *Sentinel Event Alert,* Joint Commission on Accreditation of Healthcare Organizations, (3), May 1, 1998, 2–3; *Sentinel Event Alert,* Joint Commission on Accreditation of Healthcare Organizations, (4), May 11, 1998, 2. Information about the Policy and Procedures may also be found on the commission's Web site at http://www.jcaho.org/. See also Carol Dunbar, "Lessons Learned from Sentinel Events," 12(2) *Nursing Spectrum* (1999), 14.

46. 42 U.S.C. Section 11101 *et seq.* (1986).

47. *Id.* at Section 11101.

48. Pub. L. No. 100-93 (August 18, 1987), 42 U.S.C. Sections 1396(a), 1396 v-2 (1989).

49. 42 U.S.C. Sections 11131, 11133, and 11132; 45 C.F.R. Sections 60.7, 60.9, and 60.8.

50. 42 U.S.C. Sections 11131(a); 42 C.F.R. Sections 1003.102(c)(1).

51. Kerns, Gerner, and Ryan, *supra* note 33, at 15:4. Despite protections afforded by the Act, a recent study by the Office of Inspector General indicates that hospitals are underreporting *physician* problems to the NPDB. See, for example, Laura-Mae Baldwin, L. Gary Hart, Robert Oshel, and others, "Hospital Peer Review and the National Practitioner Data Bank Clinical Privileges Action Reports," 282(4) *JAMA* (July 28, 1999), 349–355.

52. For more information about the NDB, the reader can contact the National Council of State Boards of Nursing, Inc. at 676 N. St. Clair Street, Ste. 550, Chicago, Illinois 60611-2921. The council's Web site is http://www.ncsbn.org/.

53. 42 U.S.C. Section 11112(a).

54. 745 ILCS 55/1, 553.(1990).

55. See, generally, "Defamation," in *Prosser and Keeton on the Law of Torts.* W. Page Keeton, Editor. 5th Edition. St. Paul, Minn.: West Group, 1984, 771–848 (with 1988 pocket part); Chapter 7, "Other Torts and Civil Rights."

56. Kerns, Gerner, and Ryan, *supra* note 33, 15:3.

57. *Id.*

58. 735 ILCS 5/8-2101 (1984).

59. The Medicare Web site is located at http://www.medicare.gov/.

60. Kerns, Gerner, and Ryan, *supra* note 33, at 14:25.

61. *Id.*

62. *Id.*

63. Barry Furrow, "Litigating Over Quality in Managed Care: Individual Malpractice/Negligence Claims in Arbitration and Litigation," in *Managed Care Liability: Examining Risks and Responsibilities in a Changing Health Care System.* David Leitner, Editor. American Bar Association: Tort and Insurance Practice Section, 1996, 17, *citing, generally,* Peter D. Fox. *Overview of Managed Care Trends, The Insider's Guide to Managed Care: A Legal and Operational Roadmap,* 1 National Health Lawyers Association (1990).

64. Delilah Brummet Flaum and Diane J. Romza-Kutz, "An Overview of Managed Care Organizations: Sorting Out the Alphabet Soup," in Leitner, *supra* note 63, at 1-3, 1-4.

65. Kerns, Gerner, and Ryan, *supra* note 33, at 19:7.

66. 228 Cal. Rptr. 661 (App. 2d Dist. 1986), *republished at* 192 Cal. App. 3d 1630, 239 Cal. Rptr. 810 (2d Dist. 1986), *review granted and opinion superseded,* 231 Cal. Rptr. 560, 727 P.2d 753 (Cal. 1986) *and dismissed, remanded and ordered published,* 239 Cal. Rptr. 805, 741 P.2d 613 (Cal. 1987).

67. 192 Cal. App. 3d 1630, at 1630.

68. 222 Cal. App. 3d 660, 271 Cal. Rptr. 876 (2d Dist. 1990).

69. 271 Cal. Rptr. 876, at 885.

70. Kerns, Gerner, and Ryan, *supra* note 33, at 19:7.

71. *Id.*

72. See, generally, Alan Bloom, "Who's the Boss? Controlling Liability in Managed Care," in Leitner, *supra* note 63, at 173–230.

73. *Id.*

74. Terrence Shaneyfelt, Michael Mayo-Smith, and Johann Rothwangl, "Are Guidelines Following Guidelines? The Methodological Quality of Clinical Practice Guidelines in the Peer-Reviewed Medical Literature," 281(2) *JAMA* (May 26, 1999), 1900–1905.

75. Kerns, Gerner, and Ryan, *supra* note 33, at 3:1.

76. Shaneyfelt, Mayo-Smith, and Rothwangl, *supra* note 74, at 1900 (citations omitted).

77. Susan Park Kyzer, "The Use of Clinical Pathways: Do They Improve Quality?" in McCloskey and Grace, *supra* note 1, at 303–307.

78. Sandra Mitchell, Carole Price, Mark Schneider, and others, "Legal Issues Associated with the Use and Development of Practice Guidelines," in Youngberg, *supra* note 8, at 384–398.

79. Kathleen Roman, "Practice Policies: Potential Implications for Malpractice Litigation," 15(3) *Journal of Healthcare Risk Management* (1995).

80. American Nurses Association. *Legal Aspects of Standards and Guidelines for Clinical Nursing Practice.* Washington, D.C.: Author, 1998, 8.

81. Pub. L. No. 104-191, Title II, 110 Stat. 1936 (1996).

82. Theodore LeBlang, W. Eugene Basanta, and Robert Kane. *The Law of Medical Practice in Illinois.* Volume 2. 2nd Edition. St. Paul, Minn.: West Group, 1996, 7:25 (with regular updates); Marylin Hansal, "Understanding the Need for a Corporate Compliance Program," in Youngberg, *supra* note 8, at 111–114.

83. Bureau of Health Professions' Division of Quality Assurance, Health and Human Services, "Data Bank to Combat Fraud Effective Oct. 1," *The American Nurse* (September/October 1999), 18.

84. *Id.*

85. *Id.*

86. See, generally, Hansal, *supra* note 82, 107–120; Janet Michael and Cathleen Summers, "What Should Nurses Know About Fraud and Abuse?" 5(2) *Journal of Nursing Law* (1998), 41–50.

87. Janet Haggerty Davis, "Do the Right Thing as a Compliance Officer," 12(21) *Nursing Spectrum* (1999), 21.

88. Joan Osborne, Kathleen Blais, and Janice Hayes, "Nurses' Perceptions: When Is It a Medication Error?" 29(4) *JONA* (1999), 37. See also Debra Ahmed and Suzanne Fecik, "Med Errors: The Fatigue Factor," 99(9) *AJN* (1999), 12.

89. Janet Pitts Beckmann. *Nursing Negligence: Analyzing Malpractice in the Hospital Setting.* Thousand Oaks, Cal.: Sage Publications, 1996.

90. Osborne, Blais, and Hayes, *supra* note 88, *citing* Z. Wolf, "Medication Errors and Nursing Responsibility," 4(1) *Holistic Nursing Practice* (1989), 8–17.

91. Beckmann, *supra* note 89.

92. National Coordinating Council for Medication Error Reporting and Prevention, "Recommendations to Health Care Professionals to Reduce Errors Due to Labeling and Packaging of Drug Products and Related Devices," Adopted March 30, 1998-April 1, 1999; National Coordinating Council for Medication Error Reporting and Prevention, "Solid Oral Dosage Form Identification—Room for Improvement?" 1998, April 1, 1999. Both documents are located on the council's Web site at http://www.nccmerp.org/.

93. Osborne, Blais, and Hayes, *supra* note 88, at 33 (citations omitted).

94. See, generally, David Hyman, "Consumer Protection(?), Managed Care, and the Emergency Department," in *Achieving Quality in Managed Care: The Role of the Law*. John Blum, Editor. Chicago, Ill.: American Bar Association, Health Law Section, 1997, 58–77; Mary Ellen Wurzbach, "Managed Care: Moral Conflicts for Primary Health Care Nurses," 26(2) *Nursing Outlook* (1998), 62–66.

95. Henry J. Kaiser Family Foundation. *The 1999 Survey of Physicians and Nurses*. Menlo, Cal.: Author, 1999. The report was released through a press release on July 28, 1999, on the foundation's home page on the World Wide Web at http://www.kff.org/. Copies of the questionnaire and topline data for the findings of the report can be found on the Web page or by calling the foundation's publications request line at 1-800-656-4533 (document #1503).

96. *Id.*

97. *Id.*

98. *Id.*

99. *Id.*

100. See, for example, Peter I. Buerhause, "Lucian Leape on the Causes and Prevention of Errors and Adverse Events in Health Care," 31(3) *Image* (1999), 281–286.

101. Avedis Donabedian. *The Quality of Medical Care*. D.H.E.W. Publication No. 78-1232 (P-H), Health: United States, 1978, 11.

Other Torts and Civil Rights

7

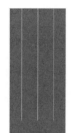

KEY PRINCIPLES

- Intent
- Intentional Torts
- Quasi-intentional Torts
- Civil Rights Act of 1871

The reader will recall that the tort of negligence and professional negligence does not require any *intent* on the part of the actor who caused injury to the victim. Rather, an actor is liable if his or her conduct does not conform with a standard of care. The law has defined other torts, however, that *do* require proof of intent, albeit in varying ways. Despite this variety, there is one unifying quality among all the other torts—the defendant's purposeful conduct interferes with an interest held by the plaintiff.[1] Because the intent of the defendant is an essential requirement in these torts, they have been identified as intentional and quasi-intentional torts. Some interests held by the plaintiff that, if violated, can result in liability include the protection of one's name and reputation (defamation), the ability to move freely without restriction as to place or time (false imprisonment), and privacy (invasion of privacy). A nurse may be involved in such suits when the nurse shares untrue information about a patient with another person, unlawfully prohibits a patient from leaving the institution, or shares private facts about the patient with others not involved in that patient's care. A nurse may also be involved as a plaintiff; that is, alleging that his or her own reputation was injured or his or her privacy invaded.

In addition to the requirement of intent, there are several other differences between negligence and professional negligence (many times referred to as negligent torts) and the other torts presented in this chapter. One difference is the damages that

may be recovered. Recall that when alleging professional negligence, the injured patient must prove that some injury occurred. In contrast, the intentional and quasi-intentional torts do not always require proof of injury or damages. The specific tort—defamation or an invasion of privacy, for example—is achieved when the required intent is present. If injury or damages take place, the extent of the injury or damages is taken into consideration by the court. If they are minimal or nonexistent, nominal damages will be awarded.

A second difference of torts other than negligent ones is that no expert witness testimony is necessary to prove the interference with the plaintiff's assailed interest. Unlike professional negligence, there is no standard of care that the health care professional—or private citizen—must meet.

In addition, punitive damages are more easily recoverable when a violation of the plaintiff's interest(s) takes place. Because the defendant's conduct is intended, assessing damages that punish that actor and deter others from engaging in the same behavior is justified.

Last, it is important to keep in mind that a defendant's actions may give rise to one or more violations of the plaintiff's interests. Thus, several violations can be alleged in a suit brought by the plaintiff, as many of the intentional and quasi-intentional torts are closely related. For example, restricting someone's freedom of movement (false imprisonment) may give rise to allegations of assault and battery as well.

Civil rights violations occur when an individual's rights are transgressed by the government or a governmental entity. Because local, state, and federal governments often maintain health care delivery systems, a patient may allege a breach of his or her civil rights under federal law. Likewise, a nurse or other health care professional may file a suit alleging a violation of a particular right protected by those same laws.

This chapter will discuss intentional and quasi-intentional torts that are most common in health care. Likewise, it will explore the Civil Rights Act of 1871, codified at 42 U.S.C. Section 1983, as it applies to health care delivery. Insofar as civil rights violations are concerned, this Civil Rights Act is only *one* way in which a person may sue for an alleged breach of rights guaranteed by the Constitution. Other avenues open to the plaintiff would include a suit alleging a violation of the Constitution itself as well as violations of other federal laws that protect civil rights.

Many of the intentional torts discussed in this chapter overlap with important constitutional rights. For example, the tort of invading one's privacy may affect one's constitutional right of freedom of speech when the action is based on a "false light" allegation.

INTENTIONAL TORTS

The concept of intent includes several basic elements. It is a state of mind about the results of a voluntary act (or the results of a voluntary failure to act) and includes not only having a desire to bring about the results but also knowing that the results are "substantially certain" to occur.[2] Intent must also exist when the act, or failure to act, takes place.[3] Insofar as tort liability is concerned, intent is not hostile or a desire "to do harm." Nor is it to be confused with motive, the reason a person acts. Rather, it is a design to cause a specific outcome that unlawfully assails the interests of another.[4]

Intent can be "transferred." For example, even though the actor intended to harm victim A but harmed victim B instead, the actor would still be liable for the injury, as the intent to harm A is transferred to meet the requisite intent to harm B.[5] This increased liability is justified because of the greater burden the law places on "intentional wrongdoers."

The requirement that the act be a voluntary one is fairly clear—liability will not exist if the conduct is not intended to bring about the result. For example, if a staff nurse faints and, in doing so, falls on a patient and injures him, the injury would not result in tort liability for assault and battery. The nurse did not *intend* to injure the patient.

> *Intentional torts most often seen in health care are assault, battery, false imprisonment . . . and conversion of property.*

Intentional torts most often seen in health care are assault, battery, false imprisonment, intentional infliction of emotional distress, misrepresentation, and conversion of property. All but conversion of property involve interference with the individual himself or herself. All, of course, require intent and the commission of a voluntary act.

Assault

Assault concerns an individual's interest in freedom from the apprehension of harmful or offensive contact.[6] There is no requirement of actual *touching* of the plaintiff; the intent to spur the victim's apprehension and the resulting fear that contact might occur satisfies this requirement. Thus, the damage or harm experienced by the individual is emotional—fright, fear, anxiety—in addition to any physical injury that may occur.[7] Therefore, the plaintiff can sue for those injuries, in addition to seeking punitive damages.

Although this tort has been described as a "touching of the mind . . .,"[8] for assault to be actionable, the victim must be aware of the threat of harmful or offensive contact. A psychiatric nurse who comes toward an unconscious patient with leather restraints has not participated in an assault because the patient was not aware (conscious) of the potential harmful contact.

Mere words alone are usually not enough to constitute an assault, and an immediate harmful or offensive contact must be perceived by the potential victim. If the same psychiatric nurse simply threatens to place a patient in full leather restraints, probably no assault has occurred. If, however, the nurse shakes the leather restraints in front of the patient and threatens to place him in restraints immediately, an assault is more probable. It is important for the nurse to keep in mind, however, that the *threat* is the important component rather than the *manner* in which it is conveyed.[9]

An assault can occur without any other intentional tort. It usually takes place, however, with the intentional tort of battery.

Battery

Battery involves an individual's interest in freedom from an affirmative, intentional, and unpermitted contact with his or her body, any extension of it (such as clothing), or anything that is attached to it and "practically identified with it."[10] Unlike assault, actual contact is essential. The intent of the defendant can be either to carry out the offensive contact *or* to cause the apprehension that the contact is immediately going to take place.[11]

In contrast to assault, however, the victim does not need to be aware that the battery has occurred. Thus an unconscious patient who is treated without his or her consent can sue for a battery, because his or her "personal integrity" is still entitled to protection.[12]

If the plaintiff experiences physical harm, the defendant will be liable for that injury. However, the defendant is also liable for contacts that create no physical harm but cause the victim to experience insult, humiliation, and anxiety. Moreover, when there is no injury to the plaintiff, nominal damages are also possible.

It is also important for the nurse to keep in mind that any consequences resulting from a battery, even if unintended and unforeseen, will be the responsibility of the actor who initiated the conduct. Furthermore, although it can be said that individuals do "consent" to "customary and reasonable" contacts as members of society (a touching of the arm or a slight bump when passing through a crowd), the court will always analyze the time, place, circumstances, and relationship of the parties when an unpermitted touching occurs.[13]

Therefore, when the nurse inserts a catheter over the patient's objections (*Roberson v. Provident House*[14]), encourages and aids a physician in performing surgery when no consent whatsoever was given by the patient (*Roberts v. Southwest Texas Methodist Hospital*[15]), initiates a game of tag with pediatric patients that results in an injury to one of the patient participants, or makes sexual advances toward a patient, he or she may be liable for assault as well as battery.

Assault and battery in medical care most often is alleged when there is a *lack of consent* for treatment, including surgery. Although a case alleging assault and battery is a perfectly viable way to seek damages for the unpermitted contact, the injured patient can seek redress by alleging lack of informed consent under a negligence theory; that is, alleging the practitioner was negligent in not providing all of the necessary information to make an informed choice about the treatment.

False Imprisonment

Freedom from a restriction of one's choice of movement is the interest infringed by this tort.

ETHICS CONNECTION 7–1

Legal issues of assault and of battery interface with moral principles of nonmaleficence, beneficence, and autonomy. The moral obligation to protect others from harm is based upon the principles of nonmaleficence and beneficence. The commitment to honor and respect the limits and boundaries of clients' space and decisions is grounded in autonomy.

Frequently, there is a tension between autonomy and beneficence. Effective nursing practice often requires that nurses cross traditional social boundaries and extend into clients' intimate space. For example, during physical assessment, nurses touch clients with their hands or with instruments such as stethoscopes. Treatment practices such as administering intravenous medications also require actions that would be impermissible in social situations. It is critically important, therefore, that nurses ask permission to intrude into intimate space, be respectful when permission is given, and honor clients' right to refuse permission.

From the perspective of the ethic of care and covenantal relationships, nurses, clients, and health care institutions have reciprocal obligations to one another (see Chapter 3). Discussions about safety usually address nurses' responsibility to clients. However, there currently is increased awareness that nurses, too, must be protected from harm not only from unsafe environmental conditions, but from clients, as well. Nurses in some areas of practice, such as emergency rooms, inpatient psychiatric settings, and community health have become more concerned about their own safety. This concern has increased as staffing in both nursing and security has declined. Some agencies have developed policies that permit nurses to refuse assignments that are potentially harmful.

An intentional restriction of movement must be against the will of the individual, for *any* length of time, however short, and the victim must be aware of the confinement.[16] Furthermore, the restraint must give the person no means to depart from the confinement, whether by physical barriers or merely through the use of force. However, moral pressure ("Stay in the hospital and clear up your sexually transmitted disease so others will not suffer from your mistake") or future threats ("I will confine you to your room if you do not eat your meal immediately") are not actionable as false imprisonment.

If the plaintiff is successful, he or she can receive monetary damages for (1) any mental or physical injury to his or her well-being, (2) lost time, (3) humiliation, (4) damage to reputation, and (5) other losses during the imprisonment (e.g., loss of property).

In the health care setting, false imprisonment is often alleged against nurses and institutions that hospitalize patients against their will, especially psychiatric nurses and hospitals. The allegations may also occur, however, when any health care delivery system keeps a patient after there is a duty to allow the patient to leave. Again, psychiatric facilities may be involved in such suits with voluntary patients, but other institutions may also commit this tort when, for example, a patient is not allowed to leave the emergency department when he or she has asked to leave and there is no duty to hold the patient, or, as was true in a 1925 case, when a hospital confined a patient for 11 hours because he did not pay his bill.[17] False imprisonment allegations can also be raised when a patient is physically or chemically restrained.

There is a distinct difference between the tort of false imprisonment and that of malicious prosecution, which is a quasi-intentional tort and will be discussed in that section.

Intentional Infliction of Emotional Distress

When a defendant's conduct is extreme and outrageous—exceeding the bounds of common decency—and it causes, or is fairly certain to cause, severe emotional distress, with or without causing concurrent physical results—this tort has been committed.[18] It is clearly based on the plaintiff's interest in protecting his or her peace of mind.[19]

As with many of the other torts discussed thus far, the context within which the extreme and outrageous conduct takes place also has bearing on the severe mental distress experienced by the plaintiff. For example, when the defendant knows about a special sensitivity of, or has a special relationship with, the plaintiff and uses it to cause the mental anguish, the specific conduct may not be of paramount importance. Rather the improper use of that knowledge or interpersonal connection to create the emotional distress is what the court evaluates.

The plaintiff in an intentional infliction of emotional distress suit may also be a family member or close associate who observes another being treated in an offensive manner. In health care, family members who observe the death of a loved one, or who see medical treatment being administered to another when they have asked that it not be continued, can sue for the mental anguish in witnessing that occurrence.[20]

Nurses are not immune from suits alleging their conduct resulted in intentional infliction of emotional distress.

Nurses are not immune from suits alleging that their conduct resulted in intentional infliction of emotional distress. In one case, a nurse was sued for handing a deceased, bloody fetus to the mother so that photographs could be taken.[21] Nurses may also be plaintiffs in such suits, however, especially in relation to conduct by their superiors or colleagues. Thus, a victim of sexual harassment or false rumors about the nurse's family spread by colleagues may file a case to seek redress for the emotional pain caused by such conduct.

Conversion of Property

Unlike the other torts discussed thus far that involve intentional interference with the individual, conversion involves an intentional interference with the *property* of another. Specifically, it requires that the defendant, with intent to affect the property in some way (e.g., exercise control over it, transfer it, alter it, or dispose of it), invades

the owner's rights in that property.[22] The plaintiff must prove that at the time of the conversion, he or she had possession, or the right of possession, of the property.

In health care, conversion can take place when a nurse takes belongings from a patient without justification. This could occur when a search of a psychiatric patient's belongings results in certain items not being returned to the patient without justification. It could also take place when a nurse removes a patient's savings bank book from his or her bedside stand. The tort is complete when the nurse wrongfully takes the property; there is no need for a demand for its return.

Misrepresentation

Misrepresentation has become a very complicated tort. This is mainly due to its flexible character and the ability to classify such conduct as the intent to deceive, as negligence, or simply as a "strict responsibility" an individual has to another.[23] It may also be viewed as a breach of an express or implied warranty in a contract.

Because of its complex nature, it will not be discussed as a tort except to state that it can easily be a component of the other intentional torts analyzed in this chapter. For example, misrepresentation by a nurse to a patient that he is drinking only orange juice when the juice contains medication can constitute a battery. It can also occur by inducing consent for one particular type of treatment that turns out to be a different medical regimen altogether. Or, if the nurse maliciously lies about a disease to a patient who is not in fact suffering from it, the patient can easily win an action for intentional infliction of emotional distress.

Defenses to Intentional Torts

Defenses to the intentional torts presented are summarized in Table 7–1. It is important to keep in mind that an additional defense not included in the table, that of the statute of limitations, can also be raised when accused of interfering with the plaintiff's interests. Generally speaking, the time period within which an injured plaintiff can sue for any of the intentional torts presented is usually 2 years from the date on which the tort occurred.

TABLE 7-1

Defenses to Intentional Torts

TORT	DEFENSES	QUALIFICATIONS	OTHER COMMENTS	EXAMPLE
1. Assault and/or Battery	Privilege	Justifiable motive	Court can inquire into motive	Nurse or patient acts in self-defense
	Mistake of law or fact	Usually goes in tandem with defense of privilege		Nurse or patient, erroneously believing he or she is being attacked, acts in self-defense
	Self-defense	Reasonable force must be used; no time to resort to other lawful remedies	No duty to retreat unless it can be done safely	Nurse in ER defends self when attacked by irate family member of patient
	Consent	Must be willingly given; no coercion or fraud used; capacity to consent must be present; no mistakes as to nature or quality of what consenting to; actor cannot exceed consent given	Consent can be manifested by conduct or words; also may be inferred; when emergency exists, consent for treatment, *absent direction to contrary*, implied	Patient, with full knowledge of procedure, gives informed consent for treatment
	Necessity	Need to interfere with property of another to protect victim or victims	Similar to privilege defense	Nurse pushes patient in clinic aside to take gun away from robber who is aiming gun at others in clinic
2. False Imprisonment	Privilege	Justifiable motive	Court can inquire into motive	Nurse places patient in seclusion room because he or she is combative and hits staff and patients
	Self-defense	Reasonable force must be used; no time to resort to other lawful remedies	No duty to retreat unless it can be done safely	See example under Privilege
	Defense of others	Defense must be reasonably necessary	May be duty to defend where a legal or social duty is established by law	See example under Privilege
	Consent	Must be willingly given; no coercion or fraud used; capacity to consent must be present; no mistake as to nature or quality of what consenting to; actor cannot exceed consent given	Consent can be manifested by conduct or words; also may be inferred	Patient agrees to go to room voluntarily until control of behavior is regained
	Necessity	Need to interfere with property of another to protect victim or victims	Similar to privilege defense	See example under Privilege

3. Intentional Infliction of Emotional Distress	Privilege	Justifiable motive	Court can inquire into motive	Nurse, to prevent bodies of dead patients from burning up in fire in morgue, places bodies in a hallway
	Self-defense	Reasonable force must be used; no time to resort to other lawful remedies	No duty to retreat unless it can be done safely	See example under Privilege
	Defense of others	Defense must be reasonably necessary	May be duty to defend when a legal or social duty is established by law	See example under Privilege
	Consent	Must be willingly given; no coercion or fraud used; capacity to consent must be present; no mistake as to nature or quality of what consenting to; actor cannot exceed consent given	Consent can be manifested by conduct or words; also may be inferred	See example under Privilege
	Necessity	Need to interfere with property of another to protect victim or victims	Similar to privilege defense	See example under Privilege
4. Conversion of Property	Privilege	Justifiable motive	Court can inquire into motive	Nurse takes possession of medications when patient returns from pass
	Self-defense	Reasonable force must be used; no time to resort to other lawful remedies	No duty to retreat unless it can be done safely	Nurse takes possession of gun patient has in bedside stand
	Defense of others	Defense must be reasonably necessary	May be duty to defend when a legal or social duty is established by law	See example under Self-defense
	Consent	Must be willingly given; no coercion or fraud used; capacity to consent must be present; no mistake as to nature or quality of what consenting to; actor cannot exceed consent given	Consent can be manifested by conduct or words; also may be inferred	Patient agrees to give nurse gun or medications upon return from pass
	Necessity	Need to interfere with property of another to protect victim or victims	Similar to privilege defense	See example under Privilege

Data from W. Page Keeton, Editor. *Prosser and Keeton on the Law of Torts.* 5th Edition. St. Paul, Minn.: West Publishing Company, 1984 (with 1988 pocket part).

QUASI-INTENTIONAL TORTS

Quasi-intentional torts are those torts in which the intent of the actor may not be as clear as with the intentional torts, but a voluntary act on the defendant's part takes place, as does the subsequent interference with an individual's interest. Common quasi-intentional torts seen in health care are defamation, breach of confidentiality, invasion of privacy, and malicious prosecution.

Common quasi-intentional torts seen in health care are defamation, breach of confidentiality, invasion of privacy, and malicious prosecution.

A quasi-intentional tort may be experienced by itself, or it may occur in combination with any of the other torts. A patient whose privacy is invaded, for example, may also sue for a breach of confidentiality and intentional infliction of emotional distress.

Defamation

Defamation includes the "twin torts" of libel (written word) and slander (spoken word).[24] The interest that is invaded is that of an individual's good name and reputation and, as such, is a "relational" interest.[25] Thus, for the tort to take place, there must be (1) a communication (publication) about the individual to a third party or parties; (2) that is so injurious that it tends to harm the victim's reputation; (3) to the point that others lower their estimation of the person and/or are deterred from associating with that person.[26]

The tort of defamation is a personal one; that is, with some narrow exceptions, only a living person may be defamed. Furthermore, "group defamation" ("All nurses are incompetent") is not actionable because, again with narrow exceptions, there is no specific, identifiable person spoken about in the particular group.

In addition, the written or spoken words must be understood as defamatory. Whether or not this has occurred is a question for the jury. The jury will evaluate various circumstances to ascertain the interpretation of the information, including whether or not the communication was intended as a joke, or that no one who heard or read the information interpreted it in a defamatory manner. This principle was illustrated in a case about a newspaper article alleged to contain defamatory statements about a representative of a nursing home. At a city council meeting, Ms. Stevens alleged that the article implied she was responsible for the nursing home's disrepair and poor maintenance. The court ruled against Stevens, holding that no reasonable person would have read the article as defamatory. Therefore, no defamation occurred.[27]

Liability for defamation can be found against the individual who initially communicates (publishes) the defamatory communication (primary publisher) and those who repeat it (republishers).

When a defamatory statement is made about a "public figure" who is of "legitimate public interest," the injured public figure must prove that the statement was made with malice; that is, that it was communicated with the knowledge that it was false *or* with reckless disregard as to its truth or falsity.[28] This requirement is based on the First Amendment protection of freedom of speech and press. The right includes the news media's ability to provide information to the public concerning public figures without undue fear of being sued for an incorrect statement. It is also based on the idea that a public figure "voluntarily" enters into public life and, as a result, has lesser protection for his or her name or reputation.

Private individuals, however, have less of an opportunity to challenge defamatory statements (e.g., no access to the news media). Greater protection is therefore afforded "nonpublic" individuals by lessening the constitutional guarantees of free speech and press for publications about them. As a result, a private person need only show that the publication was negligently done. If successful, damages for "actual injuries" can be awarded.

The damages suffered by a person whose reputation has been injured can be legion and vary considerably. They include compensatory (general or special), punitive or exemplary, and nominal damages.[29] Because determining damages can be complicated, the law has developed rules to determine injury. These rules are based on whether or not the defamatory communication is written (libel) or spoken (slander) and whether the communication is "per se" defamatory.

Libel

As has been stated, libel is defamation in writing or in some other permanent form. It may sometimes occur when the publication occurs via television or radio, especially when there is a communication from a written script. If the published communication is libelous per se, that is, clearly defamatory, the plaintiff need not offer special proof of damages. If, however, the statement is not clearly libelous to the plaintiff, then the plaintiff must plead and prove special damages suffered (e.g., loss of a job or loss of an inheritance), unless the communication fits into one of the four exceptions discussed below.

Slander

Special damages due to slander, or spoken defamation, must generally be proved by the plaintiff because of its less permanent nature when compared to libelous communications. However, there are four exceptions to this rule, and when slander alleging the following occurs (slander per se), damages are presumed:

- The plaintiff is, or was, guilty of a crime involving "moral turpitude"
- The plaintiff is suffering from a "loathsome disease"
- "Unchastity" in a woman
- Any defamatory statement bearing on the plaintiff in his or her business, trade, profession, or office[30]

A defamatory statement by a nurse can take place under almost any circumstances. When a nurse falsely told another that a former patient was being treated for syphilis and the former patient's catering business failed as a result of the statement,[31] an action was filed against the nurse. The nurse may also be a defendant in a defamation action because of statements made about nurse colleagues or physicians, especially in relation to their professional performance. The nurse may bring a defamation suit because his or her own reputation is allegedly damaged.

Breach of Confidentiality

The law on breach of confidentiality protects a patient's sharing of information with a health care provider without fear that the information will be released to those not involved in his or

---

ETHICS CONNECTION 7–3

Nurses who are employees have obligations to both their employers and their clients (see Chapter 3 for a discussion of the ethic of care as covenantal relationship). Sometimes, there is conflict between these obligations. When the standard of care or professional conduct at a given institution is not acceptable, nurses sometimes are cautious about disclosing these irregularities. Sometimes the substandard care is a shared secret that most staff know, but few disclose. Referring to this shared secret as a "white wall of silence," several nurses have disclosed that when they tried to report the substandard condition or practice, they were threatened with being fired or sued for libel.[1] Despite "whistleblowing" legislation, nurses need support from their colleagues and professional organizations to overcome this practice of suppressing rather than disclosing unacceptable conditions of patient care.

[1]New York State Nurses Association, "Clinical Network: We Ask You Answer . . ." 29(1) *Journal of the New York State Nurses Association* (1998), 18–19.

---

her care. Initially, breach of confidentiality actions were mainly brought against physicians. As the role of other health care providers, including nurses, has developed professionally and they have become legally accountable for their actions, such suits have been filed against those providers as well.

In response to the expanded roles and legal accountability of health care providers generally, many states have included the mandate of protecting patient confidentiality in medical, social work, psychology, and other practice acts. Additionally, other state and federal laws, such as Illinois' Medical Patients' Rights Act,[32] require that the confidentiality of patient information be maintained. If breached, the acts provide for financial and other remedies to the injured patient. Also, in special areas of practice, such as mental health and chemical use treatment, federal and state laws prohibit disclosure to others without the patient's consent to only a few circumstances.

In today's electronic and information age, the tort of breach of confidentiality, like the tort of invasion of privacy discussed next, takes on new legal concerns in health care. With the availability of patient information literally retrievable with a few keystrokes, protecting patient confidentiality and privacy is a constant concern. The importance of secure systems for storing patient data, rigid, carefully followed policies on access to patient care information, audit trails, and the careful guarding of user identifiers (e.g., passwords, numbers) cannot be overemphasized.[33] If these and other areas affecting patient confidentiality and privacy are not attended to, health care entities and health care practitioners, including nurses, face new and different versions of tort liability for failing to protect patients' confidentiality and privacy rights.[34]

Invasion of Privacy

Invasion of privacy is quite different from breach of confidentiality. Even so, a particular instance of conduct may give rise to allegations of a violation of each of these two protected rights.

With invasion of privacy, the interest protected is the individual's right to be free from unreasonable intrusions into his or her private affairs; in other words, "to be left alone."[35] It involves four separate possible invasions of this overall interest, which have greatly expanded the interest the tort originally protected.

Use of Plaintiff's Likeness or Name without Plaintiff's Consent for Commercial Advantage of Defendant

This violation occurs when the plaintiff's name, photograph, or other likeness is used as a symbol of his or her identity to further the product or service of another.[36] When a cosmetic surgeon used the photographs of a particular patient who had successful cosmetic surgery in a television program and department store presentation, an invasion of the patient's privacy occurred.[37] When the use does not identify the patient—for example, simply shows a hand or the back of the patient's head—no invasion of privacy takes place.

Unreasonable Intrusion into Plaintiff's Private Affairs and Seclusions

This category of invasion of privacy takes place when conduct pries or intrudes upon a person's private affairs or seclusions and is objectionable to a reasonable person.[38] The conduct can be physical intrusion by the defendant (e.g., entering one's home without consent), or it can be the result of less traditional intrusions, such as peering into the window of someone's home or eavesdropping

upon private conversations with wiretaps and microphones.[39]

It is important to note that no interference with privacy happens when one is in a public place or on a public street where there is no legal right to be left alone.

In the health care setting, this type of privacy invasion can be found actionable whenever an individual's care is observed by others, including medical, nursing, and other students, without the patient's consent.[40] It also took place when a supervisor of a former employee lifted her gurney sheet in the postanesthesia area to view the woman's abdominal incision. The patient was "helpless" and under the effects of anesthesia. No consent had been given by the patient for the supervisor to be present, much less additionally invade her privacy in the manner in which he did.[41]

Public Disclosure of Private Facts about Plaintiff

To satisfy the elements of this invasion of privacy action, (1) there must be public disclosure of *private* facts; (2) the disclosure must be objectionable to someone of ordinary sensibilities; and (3) the information disclosed must be the type that the public has no legitimate interest in knowing.[42] Information that is of public record, such as a person's divorce or a name and address, is generally not held to be private data.

A patient's right of privacy under this category may be intruded upon, for example, if the nurse or other health care provider releases information concerning the diagnosis and treatment of that patient to the press (especially when the patient is *not* a public figure). It may also occur when the discussion of an identified patient's treatment takes place during a seminar or workshop for the public.

An invasion of privacy took place when an occupational health nurse shared medical information concerning an employee's mastectomy with "numerous other employees."[43] In that Illinois case, the court held that when there is a "special relationship" between the person and the "public" with whom the information is shared (e.g., fellow employees, church members, or neighbors), dissemination to that "public" group satisfies the elements of the tort.[44]

Placing a Person in a False Light in the Public's Eye

This tort occurs when an individual publishes false facts about another—attributing views not held or actions not taken—that would be objectionable to a person of ordinary sensibilities.[45] If the information published is a matter of "public interest," malice on the part of the defendant is also required; that is, the injured party must show that the defendant acted with knowledge of the falsity of the information or acted recklessly.

In health care, this tort could occur if a picture of a patient in the hospital, but not a recipient of its contagious disease services, appeared on a brochure advertising the newly renovated infectious disease unit for the treatment of AIDS.

Malicious Prosecution

The interest protected with malicious prosecution, as with abuse of process (which will not be covered), is the interest to be free from unjustifiable criminal and civil litigation.[46] The rules regarding a violation of this interest differ in relation to whether the abusive case is a civil or a criminal one. However, certain elements must be satisfied in either instance: (1) the judicial proceeding terminated in favor of the injured party; (2) there was an absence of probable cause; and (3) there was "malice," or a controlling reason other than seeking justice, in bringing the suit.[47]

The individual who suffers because of malicious prosecution can recover for damage to reputation, mental suffering, and humiliation, as well as for reasonable expenses, including attorneys fees, in defending against the suit. Clearly, punitive damages can also be awarded, especially when a jury finds "ill will or oppressive conduct" initiated the case.[48]

It is important to keep in mind that public policy favors access to the courts. Furthermore, fear of lawsuits alleging malicious prosecution and other torts of this nature would unduly hinder their initiation. Therefore, suits that raise allegations of malicious prosecution and abuse of power are usually allowed to proceed, so long as they are initiated in good faith and with a reasonable basis.[49]

In the health care arena, a patient may bring malicious prosecution charges against a psychiatric nurse who maliciously initiates commitment proceedings against him or her.

A nurse may also initiate this kind of suit. In one such case, a registered nurse alleged malicious prosecution against her supervisor and employer for reporting her termination of employment due to unprofessional and unethical conduct to the

---

ETHICS CONNECTION 7–4

Confidentiality and privacy are central to the development and maintenance of covenantal relationships between nurses and their clients (see Chapter 3). The widespread use of electronic health databases threatens nurse-client relationships by impeding nurses' ability to maintain confidentiality and privacy. On the one hand, computer technology has benefited both nurses and clients by providing improved access to information about nursing and health care. On the other hand, this technology has led to violations of privacy and confidentiality through increased access to personally identifiable health care data. Finding the right balance between providing and restricting access to health care data is a critical challenge. Currently, laws, regulations, policies, and protocols do not adequately protect client privacy and confidentiality.[1] Until national legislation is enacted[2] to protect the public by permitting the sharing of data that are needed to improve health care and prohibiting the use of personally identifiable data, nurses must be educated to be vigilant about the storage and exchange of electronic data. The House of Delegates of the American Nurses Association (ANA) has recommended that the ANA develop a position statement about patient privacy and confidentiality of health records.[3] This statement would include the nurses' role in preserving privacy and confidentiality in this age of technology.

---

[1]North Dakota Nurses Association, "Telehealth: Issues for Nursing," 67(2) *Prairie Rose* (1998), 5.

[2]James G. Hodge, Lawrence O. Gostin, and Peter D. Jacobson, "Legal Issues Concerning Electronic Health Information: Privacy, Quality, and Liability. (Health, Law and Ethics)," 282(15) *Journal of the American Medical Association* (1999), 1466.

[3]New Jersey State Nurses Association, "ANA House of Delegates Acts on Critical Practice and Health Policy Issues," 29(6) *New Jersey Nurse* (1999), 8.

Florida Board of Nursing.[50] The nurse was not successful, however, for several reasons. One reason was the absence of malice on the part of the home health care agency and supervisor in reporting the nurse to the board.

Defenses to Quasi-intentional Torts

The defenses to quasi-intentional torts are presented in Table 7-2. As with intentional torts, the statute of limitations can be raised as an additional

TABLE 7-2

Defenses to Quasi-intentional Torts

TORT	DEFENSES	QUALIFICATIONS	OTHER COMMENTS	EXAMPLE
1. Defamation	Truth	Defendant must prove; entire statement must be truthful	If proven, an *absolute defense*	Nurse truthfully tells another patient that Mr. S. has AIDS
	Absolute privilege (or immunity)	Limited to (1) judicial proceedings and actors (judges, witnesses, attorneys); (2) legislative proceedings and actors (legislatures, witnesses, official records); (3) executive communications; (4) consent; (5) spousal communications (to each other); (6) political broadcasts	Based on protecting otherwise actionable conduct because it furthers societal purpose; privilege cannot be abused; must be knowing consent	Plaintiff's attorney calls nurse incompetent in malpractice case against nurse. Mr. S. tells nurse it is OK to tell other patient he has AIDS
	Qualified privilege	Based on interests: 1. interest of publisher	Cannot be abused or exceeded; used to protect self against defamation by another	Nurse, in response to a colleague saying she is incompetent, calls the colleague a liar
		2. interest of others	Publication justified by importance of interest; legal or moral duty may exist to share information; cannot be abused or exceeded	Former employer of nurse shares suspected drug diversion with prospective employer (*Judge Rockford Memorial Hospital*, 150 N.E.2d 202; *cert. denied*, 17 Ill. App. 2nd 365 [1958]); nurse anesthetist not slandered due to "less than desirable" reference given to prospective employer by former employer (*Gengler Phelps*, 589 P.2d 1056 [Ct. App. N.M. 1978])
		3. common interest	When publisher speaks to another who has a common interest and sharing the information furthers that interest; may be legal and/or moral duty to speak; cannot be abused or exceeded	See example in number 2 above
		4. publishing to those who may act in public interest	Good faith required; cannot be abused or exceeded	Nurse reports unprofessional conduct of physician to state medical board
		5. fair comment on matters of public interest	Extends to matters in which public has legitimate interest; cannot be abused or exceeded	Nurse writes article for newspaper on poor patient care at local hospital

Tort	Defense	Details	Conditions	Example
	Partial defenses that mitigate (reduce) damages but do not avoid liability	1. retraction	Must immediately follow the publication; must be complete and without limitation; must be in same manner as publication	Nurse writes retraction of article on poor patient care at local hospital for same newspaper
		2. evidence of plaintiff's bad reputation	Defendant must prove reputation already "bad" as to what was published	Nurse defendant introduces evidence at administrative hearing that physician had problems with unprofessional conduct in other states
2. Breach of confidentiality	Consent	Must be knowing, informed, voluntary	May be required to be in writing; cannot be abused or exceeded	Psychiatric nurse receives patient's written consent to release information about treatment to employer
	Mandatory reporting requirements	Usually found in statutes or case law; basis is, in reality, that no confidential privilege exists in the identified situations	Cannot be abused or exceeded	Nurse reports to proper authorities child abuse or neglect or presence of a communicable disease; clear, imminent danger reported to third party
	Other legal mandate to share information	Usually found in statutes or case law; also applies when required or ordered to testify in any judicial proceeding	Cannot be abused or exceeded	Nurse is subpoenaed to testify as witness in case filed by former patient alleging malpractice against physician
3. Invasion of privacy	Consent	Must be knowing, informed, voluntary	Cannot be abused or exceeded	Patient consents to nurse taking photographs of patient postoperatively
	Mandatory reporting requirements	See comments under Breach of Confidentiality	Cannot be abused or exceeded	See example under Breach of Confidentiality
	Other legal mandate to share information	See comments under Breach of Confidentiality	Cannot be abused or exceeded	See example under Breach of Confidentiality NOTE: *Truth is not a defense in invasion of privacy actions*
4. Malicious prosecution	Any of the essential elements of the tort not satisfied	1. No malice 2. Termination of suit in favor of defendant 3. Presence of reasonable or probable cause to initiate suit		Employer, with reasonable basis, reports nurse to state agency or nursing board for violation of state nurse practice act
	Guilt in fact	Must be proven by defendant; can be raised even if verdict in criminal case in favor of accused (not guilty)		

Data from W. Page Keeton, Editor. *Prosser and Keeton on the Law of Torts.* 5th Edition. St. Paul, Minn.: West Publishing Company, 1984 (with 1988 pocket part).

defense to any of the torts discussed. A defamation suit must usually be filed within one year after the cause of action occurred. For the other quasi-intentional torts, a two-year time limitation is generally the rule.

CIVIL RIGHTS VIOLATIONS UNDER SECTION 1983 OF THE CIVIL RIGHTS ACT OF 1871

Section 1983 of the Civil Rights Act of 1871

Passed after the Civil War, Section 1983 of the Civil Rights Act of 1871 protects all of the rights encompassed in the Constitution (including life, liberty, property, privacy, due process, and equal protection) as well as federal statutory and administrative rights. It does so by stating that any violation of a federal right by governmental action can be sued for through a civil action requesting damages or equitable relief (e.g., an injunction) as a remedy.

A plaintiff bringing a suit alleging a violation of Section 1983 must prove that an individual acting under color of state law deprived the plaintiff of a specific, established federal right, whether substantive or procedural; in other words, discrimination of some kind occurred. Furthermore, there must be a causal connection between the violation and the injury alleged. Also, the injury that is the basis of the suit must be a closely related result of the violation.[51] It is important to note that the Act does not apply to infringement of rights granted by state law.

A plaintiff bringing a suit alleging a violation of Section 1983 must prove . . . discrimination of some kind occurred.

Under color of state law has specific meaning in the law, and Section 1983's language is no exception. Generally this phrase means that an individual who deprives another of his or her rights is a governmental official—state or local—or a private individual whose conduct is found to be "state action" rather than private conduct.

Health Care Delivery and Section 1983

In relation to health care delivery, governmental (state) action is easily satisfied when the hospital is a local or state hospital, a public health agency, or a prison health service. It is more difficult to determine when a private entity's or health care provider's conduct satisfies the state action requirement.

Although many tests have been applied by the courts to determine if conduct characterized as private is truly state action, no one specific criterion (e.g., receipt of state financial assistance) controls. In fact, many of the reported cases filed by aggrieved plaintiffs alleging state action by a private entity or individuals have been decided in favor of the defendant—that is, finding the conduct to be "private action." Some examples include the following:

- A private hospital was not acting under color of state law for Section 1983 purposes when it reported child abuse to state authorities and placed the child under protective custody pursuant to juvenile court order.[52]
- A private hospital that denied an ophthalmologist staff privileges was not acting under color of state law when the physician could not provide facts to support his allegations that the state regulated the personnel decisions of the hospital and discriminated against him in violation of Section 1983.[53]
- A private nursing home that exerted a great deal of control over a resident's existence was not a state actor even though it received Medicare and Medicaid funds.[54]

It is important to note that in a Section 1983 action, an employer may be joined in the suit under the theory of *vicarious liability* discussed in Chapter 4. The plaintiff can do so by suing an employee of the employer individually and in his or her official role. The plaintiff can also directly name the entity, especially if the plaintiff can prove that the employer or entity violated his or her rights by the adoption of a policy ("custom or usage") that violates the statute. Under the vicarious liability theory, the plaintiff need only prove that the employer indirectly or directly acquiesced in allowing the official's conduct to continue.

Damages that can be awarded to the successful plaintiff in a Section 1983 action are intended to compensate the person for the deprivation suffered and should therefore be governed by principles of compensation.[55] Thus, they include compensatory and punitive damages as well as nominal awards. Remedies also available may include reinstatement (when, for example, an employee is illegally discharged); the closure of a facility (when, for example, conditions at a jail are found to be unconstitutional); or an injunction prohibiting continuation of the conduct found to be in violation of the law.

To envision how this civil rights law actually protects individuals' rights, the *Reed* case (Key Case 7–1, pp. 128 and 129) involving two nurses is an interesting example.

Defenses to a Section 1983 Civil Rights Action

Alleged Conduct Not Violative of Civil Rights

There are several defenses to an allegation that someone's civil rights under Section 1983 have been violated. Perhaps the most obvious is to prove that the conduct did not occur. Thus, in the *Reed* case, if the prison authorities are able to prove their conduct was not "deliberate inattention" to the incarcerated patient's medical needs but was simply "inadvertent failure to provide medical care," then that defense will be successful.

Immunity from Suit

The other defenses available to a Section 1983 case rest on the fact that the government enjoys immunity (freedom) from suit in some circumstances, as was discussed in Chapter 4. However, as a review, it is important to recall that such immunity is not absolute. Therefore, a suit may be filed if no immunity exists.

The nurse who is an employee of a governmental health care entity must also remember that any immunities granted him or her may be eliminated if the nurse acts in "bad faith" or with "malice," or otherwise abuses the immunity. In addition, many immunities are based on whether the conduct complained of was discretionary. If discretionary, immunity would exist in the absence of malice. If the conduct is ministerial, however, no immunity would be present because the individual is acting in obedience to a higher authority and without regard to his or her own judgment or discretion.[57]

ELEVENTH AMENDMENT TO THE U.S. CONSTITUTION. The Eleventh Amendment provides another form of immunity from suit by prohibiting federal court suits, either in law or in equity, against the states.[58] As a result, state treasuries are protected from being drained if there is a successful suit in federal court concerning a request for past injuries (retroactive relief) due to a violation of one's rights by state actors. However, the individual injured may be awarded other relief, such as an injunction or a declaratory judgment (nonmonetary and prospective) so that state actors comply with federal constitutional mandates.[59]

There are several exceptions to the general prohibition contained in the Eleventh Amendment. One is if the state actor is sued *personally* rather than in his or her "official capacity."[60] Only in the latter instance would the state treasury be in possible jeopardy and require application of the immunity provisions.

COMMON LAW IMMUNITIES—ABSOLUTE OR QUALIFIED IMMUNITY. As with many of the intentional and quasi-intentional tort suits discussed thus far, those involved in 1983 suits may have immunity from suit, either absolute or qualified, based on case law decisions rather than statutory law. For example, certain public officials—judges and legislators—are usually absolutely immune from suit for monetary damages under 1983 actions, but may be subject to prospective remedies sought by the plaintiff.[61]

Qualified immunity in 1983 actions rests upon whether the defendant or defendants acted in "good faith." For example, the defendant may try to prove that the conduct did not violate the plaintiff's civil rights because a reasonable person in that position would not have recognized the violation.[62] If the argument is successful, then the qualified immunity attaches, and the defendant is entitled to a dismissal of the suit.

SUMMARY OF PRINCIPLES AND APPLICATIONS

The intentional and quasi-intentional torts, as well as civil rights violations, can be a potential quagmire of liability for the nurse. In addition to the defenses already presented, the following are some guidelines for the nurse to keep in mind.

Intentional Torts

Assault and Battery

- Always make sure the patient has consented to treatment before initiating it

KEY CASE 7–1   Reed v. McBride (1999)[56]

Prisoner has several medical conditions for which no medications or food are given for days at a time

FACTS: Orrin Reed was an inmate at Westville Correctional Facility in Westville, Indiana. He had several medical problems, including paralysis, heart disease, Hunt's syndrome, hypertension, rheumatoid arthritis, and other extremity and spine crippling diseases.

According to Reed, he was denied life-sustaining medication and food for days at a time, always after his return from Wishard Memorial Hospital. When he returned to the prison, Reed alleged he was not able to get his ID badge that would allow him to receive his medications and food. As a result, he suffered "severe illness and permanent injuries," including extreme pain, internal bleeding, violent intestinal cramps, and loss of consciousness.

Reed made prison officials aware of the difficulties he was experiencing in not getting his ID badge back for days after returning from the hospital, but his letters and grievances were ignored.

Prisoner files a Section 1983 action, alleging his Eighth Amendment and Americans with Disabilities (ADA) rights were violated

Reed sued the prison officials in federal court under 42 U.S.C. Section 1983, alleging a violation of his Eighth Amendment right to be free from cruel and unusual punishment. He also alleged a violation of the Americans with Disabilities Act (ADA).

Trial court grants summary judgment motion of defendants

TRIAL COURT DECISION: The district court dismissed both of Reed's claims. Reed appealed the dismissal of his Eighth Amendment claim.

APPEALS COURT DECISION: The Seventh Circuit Court of Appeals reversed the trial court's dismissal of Reed's claim and remanded the case to that court for a trial. The appellate court held that, based on other case law concerning this issue, Reed's medical condition was "objectively serious." In addition, the court opined, withholding food from him in view of his medical condition was also objectively "serious."

Court of Appeals reverses trial decision in favor of prisoner, holding that whether conduct of prison officials was "inadvertent failure" or "deliberate indifference" to provide care is a material fact issue that trial must resolve

The court also ruled that there was a question of material fact as to whether the prison officials acted with "deliberate indifference" toward his medical condition. Because the defendants did not provide evidence that once aware of Reed's complaints, they made changes to avoid similar problems in the future, the trial court must determine whether Reed's Eighth Amendment rights were violated.

ANALYSIS: Although no nurse was a named defendant in this suit, it is clear that nurses working in the facility had to cooperate with the "noncare" of the prisoner. Did any of the nurses attempt to intervene on Reed's behalf? If so, how? Because the conduct alleged occurred over a two-year period, nurse employees would be hard-pressed to say they knew nothing of Reed's complaints.

If Reed's allegations are true, the conduct of prison officials and of any nurse employees participating in it is far from exemplary, even if it does not sink to the level necessary for a constitutional violation. Furthermore, the alleged failure to provide for the medical needs of any patient, but most certainly a prisoner who has no other options for that care, is ethically impermissible.

- If the patient refuses treatment, and there is no threat to the life or well-being of the patient, do not force treatment
- Never hold a patient down to administer medications or treatment that the patient is refusing
- Never act in a threatening manner toward a patient
- Never hit, or threaten to hit, a patient

False Imprisonment

- Never unlawfully restrict a patient's freedom
- If a patient is committed to a psychiatric or other facility, be certain all papers are properly filled out and present upon admission
- Use restraining devices (e.g., leather or posey belts) only when there is a clear clinical reason to do so and document well in the patient's record
- If a patient chooses to leave the institution against medical advice (AMA), try to talk with the patient about staying; inform the patient that Medicare and other health insurance may not pay for the hospitalization if an AMA discharge occurs, and notify proper persons (doctor, nurse manager). If the patient refuses, ask him or her to sign the appropriate form. If he or she does not do so, simply let the patient go, document the incident well, and notify the proper individuals in the institution of the patient's leaving

Intentional Infliction of Emotional Distress

- Always think before acting or speaking to patients and their families or significant others
- Remember that when injury or death to a loved one occurs, friends and family are vulnerable and must be treated with an increased sense of empathy

Conversion of Property

- Always ask a patient or family member if belongings can be removed, stored, or otherwise disposed of
- Any belongings that are removed, stored, or disposed of should be properly documented in the patient's medical record or on other appropriate forms
- Any patient belongings taken home by friends or family members should be documented in the patient's medical record
- Never remove a patient's belongings without his or her consent

Quasi-intentional Torts

Defamation

- Always be sure that what you are saying about a patient is the truth

- If you must share information about a patient or another person and you may enjoy an absolute or qualified privilege to share what might be defamatory, be certain not to abuse or overstep the privilege
- When disciplining a nurse colleague or discussing something sensitive with a patient, be sure to do so in private so that what is discussed is not published to a third party
- When asked to write a reference for a nurse colleague, be sure to adhere to the institution's policy concerning references. If uncertain about what you are sharing about the colleague, sending the reference to the nurse for review and asking him or her to send it on to whoever is asking for it will avoid any publication by the nurse giving the reference
- Never repeat information received unless you know it to be true
- Always adhere to the institution's policies concerning speaking with reporters or other news media personnel

Breach of Confidentiality

- Adhere strictly to any obligations to maintain patient confidentiality
- Do not discuss patients with those not involved directly with their care
- Adhere to institution policies concerning confidentiality, especially in relation to information given over the phone about the patient and in speaking to reporters or other news media
- If practicing in an area of nursing where special mandates concerning confidentiality exist—psychiatric nursing, for example—continually review and adhere to the obligations to maintain confidentiality

Invasion of Privacy

- See guidelines for Breach of Confidentiality, above
- Always obtain consent for any photographs or use of the patient's name before disclosing either to another person
- Provide patient care in a respectful and dignified way
- Always ask the patient if observers of any kind can be present before care or treatment is initiated

Malicious Prosecution

- Never initiate, or get involved in, a suit against another, including a patient, if there is no reasonable basis to do so

Section 1983 Civil Rights Violations

- The nurse who is an employee of a local, state, or governmental health care delivery system must take great care to protect the patient's civil rights

- If an absolute or qualified privilege exists, the nurse must make sure that no abuse of the privilege occurs

- Good faith and knowledge of what a reasonable person would have known concerning the federal right are two tests that should also be kept in mind concerning the application of a qualified privilege

TOPICS FOR FURTHER INQUIRY

1. Analyze at least two reported cases naming a nurse as a defendant in a breach of nurse-patient confidentiality. If possible, use one case that involves a breach with electronic patient information. Compare and contrast the manner in which the breach occurred and any defenses raised by the nurse. Suggest how the nurse in each case might have handled the situation differently to avoid the breach of confidentiality.

2. Develop a patient care policy for obtaining consent for treatment with the specific concern of avoiding assault and battery allegations against a nurse who must provide care for patients in the institution or agency.

3. Write a research paper comparing and contrasting libel with slander. Focus specifically on how a nurse might be involved in libeling or slandering a colleague or libeling or slandering a patient. Discuss specific guidelines the nurse should follow to avoid these intentional torts.

4. Develop an interview instrument to question several nurses about their respective understanding of intentional or quasi-intentional torts. Utilize a situation-specific format that requires the nurse being interviewed to identify a particular tort or torts. Analyze the results and make suggestions for how to increase nurses' understanding of the tort or torts included in the interview instrument.

REFERENCES

1. W. Page Keeton, General Editor. *Prosser and Keeton on the Law of Torts.* St. Paul, Minn.: West Publishing Company, 1984, 33 (with 1988 pocket part)
2. *Id.* at 34.
3. *Id.*
4. *Id., citing Baldinger v. Banks,* 201 N.Y.S. 2d 629 (1960); *Restatement of Torts,* Section 13, Comment e (1977).
5. Henry Campbell Black. *Black's Law Dictionary,* 7th Edition. St. Paul, Minn.: West Group, 1999, 814.
6. Keeton, *supra* note 1, at 43.
7. *Id.*
8. *Id., citing Kline v. Kline,* 64 N.E. 9 (1902).
9. Keeton, *supra* note 1, at 45, *citing* Seavy, "Threats Inducing Emotional Reactions," 39 *North Carolina Law Review* 74 (1960).
10. Keeton, *supra* note 1, at 39, *citing Restatement of Torts,* Sections 13 and 18.
11. *Id.*
12. Keeton, *supra* note 1, at 40.
13. Keeton, *supra* note 1, at 41–42.
14. 576 So. 2d 992 (1991).
15. 811 S.W.2d 141 (1991).
16. Keeton, *supra* note 1, at 47.
17. *Gadsen General Hospital v. Hamilton,* 103 So. 553 (1925).
18. Keeton, *supra* note 1, at 60, 64.
19. *Id.* at 56.
20. See, for example, *Austin v. Regents of the University of California,* 152 Cal. Rep. 420 (1979); *Grimsley v. Sampson,* 530 P.2d 291 (1975); *Strachan v. John F. Kennedy Memorial Hospital,* 538 A.2d 346 (N.J. 1988).
21. *Brown v. Philadelphia College,* 674 A.2d 1130 (1996).
22. Keeton, *supra* note 1, at 92–93.
23. Keeton, *supra* note 1, at 727; see also Nancy J. Brent, "Exaggerating the Capability to Provide Care in the Home: More Than Just Puffery?" 16(5) *Home Healthcare Nurse* (May 1998), 320–322.
24. Keeton, *supra* note 1, at 771.
25. *Id., citing* Green, "Relational Interests," 31 *Illinois Law Review* 35 (1936).
26. *Restatement (Second) of Torts,* Section 559, Comment e.
27. *Stevens v. Morris Communication Service,* 317. S.E.2d 652 (1984).
28. *New York Times v. Sullivan,* 376 U.S. 254 (1964).
29. Keeton, *supra* note 1, at 842.
30. Keeton, *supra* note 1, at 789–793.
31. *Schlessler v. Keck,* 271 P.2d 588 (Cal. 1954).
32. 410 ILCS 50/0.01 *et seq.* (1993). The federal government is so concerned about health care information and privacy that Congress is considering several bills to protect personal health care data. Carole P. Jennings, "Who's Minding Your Healthcare Information?" 12(17) *Nursing Spectrum* (1999), 25. For the latest information on bills pending, or bills passed, concerning health care information and privacy, the reader should check www.congress.gov.
33. See, generally, Gary Scott Davis, Nanette Wernstrom, and Michael Levisnon, "Changing Confidentiality: The Effects of Technology and Health Care Reform on Patient Information," in *1998 Health Law Handbook.* Alice Gosfield, Editor. St. Paul, Minn.: West Group, 1998, 267–282; "Computerized Medical Records," in William Roach and the Aspen Health Law and Compliance Center. *Medical Records and the Law.* 3rd Edition. Gaithersburg, Md.: Aspen Publishers, 1998, 290–327.
34. "Electronic Medical Information: Privacy, Liability & Quality Issues," 25(2 & 3) *American Journal of Law & Medicine* (1999) (Symposium Issue).
35. Keeton, *supra* note 1, at 851.

36. *Id.* at 853.
37. *Vassiliades v. Garfinkle's Brooks Brothers,* 492 A.2d 580 (D.C. App. 1985).
38. Keeton, *supra* note 1, at 855.
39. *Id.*
40. See, for example, *Melvin v. Burling,* 490 N.E.2d 1011 (3rd App. Dist. 1986), *appeal denied* October 2, 1986.
41. *Vernuil v. Poirer,* 589 So. 2d 1202 (1991).
42. Keeton, *supra* note 1, at 856–857, *citing* Prosser and *Restatement (Second) of Torts,* Section 652D, Comment d (1977).
43. *Miller v. Motorola,* 560 N.E.2d 900 (App. Ct. 1st Dist. 1990).
44. *Id.* at 903.
45. Keeton, *supra* note 1, at 863–865.
46. *Id.* at 870.
47. *Id.* at 871.
48. *Id.* at 888.
49. Robert Miller, "General Principles of Civil Liability," in *Problems in Hospital Law.* 7th Edition. Gaithersburg, Md.: Aspen Publishers, 1996, 287.
50. *Northwest Florida Home Health Agency v. Merrill,* 469 So. 2d 893 (Fla. App. 1st Dist. 1985).
51. Ralph Chandler, Robert Enslen, and Peter Renstrom. *Constitutional Law Handbook: Individual Rights.* 2nd Edition. St. Paul, Minn.: West Group, 1993, 273 of May 1999 pocket part, *citing Albright v. Oliver,* 114 S. Ct. 807 (1994).
52. *Young v. Arkansas Children's Hospital,* 721 F. Supp. 197 (E.D. Ark. 1989).
53. *Pao v. Holy Redeemer Hospital,* 547 F. Supp. 484 (D.C. Pa. 1982).
54. *Hoyt v. St. Mary's Rehabilitation Center,* 711 F.2d 864 (8th Cir. 1983).
55. *Carey v. Piphus,* 435 U.S. 247 (1978).
56. 178 F.3d 849 (1999).
57. Henry Campbell Black. *Black's Law Dictionary.* 7th Edition. St. Paul, Minn.: West Group, 1999, 753. For an interesting case filed by a Utah prisoner against a nurse practitioner and the Utah prison medical administrator in which the nurse's and the medical administrator's defense of immunity did not apply, see *Bott v. Deland et al.,* 922 P.2d 732 (1996).
58. U.S. Constitution Amendment XI.
59. *Ex Parte Young,* 209 U.S. 123 (1908).
60. Keeton, *supra* note 1, at 1044, *citing Kentucky v. Graham,* 473 U.S. 159 (1985).
61. *Pulliam v. Allen,* 466 U.S. 522 (1984).
62. Keeton, *supra* note 1, *citing Harlow v. Fitzgerald,* 457 U.S. 800 (1982).

Administrative Law

8

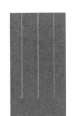
KEY PRINCIPLES

- Administrative Procedure Act
- Delegation of Authority to Administrative Agency
- Rulemaking
- Rulemaking Procedure
- Due Process
- Property Interest
- Liberty Interest
- Judicial Review

Administrative law is defined as the body of law—statutes, agency-made law (rules, regulations, orders, and decisions), and legal principles governing the acts of agencies—that governs the organization and operation of administrative agencies.[1] Administrative agencies, whether state or federal, are created by respective state or federal (Congress) legislatures, which then delegate the responsibility of carrying out particular pieces of legislation, such as statutes, that are specific to the agency. In the health care field, and in nursing specifically, administrative law and administrative agencies have a great impact on the delivery of health care and on nursing practice.

The character, role, and powers of administrative agencies are varied and complex. Although an agency is created by a particular legislature with defined powers and roles, the ability of the agency to carry out those roles is also further defined. This further definition is found in the agency's authority to promulgate its own rules and regulations to enforce its responsibilities and is called formal or informal rulemaking. Furthermore, administrative bureaus also function as enforcers of the legislation they are empowered to oversee, often in a trial-type hearing. As a result, an administrative agency is often involved in sanctioning, limiting, or eliminating rights granted to citizens by the legislation when violations of an act occur. One such example is when a professional licensee (registered nurse or licensed practical nurse) is disciplined. Rulemaking and enforcement roles are usually governed by the state or federal Administrative Procedure Act.

Other functions, however, although required to conform to certain rules of law and court decisions, are less readily defined. An example of such a role would be settlement powers of the agency.

This chapter will present a broad overview of administrative law and process and briefly discuss administrative agencies that most directly affect the health care field generally and nursing specifically. Although the focus will be primarily federal in nature, some discussion of state laws will occur.

ESSENTIALS OF ADMINISTRATIVE LAW

Origins and History of Administrative Law and Agencies

Administrative law deals with the body of law of governmental or public agencies, whether federal, state, or local. Most commentators mark the beginning of administrative law with the establishment of the Interstate Commerce Commission (ICC) in 1887.[2] The Interstate Commerce Commission, like other early administrative agencies, was "regulatory" in nature, meaning that its primary purpose was to control the growth of large corporations and ensure that no undue influence or power was vested in a few companies. As the nation developed, other types of administrative agencies appeared, and their respective characters reflected what was happening in the country at the time. For example, when the country focused upon social reform for its citizens, administrative laws and bureaus concentrated on benefit programs such as Medicare, unemployment insurance, and worker's compensation.[3]

Administrative law deals with the body of law of governmental or public agencies, whether federal, state, or local.

Despite the specific focus of an administrative agency, administrative bureaus became, and still are, a vital piece of the overall picture of a government's ability to function. Without them, the local, state, and/or federal government would virtually be at a standstill.[4] In addition to being a necessary vehicle for carrying out the goals of government, administrative agencies also serve other important goals that include managing issues with citizens fairly and in accordance with due process protections and deciding issues as accurately as possible by utilizing the best method to do so (trial-type hearing or informal notice, for example).

Essentially, two basic types of administrative agencies have emerged. The first, an executive department, agency, or bureau, is organized with a secretary appointed by the president as the head. Because these agencies are directly under the control of the president, he or she has the power to appoint and remove agency heads.

The second type of administrative agency is the commission or board, a more independent body in the sense that the head of a commission is appointed for a fixed term. As a result, it is more difficult to remove commission heads unless there is a just reason for doing so. Furthermore, the commission is formed for a specific purpose, its members are appointed because of their expertise in a certain area, and, like the commission head, they cannot be removed from their position unless there is a clear reason to do so. An example of a commission is the National Labor Relations Board, which administers the National Labor Relations Act.

Delegation, Accountability, and Control of Administrative Agencies

The U.S. Constitution (and respective state constitutions) establish and protect a tripartite system of government—the legislative, executive, and judicial branches—to provide a system of checks and balances on the powers of each branch.

Because specific powers and responsibilities are given to each branch of government, when the delegation of those powers and/or responsibilities to a governmental agency occurs, the delegation can raise serious constitutional questions.

Delegating powers and/or responsibilities to administrative agencies has always been controversial. Even so, the very language of the U.S. Constitution, Article I, Section 1 and Section 8, Paragraph 18, has been used to support the need for delegation to administrative agencies.[5] In addition, many cases decided by the federal courts support the ability of Congress to delegate to federally created administrative organizations.[6]

Accordingly, administrative agencies have been delegated powers through the so-called Delegation Doctrine that reflect the powers of all three branches of the government; that is, legislative powers (to pass rules and regulations to which affected people and organizations must adhere or face civil and criminal penalties), judicial powers (to hear and resolve disputes when an alleged violation of an act or its rules and regulations occurs), and executive powers (to investigate, subpoena, and prosecute alleged violations).[7]

Despite the determination that delegation can occur, the judicial branch of the government—the courts, both federal and state—stands ready to carefully analyze and decide the propriety of any delegation of power to an agency that is challenged, including its constitutionality.

The reins can be applied to administrative agency functioning in many ways. One very strong control is "legislative oversight," whether formal or informal,[8] whereby Congress or a state legislature determines that an agency has overstepped its responsibilities. If that determination occurs, for example, the legislative body may "restructure" the agency.

A second means of control over administrative bureaus is by controlling the staff and employees of the agency.[9] When the president of the United States or governor of a particular state exercises his or her power to appoint heads of executive agencies, for example, it is a powerful way to ensure accountability and adherence to agency policy. Likewise, Congress, although it cannot make appointments to agencies, can establish qualifications for agency offices. These confirmation hearings can become very effective tools for ensuring that the person confirmed for a particular office will adhere to the mandates of the agency's delegated powers and responsibilities.[10]

A third effective means of control over administrative bureaus is "executive oversight," usually in the form of an executive order.[11] Other methods include the ability of the president to reorganize the agency and to control litigation involving administrative agencies through the Justice Department. Federal administrative bureaus must be represented by the Justice Department; if the department refuses to defend or represent an agency policy, the practical effect of that refusal is that the policy is without force.[12]

Similarly, state agencies are represented by the state attorney general's office. Again, if there is a decision to represent a particular state agency in a certain situation or, conversely, to settle a suit filed by a plaintiff, that decision effectively represents either support or nonsupport of the agency's performance.

ESSENTIALS OF ADMINISTRATIVE PROCEDURE

The Administrative Procedure Act

The federal or state Administrative Procedure Act is a statute that governs practice and proceedings before respective federal and state administrative agencies. The federal Act was passed in 1946 to provide minimum standards of procedures that all federal agencies were to follow. It also became a model for state legislatures contemplating their own acts. Areas included in the federal statute are (1) definitions of terms used; (2) access to, and publication of, agency rules, opinions, (public) records, and orders; (3) rulemaking powers; (4) obligations of agencies to protect the privacy of individuals involved in administrative procedures (Privacy Act); (5) the requirement that specified agency meetings and proceedings be "open" (Government in the Sunshine Act); (6) adjudicatory practice and procedure (hearings, sanctions, and decision-making process; and (7) judicial review.[13]

Most states have adopted state administrative procedure acts that contain sections similar, if not identical, to those in the federal law.

> *The federal or state Administrative Procedure Act is a statute that governs practice and proceedings before respective federal and state administrative agencies.*

Rulemaking

The process of rulemaking is a way for an administrative agency to deal with its responsibilities in carrying out a particular piece of legislation with clarity and efficiency. Rather than exercise its adjudicatory power and issue an *order* each and every time there is an alleged violation of the act or its rules and regulations (which would apply only to those specific individuals or organizations), an adopted rule or regulation, if clear and well drafted, can provide guidance to the greatest number of individuals and organizations expected to comply with the particular act.

The Administrative Procedure Act defines the types of rules that can be passed, the process of rulemaking, and its scope. The types of rules that an agency is authorized to promulgate are (1) *legislative rules,* which have "the force and effect of law," are considered "binding" on all those affected by them, and must be adopted pursuant to established, "formal," or at a minimum, "informal," rulemaking process; (2) *interpretive rules,* which indicate the agency's opinion on the act it administers; these are exempt from the rulemaking process, but must be published; and (3) *procedural rules,* which regulate the agency's own practices and procedures, are legally binding on the agency (moreover, if not followed, can be challenged by persons adversely affected by the noncompliance), and, although also exempt from the rulemaking procedure, must be clearly articulated and published.[14]

There are two types of rulemaking procedures authorized in the Administrative Procedure Act—"informal" (or "Notice and Comment" rulemaking) and "formal." The two types are summarized in Table 8–1. All federal agencies are required to follow these procedures. State agencies usually adopt similar informal and formal rulemaking procedures. However, publication would occur in the

TABLE 8–1	
Informal and Formal Rulemaking Procedures Authorized by the Federal Administrative Procedure Act	
INFORMAL	**FORMAL**
1. Publish draft in *Federal Register*	1. Publish draft in *Federal Register*
2. Public can submit written comments concerning draft	2. Provide informal rulemaking hearing for oral public comment or, if authorized by another act, trial-type hearing may be required
3. Review comments and revise draft, if necessary	3. Review oral comments and revise draft, if necessary
4. Publish final rule in *Federal Register* 30 days before effective date	4. Publish final rule in *Federal Register* 30 days before effective date; if trial-type hearing, hearing officer enters order that contains findings of facts based on evidence presented in the hearing
5. Include final regulation in *Code of Federal Regulations*	5. Include final regulation in *Code of Federal Regulations*

Data from 5 U.S.C. Sections 552, 553, 554 (1946).

particular state registry and code. For example, the State of Illinois utilizes the *Illinois Register* and the *Illinois Administrative Code.*

Protection of Individual Constitutional Rights

Due Process

In administrative law and procedure, due process protections are important to the individual or organization because the administrative agency, again an arm of the federal or state government, cannot deprive a citizen of "life, liberty, or property" without due process of law.[15] Although a threat to one's life is usually *not* an issue in administrative actions, liberty or property rights *are* often the central issues. Thus the Administrative Procedure Act, and its state counterparts, grant clear procedural protections to those individuals or organizations who face an infringement of liberty or property.

In administrative law and procedure, due process protections are important to the individual . . . because the administrative agency . . . cannot deprive a citizen of "life, liberty, or property" without due process of law.

Property Interest

A property interest is liberally construed by the courts and defined in diverse ways based on

the context in which it arises. In administrative law, property interest is interpreted to be any "legitimate claim of entitlement" to a benefit that may be adversely affected by an administrative action.[16] An example of a property interest in the context of administrative law is the possession of an occupational license to practice one's profession (e.g., RN or LPN).

Liberty Interest

Liberty interests are also liberally construed and defined in diverse ways by the courts. In criminal law, this interest clearly encompasses a potential restriction of movement if incarceration is contemplated as punishment. In administrative law, however, this interest has been expanded to also include "the right of the individual to contract, to engage in any of the common occupations of life, to acquire useful knowledge, to marry . . . and generally to enjoy those privileges long recognized . . . as essential to the orderly pursuit of happiness by free men."[17] An example of a liberty interest in the context of administrative law is the possession of an occupational license in good standing. If an RN or LPN is disciplined in a manner inconsistent with procedural protections, for example, his or her "freedom" to reinstate the license to one in good standing (not disciplined) is jeopardized. Likewise, the registered nurse or licensed practical nurse's ability to obtain licensure in another state ("freedom" to obtain licensure) is also threatened.

When a property or liberty interest is potentially at risk by an administrative agency action, the Administrative Procedure Act requires that the protections listed in Table 8–2 be afforded the individual or organization.

TABLE 8-2

Due Process Rights Required by Federal Administrative Procedure Act When Protected Rights Threatened

RIGHT	SPECIFICS OF RIGHT	EXCEPTIONS
1. Notice	1. Inform party of action; time, place, and nature of hearing; basis of agency authority to take action	1. Need for immediate action to protect public from harm; or if a statute or "common law" already provides "process due"
2. Trial-type hearing	2. Present testimony; cross-examine witnesses; present evidence	2. If decision of agency "nonlegal" in nature; or if controversy can be decided by agency without hearing and denial of due process
3. Counsel	3. Attorney can "advise, represent, and accompany" party	3. If party is not compelled to appear before agency; if party cannot afford lawyer
4. Unbiased decision	4. Body or person making determination must not have direct or indirect conflict with merits of case	4. None
5. Complete record of decision	5. Record must set out "findings, conclusions, and basis of both from testimony and exhibits"	5. None

Data from 5 U.S.C. Sections 554, 555, 556 (1946).

Judicial Review

Judicial review is a means by which parties affected by an agency decision can challenge the decision if they believe it is arbitrary (unreasonable), not based on the law, illegal, or not based on the agency's power, procedures, or policies.[18] To do so, however, the party seeking review of an agency decision in the courts must meet certain requirements enumerated in the Administrative Procedure Act and delineated by many court decisions. They include "standing" to challenge the decision ("suffering legal wrong . . . or adversely affected or aggrieved . . . by agency action"[19]) and, with specific exceptions (e.g., when a party is challenging the jurisdiction of the agency to bring the action), a *final* administrative decision must have taken place for court review to occur. This latter requirement is often referred to as the exhaustion of administrative remedies rule. This rule is strictly adhered to by the courts, and the party seeking review must show that all agency appeal and review procedures have been used before seeking the court's decision.

The scope of the court's review is to include "relevant questions of law, interpret relevant constitutional and statutory provisions, and determine the meaning or applicability of the terms of an agency action."[20] The court is empowered to order an agency to act when the agency's action is "unlawfully withheld or unduly delayed." The court can also declare unlawful and set aside any agency "action, findings, and conclusions" found to be arbitrary, capricious, or an abuse of discretion, unconstitutional, in disregard of procedures required by law, or exceeding statutory authority, jurisdiction, or limitations.[21]

Other Aspects of Administrative Procedure
Information Gathering

For an agency to carry out whatever powers it has been delegated, it must have information upon which to rely when carrying out its responsibilities. Because the governmental agency or commission is an "arm" of the government, it is constrained by constitutional mandates when seeking out whatever information it needs from private individuals or entities, especially when the request for information is challenged. Thus, the Fourth, Fifth, *and* Fourteenth Amendment protections must be respected by the administrative bureau when it attempts to gather facts and evidence upon which to take action.

THE ABILITY TO ISSUE SUBPOENAS. An administrative organization generally has the power to issue subpoenas when seeking information, but the power is not unlimited. Rather, it is limited by four main constraints: (1) the inquiry must be within the powers of the agency and done for a lawful purpose or reason; (2) the information asked for must be "relevant" to the lawful purpose or reason; (3) the inquiry must be sufficient and not unrealistically "burdensome"; and (4) the information requested cannot be privileged information (e.g., information obtained by the nurse from a patient during the course of providing patient care is generally treated as privileged by state law).[22]

THE ABILITY TO COMPEL TESTIMONY. An administrative bureau may request that an individual testify about a matter that may have criminal law ramifications. For example, a nurse appearing before the licensing authority for an alleged violation of the nurse practice act may admit to behavior that is a violation not only of the practice act but also of the criminal statutes. If that is the case, the individual can refuse to incriminate himself or herself by relying on the Fifth Amendment's protections.[23]

Second, the protection against self-incrimination is *personal* in nature and does not extend to an organization, corporation, or association.[24] Thus the nurse entrepreneur who has formed her own nurse registry, is an officer or principal in that agency, and is asked to produce agency records when accused by the Office of the Inspector General of fraudulently billing Medicare cannot raise the Fifth Amendment as a protection. Furthermore, the nurse cannot rely on the fact that the records may incriminate her; by producing the nurse agency records, she is, as the record custodian, not performing a *personal* act. Rather, she is performing an act of the entity.[25]

Last, it is important to note that even if testimony given in an administrative hearing may be self-incriminating from the criminal law perspective, an individual may be forced to testify against himself or herself if granted immunity from prosecution. The immunity granted may be "use immunity" (prevents the testimony "and its fruits" from being used in connection with future criminal law prosecution) or "transactional immunity" (prevents prosecution for any event or transaction to which the testimony relates).[26] In either case, the immunity would not prevent prosecution with *new* information obtained from sources independent of the compelled testimony, nor does it allow the individual any grant of immunity in the administrative hearing itself.[27]

THE ABILITY TO CONDUCT INSPECTIONS AND SEARCHES. Generally the constitutional prohibitions against warrantless searches apply to administrative agencies; that is, a warrant is generally required.[28] However, the U.S. Supreme Court has established some important exceptions to that general rule for administrative agencies. To begin with, so long as the search or inspection is based upon valid statutory authorization for the agency to conduct the search, there is no need to establish probable cause in the same manner that is required in criminal law, and a warrant is not required unless entry into the place to be searched is denied.[29]

Other exceptions to obtaining a search warrant include (1) when a particular type of business is heavily licensed/regulated by the administrative agency[30]; (2) when an emergency exists[31]; (3) when valid, voluntary consent is given, whether express or implied (e.g., not objecting to an inspection)[32]; and (4) when the space or area to be searched is considered to be "in open view"; that is, consisting of what is "in plain view," so long as the inspector is legally on the premises, or consisting of "open fields," meaning outdoor property, even if privately owned.[33]

Examples of administrative searches or inspections that a nurse might experience include inspections by the Occupational Safety and Health Administration (OSHA) because, for example, a complaint had been filed with the local agency office concerning violations of the employer's duty to provide a healthful and safe workplace. Or, an inspection by state or local licensing officials may take place concerning whether the health care delivery entity complies with that agency's licensing rules and regulations. In either case, the inspection might also involve the testing of materials found within the health care delivery system. For example, if a complaint alleged unhealthy air due to the presence of some toxin, samples could be taken by the inspector.

Examples of administrative searches or inspections that a nurse might experience include inspections by the Occupational Safety and Health Administration (OSHA) . . . concerning violations of the employer's duty to provide a healthful and safe workplace.

Administration of Benefit Programs

Federal programs (e.g., Social Security Disability) and state programs (e.g., workers' compensation) that provide financial benefits to citizens must be able to expeditiously handle large volumes of applications for benefits and administer awards to those who are eligible. Thus the administrative agency charged with these responsibilities makes unceremonious decisions concerning coverage on a daily basis. Some of the programs, such as the Social Security Disability program, do provide an "appeal" procedure, which includes a trial-type hearing before an administrative judge if benefits are initially denied. Even so, most of the initial decisions concerning coverage are made by first-level agency employees without a hearing, and they are not challenged by the applicant for many reasons, including a lack of information concerning the appeal process and a lack of financial resources.

Summary Administrative Powers

Most administrative agencies have the power to act swiftly when an immediate threat to the public's health or safety exists. The Food and Drug Administration, for example, is empowered to confiscate any drug on the market that is adulterated or misbranded in violation of the Food, Drug, and Cosmetic Act.[34] Likewise, state licensing authorities often have the ability to suspend a license without a hearing when there is a need to protect the public's well-being.[35] Despite the authority to take these actions, the administrative procedure statute allowing summary powers or, if no protections are present in the law, due process mandates, requires a postsuspension trial-type hearing within a certain time period so that the organization or individual has an opportunity to defend against the agency action.[36]

Settlement of Issues without Full Hearing

Because administrative agencies would be hopelessly inefficient if each were required to determine legal issues only through a trial-type hearing or some other more formalized process, administrative bureaus generally can use other methods of resolving conflicts. Those methods include negotiation, settlement, consent orders, and "alternative dispute resolution."[37] In addition to benefiting the agency, such methods often benefit the individual or organization alleged to have violated some

provision, rule, or regulation of the agency because a resolution involves less cost, less time, and perhaps less emotional strain to the respondent.

For example, if a union files a complaint with the National Labor Relations Board (NLRB) accusing an employer of committing an unfair labor practice, the employer can enter into a consent order with the board to resolve the issues. Although the consent order will contain allegations, stipulations, and the specific terms of the agreement, there is no formal admission by the employer as to the allegations. Even so, once signed, the consent order has the same effect as a final agency order.[38]

Additional Considerations

Many of the additional aspects of administrative procedure overlap with those already discussed. They include, for example, the ability to issue advisory opinions and declaratory orders; to supervise businesses over which the agency has jurisdiction; and to award contracts and grants.[39]

Accountability of Agencies to the Public

Thus far, the discussion of administrative procedure has centered on the agency and its processes in getting its work done in a fair and equitable manner. There is another very important part of administrative procedure, however, which is the public's power to ensure that the administrative bureau is performing as mandated by federal and state law. Three important tools available to the public to determine agency compliance are the Privacy Act (and comparable state law, if any), the Freedom of Information Act (and comparable state law), and the Government in the Sunshine Act (and comparable state law). It is important to note that although the titles of these three acts sound as though they are separate pieces of legislation, in the federal system they are all contained in the Administrative Procedure Act.

The Privacy Act

The Privacy Act[40] amended the Administrative Procedure Act because Congress was concerned that the privacy of individuals may be threatened by the "gathering, maintenance, use and dissemination" of personal information by federal agencies, especially when advanced technology, such as computers, is used to compile and use such information.[41] Furthermore, Congress stated that because the right of privacy is a personal and fundamental right protected by the Constitution of the United States, regulations concerning the personal information obtained and its use must be established.[42] The Office of Management and Budget was instructed to develop guidelines in accordance with the act.

Basically the Act provides that no disclosure of any record in a (federal) system of records can occur except with the written request of, or consent of, the individual.[43] Exceptions to this general rule include disclosure to officers and employees of the agency who maintain the records and who have a need for the information to perform their duties; release required under the Freedom of Information Act; disclosure to a person who shows "compelling circumstances" that affect the health or safety of an individual, so long as notice of the disclosure is sent to the last known address of that individual; release pursuant to a valid order of a court of competent jurisdiction; and disclosures for use in statistical research or reporting of statistics, so long as the individual cannot be identified.[44]

Furthermore, the Act requires that each agency (1) maintain an "accounting" of disclosures made; (2) when possible, obtain information from the subject (individual) himself or herself when the potential for adverse decisions for benefits under federal programs may flow from the information gathered; and (3) among other things, make an effort to ensure prior to release for any purpose, other than a Freedom of Information Act request, that the records are accurate, timely, and relevant for agency purposes.[45]

. . . The [federal Privacy] Act provides that no disclosure of any record in a (federal) system of records can occur except with the written request of, or consent of, the individual.

Another important provision of the Privacy Act is the ability of any individual, upon request, to have access to, review of, and copies of records about him or her contained in the agency's sys-

tem.[46] Upon receiving such a request, the agency, pursuant to its established procedures, is required to search its system of records and produce nonexempt information to the requesting person. The agency *should* acknowledge the request within 10 business days and provide access within 30 days, unless "good cause" for further delay is shown. If the information is reproduced for the individual, the agency can charge for that reproduction, but not for its search.[47]

If a request is denied by the agency, an appeal process *can* be established by the agency, but no administrative appeal is mandated by the Act. In either case, the aggrieved individual can seek judicial review of the denial. If an appeal process is provided by the agency, it must be exhausted before seeking a court's decision concerning the denial.[48]

The Act also provides for the individual to amend and correct agency records that are inaccurate, untimely, not relevant, or not complete.[49] The person can also seek judicial review of any denial by the agency to allow corrections. In this instance, the agency *must* provide an agency appeal process.[50]

Exceptions to an individual's ability to obtain access to his or her records consist of two general categories that have been described as those involving agency "discretion" and those that must be published in the Federal Register before being effective[51]: *general exceptions* (exemptions) and *specific exceptions.* Examples of the general exceptions include CIA records and any records kept by an agency that has criminal law enforcement as its main purpose.[52] Specific exemptions include "material required by statute to be maintained and used solely as statistical records. . . . and investigatory material compiled for law enforcement purposes" not included in the general exemption category.[53]

Other aspects of privacy are also governed by the Privacy Act. Because Social Security numbers can provide access to a wealth of information about an individual, since 1975 Social Security numbers cannot be required by a federal, state, or local government without notifying the individual (1) whether the disclosure is mandatory (required by federal law) or voluntary; (2) what the number will be used for; and (3) the authority for requesting the number.[54] In addition, generally no governmental entity can deny an individual a right, benefit, or privilege under federal law because the individual refuses to provide his or her Social Security number.[55]

Also, under the Computer Matching and Privacy Protection Act of 1988,[56] Congress amended the Privacy Act to regulate the sharing of private information about individuals between agencies through, among other things, the establishment of a "matching agreement" stating that data obtained may be subject to verification and disclosure through agency computer-matching programs.[57] Because computer matching consists of "side-by-side comparisons" of different agencies' data banks and information about a particular individual or individuals, the matching agreements are aimed to prevent agency abuse of access to personal information listed in the data banks.[58]

The Freedom of Information Act

The Freedom of Information Act (FOIA)[59] makes "all" agency records available to any member of the public who requests them unless the records are exempt from disclosure.[60] Exempt agencies include Congress, the federal courts, and those divisions within the presidential Executive Office whose only function is to advise and assist the president (e.g., the chief of staff).[61]

The Freedom of Information Act (FOIA) makes "all" agency records available to any member of the public who requests them unless the records are exempt from disclosure.

Agency records that must be made available (either for inspection and copying or release) from applicable agencies have been interpreted by the courts to include documents or any other materials that contain information (e.g., audio or computer tapes) that were "created or obtained by the agency and, at the time of the request, are in the possession and control of the agency."[62] If no record exists, the Act does not require the administrative agency to create one. Furthermore, if a record exists but is not in the possession of the agency when access is sought, there is no duty to obtain it.

Some agency records are exempt from mandatory release to the public. The act contains nine

---

ETHICS CONNECTION 8–1

Changes in privacy statutes and regulations are examples of how ethics and law mutually influence one another. Federal statutes and regulations are limited in their protection of privacy. These statutes and regulations give federal agencies "substantial administrative discretion to disclose data without individual consent."[1] They are more concerned with transmission of government-held health information than with disclosure of private-sector health information data. Currently, efforts are being made to develop more comprehensive federal protection of health care information than present law offers. For example, the U.S. Department of Health and Human Services has provided Congress with key principles about the protection of health information, and Congress has debated health information privacy bills.

States vary in the degree to which they safeguard health information privacy. Some states have crafted legislation that is more restrictive than federal legislation; others have statutes that are less comprehensive than their federal counterparts. State statutes range from a focus on government-held data to "super-confidentiality" statutes for selected health data or diseases, such as mental illness or human immunodeficiency virus and/or acquired immunodeficiency syndrome (HIV/AIDS). This area of legislation concerned with health care privacy and disclosure reveals the tension between what is good for the individual and what is good for society (see Chapter 3 for a discussion of related ethical theories).

[1]James G. Hodge, Lawrence O. Gostin, and Peter D. Jacobson, "Legal Issues Concerning Electronic Health Information: Privacy, Quality, and Liability. (Health, Law and Ethics)," 282(15) *Journal of the American Medical Association* (1999), 1466.

---

exceptions. Among these are (1) national security information; (2) internal agency personnel rules and practices; (3) information clearly exempted from disclosure by statutes other than the Freedom of Information Act; (4) personnel, medical, or other files that would constitute a clear "unwarranted invasion of privacy"; and (5) records or information gathered for law enforcement purposes, if the disclosure would be harmful under several situations listed in the act.[63] The Act also states that if an exemption does apply to a request for records, that information should be deleted and the remainder of the record released.

The procedures for obtaining access to agency records are clearly spelled out in the Act and in the *Federal Register*. The request should be in writing and "reasonably describe" the information sought. Although there is no need to justify a reason for the request, in some instances it may be helpful to do so; for example, when seeking a waiver of any fees that may be charged for the records request.[64] The request should also specify that the agency is expected to make an "agency determination" within the time frames spelled out in the Act; that is, within 10 working days of receipt of the request and within 20 working days of receipt of an appeal letter to contest the agency determination to the initial request.[65]

If the internal agency appeal process does not prove successful for the person requesting agency records, it is possible for that individual to seek help from the representative or senator in his or her district, although congressional members have no more power under the act than other persons.[66] Another option is to seek judicial assistance by filing a suit for injunctive relief (asking the court to require the agency to release the requested records) and other relief. Such suits are costly and time consuming but may be successful if the specific situation is favorable to the plaintiff. In either case, all internal agency appeals must be exhausted before outside help or review is sought.

In 1996, the Electronic Freedom of Information Act Amendments were passed.[67] All agency materials subject to the act created on or after November 1, 1996, must also be made available to the public by computer telecommunications. If an agency does not have computer capabilities, the agency records must be made available in some other electronic form.[68]

State Freedom of Information Acts are very similar in structure to the federal law; that is, they contain a general mandate that records be made available to the public; some records are exempt from disclosure; time guidelines for agency response are listed; and the appeal process is spelled out.[69]

A nurse who is interested in obtaining records about himself or herself from a federal agency may be confused as to which act to utilize—the Privacy Act or the Freedom of Information Act. There are clear benefits and drawbacks to both, and they are listed in Table 8–3.

The Government in the Sunshine Act

The Sunshine Act[70] was passed by Congress to ensure that the government conducts the public's business in public.[71] It requires that federal agencies (and any subdivision authorized to act on behalf of an agency) subject to the Freedom of Information Act and headed by a "collegial" body of two or more members (the majority appointed by the president, with the advice and consent of the Senate) must hold their meetings "in the open."[72] Access to any agency meeting covered under the Act must be afforded to the public.

Ten narrow exceptions to the general rule of open meetings are enumerated in the Act. These include meetings that (1) relate solely to the internal personnel rules and practices of the agency; (2) accuse any individual of a crime; (3) formally censure a person; (4) would disclose information of a personal nature that would result in unwarranted invasion of personal privacy; and (5) prematurely disclose implementation of a proposed agency action, thus frustrating its implementation.[73] The Act requires the agency to carry out its nonexempt agenda items in the open.

The Act also contains procedures for administrative bureaus to follow when closing a meeting or portion thereof; notice requirements concerning meeting dates and times; maintaining minutes of *all* agency meetings; and procedures for challenging an agency action carried out in violation of the act.[74]

State laws concerning open governmental meetings are very similar to the federal law. In fact, it may be that many of these state laws served as models for the federal legislation, because when the Sunshine Act was passed in 1972, 49 states had passed open-government laws, and 39 had constitutional provisions concerning open government.[75]

Nurses may need to ensure that a federal or state agency conducts its business in conformity with such public meeting acts, not only as private citizens but as health care professionals as well. If, for example, the state board of nursing considers an amendment to the state nurse practice act in a closed meeting rather than an open one if required by the act, or does not keep minutes as mandated, those actions can be challenged in the courts. Such challenges cannot be made in an irresponsible or careless manner, but the opportunity to contest an agency's action lies at the very heart of ensuring that agency's accountability to the public.

PRIVACY ACT	FOIA
1. Applies to U.S. citizens, permanent resident aliens	1. Applies to "any person"
2. Access to records kept by agency in its control and identifiable in some way (name, number, symbol)	2. Access to "any" agency records
3. Broader exemptions for most exempt records	3. Not as inclusive categories for exemptions
4. Does not specify time limits for agency response	4. Specified time limits for agency response
5. Does not mandate appeal procedures	5. Appeal procedures established
6. Agency can charge for copying, but not search, of records	6. Agency can charge for copying records

Data from Allan Robert Adler, Editor. *Litigation Under the Federal Open Government Laws.* Wye Mills, Md.: American Civil Liberties Union, 1997.

SELECTED ADMINISTRATIVE AGENCIES THAT AFFECT HEALTH CARE

Federal Agencies

Numerous federal agencies affect health care. Because federal law most often preempts state law, familiarity with the following selected federal agencies is important:

- The Department of Health and Human Services—Social Security Administration
- The Department of Health and Human Services—Food and Drug Administration
- The Occupational Safety and Health Administration (OSHA)
- The Drug Enforcement Administration (DEA)
- The Department of Justice
- The Equal Employment Opportunity Commission (EEOC)
- The National Labor Relations Board (NLRB)
- The Department of Labor

State Agencies

As has been discussed throughout this chapter, many states have counterparts to the federal agencies listed above, and additional state administrative bureaus affect health care delivery. They include:

- Department of Public Health
- Board of Nursing or other body that regulates professions and occupations in the state
- State Labor Department

- Department of Protective Services (child abuse, elder abuse)
- Department of Aging
- Workers' Compensation Board
- Civil Rights Commission or Board
- Board of Education (school nursing)
- Department of Public Aid
- The Insurance Board or Commission
- Department of Alcohol and Substance Abuse
- Department of Human Rights

ETHICS CONNECTION 8–2

Nurse practice acts are the "foremost legal statute[s] regulating nursing."[1] These acts are intended to protect the public. They define nursing and establish the scope of nursing practice. As nursing and health care change, nurse practice acts also change to reflect contemporary practice. Recent changes in most nurse practice acts reflect advanced practice in nursing, including prescriptive authority. These changes occurred, in large part, because nurses and nursing organizations worked with legislators, consumer groups, and others to craft nurse practice acts that better reflect nursing's service to the public. This direct involvement of nurses and nursing in influencing legislation at the state level is an example of nurses' moral responsibility to "participate in the profession's efforts to implement and improve standards of nursing."[2]

[1]Margaret A. Burkhardt and Alvita K. Nathaniel. *Ethics & Issues in Contemporary Nursing.* Detroit: Delmar Publishers, 1998.
[2]American Nurses Association. *Code for Nurses with Interpretive Statements.* Kansas City, MO: Author, 1985.

SUMMARY OF PRINCIPLES AND APPLICATIONS

Administrative law can be complex and confusing. In addition, because it is not governed by the more traditional rules that define civil and criminal law, it is often feared by those who must occasionally deal with it. Nurses have more exposure to administrative law than other individuals, mainly through their professional roles and responsibilities. Keeping certain guidelines in mind can be helpful in successfully getting through the administrative maze should that need arise. Those guidelines include:

- Consulting the federal and state Administrative Procedure Act

- Asking for agency accountability for agency actions

- Utilizing access to agency record laws

- Retaining counsel experienced in administrative law when representation or advice is needed

- Attending federal or state agency meetings, especially those that affect health care delivery

- Advising congressional and state legislative representatives of needed changes in the respective laws dealing with regulatory agencies

- Educating the public, especially patients, on their rights and responsibilities under administrative laws that affect them and the delivery of health care

TOPICS FOR FURTHER INQUIRY

1. Develop a questionnaire to determine RNs' understanding of the Privacy Act and the Freedom of Information Act. Also ascertain whether or not the nurses surveyed have used either or both to obtain information about themselves, others, or a governmental agency. Analyze the data obtained, and if possible, utilize a similar questionnaire to obtain the same information from another professional group. Compare and contrast the data for the two groups.

2. File a Freedom of Information Act request under either the federal or state statute for specific information and report on the success or failure experienced. Analyze how the procedure worked (if so) or where it could be improved.

3. Attend a public meeting in which proposed rules are being discussed by an agency, preferably an agency affecting nursing. Identify who provides testimony and whether or not the agency considered that testimony in the drafting of the final rule.

4. Write a paper comparing and contrasting due process rights protected in administrative hearings with those protected in criminal proceedings. Utilize actual reported cases in analyzing the differences and similarities. If possible, utilize cases involving a nurse or another health care provider.

REFERENCES

1. Henry Campbell Black. *Black's Law Dictionary.* 7th Edition. St. Paul, Minn.: West Group, 1999, 46.
2. Lawrence Friedman, "Administrative Law and Regulation of Business," in *A History of American Law.* 2nd Edition. New York: Touchstone Books, 1985, 439.
3. *Id.* at 454–463.
4. Alfred Aman and William Mayton. *Administrative Law.* St. Paul, Minn.: West Group, 1998, 7.
5. This article and its sections read: "All legislative Powers herein granted shall be vested in a Congress of the United States, which shall consist of a Senate and House of Representatives. . . . The Congress shall have power . . . (18) To make all laws which shall be necessary and proper for carrying into Execution the foregoing Powers, and all other Powers vested by this Constitution in the Government of the United States, or in any Department or Officer thereof." U.S. Constitution, Article I, Section 1, Section 8 (18).
6. See, for example, *Field v. Clark,* 143 U.S. 649 (1892); *United States v. Grimaud,* 220 U.S. 506 (1911); *Crowell v. Benson,* 285 U.S. 22 (1932); *Amalgamated Meat Cutters v. Connally,* 337 F. Supp. 737 (D.D.C. 1971).
7. George D. Pozgar. *Legal Aspects of Health Care Administration.* 7th Edition. Gaithersburg, Md.: Aspen Publishers, 1999, 9–13.
8. *Id.*
9. See, generally, Aman and Mayton, *supra* note 4, at 1–39.
10. *Id.*
11. *Id.* at 559–601.
12. 28 U.S.C.A. Section 516 (1966).
13. 5 U.S.C. Section 551 *et seq.* (1946).
14. Administrative Procedure Act, *supra* note 13, at 552, 553, and 554.
15. Amendment V, U.S. Constitution (1791); Amendment XIV, U.S. Constitution (1868).
16. *Board of Regents of State Colleges v. Roth,* 408 U.S. 564 (1972).
17. *Id., quoting Meyer v. Nebraska,* 262 U.S. 390, 399 (1923).
18. Pozgar, *supra* note 7, at 10–12.
19. 5 U.S.C. Section 702 (1946).
20. *Id.* at Section 706.
21. *Id.*
22. 5 U.S.C. Section 555(c).
23. See, generally, Robert A. Griffith, "Defending Physicians Before Boards of Registration in Medicine," in *1994 Health Law Handbook.* Alice Gosfield, Editor. St. Paul, Minn.: West Group, 1994, 355–374; Aman and Mayton, *supra* note 4, at 714–722.
24. See *In re Zisook,* 430 N.E.2d 1037 (1982), *cert. denied,* 457 U.S. 1134 (1981); *Bellis v. United States,* 417 U.S. 85 (1974); *Fisher v. United States,* 425 U.S. 391 (1976).

25. *Braswell v. United States,* 487 U.S. 99 (1988). See also Aman and Mayton, *supra* note 4, at 714–722.

26. Black, *supra* note 1, at 754. In the federal system, any immunity granted must be for testimony "necessary to the public interest" (18 U.S.C. Section 6004) and the attorney general must approve the immunization before it is granted.

27. Black, *supra* note 1, at 754.

28. *Camara v. Municipal Court,* 387 U.S. 523 (1967); *See v. Seattle,* 387 U.S. 541 (1967).

29. Mark Rothstein. *Occupational Safety and Health Law.* 4th Edition. St. Paul, Minn.: West Group, 1998, 281 (with 1999 pocket part). See also *United States v. Blanchard,* 495 F.2d 1329 (1st Cir. 1974); *Camara* and *See, supra* note 28.

30. *United States v. Biswell,* 406 U.S. 311 (1972). In this case, the business involved was a pawn shop. Because the shop sold guns, the warrantless search, based on the Gun Control Act of 1968, was upheld. The Court reasoned that, among other things, the pawn shop owners waived their Fourth Amendment rights and gave their implied consent to warrantless administrative searches. Rothstein, *supra* note 29, *citing* 3 Wayne LaFave, *Search and Seizure,* Section 10.2 (1987) and Rothstein and Rothstein, "Administrative Searches and Seizures: What Happened to *Camara* and *See?*" 50 *Washington Law Review* 341 (1975).

31. Rothstein, *supra* note 29, at 282–283.

32. *Id.* at 283–284, *citing Stephenson Enterprises v. Marshall,* 578 F.2d 1021, 1023–1024 (5th Cir. 1978).

33. Rothstein, *supra* note 29 at 285–286, *citing See v. Seattle, supra* note 28, at 545 and *Air Pollution Variance Board v. Western Alfalfa Corp.,* 416 U.S. 861 (1974).

34. 21 U.S.C. Sections 301, 331, 334 (1938).

35. See, for example, 255 ILCS 65/20-135 (1998). This Illinois Nursing and Advanced Practice Nursing Act's section provides for temporary suspension of a license without a hearing when there is an immediate danger to the public from the licensee's conduct.

36. The Illinois Nursing and Advanced Practice Nursing Act, for example, mandates a hearing within 15 days after the suspension and is to be completed "without appreciable delay." *Id.*

37. Rothstein, *supra* note 29, at 422–428.

38. *NLRB v. Ochoa Fertilizer Corp.,* 368 U.S. 318, 322 (1961).

39. Aman and Mayton, *supra* note 4, at 256–306.

40. The Privacy Act of 1974, Pub. L. No. 93-579, 88 Stat. 1896 (September 27, 1975), codified at 5 U.S.C. Section 552a.

41. Section 2 of Pub. L. No. 93-579, *Congressional Findings and Statement of Purpose, cited in* 5 U.S.C. Section 552a (Historical Note), 204.

42. *Id.*

43. 5 U.S.C. Section 552a(b) (1974).

44. *Id.*

45. 5 U.S.C. Sections 552a(c) and 552a(e)(1)–(11).

46. 5 U.S.C. Section 552a(d)(1).

47. 5 U.S.C. Section 552a(f)(1)–(5).

48. Allan Adler and Henry Hammitt, "The Privacy Act," in *Litigation Under the Federal Open Government Laws.* Allen Adler, Editor. 20th Edition. Wye Mills, Md.: American Civil Liberties Union Foundation, 1997, 297, 305.

49. 5 U.S.C. Section 552a(d)(2), (f)(4).

50. 5 U.S.C. Section 552(a)(d)(3).

51. Adler and Hammitt, *supra* note 48, at 299.

52. 5 U.S.C. Section 552a(j)(1) and (2).

53. 5 U.S.C. Section 552a(k)(1)B(7).

54. Adler and Hammitt, *supra* note 48, at 312–313.

55. *Id.*

56. Pub. L. No. 100-503, 5 U.S.C. Section 552a(o).

57. *Id.*

58. Adler and Hammitt, *supra* note 48, at 314–316.

59. 5 U.S.C. Section 552 *et seq.* (1966), as amended.

60. Allan Adler, "Overview of the Freedom of Information Act," in *Litigation Under the Federal Open Government Laws, supra* note 48, at 1.

61. Katherine Meyer and Allan Adler, "Agency," in *Litigation Under the Federal Open Government Laws, supra* note 48, at 191–192.

62. Katherine Meyer, Allan Adler, and Elaine English, "Agency Records," in *Litigation Under the Federal Open Government Laws, supra* note 48, at 194.

63. 42 U.S.C. Section 552 (b)(1)–(9).

64. Allan Adler, "Administrative Process," in *Litigation under the Federal Open Government Laws, supra* note 48, at 20.

65. 42 U.S.C. Sections 552(a)(6)(A)(i); 552(a)(6)(A)(ii).

66. Adler, *supra* note 64, at 31.

67. These amendments were incorporated into the original Freedom of Information Act.

68. Adler, *supra* note 60, at 3.

69. See, for example, 70 ILCS 405/11 *et. seq.* (1984).

70. Pub. L. No. 94-409, Section 2, Stat. 1241, 42 U.S.C. Section 552b (1977).

71. S. Rep. No. 354, 94th Cong., 1st Sess. 1, *reprinted in Government-in-the-Sunshine Source Book: Legislative History, Texts, and Other Documents,* Committees on Government Operations, U.S. Senate and House of Representatives, 94th Cong., 2nd Sess. (1976).

72. 5 U.S.C. Section 552b(a)(1).

73. 5 U.S.C. Section 552b(c)(1)–(10).

74. 5 U.S.C. Section 552b(d)(1)–(m).

75. S. Rep. 354, *supra* note 71, at 7.

Criminal Law

9

KEY PRINCIPLES

- Misdemeanor
- Felony
- Actus Reus
- Mens Rea
- Classification of Crimes
- Beyond a Reasonable Doubt
- Bail
- Plea Bargain
- Presumption of Innocence
- Constitutional Protections of the Individual
- *Miranda* Warning

A nurse may be involved as a defendant in the criminal justice system in one of two ways: either as a private citizen or as a professional. In either instance, the nurse has allegedly violated the state or federal criminal laws, and if those allegations are proven beyond a reasonable doubt (the standard of proof in criminal actions), the nurse is found guilty of the crime. In criminal cases, unlike civil cases in which monetary compensation is sought for injuries or damages sustained, a guilty verdict brings with it some sort of punishment. The form of the punishment varies according to the crime, but some examples include fines, incarceration, and the death penalty.

In addition to some sort of sanction, criminal law is also very different from civil law because of the plaintiff who initiates the suit. With *civil* law, a private person or entity initiates the suit. The plaintiff in criminal cases, however, is always the state or federal government and its respective citizens, represented by the prosecutor (called the U.S. attorney in the federal court system and the district attorney, county attorney, prosecuting attorney, or state's attorney in the state system).[1] This person, with the help of law enforcement officers, is able to bring the case against the accused. The prosecuting attorney's responsibility is to ensure that when the public's safety or welfare is threatened or has been harmed, the guilty party is punished in some way for that behavior. Theories of punishment, and their specific effect on transgressors, have been the subject of much study in criminal law. Some include prevention of further criminal acts by the particular criminal ("particular deterrence"); prevention of further criminal acts by others who may be contemplating similar conduct ("general deterrence"); education of the public as to what conduct is good and bad; and retribution, making the offender "pay" for what he or she has done.[2]

This chapter will provide an overview of the criminal law and criminal justice system and its application to nurses and nursing practice, regardless of specialty area of practice or the health care delivery setting in which the nurse practices. It is important to keep in mind, however, that the information presented also applies to the nurse, or any other person, as a private citizen, that is, when not functioning in his or her professional role.

ESSENTIALS OF CRIMINAL LAW

As is the case with other types of law, criminal law did not develop, nor does it exist, in a vacuum. Rather, it is a creature of the state or federal legislature, both of which determine what kinds of behavior are criminal and what the punishment will be for a violation of the criminal statute or code.[3] In addition, behavior that violates criminal law may also violate respective civil or administrative statutes. For example, a nurse who falsifies narcotics records to "cover up" diversion of controlled substances from the employer may face not only criminal charges of forgery but also disciplinary action by the state nursing board or regulatory agency. Unlike civil law, and to a lesser extent administrative law, criminal law clearly involves all three branches of the government—legislative (passing laws), judicial (trying cases and hearing appeals, as well as determining sentences for those found guilty), and executive (issuing pardons and executive orders).

The criminal law cannot function without acknowledgment of constitutional (both federal and state) and jurisdictional limitations placed upon it. Constitutional limitations affect the power to pass laws that define criminal conduct (e.g., if the statute is vague or overly broad it will not be upheld), require treating an individual the same as others similarly situated unless there is a reasonable basis to do otherwise (equal protection), require clarity in informing the public what conduct is prohibited, and prohibit "ex post facto" laws (making conduct a crime after it has occurred) and violation of rights guaranteed by the Bill of Rights (see Table 9–1), to name a few.[4]

Jurisdiction is generally defined as the ability of the court to acknowledge and decide cases.[5] In constitutional terms, jurisdiction is limited in many ways. One important limitation deals with whether the federal or state government has the authority to prosecute a particular crime. An 1872 case[6] divided the powers of the government into four classes: (1) those belonging exclusively to the states; (2) those that can be exercised only by the federal government; (3) those that may be exercised concurrently and independently by both; and (4) those that the states can exercise, but only until Congress decides to exercise control over them.[7]

Thus, in any area involving criminal law where the federal government has taken control or "preempted" state law, it will be the federal government that will prosecute that alleged violation. An example would be any alleged violations of the many Medicare/Medicaid antifraud and abuse statutes. Conversely, when there is independent and concurrent jurisdiction, either the state or federal prosecutor may initiate criminal proceedings, so long as the state law does not conflict with the federal law. An example is in the area of controlled substances and their illegal possession and trafficking. In contrast, an example of a criminal law exclusively within state jurisdiction is practicing a particular licensed profession without the requisite license.

Constitutional Protections

Because any action taken against a person alleged to have committed a crime is carried out by the state or federal government, clear constitutional mandates protect the individual against arbitrary action by agents of the government, whether they be law enforcement officers or attorneys. Table 9–1 summarizes those protections mandated by the U.S. Constitution and case law interpreting the Constitution. State constitutions may provide additional protections but cannot limit those granted by the federal government.

Actors

Whenever criminal conduct is alleged, all three branches of the government are involved in the case, from its initiation until its completion. Thus, various actors and roles exist throughout the process. State or federal law enforcement officers initiate the prosecution of an alleged offender by investigating him or her, and if adequate evidence is available, arresting the person alleged to have committed the crime. In the federal system, law enforcement officers may be agents of the Federal Bureau of Investigation (FBI) or the Drug Enforcement Agency (DEA). State officers include state and local police.

Prosecutor

Those who prosecute the case wield great power in the criminal justice system because of

TABLE 9–1

Constitutional Protections of the Individual

RIGHT PROTECTED	SOURCE
Due process of law for government taking life, liberty, and property	5th Amendment (federal); 14th (states)
Establishment and exercise of religion, freedom of speech and press, peaceful assembly, and petition government for redress	1st Amendment
No unreasonable searches or seizures of self or property; search warrants issued upon "probable cause" only; illegally seized evidence excluded from trial	4th Amendment; *Draper v. U.S.; Stone v. Powell*
No self-incrimination or double jeopardy	5th Amendment
Counsel, speedy and public trial, impartial jury, notice of accusations, confront and cross-examine adverse witnesses, "compulsory process" for obtaining favorable witnesses	6th Amendment
No cruel or unusual punishment	8th Amendment

From: *Draper v. United States,* 358 U.S. 307 (1959); *Stone v. Powell,* 428 U.S. 465, *on remand,* 539 F.2d 693, *rehearing denied,* 429 U.S. 874. The right against self-incrimination protects one speaking about his or her involvement in a crime and thus is "testimonial" in nature. The Supreme Court has ruled in many cases that it does not extend to the production of physical evidence, such as blood or hair samples. See, for example, *Schmerber v. California,* 384 U.S. 757 (1966); *Doe v. United States,* 487 U.S. 201 (1988). In *Baldwin v. New York,* 399 U.S. 66 (1970), the U.S. Supreme Court held that the right to trial by jury guaranteed by the Sixth Amendment was applicable to those crimes involving a potential sentence of greater than 6 months in prison, or "serious" crimes. *Blanton v. North Las Vegas,* 109 S. Ct. 1289 (1989).

their ability to decide what cases will go to trial, what charges will be the basis of the trial, and whether or not a plea bargain will take place.[8] Federal and state prosecutors work closely with law enforcement officers and the other actors in the criminal justice system to ensure success with the case for which they are responsible.

Defense Attorney

The defense attorney also plays an important role in the criminal justice system. The attorney may be privately hired or may be appointed by the court (public defender) when the accused is indigent and unable to afford an attorney.

Judge

The judge is a pivotal actor in any judicial system, and the criminal justice system is no exception. In addition to presiding over the trial, ruling on issues of law and determining sentence in jury trials, the judge is involved in pretrial determinations such as setting bail. If there is no jury and a bench trial occurs, then the judge (or federal or state magistrate for some crimes of a less serious nature) determines the innocence or guilt of the accused.

Jury

There are two types of juries in criminal law: the grand jury and the trial jury. In either case, the membership is theoretically to be composed of "impartial" individuals who represent a "cross section of the public."[9] Grand juries exist in most federal and state systems, and their role is to determine if there is adequate evidence to bring the accused to trial. In contrast, the trial jury's role is to determine issues of fact in the trial and determine the guilt or innocence of the defendant.

There are two types of juries in criminal law: the grand jury and the trial jury.

Defendant

The defendant in a criminal trial is the individual accused of committing a certain crime or crimes. The defendant can be an individual, individuals, a corporation, a governmental agency, or the federal or state government itself.

Probation Officer and Other Personnel

One additional person with an important role is the probation officer, whose job it is to supervise the defendant who is placed on probation as a result of a determination of guilt or as a condition of release from jail or prison. The probation officer is mandated to report to the court regularly on the success of the probationer with the terms and conditions of the probation and must surrender the probationer to the court if those conditions are violated.[10]

Other actors in the criminal justice system include the court personnel discussed in the chapter on the judicial system.

Classification of Crimes

Crimes are classified in a manner that reflects the particular societal interest protected. Examples of interests protected include the integrity of the state or federal government (e.g., bribing a public official, perjury); public safety (e.g., assault, murder, and kidnapping); property (e.g., burglary, robbery, and theft of services); and honesty (e.g., forgery and falsification of legal documents and business records).[11]

Types of Crimes

There are essentially two types of crimes: misdemeanor and felony. A misdemeanor is a criminal offense punishable by a fine or imprisonment (usually a year or under) or both. Misdemeanors are considered less serious offenses than felonies. Examples of misdemeanors include breaching patient confidentiality, failing to report suspected or actual child abuse to the proper authority, and disseminating any false information concerning the existence of any sexually transmitted disease.

There are essentially two types of crimes: misdemeanor and felony.

A felony is a more serious offense than a misdemeanor and is therefore punishable by imprisonment for more than a year or by death. Examples of felonies include murder, diversion of controlled substances from a health care facility, and aggravated unlawful restraint.

Grades of Crimes

The state or federal statutes may also utilize different grades of crimes, such as Class A or Class B misdemeanors or felonies. The grading of the crimes reflects the seriousness of the offense and also aids the judge in sentencing the offender once the defendant is found guilty of the crime.

Components of Crimes
Act ("Actus Reus") and Intent ("Mens Rea")

In criminal law, a bad thought in and of itself cannot constitute a crime. Thus, any conduct that is allegedly criminal must consist of a criminal act (or a failure to act when there is a duty to do so, as when a nurse does not report suspected child abuse or neglect to the proper authorities), *and* criminal intent.

Intent traditionally has been defined to include consciously desiring a certain result as well as knowing a result is "practically certain" to occur as a result of certain conduct, regardless of the desire for a certain result.[12] Modern legal theory distinguishes intent from knowledge and calls it purpose or acting purposely.[13] Thus, crimes may require an individual to act intentionally or purposely, or they may require that the perpetrator knowingly or intentionally cause a specific result by his or her act or failure to act.[14]

It is also important to note that not all crimes require the intent or knowledge component to be applied exactly as discussed above. An individual can commit a criminal act by reckless conduct, reckless omission to act, or recklessly causing a particular result.[15] If a nurse acts in a reckless or indifferent manner and does not intervene when a patient is short of breath, for example, and a death occurs, the nurse might be charged with involuntary manslaughter. Similarly, if an individual acts with unreasonable risk of harm to another and that conduct is "grossly negligent" or defined as "willfully and wantonly negligent," then a charge of criminal negligence may be sustained (e.g., negligent homicide).

Other Acts

An individual may be found guilty of a crime not only when he or she is directly violating a criminal statute, but also when involved in criminal conduct in a more ancillary manner. Traditionally called party to the crime, but now given the name accomplice, this person can act in three main ways: (1) a principal in the second degree; (2) an accessory before the fact; and (3) an accessory after the fact.[16] Regardless of the terminology, however, the main focus is to evaluate two issues: (1) whether the accomplice gave assistance or encouragement to the principal or failed to carry out a legal duty to prevent the crime; and (2) whether the accomplice acted with the intent to encourage or aid the commission of the crime.[17]

A nurse may be involved as a principal in the second degree if, for example, he or she "aids and abets" the unauthorized practice of nursing by one who is not licensed as a nurse. If the nurse leaves the narcotics keys in a prearranged place for a nurse colleague so the latter can obtain controlled substances from the hospital narcotics supply, a charge of accessory before the fact may be possible.

If a nurse alters patients' narcotics records to indicate narcotics were given by a nurse colleague when the nurse colleague did not administer those drugs, the nurse's conduct may give rise to a charge of being an accomplice after the fact.

In addition to being named an accomplice, an individual may also become involved indirectly in a crime if a conspiracy takes place. A conspiracy is defined as an agreement between two or more individuals to intentionally carry out an act that is unlawful or to carry out a lawful act by unlawful means.[18] An example of a conspiracy is when two or more individuals or entities, or both, agree to limit the ability of a nurse-midwife to obtain admitting privileges on the staff of a particular hospital, in violation of the federal antitrust laws. This topic is discussed at length in Chapter 22.

Causation

Causation is just as important in the criminal law as it is in civil law. When criminal conduct is alleged, the prosecutor must be able to prove that the conduct of the accused was the "legal" or "proximate" cause of the specific result.[19] In the criminal law, the standard is phrased as the "but for this conduct, this result would not have occurred" test. It is also possible that an individual can be found guilty of a particular crime when his or her intended or reckless behavior does not specifically comply with that standard. In the latter example,

any variation in the actual result must be similar to, or create a risk of happening similar to, what the accused originally had in mind for causation to exist.[20] For example, if a nurse participates in an abusive search of a nursing home resident's pockets for missing money, and the resident's death results, the nurse can be found guilty of willfully violating state criminal law prohibiting such conduct even though such searches took place frequently.[21]

Application of Components to Selected Cases and Crimes

MURDER. Once defined simply as the killing of a human with malice aforethought,[22] murder is now defined by types: intent-to-kill murder, intent-to-do-serious-bodily-injury murder, depraved-heart murder, and felony murder.[23] Categories of murder may also be further delineated by degrees—first-degree and second-degree murder, for example—to provide guidelines for punishment. Unless the murder is justified (for example, in defending oneself), it is subject to prosecution. Theoretically, a nurse may be charged with any type of murder, depending on the circumstances. Table 9–2 lists selected murder prosecutions against nurses in the United States.

MANSLAUGHTER. Manslaughter was once defined as the unlawful killing of another without malice aforethought.[28] Now, however, it is defined

---

TABLE 9–2

Selected Murder Prosecutions Against Nurses

CASE	PROFESSIONAL INVOLVED	ALLEGATIONS	OUTCOME
Jones v. Texas[24]	LVN	Injecting children with medication (Anectine) that caused seizure or death; Jones charged with 1 count of murder and 7 counts of causing injury to other children	Trial court conviction of murder, with sentence of 99 years in prison; appeals court upheld trial court conviction
Rachals v. State[25]	RN	Injecting patients with medication (potassium chloride) that caused cardiac arrest; Rachals charged with 6 counts of murder and 20 counts of assault	Trial court convictions on murder counts; appeals court upheld trial court convictions
United States v. Narcisco and Perez[26]	RN (2)	Injecting patients with medication (Pavulon) that caused cessation of breathing on 51 occasions during a 6-week period; both nurses charged with 1 count of murder and 3 counts of assault	Trial court convicted both nurses; appeals court overruled trial court convictions on due process violations
Indiana v. Orville Lynn Majors[27]	LPN	Injecting patients with potassium chloride and Epinephrine that caused death; Majors charged with 7 counts of murder	Trial court convictions on 6 of the 7 counts; appeal will be filed

From: Beatrice Yorker, "An Analysis of Murder Charges Against Nurses," 1(3) *Journal of Nursing Law* (1994), 35–46; Janan Hanna, "Ex-Nurse Guilty in 6 Hospital Deaths," *Chicago Tribune,* October 18, 1999, 1, 13.

perhaps less distinctly as homicides not bad enough to be murder but too bad to be no crime whatever.[29] Categories of manslaughter include voluntary manslaughter (killing another in the heat of passion or when provoked),[30] involuntary manslaughter (killing another when committing a crime or when criminally negligent),[31] or criminal-negligence involuntary manslaughter (conducting oneself in a lawful manner but without proper care or necessary skill).[32] A nurse may be charged with any of the three categories of this crime depending on the circumstances. An example of circumstances that gave rise to allegations of manslaughter against three Colorado nurses is the case of Miguel Angel Sanchez.

Miguel Sanchez was born on October 15, 1997. Because his mother had been treated in the past for a sexually transmitted disease, the infant's physician prescribed an oil-based penicillin to be given by intramuscular injection. The route of administration was unclear, and the pharmacist checked the package insert of the medication without success.[33] The pharmacist filled the prescription, but "mistakenly" did so with 10 times the amount the physician prescribed. Even so, the pharmacist labeled the medication to be given IM.[34]

When Miguel's primary nurse received the medication for injection IM, she was concerned about the amount of medication and the number of times she would need to inject the infant in order to administer it. She expressed her concerns to her supervisor and to the pediatric nurse practitioner. Neither contacted the pharmacist or the doctor about the primary nurse's concerns. Instead, the pediatric nurse practitioner decided to change the route of administration from IM to IV. The supervisor then administered the IV penicillin to Miguel. Miguel died three hours later due to the formation of blood clots in his lungs. He was one day old at the time of his death.

Criminal negligence homicide charges were brought against all three nurses. The two nurses involved in changing the route of administration and the administration of the medication pled guilty to the criminal negligence homicide charges.[35] Miguel's primary nurse, who was not involved in the changing of the order or in the administration of the penicillin (she was not present when the penicillin was given), pled not guilty, and a jury acquitted her of all charges.

The nursing supervisor and the pediatric nurse practitioner received a sentence of two years of criminal probation and community service.[36]

Nurses and other health care professionals have also been involved in both criminal and civil cases over the removal of life support systems, including food and/or fluids. Several of these cases are discussed later in this chapter in the section Special Considerations.

ASSAULT AND BATTERY. Once classified as common law crimes (developed as a result of case law), assault and battery are now statutory crimes in all American jurisdictions.[37] The two are distinguishable by determining whether physical contact between the perpetrator and the victim occurred. An assault takes place when a person is fearful a battery may take place, but no actual touching occurs. A battery, on the other hand, requires that an offensive touching or bodily injury actually take place.[38] The two causes of action are further distinguished by degrees in many jurisdictions; in other words, simple assault, or aggravated battery (e.g., battery with intent to kill), or criminal-negligence battery.

A nurse may be charged with assault and battery when death of a patient occurs[39]; when unnecessary or unreasonable force is utilized against a patient (especially against an elderly patient in some jurisdictions)[40]; when a nurse, with a duty to act, simply omits that duty;[41] or when the nurse's conduct is directed against someone other than a patient.[42]

An assault takes place when a person is fearful a battery may take place, but no actual touching occurs. A battery . . . requires that an offensive touching or bodily injury actually take place.

FRAUD. Conduct constituting fraud, and possibly other related crimes (such as false pretenses and forgery), involves an individual falsely representing a fact (by conduct, words, false or misleading allegations) or concealing what should have been disclosed to another person. The intent is to deceive the person and cause him or her to act upon the information to his or her legal detriment.[43] Although the actual conduct alleged to be fraudulent may not involve property in the traditional sense, fraud is a crime against property as opposed to a crime against a person, such as murder.

In health care, fraudulent conduct can take place in a number of ways. One fairly common example is falsification of medical records, either by entering information that is clearly false (e.g., recording treatments that did not take place) or by signing another nurse's name on the narcotic record as the nurse who gave a particular narcotic when that nurse did not administer it.

When the falsification of the medical record takes the form of making false claims to Medicare to obtain payment for services not actually rendered, criminal penalties may apply under federal law.[44] If such false claims are made to other third-party payers, whether public or private, additional criminal charges may be brought against the nurse.

Other examples of fraud include utilizing the U.S. mail to carry out a fraudulent business activity (such as a school for practical nurses),[45] and practicing professional or practical nursing with a fraudulently obtained license, diploma, or record.[46]

Defenses to Crimes

The defendant in a criminal case can raise several defenses to contest the allegations against him or her. For example, when criminal intent is a component of the crime, the defendant can attempt to deny the presence of that mental state. When intent is not an essential element, as in strict liability crimes, the mental state defense would not be helpful.

The Insanity Defense

The insanity defense has undergone radical changes throughout its history. Generally, its purpose is not an acquittal (finding of not guilty) and subsequent release of the defendant. Rather, the successful insanity defense provides a particular verdict (such as not guilty but mentally ill or not guilty by reason of insanity) that results in involuntary treatment in a mental institution.[47] The defense has been identified by various names: the *M'Naghten rule* (during the commission of the crime, the defendant did not know he was doing wrong, could not control his conduct because of mental illness or disease, or did not know the "nature and quality of the act he was doing")[48]; the *Durham rule* (the crime was the result or "prod-

uct" of a mental disease or defect)[49]; and its most current rule, the *American Law Institute (A.L.I.) Substantial Capacity Test* (a person is not responsible for criminal conduct if, at the time of the criminal act resulting from a mental disease or defect, but not repeated criminal or otherwise antisocial conduct, the person lacked the substantial capacity to either appreciate the wrongfulness of his or her conduct or to conform to the requirements of the law).[50]

The use of the insanity defense has been the subject of much controversy and debate.[51] It is still a viable defense to many crimes, however, and will most likely continue to be unless there is a major change in the criminal justice or mental health system.

If the existence of a mental disease or defect inhibits the defendant in understanding the proceedings against him or her or prevents assistance with the attorney's defense against the charges (called incompetent to stand trial), then the defendant may not be tried, convicted, or sentenced until treatment renders him or her capable to stand trial. Similarly, if the defendant's mental illness does not allow an understanding of the nature and purpose of a death sentence, then that punishment cannot occur until such understanding is present. As with the insanity defense generally, this protection has been the subject of dispute for some time.[52]

The Chromosome and Automatism Defenses

Two additional defenses that are separate from the insanity defense, but are often discussed along with it, are the XYY Chromosome Defense and the Automatism Defense.[53] The former involves the presence of a chromosomal abnormality (the "super male" or XYY configuration) that supposedly results in increased likelihood of antisocial or criminal conduct.

The automatism defense, on the other hand, basically rests on the fact that because the criminal behavior happened in an unconscious or semiconscious state, it could not be the result of a voluntary act. Examples of conditions that might give support to this defense include epilepsy, premenstrual syndrome (PMS), and post-traumatic stress disorder (PTSD).[54]

The Intoxication Defense

When a criminal defendant raises this defense, he or she is stating that because of the voluntary or involuntary presence of drugs or alcohol, the required intention to commit the crime, or knowledge that the behavior was illegal, was nonexistent. This defense, of course, is helpful only when the mental state of the accused is a component of the crime (e.g., forgery, when the prosecution must prove intent to defraud).[55] It would not be helpful, however, when being under the influence of drugs or alcohol was an essential element of the crime, as in driving under the influence (DUI) cases.

In today's society, drug addiction and chronic alcoholism are often more the rule than the exception. As a result, this defense is receiving much scrutiny by the criminal justice system as a whole, especially when the defendant argues that the criminal act was the result of addiction or alcoholism. That argument has received varying responses, the most successful under the U.S. Constitution's Eighth Amendment prohibition against cruel and unusual punishment.[56] When addiction or alcoholism is not successful as a defense against a crime, it *may* serve to mitigate (reduce) the punishment imposed. In addition, chemical use is currently viewed as a disease. Thus, requiring evaluation, treatment, and rehabilitation as part of the criminal's sentence or probation may be helpful in reducing the possibility of future use and the commission of future crimes due to chemical substances.

The Infancy Defense

Briefly, this common law defense squarely rests on three basic presumptions, although their application to specific instances of criminal conduct by minors has not been as easily resolved, especially since some legislatures have modified the assumptions by statute. Children 7 years old and younger are absolutely presumed to be without criminal capacity; those 7 to 14 have a rebuttable presumption (one that can be overturned if sufficient proof is presented) of criminal incapacity; and those minors 14 years of age and over are seen as fully responsible for their actions.[57] All states provide for the establishment of juvenile courts, which may have exclusive, or specified, jurisdiction over crimes committed by minors.

The Entrapment Defense

The entrapment defense can be used only against law enforcement officers or individuals cooperating with law enforcement officers or agencies. The essence of this defense is that the law enforcement officer or agency oversteps their role in "encouraging" another to commit a crime and instead initiates the criminal act and convinces an otherwise uninterested individual to participate in that crime.[58] Moreover, the "otherwise uninterested individual" cannot have a predisposition to commit the crime. If he or she does have a propensity to engage in the proposed criminal conduct, and the law enforcement officer or agent simply provided the means for that crime to occur, then the defense will not be successful.

The Mistake or Ignorance Defense

This defense has been categorized into two specific types: mistake of fact and mistake of law. The former allows the defendant to nullify any criminal intent requirement of a crime, and the latter, in some instances, allows an individual to raise ignorance as to the existence of the law or a belief that the conduct was not prohibited by law.

Usually, ignorance of the law is not a successful defense in the criminal law. However, a mistake of fact may be helpful in defending against criminal charges. Suppose the death of a patient occurs because a nurse mistakenly injected what she thought was a certain medication prepared and labeled in the pharmacy, but which turned out to be another medication altogether—one to which the patient was allergic. No liability would exist because intent (mens rea) is an essential element of the crime of murder. Since the nurse had no intent to kill the patient, she would have no criminal liability.

The Necessity Defense

Based on the public policy premise that an individual in an emergency may be confronted with two choices (two "evils")—one to conform to the law and the other to break it—and either of them will produce a harmful result, this defense allows the individual to commit the crime, which is seen as the lesser of the two harms, and escape liability.[59] In other words, the criminal conduct is justified (or "necessitated") by the situation. Sometimes this defense is coupled with two others, the defense of others and duress.

Suppose an ED nurse, for example, is confronted with an individual who points a gun at a patient taken hostage and demands that she "get drugs" for him or he will "blow the patient's head off and kill everyone in the ED." If she stabs and kills the perpetrator with one of the ED instruments, the nurse may be able to successfully utilize one or more of these defenses against murder charges. Or, if a nurse trying to save a life in an emergency situation administers a medication without an order, he or she may well be able to avoid any criminal charge of practicing medicine without a license because of the "necessity" of the situation.

It is important to note that the effective use of any of the defenses discussed in this section requires weighing certain factors. The factors include the harm done, intent to avoid the greater harm at the time of the incident, determination by the court that the individual did *indeed* avoid the greater evil, and determination that the individual had no part in bringing about the situation in which he or she was required to make a choice.[60]

The Self-Defense Defense

Self-defense allows a person who is not an aggressor to use *reasonable* force against another when of the belief that he or she is in immediate danger of unlawful bodily harm and that the use of force is necessary to avoid the bodily harm.[61] Generally the amount of force that can be used by the potential victim depends on the circumstances. Deadly force against the aggressor is justified when the person reasonably believes that deadly force (which can cause death or serious bodily injury) may be inflicted.[62]

Nurses may be involved in situations that require self-defense when, for example, the nurse is attacked by a violent patient or an unruly family member.

Nurses may be involved in situations that require self-defense when, for example, the nurse is attacked by a violent patient or an unruly family member. It may also occur, as was discussed in the case *People v. Clark*,[63] when a nurse or licensed practical nurse attempts to defend herself against an alleged beating by a hospital security guard. These types of situations are always difficult ones, for the nurse may be charged with some sort of criminal conduct when the self-defense occurs in

a patient care situation. The court would probably evaluate the following factors in determining whether or not the actions taken by the nurse were truly self-defense: the details of the incident, whether the nurse immediately reported the incident to superiors, if the incident was documented in the patient record, if the nurse left or attempted to leave the scene, and whether the nurse attempted to obtain help from others, such as the police or hospital security.

ESSENTIALS OF CRIMINAL PROCEDURE

Criminal procedure is defined as the rules governing the process under which crimes are investigated, prosecuted, adjudicated, and punished.[64] It begins with the investigation of alleged criminal activity and terminates with the release of the offender, whether by return of a not guilty verdict and release of the individual, by a guilty verdict and completion of the sentence imposed, or by dismissal of the charges. Whatever the ultimate outcome of a case, the procedural aspects of criminal law must conform to state and federal constitutional mandates presented in Table 9–1. If they are not adhered to, the criminal defendant can challenge any part of the procedural process as a violation of those constitutional protections.

Pretrial Steps

Once a crime is reported to the police, the various phases of criminal procedure begin. It is important to note that the steps will be discussed in a sequential order, but in reality, several may be going on simultaneously.

Investigation

The investigation of a crime involves much footwork and results in the apprehension of a particular individual or individuals. When a specific individual's involvement in a crime is suspected, the investigation focuses on that particular person. The focus on a particular suspect may occur before arrest and booking of the individual. *When* the investigation takes place is important, for if the individual is questioned about the crime when "in custody" (in other words, involved in a custodial interrogation when he or she is not free to leave), the suspect has clear protections based on Fourth, Fifth, Sixth, and Fourteenth Amendment rights. Furthermore, the individual must be reminded of his or her rights by being given a *Miranda* warning to avoid a coerced confession.

The U.S. Supreme Court, in its *Miranda v. Arizona*[65] decision, scrutinized custodial interrogation proceedings and practices. The opinion blended the Fifth Amendment right against self-incrimination with the Sixth Amendment's guarantee of the right to counsel before trial.[66] The Court held that, at the time of arrest and *before* interrogation by law enforcement officers, the arrested person must be told (1) of the right to remain silent; (2) of the right to consult with an attorney and to have the attorney present during the interrogation; (3) that anything that is said can and will be utilized against him or her in court; and (4) that if he or she is unable to afford an attorney, one will be provided. Furthermore, the Court held that if this warning is not given to the arrestee, any statements made by the accused are inadmissible at trial.[67]

The U.S. Supreme Court, in . . . Miranda v. Arizona . . . blended the Fifth Amendment right against self-incrimination with the Sixth Amendment's guarantee of the right to counsel before trial.

In addition to being interrogated, a suspect or an arrestee may be asked to participate in other investigative procedures including a lineup, provide writing samples, and provide blood or hair samples. In some instances, the suspect's attorney must be present during these procedures.

During the investigation phase, physical evidence may also be of importance in linking the suspect to criminal conduct. Therefore, searches of the individual and the individual's home or office, for example, and the confiscation of matter, such as a weapon or documents, may occur. The investigators must adhere to the federal and state constitutional mandate that protects an individual against unreasonable and unwarranted searches and seizures.

Briefly, the mandate generally requires that searches and seizures occur only after a warrant has been issued by a neutral party (e.g., a judge or magistrate) upon probable cause.[68] Some excep-

tions to the general rule of a warrant are when there is probable cause *and* an urgent situation exists (that is, when delaying the search and seizure to obtain a warrant would endanger the success of the search or pose a threat of harm to the investigators) and when valid consent for the search has been obtained. If evidence is obtained in violation of the individual's Fourth Amendment rights, it is inadmissible at trial. This is known as the exclusionary rule or the fruit of the poisonous tree doctrine. The rule has been the subject of much debate and criticism, mainly because it is seen as rewarding criminal defendants.[69] Even so, it probably will survive in the criminal justice system until a better alternative is found to replace it.[70]

A nurse who is, or may be, the focus of any investigation involving potential criminal liability must be very careful to protect his or her constitutional rights. The investigation may be conducted by police, state investigators from the licensing body (who are also police officers), or employer security personnel. To begin with, the nurse should not speak to any of these individuals without seeking advice from an attorney who is knowledgeable about criminal law *and* practice issues. Furthermore, no statement should be given to law enforcement officers unless the attorney is present.

A nurse who is, or may be, the focus of any investigation involving potential criminal liability must be very careful to protect his or her constitutional rights.

If the nurse is asked to talk with any of these individuals, he or she should first ascertain whether or not an arrest is occurring or he or she is being detained. If neither is the case, the nurse should indicate that no interview or search will occur, and the nurse should leave. If the request occurs in the nurse's home, he or she should state the reasons for the position and ask that the investigators leave the home or the premises.

If, on the other hand, the nurse is informed he or she is being detained because of "reasonable suspicion" of being involved in a crime, or is being arrested, the nurse should not resist the detention or arrest but clearly request an attorney's presence and advice and inform the investigators that no statement will take place until that request is granted.

Likewise, if the law enforcement officers ask to search any belongings, such as the nurse's locker or home, or to conduct a body search, the nurse should ask if a search warrant has been obtained. If the investigators have no search warrant, the nurse is justified in refusing to participate in that search. If it takes place without the warrant, the nurse may have a basis for excluding any evidence obtained during that "illegal search," under the exclusionary rule. Of course, if the law enforcement officers can prove that the search or seizure was necessary even though no warrant existed (e.g., concern that if the locker were not inspected at that time, any potential evidence might be removed from it), then the evidence may be used against the nurse.

It is important to note that if the nurse, in an attempt to "cooperate" with the investigators, validly consents to a search without a warrant, then the law will not exclude any of the evidence obtained. The valid consent is seen as a waiver of the right to be searched only upon the issuance of a warrant.

In the workplace, nurses are not always initially investigated or questioned by the police but are sometimes examined by the employer's security staff or by a middle-level nurse manager or nurse executive. If the employer is a governmental entity (e.g., Veterans Administration or county institution), constitutional protections exist for the nurse employee. If employed by a private entity, however, these individuals are considered *private* actors and are not constrained by the constitutional mandates discussed thus far. As a result, the nurse needs to be clear that information given to internal staff members most often is shared with appropriate law enforcement personnel and can be used against the nurse in the criminal action as well as institutional disciplinary proceedings. The need for legal counsel, not only for advice but also for presence during any and all meetings with hospital administration, when possible, is imperative.

Grand Jury Indictment or Written Complaint and Information

When a crime involves a violation of federal law that is a felony, the Fifth Amendment requires that a grand jury be convened, and its role is to determine if there is "probable cause" to go forward with the prosecution of the suspect. Named so because of its size (usually more than 12 but no more than 23 members, as compared to a trial [petit] jury of 12 members), a grand jury has subpoena powers as well as the power to require witnesses to testify before it. If it determines that the suspect should be prosecuted, the grand jury issues an indictment (or "true bill") that formalizes, in writing, the accusations against the individual, and if the suspect has not yet been arrested, an arrest warrant is issued by a judge. If, on the other hand, the jury finds there is not probable cause to prosecute, then the case is dismissed with a "no bill."

Twenty states utilize the grand jury system.[71] The grand jury is not required in the state system, however, and many states employ another form of determining probable cause, the written complaint and information.

With this approach, law enforcement personnel share the results of their investigation with the state prosecutor through a complaint, which is a sworn statement listing the crimes committed and the evidence to support the charges. Then, most often, an arrest warrant is issued, the suspect is arrested, and an information—a formal, written accusation of the charges against the defendant—is drafted so that the arrestee can begin to develop his or her defense against the charges.

The determination of the grand jury and the decision by the prosecutor either to drop the charges or to go forward with the criminal case are called the preliminary hearing phase.

Arrest and Booking

An arrest occurs when a person is taken into custody by legal authority in response to a criminal charge.[72] As was discussed above, it usually occurs after an arrest warrant has been issued by a judge pursuant to an indictment or complaint. However, an arrest can occur without a warrant if there is probable cause that a crime is being committed or had been committed. In any of the circumstances, however, the individual arrested is truly in custody, and a *Miranda* warning must be given by the law enforcement agents.

The booking procedure involves recording identifying and other information (e.g., name, address, age) about the person arrested in the police log or blotter. Also included, of course, is the crime committed. Booking also includes fingerprinting and photographing the arrestee.

Setting Bail

Because an alleged violation of criminal law, whether a misdemeanor or felony, results in an arrest and possible incarceration, a hearing is held to determine if bail can be set. Bail is used to ensure that the accused will remain in the state and be present in court for the trial of the alleged crime(s). Bail consists of money, and can be cash. Bail may also be arranged through a bail bondsman, where the accused enters into a contract with that bondsman to post the amount of the bail for a percentage of the bail amount. If the accused does not show up for court, or flees the state, then the court is paid the amount of the bond, and the defendant forfeits the money.

The amount of the bond is determined by many factors, including the type of crime and the accused's prior criminal record, if any, and threat to public safety.[73] Sometimes the defendant is released on a personal recognizance bond because of his or her integrity and the court's belief that he or she will comply with all the proceedings.

In other instances, bond is not available at all, especially when the crime is a heinous one, such as the rape and murder of a child or elderly person. If bond is denied, the accused remains in the custody of law enforcement officers.

Arraignment

The arraignment is the first formalized court appearance for the accused in which he or she is informed of the charges, is informed of his or her rights, and is asked to plead guilty or not guilty to the charges. Most often, defendants plead not guilty at this pretrial stage. If a not guilty plea is made, the prosecutor is then required to prove every charge the defendant is accused of at trial.

If, however, the defendant pleads guilty, the judge must ascertain that he or she is doing so voluntarily and clearly understands the ramifications of the plea, for doing so waives all of the constitutional rights that would otherwise protect the defendant, including, of course, the right to a jury trial. If the judge accepts the guilty plea, then no trial occurs, and the defendant's sentence is decided and carried out.

Discovery, Motions, and Plea Bargaining

If the defendant has entered a not guilty plea during the arraignment and the case is to proceed to trial, a discovery period usually takes place during which the accused's attorney is given information in the possession of the prosecutor concerning the defendant and the crimes charged. Although state laws concerning discovery may vary, most provide for "reciprocal discovery," meaning that an exchange of information from both the prosecution *and* defense takes place.

The federal rules of criminal procedure clearly allow for ample discovery. Furthermore, under the *Brady* decision[74] and subsequent cases,[75] the U.S. Supreme Court has held that a prosecutor is required to provide the defense attorney with evidence "favorable to (the) accused" and "material to . . . guilt or punishment." If such existing evidence is not given to the defense, the accused's due process rights are violated. Examples of evidence that constitute discovery include statements to police officers, lists of property belonging to the defendant, reports of scientific tests or comparisons, and witness statements.

Also important at this step in the pretrial phase is the opportunity for defense counsel to attempt to exclude evidence that has been obtained in violation of his or her client's constitutional rights. Examples might include a statement of the defendant obtained without the required *Miranda* warning, evidence seized in violation of the accused's Fourth Amendment rights, and lack of assistance of counsel at any "critical stage" of prosecution. Or challenges may be made on the basis of imperfections in the statutory law under which the accused is charged; for example, that the statute is vague or that it violates the individual's other constitutional guarantees, such as freedom of religion or assembly.

It is important to note that in many states, criminal procedure statutes require the defendant to raise any defenses he or she may decide to use at trial at this time. Thus, if the defense decides to use the *necessity defense,* for example, it must be disclosed now, or its use may be barred at trial.

Plea bargaining also can take place at this time, although it may realistically occur during any of the procedural phases. Plea bargaining is the process in which the accused, through his or her attorney, agrees to plead to a lesser offense (or one of multiple charges) in exchange for a concession by the prosecutor.[76] The final settlement is subject to court approval, either during its negotiation or before it will officially be accepted by the court. The accused can plead guilty to a lesser crime (one less serious than the one he or she is charged with), called a *charge bargain,* or plead guilty to some of the counts of a multicount complaint or indictment and, in return, receive a lesser sentence, called a *sentence bargain,* or both.[77]

Many factors enter into the decision to engage in the controversial practice of plea bargaining on both the prosecution and defense sides. They include saving time by resolving a case without many hours of preparing for and participating in a lengthy trial; achieving desirable outcomes in which the prosecuting attorney is assured a conviction and the accused is guaranteed a lesser sentence than is probable at trial[78]; and saving taxpayers' dollars by avoiding unnecessary appeals of trial decisions.

Trial

The Sixth Amendment of the U.S. Constitution guarantees the criminal defendant certain rights during the trial (see Table 9–1) that make the criminal trial very different from a civil one. For example, the accused does not have to testify in his or her own defense unless the defendant and the attorney decide to do so. A presumption of the innocence of the defendant is also unique to a criminal trial. More accurately described as an assumption,[79] this principle states that simply because an individual is charged with a crime does not mean he or she is guilty of that conduct. The presumption requires that the prosecuting attorney meet his or her burden of proof—both in presenting evidence and establishing the guilt of the accused—"beyond a reasonable doubt."

A presumption of the innocence of the defendant is . . . unique to a criminal trial.

The burden of proof is higher in a criminal case and requires the prosecution to prove each and every element of the crime(s) charged beyond a reasonable doubt. Reasonable doubt has been difficult to define but is often described as not possessing, to moral certainty, a conviction of the truth of the charge(s) against the defendant.[80] This standard is much higher than in civil trials or

administrative proceedings because the verdict of guilty in a criminal trial results in punishment that may include incarceration or death. Since deprivation of life, liberty, and property are constitutionally protected interests, a high degree of proof is necessary before these interests can be taken from the individual. Furthermore, in all but a few states, the jury must return a unanimous verdict in support of the defendant's guilt or innocence.[81]

The trial itself follows a format similar to civil trials in that there is:

1. Jury selection (voir dire)
2. Opening statements by each attorney
3. Presentation of the prosecutor's case (with cross-examination by defense counsel)
4. Presentation of the defense case (with cross-examination by the prosecutor)
5. Closing arguments
6. Jury instructions by the judge
7. Jury deliberation
8. Verdict

Sentencing

If the defendant is acquitted by the jury, the case is over, and the government is not able to retry the case. If, however, the defendant is found guilty, a sentencing hearing is held after the trial itself. The sentence imposed is usually dictated by Congress or the state legislature, thus allowing the judge little, if any, deviation from those guidelines. Furthermore, parole board decisions also are often carefully delineated in sentencing statutes.[82]

Post-trial Steps

Clearly, either before or after sentencing takes place, the criminal has many options to challenge his or her conviction and/or sentence. Some of those options include a motion for a new trial (alleging some violation of constitutional or other rights); an appeal of the decision of the state or federal trial court in which, if successful, the conviction may be overturned or a new trial ordered in certain situations; and filing a *writ of habeas corpus* ("you have the body"), which asks the court to immediately release the individual because he or she is being illegally imprisoned or detained. The court determines if the imprisonment is illegal and, if so, if the individual should be released.

The court's decision concerning the writ can also be appealed.

SPECIAL CONSIDERATIONS

Generally, the criminal law has not been utilized to regulate nursing or medical practice. Early cases that did involve criminal allegations against health care providers focused on liability for withdrawing or withholding treatment from patients.[83] Although liability for withdrawing or withholding treatment is still a concern, the special circumstances in which criminal conduct has been alleged against health care professionals, including nurses, have changed. Additional areas of special concern include practicing a profession without a license and the criminalization of professional negligence.

Withdrawing and Withholding Treatment

Several early cases concerning the removal of life-sustaining treatment and their impact, albeit somewhat indirectly, on criminal liability are important to mention briefly here (these, and other cases, are discussed at greater length in Chapter 13, Issues in Death and Dying). In two early cases, *In the Matter of Karen Quinlan*[84] and *In the Matter of Shirley Dinnerstein,*[85] respective civil courts held there would be no civil or criminal liability for any participant involved in the removal of life-sustaining treatment in consultation with the physician (whose decision is made with "skill and care" and based on accepted medical standards), the patient and/or his legal representative, the family, and, clearly the case in *Quinlan,* an ethics committee. Furthermore, the courts held that no prior judicial approval of a decision based on those guidelines was necessary.[86]

In Re Claire Conroy[87] involved the New Jersey Supreme Court's decision that an incompetent patient's feeding tube could be removed under specific guidelines drawn by the court. This reversed the lower appellate court's ruling that removal of the nasogastric tube would be unlawful and tantamount to killing her.[88] Also, in *John F. Kennedy Memorial Hospital v. Bludworth,*[89] the Supreme Court of Florida upheld the right of a terminally ill, comatose patient's choice to terminate treatment (in this case, a ventilator) through his "living" or "mercy" will. The court echoed the *Quinlan* and *Dinnerstein* decisions in holding that any individual, including a guardian, who participates in

a good-faith decision to cease treatment will not be held civilly or criminally liable for that decision, and that prior judicial approval for it is not necessary.[90]

These and other cases do not provide *absolute* immunity from civil or criminal liability for decisions to withhold or withdraw treatment, for despite the best intentions of all of the individuals involved, disagreements concerning decisions to discontinue treatment may arise. Moreover, there may be questions as to the "good faith" of one or more individuals who participate in such decisions. Furthermore, there will be no protection from criminal charges when a nurse or other health care provider decides on his or her own to withhold or withdraw treatment, particularly with no input from the patient, the legally recognized surrogate decision maker, and/or the family. Also, one must keep in mind that all of the cases discussed here were decided before the U.S. Supreme Court's decision in *Cruzan,* which has potentially far-reaching and yet unforeseen implications, both civilly and criminally.

Even so, the nurse who is involved with carrying out decisions to withhold or withdraw treatment can be somewhat comfortable in relying on these decisions in relation to criminal liability. However, the suggested guidelines are important to adhere to. They include obtaining written orders for any care decisions to withdraw or withhold treatment and physician documentation of the reasons for the decision to cease treatment; including the patient, or his legal representative, in such decisions; making any advance directive a part of the patient's medical record; informing the patient and family of any decisions that are made; assuring adequate nursing documentation of the patient's care; utilizing ethics committees to confirm decisions to terminate treatment; and never making a unilateral decision to withdraw or withhold treatment from a patient. If possible, the nurse should participate as a member of an ethics committee, including, if possible, a nursing ethics committee, to provide invaluable input that aids in reasoned decision making in patient/client care based on clear consideration of ethical dimensions.[91]

Practicing a Profession Without a License

State practice acts make the practice of a particular profession—nursing, medicine, and pharmacy, for example—without a license a criminal

ETHICS CONNECTION 9–1

Withholding and withdrawing medically futile treatment usually is grounded in the moral principles of respect for autonomy and beneficence. Although ethical practices concerned with withholding or withdrawing treatment are reasonably clear in situations of medical futility, emotional responses and personal values almost always complicate the decision making. As with so many other ethical practices, clear, unambiguous communication is central to making a decision to withhold or withdraw treatment and to following through with the decision. When the client has been clear about his or her treatment preferences and has had a conversation about those preferences with the surrogate decision maker, other family members, and attending physician, there is less likelihood that the legal system will be centrally involved in decision making. However, when the client does not have an advance directive, or has indicated a treatment preference but has not discussed it with the family, dissension frequently results. Conflicts occur both within and between the family and health care team. Such dissension, if not resolved, leads to civil and/or criminal charges much more often than when all concerned parties agree with the decisions.

Conflict between personal and professional moral values is present in many situations when treatment is to be withheld or withdrawn.[1] Nurses need to be aware of current ethical knowledge and practices regarding medical futility and withholding and withdrawing treatment. Refusing to abide by a morally acceptable decision creates unnecessary and unacceptable distress for the client and family. For example, an attending physician whose religious beliefs require that he never withhold or withdraw treatment refused to withhold parenteral nutrition from a dying client. The client had been clear that he did not want any intravenous or other life-prolonging treatments. The attending physician, however, disagreed and verbally threatened the family and nurses with criminal charges, saying that they would be "guilty of homicide" when the client died. When the client's or surrogate's decision is morally acceptable and in agreement with professional codes and values, but conflicts with the individual practitioner's personal values, the practitioner must be prepared to withdraw from the case so that another may provide care.

[1]Margaret A. Miller and Margaret R. Douglas, "Presencing: Nurses Commitment to Caring for Dying Persons," *International Journal of Human Caring* (1999), 24–31.

offense.[92] Likewise, hiring someone to practice a specific profession without a valid, current license is also a crime. Moreover, aiding and assisting another to practice a licensed profession without a valid, current license is also considered criminal conduct. Some state statutory schemes make a first offense a misdemeanor with subsequent or second convictions a felony.[93]

State practice acts make the practice of a particular profession . . . without a license a criminal offense.

Nurses in advanced practice—nurse-midwives, nurse practitioners, nurse anesthetists, and clinical specialists—probably are most likely to be included in a criminal suit alleging the unlicensed practice of *medicine* because of their very independent and nontraditional roles and responsibilities. This was clearly the situation in the *Sermchief* case, discussed in Chapter 21, in which the nurse practitioners were functioning pursuant to physician-developed protocols for prescribing medications and performing other functions in rural obstetric and gynecologic clinics throughout Missouri. Although the Missouri Supreme Court decided in favor of the nurse practitioners and the physicians, this challenge to advanced practice continues today in many states across the country.

Nurses who are in advanced practice, those who are asked to perform nontraditional care in any health care delivery setting, and those who decide to initiate their own practice as an entrepreneur need to be aware of the potential criminal liability resulting from their expanded practice. To avoid unnecessary inclusion in a suit alleging the unauthorized practice of a particular profession, the nurse must know the state nurse practice act and its rules and regulations intimately. By conforming to both, the nurse can stay well within the scope of practice of *nursing* and his or her specialty. Furthermore, it is important for the nurse to be familiar with other state practice acts, including the medical practice act, pharmacy registration act, physical therapy practice act, and psychologist registration act to avoid an unknowing, but nonetheless clear, violation that may result in criminal liability for the nurse.

In addition, nurse administrators or nurse executives who hire nursing staff need to ensure that each nurse considered for a position, whether an RN, an LPN, or a nurse with a specialty license, such as a nurse-midwife, has a valid and current license. If the state nurse practice act requires certain certification or credentialing for advanced practice, those additional criteria should also be checked.

Each RN or LPN must adhere to renewal periods for the license and ensure that the license (and any required credentialing) does not expire. If expiration occurs, the nurse should not practice nursing until the license is renewed. Likewise, if the nurse moves to a new state and applies for licensure through endorsement, no nursing practice should occur until a valid license has been issued or, if the state practice act allows, until a temporary permit has been obtained.

Criminal Law and Professional Negligence

Health care professionals, including nurses, increasingly face criminal charges for patient clinical injuries or deaths once seen only as professionally negligent.[94] Although criminal cases have been brought against health care providers for such injuries or deaths—most notably physicians since 1894[95]—recently, registered nurses[96] and a "physician-directed" corporation have been involved in criminal cases where a serious injury or the death of a patient has occurred.[97]

Situations resulting in criminal charges include failure to provide care in an emergency department to an 11-month-old boy, resulting in the infant's death[98]; a "botched" liposuction procedure that resulted in the death of a 43-year-old woman[99]; and endangering the welfare of a stroke patient, alleged against three New Jersey nurses whose conduct resulted in the death of the 74-year-old patient.[100]

The charges brought against these, and other, health care professionals include murder,[101] manslaughter,[102] and willful neglect.[103]

Various explanations have been given for the increase in prosecuting what was once seen only as professionally negligent conduct. They include (1) "failure" of health care professions to "police" their own members; (2) "failure" of regulatory boards (e.g., boards of nursing and boards of medicine) to discipline licensees who violate practice

acts; (3) criminal statutes that are too general and too vague; and (4) prosecutors' wide discretion in bringing criminal charges against health care providers when serious injuries or deaths occur in the provision of health care.[104]

Nurses, other health care practitioners, and respective professional organizations have been critical of the increase in criminal cases against health care providers.[105] The criticisms are varied and include, for example, the "singling out" of nurses when the real problems are short-staffing, overworked staff, and other "system failures."[106] Moreover, others argue that when a serious patient injury or death occurs, the conduct should be evaluated by the appropriate state board. Those regula-

---

tory boards, the argument continues, are set up to deal with unsafe and/or negligent practice, so that when "punishment" is necessary, discipline imposed by the regulatory boards should suffice.

It is certain that the controversy surrounding the use of the criminal law when professional negligence results in a patient injury or death will not be easily resolved. However, it is clear that the nurse must be ever vigilant in his or her duties of protecting the patient's safety and well-being within the legal and ethical parameters of that role. Because accountability is something all health care professionals must accept, the potential of criminal liability for "fatal errors" and "clinical mistakes" may be difficult to escape.[107]

ETHICS CONNECTION 9–3

"The nursing profession is committed to the welfare and safety of all people."[1] Error in medicine and health care is a national problem that is a serious threat to human safety and welfare. It is often the case that such error occurs because of institutional system problems that are not solely the responsibility of the professionals who have made the errors. It is immoral both to place clients at unnecessary and unacceptable risk and to penalize individual professionals for organizational problems. As health care becomes more complex, staffing becomes more minimal, and patients' length of stay becomes shorter, nurses are at ever greater risk of making errors that may be considered negligent. This creates a serious problem for both the public and for the nursing profession.

Working toward reduction of systematized error in health care is a critical priority. Professional organizations such as the American Nurses Association recognize how important it is to work toward the prevention of error in a systematic, national way. Although protection of the public is the primary reason for addressing error prevention, protection of nurses is a consideration as well. There is an increasing tendency to bring criminal charges against nurses who have been accused of professional negligence. It is morally unjust for individual nurses to bear a disproportionate burden of punishment for errors that have arisen partly or primarily from institutional problems.

[1]American Nurses Association. *Code for Nurses with Interpretive Statements.* Kansas City, Missouri: Author, 1985.

SUMMARY OF PRINCIPLES AND APPLICATIONS

Although nurses are more frequently involved in civil suits, it is clear that the possibility exists for the RN or LPN to be a defendant in a criminal case. Because inclusion in a criminal case has far-reaching implications, including the possibility of incarceration, it is vital that the nurse be ever mindful of professional and personal conduct that might result in criminal liability. Furthermore, if the nurse becomes the target of a criminal investigation or is named in a criminal suit, the following guidelines can be helpful:

- Retain an attorney who concentrates his or her practice in criminal law and who is familiar with practice issues

- Remember the constitutional protections afforded any individual who is accused of a crime, and exercise them

- Any statement made to a law enforcement officer can be used against the speaker

- Statements made to health care delivery system security personnel can be turned over to law enforcement agents

- Criminal liability may exist as a result of state *and* federal laws, so an understanding of both is essential

- The elements of a crime include an act, intent, and causation

- There are defenses to criminal conduct that may help in reducing a criminal charge or result in an acquittal

- Substantive and procedural protections afforded a person through the criminal justice system include the right to counsel at any "critical stage" of the proceedings, which includes a detention or arrest

- If asked to speak to any law enforcement person when suspected of a crime or criminal conduct, remember that a *Miranda* warning must be given to anyone detained, in custody, or arrested. Under no circumstances should the nurse "volunteer" information. If not being detained, or not in custody, or not arrested, the nurse has a right to leave

- When involved in decisions about withdrawing or withholding treatment, obtain written orders from the physician and provide good documentation concerning the care given and care not given pursuant to those orders

- Never practice nursing without a current and valid license

- Verify that nursing staff have current and valid licenses

- Provide patient care consistent with standards of practice

TOPICS FOR FURTHER INQUIRY

1. Analyze any cases filed against nurses involving the practice of nursing in the state in which you practice. Determine the differences and similarities of the charges against the respective nurse defendants. Based on the analysis, identify guidelines that could help nurses avoid future potential allegations of criminal conduct.

2. Critically evaluate one of the defenses to a crime. Attempt to use a reported case against a nurse involving the practice of nursing. If none is available, a "case" can be created. In either event, focus on such issues as whether the defense would aid the nurse defendant and why. What might be the potential difficulties in using the defense based on the case being evaluated? Suggest other possible defenses.

3. With the consent of the facility and following privacy and confidentiality mandates, analyze the documentation done in patient medical records when medical care is withdrawn or withheld. Areas to evaluate include documentation of the existence of an advance directive; whether or not the advance directive is included in the chart; documentation by physician of orders consistent with the advance directive; if no advance directive exists, how the patient's consent for refusal of treatment was recorded.

4. Write a position paper on the presumption of innocence. Include ways to improve the presumption or why it should be eliminated altogether.

REFERENCES

1. Lawrence Baum. *American Courts: Process and Policy*. 4th Edition. Boston: Houghton Mifflin Company, 1998, 168–169.
2. Wayne LaFave and Austin Scott. *Criminal Law*. 2nd Edition. St. Paul, Minn.: West Group, 1986, 22–29 (with 1999 pocket part) (Hornbook Series).
3. Baum, *supra* note 1, at 6.
4. LaFave and Scott, *supra* note 2, at 90–190.
5. Henry Campbell Black. *Black's Law Dictionary*. 7th Edition. St. Paul, Minn.: West Group, 1999, 855.
6. *Ex parte McNiel,* 80 U.S. (13 Wall.) 236 (1872).
7. *Id.*
8. Baum, *supra* note 1, at 168–169.
9. Henry Abraham. *The Judicial Process*. 7th Edition. New York: Oxford University Press, 1998, 122.
10. Black, *supra* note 5, at 1220.
11. LaFave and Scott, *supra* note 2, at 29–37.
12. *Id.* at 216–217.
13. *Id.* at 218–220.
14. *Id.* at 216–220.
15. *Id.* at 231–233.
16. *Id.* at 569–573.
17. *Id.* at 576.
18. *Id.* at 525.
19. *Id.* at 277.
20. *Id.* at 279.
21. *People v. Coe,* 501 N.Y.S.2d 997 (Sup. 1986).
22. Black, *supra* note 5, at 1038.
23. LaFave and Scott, *supra* note 2, at 612–632.
24. 716 S.W.2d 142 (Tex. App. 1986).
25. 364 S.E.2d 867 (1988).
26. 446 F. Supp. 252 (1977).
27. Cause No. 83 CO 1-971 2-CF-0074 (Vermillion County). Additional information about this case can be found at www.courttv.com/
28. LaFave and Scott, *supra* note 2, at 652.
29. *Id.*
30. Black, *supra* note 5, at 976.
31. *Id.*
32. LaFave and Scott, *supra* note 2, at 668–669.
33. Nancy J. Brent, "Criminal Indictments in Denver: Could It Happen to You?" 11(22) *Nursing Spectrum* (1998), 12 (citations omitted).
34. Paul R. Van Grunsven, "Medical Malpractice or Criminal Mistake?—An Analysis of Past and Current Criminal Prosecutions for Clinical Mistakes and Fatal Errors," 2(1) *DePaul Journal of Health Care Law* (1997), 34.
35. Brent, *supra* note 33, at 12.
36. *Id.* The deferred judgment against the two nurses will be dismissed if they successfully complete their sentences, resulting in a "clean" record for both of them. In addition to the criminal sentence, the Colorado Board of Nursing suspended both licenses for one year. When the licenses are reinstated, the licenses will be placed on probation for a two-year period.
37. LaFave and Scott, *supra* note 2, at 684.
38. *Id.* at 685.
39. *Commonwealth v. Knowlton,* No. 84-7322 (Mass. 1984), *reported in National Law Journal,* October 29, 1984, at 13. This case involved a nurse who allegedly turned off a patient's respirator while caring for the patient in his home. The patient died, and the nurse was charged with assault and attempted murder. The jury returned a verdict of not guilty. Also, in *People v. Nygren,* 696 P.2d 270 (Colo. 1985), a nursing home, its director of nursing, and charge nurse were charged with second-degree assault for giving a patient Thorazine that was not ordered for that patient and was used to sedate him. The patient died as a result of the injection.
40. See, for example, S.H.A. 720 ILCS 5/12-4.6 (1989), which provides for the crime of Aggravated Battery of a Senior Citizen. The crime is a Class 2 felony.
41. For example, if a nurse or other health care provider fails to warn a blind patient that he or she is walking toward an open window, and the patient falls out of the window and is injured, the nurse could be charged with intentionally or recklessly causing that battery. LaFave and Scott, *supra* note 2, at 686.
42. For example, in *People v. Clark,* 474 N.Y.S.2d 409 (N.Y. City Criminal Ct. 1984), a licensed practical nurse was charged with assault in the third degree, criminal trespass, and menacing stemming from her refusal to show a hospi-

tal security guard her identification card when asked. In addition to refusing to show her ID, Ms. Clark also swore at the guard and kicked him. Although the case was ultimately dismissed because of a pending civil suit brought by the nurse against the security guard for injuries he inflicted upon her, it stands as an example of how a nurse may be involved in an assault case for conduct other than that involving the care of a patient.

43. Black, *supra* note 5, at 670–672.
44. 42 U.S.C. Section 1395nn *et seq.* (1977). These amendments are called the *Medicare and Medicaid Anti-Fraud and Abuse Amendments of 1977.*
45. *Adams v. United States,* 347 F.2d 665 (1965), *cert. denied,* 382 U.S. 975 (1965).
46. S.H.A., 225 ILCS 65/10-5 (1998).
47. LaFave and Scott, *supra* note 2, at 304.
48. *Id.* at 311.
49. *Id.* at 323.
50. American Law Institute. *Model Penal Code* Section 4.01 (1955).
51. See, for example, Richard Bonnie, Norman Paythress, Steven Hodge, John Monahan and Marlene Eisenberg, "Decision-Making in Criminal Defense: An Empirical Study of Insanity Pleas and the Impact of Doubted Client Competence," 87 *Journal of Criminal Law and Criminology* (1996), 48–82; Randi Ellias, "Should Courts Instruct Juries as to the Consequences to a Defendant of a 'Not Guilty by Reason of Insanity' Verdict?" *Journal of Criminal Law and Criminology* (1995), 1062–1116.
52. See, for example, Alaya Meyers, "Rejecting the Clear and Convincing Evidence Standard for Proof of Incompetence," 87 *Journal of Criminal Law and Criminology* (1997), 1016–1077.
53. LaFave and Scott, *supra* note 2, at 377–387.
54. *Id.* at 383.
55. *Id.* at 389.
56. *Id.* at 395–398. Some of the cases dealing with this issue are *Robinson v. California,* 370 U.S. 660 (1962) (one cannot be convicted of a criminal offense for "being addicted to the use of narcotics"—often called the "Status Case"), and *Powell v. Texas,* 392 U.S. 514 (1968), *rehearing denied,* 393 U.S. 898 (1968).
57. LaFave and Scott, *supra* note 2, at 398.
58. *Id.* at 420.
59. *Id.* at 441–443.
60. *Id.* at 441–450.
61. *Id.* at 454.
62. *Id.*
63. See note 42, *supra.*
64. Black, *supra* note 5, at 382.
65. 384 U.S. 436 (1966), *rehearing denied,* 385 U.S. 890 (1966).
66. Ralph Chandler, Richard Enslen, and Peter Renstrom. *Constitutional Law Deskbook: Individual Rights.* 2nd Edition. St. Paul, Minn.: West Group, 1993, 370 (May 1999 pocket part).
67. *Miranda v. Arizona, supra* note 65. In 1968, Congress enacted a new law based on *The 1968 Crime Control Bill,* which allows some confessions and statements to be admitted into evidence when the suspect was not given the *Miranda* warning, so long as the statements "were not coerced." The decision as to whether to allow the statements into evidence was given to the judge hearing the case. "Death of the Miranda Rule," 4(2) *USCA Advantage* (1999), 8. In a recently decided case, the Fourth Circuit Court of Appeals reversed a federal district court decision barring the defendant's confession from being introduced into evidence. The appeals court held that if the defendant's statement was voluntary, it was admissible, even in the absence of his being given his *Miranda* rights. *Id., citing (U.S. v. Dickerson,* 1999 WL 61200). On June 26, 2000, the U.S. Supreme Court, in a 7-2 decision, overruled the Fourth Circuit Court of Appeals, holding that the *Miranda* warning is a right based in the U.S. Constitution. Jan Crawford Greenburg, "High Court Upholds Miranda Warning," *Chicago Tribune,* June 27, 2000, 1, 14.
68. Chandler, Enslen, and Renstrom, *supra* note 66, at 703.
69. *Id.* at 652.
70. *Id.*
71. Henry J. Abraham. *The Judicial Process: An Introductory Analysis of the Courts of the United States, England and France.* 7th Edition. New York: Oxford University Press, 1998, 113.
72. Black, *supra* note 5, at 72.
73. *Stack v. Boyle,* 342 U.S. 1 (1951); *United States v. Salerno,* 107 S. Ct. 2095 (1987).
74. *Brady v. Maryland,* 373 U.S. 83 (1963).
75. *United States v. Agurs,* 427 U.S. 97 (1976); *United States v. Bagley,* 473 U.S. 667 (1985).
76. Black, *supra* note 5, at 798.
77. Baum, *supra* note 1, at 180–182.
78. Baum, *supra* note 1, at 183–187.
79. LaFave and Scott, *supra* note 2, at 58.
80. Black, *supra* note 5, at 1272–1273.
81. Baum, *supra* note 1, at 192.
82. *Id.* at 197–210.
83. See, as examples, *State v. Shook,* 393 S.E.2d 819 (1990); *Barber and Jejdle v. Superior Court,* 195 Cal. Rptr. 484 (Cal. App. 2 Dist. 1983).
84. 355 A.2d 647 (N.J. 1976).
85. 380 N.E.2d 134 (Mass. 1978).
86. The *Quinlan* case dealt with the removal of a ventilator, while *Dinnerstein* focused on whether or not a Do Not Resuscitate (DNR) Order would result in liability.
87. 486 A.2d 1209 (N.J. 1985).
88. George Pozgar, *Legal Aspects of Health Care Administration.* 7th Edition. Gaithersburg, Md.: Aspen Publishers, 1999, 405–408.
89. 452 So. 2d 921 (Fla. 1984).
90. *Id.* at 926.
91. See Margo Zink and Linda Titus, "Nursing Ethics Committees: Do We Need Them?" in *Current Issues in Nursing,* 5th Edition, Joanne McClaskey and Helen Grace, Editors. St. Louis, Mo.: Mosby–Year Book, Inc., 1997, 640–646; Charlotte McDaniel, "Hospital Ethics Committees and Nurses' Participation," 28(9) *JONA* (1998), 47–51.
92. See *Hunter v. State,* 676 A.2d 968 (1996).
93. See, for example, The Illinois Nursing and Advanced Practice Nursing Act, S.H.A. 225 ILCS 65/10-5, 65/20–70(b) (1998).
94. See Martin B. Flamm and Judith Ann Gic, "The Criminalization of Health Care Practice," in 1998 *Wiley Medical*

Malpractice Update, Levin A. Shiffman, Editor. New York: John Wiley, 1998, 247–280.

95. *Id.* at 247.

96. The case of Miguel Sanchez, discussed earlier in this chapter, is one such case. See also Paul Van Grunsven, "Medical Malpractice or Criminal Mistake? An Analysis of Past and Current Criminal Prosecutions for Clinical Mistakes and Fatal Errors," 2(1) *DePaul Journal of Health Law* (1997), 1–54.

97. *Einaugler v. Supreme Court,* 918 F. Supp. 619 (1996).

98. *People v. Wolfgang Schug, M.D.;* Van Grunsven, *supra* note 96, at 37–42.

99. The case of Dr. Patrick Chavis; Van Grunsven, *supra* note 96, at 42.

100. Van Grunsven, *supra* note 96, at 37. The nursing home failed to contact the physician when the patient's status deteriorated. The patient "bled to death" as a result of the improper administration and monitoring of Coumadin. All of the nurses were indicted on charges of endangering the welfare of an elderly person in their care, but the judge in the case "dismissed" the charges against them because it was a first offense for them and they were "unlikely" to make the same mistake again. At the time the article was published, a civil case was filed against the nurses, and the state ombudsman was urging the New Jersey Board of Nursing to discipline the nurses.

101. *People v. Protopappas,* 246 Cal. Rptr. 915 (1998).

102. *Gian-Cursio v. State of Florida,* 180 So. 2d 396 (1965), *writ dismissed,* 196 So. 2d 105 (1966), *cert. denied,* 389 U.S. 819 (1967).

103. *Einaugler v. Supreme Court, supra* note 97.

104. Van Grunsven, *supra* note 96.

105. See, as examples, Sandra Plum, "Three Denver Nurses May Face Prison in a Case That Bodes Ill for the Profession," 7(2) *Revolution—The Journal of Nurse Empowerment* (1997), 11–12; Leah Curtin, "When Negligence Becomes Homicide," 38(7) *Nursing Management* (1997), 7–8 (editorial opinion); Susan Laughlin, "Criminal Charges for Clinical Errors, Advanced Practice Nurse Liability," 5(2) *Journal of Nursing Law* (1998), 65–73.

106. Jean Burgmeier, RN, "Error-Proof the System," 28(10) *Nursing Management* (1997), 1097 (letters section).

107. See Robert Grant, 17th Judicial District Attorney, "To the Members of the Nursing Community," 28(10) *Nursing Management* (1997), 1097 (letters section); Nancy J. Brent, "Criminal Indictments in Denver: Could It Happen to You?" 11(22) *Nursing Spectrum* (1998), 12–13.

Contract Law

10

KEY PRINCIPLES

- Contract
- Assignment and Delegation of a Contract
- Statute of Frauds
- Rules of Contract Interpretation
- Parol Evidence Rule
- Breach of Contract
- Completion of Contract
- Good Faith/Fair Dealing

In addition to potential civil liability under tort law or civil rights violations, liability under contract law may also exist for the nurse or other health care professional. An injured patient can bring a suit alleging many possible causes of action. Against a nurse anesthetist, for example, a count alleging a breach of contract for misrepresenting the services to be rendered to the patient could accompany a count alleging negligence in the administration of the anesthesia.

Although the wrong allegedly suffered by the patient under contract law may be very different from that under tort law, many times the distinctions between the two become blurred because of the law's sometimes confusing treatment of the two areas of liability. For instance, in the example above, in addition to alleging negligence in the administration of anesthesia because an injury occurred, the patient could also allege a breach of contract for the same injury because of the nurse anesthetist's failure to provide services with reasonable skill and care.[1]

Despite the blending of the two types of civil actions, the reader should try to keep the two separate by remembering that tort law involves obligations imposed by law to avoid injuries to another.[2] Contract law, in contast, deals with promises, either present or future, and the enforcement of them when a legal right has been created.[3] Therefore the nurse anesthetist in the example above could not legally contract with the patient not to exercise due care in the provision of anesthesia services because the law of torts has established obligations the nurse anesthetist can not alter in a contract. She could, however, contract to provide the services for a specific fee and on a specific date.

Contract law . . . deals with promises . . . and the enforcement of them when a legal right has been created.

Contract law is an important area of law for the nurse to be familiar with because it is often utilized by the nurse employee, nurse manager, or nurse entrepreneur in relation to respective rights and responsibilities within the job or business setting. For example, the nurse employee may allege a breach of an express or implied contract of employment when discharged from a position. Or a nurse entrepreneur may allege failure on the part of an independent contractor to provide services for the business the nurse has founded.

This chapter will address the basic principles of contract law and relate those principles to the delivery of health care in various settings and to the nurse who experiences a breach of his or her contract rights. Because the delivery of health care is a service, this chapter will not focus on contracts concerning goods. As a result, the Uniform Commercial Code (UCC), a uniform law adopted by states to cover the sale of goods in the state, will not be covered in any detail. Knowledge of this law, however, would be important if the nurse entrepreneur is involved in any way in the sale of goods or products in his or her business.

ESSENTIALS OF CONTRACT FORMATION

Elements of a Contract

A contract is a voluntary agreement between two or more individuals that creates an obligation to do or not do something and that creates enforceable rights or legal duties.[4] For a contract to be valid, certain elements must be present: (1) capacity to enter into the agreement; (2) mutual assent (includes an offer and acceptance); (3) legal consideration; and (4) no defenses that would void the agreement.[5]

Contracts exist in many forms, and the forms may overlap. For example, they may be (1) oral, (2) written, (3) express, (4) implied or quasi contracts, (5) unilateral, (6) bilateral, (7) void, (8) voidable, (9) adhesion (form), and (10) unenforceable.[6]

Generally a contract is entered into for the benefit of the two or more individuals who are parties to it. However, a contract can also be for the benefit of a third party. The third person, who is not directly involved in the formation of the contract, may have enforceable contract rights nonetheless.[7]

For example, assume agency A owed money to a nurse for nursing services rendered through that agency. Because of difficult financial times, the agency decides to enter into a contract with nurse agency B. The contract specifically requires agency B to hire the nurse and "perform agency A's obligations" (payment of the money owed) to the nurse. If agency B did not pay the money owed to the nurse as it contracted to do, the nurse would have the right to sue for the money owed. The nurse would be a third party beneficiary to that contract in addition to being able to assert basic contract rights against agency A.[8]

Assignment and Delegation of Contract

If a valid contract is formed, one party may attempt to assign the rights under the contract to another. For example, a nurse who is under a contract of employment can "assign" the money to be received under the contract to her parents. The nurse continues to perform the work required by the terms of the contract, but transfers the right of payment under the contract to the parents. Generally one can assign whatever one wishes under a contract so long as there is no prohibition of assignment.[9]

Contracts may be delegated as well. A delegation most often occurs when the *duties* or responsibilities contracted for are transferred to another.[10] If a nurse educator, for example, contracts with a particular organization to do a full-day seminar, but cannot teach the program because of illness, he or she can substitute another colleague to do the program. However, if the contract restricted delegation to another, then the nurse educator would not be able to use a replacement. Instead, the nurse would have to reschedule the date of the seminar to fulfill the contract.

Questions Concerning the Validity of a Contract

Capacity to Enter into Agreement

For a contract to be valid and enforceable, the parties entering into it must have the legal qualifications to enter into the agreement. They must understand the nature of the contract, its effect, and their obligations under it. Although adults—persons who are 18 years of age and older—are presumed to possess the capacity or competency to enter into contracts, in certain situations the presumption may be defeated.

An adult's condition might affect his or her cognitive ability to enter into and carry on a contract. For example, someone who has an IQ of 50 may not be able to appreciate the legal ramifications of entering into a contract to sell a house or perform certain personal services. Or, someone who enters a contract when under the influence of a chemical substance or medication may not have the full mental capacity to do so at that time.

If an individual has been declared incompetent (also called, in some states, legally disabled) and a guardian appointed for the person (ward), his or her capacity to enter contracts may be affected. If a guardian over the person's estate or finances has

been found to be necessary by the court, then clearly the ward would not be able to enter into any contracts concerning the sale or purchase of property, goods, or services. Likewise, a patient who signs an agreement to pay for care provided by a health care delivery system when such decisions have been turned over to the person's guardian does not enter into a valid and enforceable contract.

Some states have incorporated into their criminal statutes the suspension of a prisoner's civil rights upon conviction and until the sentence imposed by the court is completed. If so, then a prisoner cannot enter into a contract during that time period because he or she has lost the ability to do so by law. Other states limit the loss of a criminal defendant's civil rights and specify when and how they are restored. Illinois, for example, presumes that a criminal defendant retains his or her civil rights, except the right to vote, during incarceration.[11]

Other losses due to the conviction, such as suspension or revocation of a license (for example, a nursing license), can be restored after sentencing and after any probation has been completed, so long as the agency responsible for the licensing does not find the restoration to be contrary to the public interest.[12]

Generally a minor (or an "infant," the term most often used in state statutes) does not possess the legal capacity to enter into a contract. Thus, until the minor reaches the age of majority—or adulthood—he or she would not be able to enter into a contract of any kind. Almost every state sets the age of adulthood at 18 years.[13]

Exceptions exist in most states to the general rule that a minor is unable to enter into a contract.

Exceptions exist in most states to the general rule that a minor is unable to enter into a contract. The exceptions may include a minor judicially declared an "emancipated minor" under state law,[14] or a minor parent who enters into a health care arbitration agreement on behalf of a minor child.[15]

Mutual Assent

Assent is legally defined as approving, ratifying, and confirming something.[16] Assent requires active participation by the party assenting to the issue or situation at hand. Therefore, mutual assent requires the parties to approve, ratify, and confirm something.

In relation to contract law, mutual assent has been termed a "meeting of the minds." It is composed of an offer and the acceptance of the offer.

OFFER. An offer is a conditional promise (written or oral) to do a specified thing or to refrain from doing a specific thing in the future, should the other party (the offeree) accept the offer.[17] Generally an offer can be revoked at any time before acceptance so long as notice is given to the offeree. It can also be revoked if not accepted by the offeree within the time period set by the individual making the offer. If no time is set, the offer is considered revoked if not accepted within a reasonable amount of time.

ACCEPTANCE. Acceptance occurs when there is a voluntary, clear, definite communication to accept the offer as specified by the offeror, thereby creating the legal relationship of a contract.[18] The offer may need to be accepted in the same manner that the offer was communicated to the offeree. For example, if a nurse executive receives a proposed written severance agreement upon termination and is asked to give his or her written acceptance or rejection on a date certain, the response must be in writing. Responding in any other manner would not conform with the terms of the agreement. Rather, any other response would be a counteroffer, and no agreement would be reached on either "offer" until acceptance by both parties took place.

It may be that the proposed contract terms do not specify a manner of acceptance. If so, any form of communication of acceptance—words, a writing, or conduct—can satisfy this requirement. The nurse executive in the example above could then accept the proposed severance agreement by, for example, informing the employer of acceptance and tendering her resignation. It is important to note, though, that silence—not responding in any way—is not usually considered to be acceptance of a contract.[19]

Legal Consideration

Consideration is the cause, motive, "bargained for exchange," the *quid pro quo* (something for something) that motivates a person to enter into a contract.[20] Consideration includes both parties giving something of value. For example, a nurse faculty member is hired to provide academic in-

struction to students in a particular university and to forgo other faculty positions at other colleges. The university, in turn, agrees to pay the nurse faculty member a salary commensurate with his or her qualifications and retain the faculty member for a certain period (e.g., a year contract of employment at a specific rank).

Consideration is *not* the same as a gratuitous promise to do something or to give something, because the one to whom the promise is made is not giving up anything of value. Furthermore, consideration does not exist when (1) past consideration is used for a future agreement; (2) a party to the contract agrees to do something he or she is already legally obligated to do; (3) the consideration is illegal or immoral; or (4) the consideration is inadequate, that is, not reasonable in light of what is contracted for.[21]

No Defenses That Would Void the Agreement

If a contract is to be valid and enforceable, there should be no successful challenges (defenses) to its formation. If a defense is raised, the court will determine its validity and then determine what impact the defense has on the contract itself. If a defense is found to exist, the court can declare the contract (1) void (having no legal or binding effect), (2) voidable (void at the election of the wronged party), (3) unenforceable, or (4) unconscionable.[22]

If a contract is to be valid and enforceable, there should be no successful challenges (defenses) to its formation.

DEFENSES TO CONTRACT FORMATION. The challenges (defenses) that can be raised to question whether or not a contract was legally formed are varied and complex. Moreover, several challenges may be raised concerning one contract. Table 10–1 lists most of the defenses that one or both parties to a contract may use in an attempt to avoid the obligations of the agreement.

Contract Interpretation
Rules of Interpretation

The law has adopted guidelines to clarify a contract when there is a challenge to its language.

TABLE 10–1

Defenses to Contract Formation

DEFENSE	COMMENT
No capacity to enter into contract (minor, mental illness)	Depending on circumstances, court may void entire contract or may make portions voidable; court will also look to nature of transaction
Undue influence	One party unfairly influences the other into contracting and other could not use free choice; often found in "fiduciary relationships" (e.g., where professional-client relationship exists, and client places trust and confidence in professional)
Duress	Party enters into contract because of improper express, implied, or inferred threat
Mistake	Most successful if mutual; less so if unilateral
Misrepresentation	Defined as a claim that is not consistent with the facts; it must be substantial and cause the other to enter into the contract
Fraud	Person who is fraudulent must make misrepresentation with intent to have other rely on it and with knowledge that it was false
Unconscionability	Raised when there is a question as to the ability of one of the parties to understand the terms of the contract as a whole; also used when the contract itself, or portions of it, are harsh or onerous; can be used when one party's capacity to enter into contract is questionable or when one party lacks equal bargaining power
Illegality/Violation of public policy	Used when contract is not in public's best interest or is illegal; examples include a contract to commit a criminal act, or an agreement that a health care consumer must waive the right to sue for any injuries suffered as a result of care and waiver is required *prior* to receiving care

Data from: John Calamari and Joseph Perillo. *The Law of Contracts*. 4th Edition. St. Paul, Minn.: West Group, 1998 (with updates).

These general guidelines are (1) a contract will be interpreted as a "whole," with specific clauses given less weight than the contract's general intent; (2) words in the contract will be given their "ordinary meaning"; (3) technical words and terms will be given those meanings when the contract covers a particular technical area (unless a different intent is clear in the contract); (4) custom and usage in the particular business and location where the contract is formed or performed are given considerable weight; (5) form ("adhesion") contracts will be scrutinized more closely than a typed or written contract drafted jointly by the parties, since adhesion contracts usually protect the interests of the drafter only rather than the interests of both parties.[23]

Good Faith/Fair Dealing

The duty of good faith and fair dealing to perform and enforce the contract is an implied term of all contracts.[24] Therefore, all parties to a contract are expected to conduct themselves accordingly once the contract has been entered into. Examples of bad faith and unfair dealing include not performing obligations diligently or performing them poorly, and failing to cooperate when the other party's obligations under the contract require one's participation.[25]

> *The duty of good faith and fair dealing to perform and enforce the contract is an implied term of all contracts.*

Many times the presence of bad faith and unfair dealing is alleged when a breach of the contract occurs. In fact, some jurisdictions recognize bad faith and unfair dealing as not only a contract action but also a tort action.[26] The court may also utilize the finding of bad faith or unfair dealing to support a finding that a breach has effectively taken place, even though that is not initially alleged.[27]

Parol Evidence Rule

The parol evidence rule of contract interpretation is very important when challenging a contract and its terms. In its simplest form, the rule states that when a contract, will, or trust is a written one that both parties intend to represent the entire declaration of their agreement, the written document is legally binding on the parties. No other oral or written agreements (called "extrinsic"

ETHICS CONNECTION 10–1

Not only must nurses be careful to stay within the boundaries of their competence and expertise in relation to clients, they must be careful about not overextending or representing their knowledge and skills to one another. It is easy, for example, for nurse managers and educators to overstep their contractual boundaries with staff or students and practice counseling. In a situation that did not lead to litigation but certainly is immoral from the prespectives of respect for autonomy,[1] nonmaleficence, and beneficence, a director of nursing (DON) told a nurse to "kick her husband out" of a faltering marriage. The nurse followed the advice of the DON, then blamed the DON for the marriage breakup and resigned from her position as a staff nurse.

[1]Karen L. Bonn, 48(3) *Nursing Homes Long Term Care Management* (1999), 72.

---

agreements) made prior to, or contemporaneously with, that written contract can be used to modify or add to its terms.[28] For example, a nurse who attempts to challenge a contract because a salary increase did not take place will find it difficult to do so by relying on an earlier written promise concerning the salary when that promise did not end up in the final, written contract of employment.

The rule does not, however, forbid the use of prior written or oral evidence to challenge matters other than the contents of the contract. Therefore the nurse could use the earlier written promise as evidence that the employment agreement was affected by fraud, duress, mistake, misrepresentation, or prior custom or use.[29]

Statute of Frauds

The Statute of Frauds (originally an English law) requires that certain contracts be in writing and signed by the party who must perform them. Its purpose is to ensure reliable, objective evidence of agreements. This is of particular importance after a substantial amount of time has passed since the contract was entered into and accurate recollection of its terms may have faded.

The Statute of Frauds . . . requires that certain contracts be in writing and signed by the party who must perform them.

States in the United States that have adopted the principles of the Statute of Frauds in their respective statutes specify the *types* of contracts that must be in writing.[30] They are (1) an "agreement" in consideration of marriage; (2) a contract for the sale of goods amounting to a specific price or more, or having a "value" of a specified amount; (3)· a promise to pay for the "debt, defaults or miscarriages" of another; (4) an "agreement" that cannot be performed within 1 year; and (5) a contract for the sale of interest in real estate, including a lease agreement, for more than 1 year.[31]

The requirement of a written instrument may be satisfied by a formal contract or a "written memorandum" that is sufficiently clear as to the subject matter of the contract and its terms.[32] In addition, the memorandum need not be one single document, but may consist of several documents.[33] The several documents must be referred to within the main or initial writing (called incorporating by reference).

The Statute of Frauds can affect a nurse in many ways. It may be used, for example, to defeat a nurse fired after 6 months of employment who claims that he or she had been offered a 5-year contract, when there is no written document supporting the nurse's claim. Or, if a nurse entrepreneur enters into an agreement to purchase real estate on which to eventually open a clinic, the agreement must be in writing to be valid under the Statute of Frauds.

COMPLETION OF CONTRACT

A contract can be ended in several ways. The most obvious is when the contract is performed; that is, the contract is adhered to, performance occurs, and the obligations under the contract are met. The result then is termination of the contract; no further obligations under the contract exist.

Sometimes, however, there is a need to end a contract because of problems that arise among and between the parties. For example, a contract that is impossible to perform is not seen as realistically enforceable. If the nurse lecturer, for example, contracted to do a 3-day workshop in a foreign country and war broke out in that country the day the nurse was to leave for the workshop, enforcing the contract would be foolish at best.

However, the nurse lecturer and the organization could renegotiate their agreement, thus ending the initial contract and entering into another. This is called accord and satisfaction.

The nurse lecturer and the entity may decide, however, that because of the unpredictability of the war, it would be unwise to end the initial contract and enter into another. They agree, then, to rescind the contract and end their respective obligations under it by treating it as though it never existed.[34] The two parties can do so because there are no third parties who have a vested interest in the contract or irrevocable assignments under it.

BREACH OF CONTRACT

A breach of contract occurs when one party to a contract fails to perform, without a legal justification, any major promise or obligation under the contract.[35] One may breach a contract simply by failing to perform one's obligations or in other ways, such as making it impossible for the other party to perform his or her obligations or by declaring that one's obligations will not be carried out ("repudiation"). When the breach occurs, the nonbreaching party can sue for any damages, so long as that party can show that *but for* the breach, he or she is willing and able to perform the contract.

Table 10–2 lists the types of remedies the nonbreaching party can seek in a suit alleging a breach of contract.

An interesting example of a nurse alleging a breach of employment contract is presented in Key Case 10–1.

SPECIAL CONSIDERATIONS

Express or Implied Promises Given in the Delivery of Health Care

One way contract law principles can be applied to the delivery of health care is by incorporating implied rules of conduct for the health care provider. When a nurse psychotherapist undertakes therapy with a depressed client, and recovery does not occur because of an alleged fault on the part of the nurse, the court may impose an implied contractual provision that governs the relationship. For example, an applicable provision might be that the nurse must provide therapy with the required skill and care in exchange for the client's payment of the fee. Therefore, if the nurse fails to provide such skill and care, the client can recover

TABLE 10–2

Breach of Contract Remedies

REMEDY	COMMENTS	EXAMPLE
Compensatory damages	Monetary amount that covers losses suffered by injured party; nonbreaching party must minimize losses, if possible, until contract dispute resolved	Nurse owns temporary nurse agency and has a contract with hospital; hospital does not abide by contract; agency must try to enter into contract with another hospital; agency also seeks attorney fees, punitive damages, and any other damages spelled out in contract ("liquidated damages")
Specific performance	Nonbreaching party asks that contract be carried out; court grants when goods are unique and not personal services; often requested when compensatory damages not adequate	Nurse-inventor does not deliver designed surgical instrument to manufacturing company; company sues for delivery
Injunction	Equitable remedy; court does not have to allow; can be prohibitory or mandatory injunction	Manufacturer asks court to prohibit nurse from giving instrument to other companies, or require nurse to deliver it to them
Reformation	Equitable remedy; court can amend or remodel contract based on real or original intent of contract	Court rules hospital in first example must use agency for 3 more months

Data from: Henry Campbell Black. *Black's Law Dictionary.* 7th Edition. St. Paul, Minn.: West Group, 1999.

KEY CASE 10–1   McCullough v. Visiting Nurse Service (1997)[36]

Nurse is hired as a part-time, at-will employee

FACTS: In 1991, Christine McCullough, RN, was hired by the VNA of Southern Maine, Inc. on a part-time basis. McCullough signed a number of documents when she applied for employment and after she was hired. The documents clearly stated that she was an at-will employee and could therefore be terminated from her position at the will of the employer, with or without cause. At least one of the documents signed by nurse McCullough also stated that any change in the at-will employment relationship would need to be in writing and signed by both Ms. McCullough and the president of the VNA.

In June of 1992, McCullough was issued a verbal warning for failure to properly flush a patient's infusion line. In March of 1994, McCullough was accused of failing to add ordered medications to a patient's infusion line. Although the incident report was made out by nurse McCullough's supervisor and filed according to agency policy, the supervisor did not issue a written warning. When the incident report was reviewed by the VNS home health director, she decided that McCullough should receive a formal warning. After the two incidents, the VNS decided to terminate her employment.

After two patient care incidents, the nurse is terminated from her position

McCullough filed a grievance over her termination and the VNS agreed to review the decision to terminate her. The VNS found that the 1992 incident was not entirely Ms. McCullough's fault and held that "counseling" rather than termination was a more appropriate discipline after the second incident.

The nurse's grievance over her termination results in an offer of reinstatement and back pay

The VNS offered to reinstate nurse McCullough and give her "back pay." Ms. McCullough declined the offer and instead brought a lawsuit against the VNS alleging a breach of her employment contract and defamation.

Nurse rejects offer and sues for breach of contract and defamation

TRIAL COURT DECISION: The Superior Court of York County, Maine, granted the VNS's motion for summary judgment against McCullough. Ms. McCullough appealed the trial court decision.

Trial court dismisses case

SUPREME COURT OF MAINE DECISION: The Maine Supreme Court affirmed the judgment of the trial court. The court clearly held that Ms. McCullough was an at-will employee. The court also found that nothing the employer did created an employment contract for a definite period of time. The court also opined that exceptions to the at-will employment doctrine are carefully evaluated, and only in clear instances of contract formation will an exception be made.

Supreme Court of Maine upholds dismissal of case

The court rejected Ms. McCullough's allegations of defamation as well.

ANALYSIS: This case illustrates the importance of being able to show that some kind of contract was entered into between two parties before an appellate court will return a case to the trial court for a trial. The contract that exists does not need to be an express, written contract, however. In employment situations, implied contracts can govern the employer-employee relationship. Implied contracts can be formed when, as an example, the employer gives an oral promise that an employee is "hired for life" or "for at least 1 year." Here, however, no such promises, nor any other conduct, by the VNS supported the formation of a contract. As a result, Ms. McCullough

KEY CASE 10–1	McCullough v. Visiting Nurse Service (1997)[36] *Continued*

could be terminated because no contract of employment was ever entered into by the VNS and the nurse.

At-will employment and defamation will be discussed in greater depth in Chapters 16 and 7 respectively.

ETHICS CONNECTION 10–2

As nurses become more involved in providing or teaching clients about nonallopathic or complementary therapies, they must be wary of making claims about the benefits of the therapies that may not be realized. Making claims that are not fulfilled may not only be a breach of contract from the legal perspective; it also is unethical to make such claims. Making unwarranted claims for therapy outcomes violates the moral principle of promise keeping and also may cause harm, thus violating the moral principle of nonmaleficence. In this era of demonstrating outcomes of therapy, it is difficult to refrain from making claims of healing or improving health. Nevertheless, practitioners of complementary therapies, such as Therapeutic Touch, know that healing is so complex that an intended outcome cannot be predicted with a reasonable level of confidence. They refrain from telling the patient what outcomes will be.

any amounts paid out pursuant to that treatment and the resulting breach (e.g., fees paid to the nurse for therapy). These types of damages are compensatory damages—those compensating the client/plaintiff as a result of the implied agreement.

A second way in which contract law can be applied to health care delivery is when the health care provider makes an express promise or warranty to the patient. Using the above example, if the nurse psychotherapist promises to cure a client's depression and that does not happen, the court may find an express contract. As with implied contract theory, damages would be based on any money the plaintiff expended as part of the express agreement.

It is important to note that generally the law is not fond of finding express contracts in the context of health care delivery.[37] Because much of what a health care provider says to a patient concerning his or her treatment is more in the form of opinion, reassurance, and optimistic prediction rather than a clear contract, the law requires the patient-plaintiff to clearly prove all the elements of the formation of an express contract.[38] Even so, the nurse is well advised to proceed cautiously when discussing health care treatment and results with patients.

Witnessing Special Contracts of Patients

No one comes into a hospital or other health care delivery system for care because he or she is well. Rather, consumers of health care are in need of health care services, whatever their nature. At times the condition requires extensive treatment, and the survival of the individual may be in question. As a result, many times nurses are asked to witness various documents that patients deem necessary to complete in the event their condition worsens, they become unable to speak for themselves, or they die.

The documents most often needed by patients include a testamentary will to dispose of property, advance directive(s) for health care (living will, durable power of attorney, or medical directive), and an advance directive for financial decisions. To ensure their validity and attest to the testator's or declarant's soundness of mind when executing the documents, witnesses are helpful, sometimes required. Although it might seem natural, even helpful, for the nurse to witness these documents, it is prudent for the nurse to think carefully about doing so.

Although it might seem natural, even helpful, for the nurse to witness . . . documents, it is prudent for the nurse to think carefully about doing so.

ETHICS CONNECTION 10–3

Express or implied promises regarding health care delivery are made between nursing and society as well as between individual nurses and other parties, such as clients or employers. *Nursing's Social Policy Statement*[1] is a statement of the profession's social contract. The nurse-patient relationship is an example of an implied contract between individual nurses and their clients.[2] From the moral perspective of covenantal relationships, nurses who are employees are parties to very complicated implied contracts.[3] Such nurses have responsibilities to both their employers and their clients. This dual commitment frequently creates moral tension for nurses, who often are characterized as working in "the in between." When the institutional culture and ethical policies and practices are congruent with the *American Nurses Association's Code for Nurses with Interpretive Statements*[4] and the nurses' own moral values, there is little conflict between the implied contracts to the employer and to the client. When, however, the employer and the client have competing claims on the nurse's fidelity, the nurse is in a very difficult moral position. In such situations, fulfilling the obligations of one implied contract will make it impossible for the nurse to fulfill the obligations of the other. For example, a nurse employee of a community hospital may know that a patient who requires neurosurgery would be more competently treated at a competing medical center but probably will not disclose that fact to the client for fear of reprisal from her employer. In a classic 1980s study of nurses' freedom to be moral agents, Yarling and McElmurry[5] found that nursing students reported that they would probably respect institutional lines of authority rather than advocate for a client when whistleblowing was morally required. The forthcoming revision of the *Code for Nurses* supports nurses' primary responsibility to clients rather than to competing institutional or other interests. If the *Code,* as currently proposed, is adopted, nurses will have clearer moral accountability to their clients. The competing claims of antagonistic implied contracts should then be minimized as a result of a clearer statement of nurses' moral obligations to clients.

[1] American Nurses Association. *Nursing's Social Policy Statement.* Washington, D.C.: Author, 1995.

[2] Margaret A. Burkhardt and Alvita K. Nathanial. *Ethics and Issues in Contemporary Nursing.* Detroit: Delmar Publishing, 1998.

[3] See Chapter 3 for discussion of covenantal relationships and conflict.

[4] American Nurses Association. *Code for Nurses with Interpretive Statements.* Kansas City, Mo., 1985.

[5] Rod Yarling and Beverly McElmurry, "The Moral Foundation of Nursing." 8(2) *Advances in Nursing Science* (1986), 63–73.

First of all, the nurse must check his or her institution or agency's policy concerning the witnessing of personal documents. Generally, most health care delivery systems have adopted a position that nursing staff should not do so. This prohibition may be based on state laws that restrict health care employees, including nurses, from witnessing certain documents. Such a policy may seem contrary to a policy that allows the nurse to witness a patient's signature on a consent, or refusal of consent, form for treatment. However, upon closer analysis, the distinction is somewhat logical because of the nature of the personal documents.

The testamentary will, for example, is clearly not something that is within the purview of nursing care. Furthermore, it is a highly personal document. Therefore, the rationale goes, the nurse need not be involved in its execution.

Although an advance directive is intimately connected to the delivery of health care, it is generally agreed—in fact, even mandated in some state statutes—that a health care provider *providing* care to a patient *should not* witness the signing of an advance directive. This prohibition eliminates any contest as to the influence the health care provider or the institution may have had on the patient in executing the advance directive.

If the nurse decides to witness a will or advance directive and the witnessing is not contrary to the employer's policy or statutory law, then it is important for the nurse to understand that he or she may be called upon to testify to the following, and other issues, should the signing of the document be brought into question:

- In the case of a will, did the testator sign the document in the nurse's presence?
- What was the testator or the declarant's state of mind when signing the will or advance directive?
- Who, if anyone, was also present when the signing took place?
- What, if anything, did the testator or declarant say about the document and what he or she was asking the nurse to do?
- Did the testator or declarant seem to freely sign the document or was he or she coerced or under duress?
- Who took possession of the document once it was signed?

Also important for the nurse would be the necessity of documenting in the patient's record the event, who was present, the observed state of mind of the patient, and any comments made by the patient before, during, or after the document was signed.

SUMMARY OF PRINCIPLES AND APPLICATIONS

Contract law permeates a large part of health care delivery, whether directly or indirectly. It influences a nurse's purchase of professional liability insurance and governs a nurse's relationship with his or her union, as examples. Although it does not always receive the attention it may deserve in comparison with other areas of health care law, such as professional negligence or refusal of treatment, it is nonetheless a key area of concern for the nurse. Furthermore, contract law can be a valuable tool for challenging employment and other decisions that are adverse to the nurse's interest if an express or implied contract governs the situation. Therefore the nurse should remember the following:

- To be valid, a contract must be formed with the capacity to enter into it, a "meeting of the minds," legal consideration, and no defenses that would void it

- A contract can exist in many forms, including oral, written, express, implied, unilateral, bilateral, and adhesion

- The Statute of Frauds requires that certain contracts must be in writing, and if they are not, no contract will be found to exist

- Rules of contract interpretation exist to help the court decide on the validity of a contract's terms

- A contract is not fulfilled if a breach of the contract occurs. When that happens, possible remedies against the breaching party include money damages (compensation), specific performance, reformation of the contract, or an injunction

- Good faith (or fair dealing) is an implied term of all contracts

- The presence of certain factors—incapacity, minority—may render the contract void, voidable, unenforceable, or unconscionable

- Defenses to contract formation include duress, fraud, mistake, and undue influence

- The nurse must take care not to warrant or expressly state a specific cure, result, or outcome when providing care to patients

- Witnessing patient contracts—testamentary wills or advance directives—may be against agency policy and state law

- If a nurse believes that his or her express contract is breached, or an implied one is not adhered to, the nurse should seek advice from an attorney and determine if the principles of contract law can aid the nurse in obtaining a remedy for the unfulfilled arrangement

TOPICS FOR FURTHER INQUIRY

1. Analyze at least two employment contracts for health care providers. If possible, one should be for a nurse. Identify the various provisions in the contract, including provisions for a breach of contract, termination of the contract, and remedies specified (e.g., suit, arbitration, injunctive relief). Suggest additions to the contracts that might be beneficial to the health care provider. Draft language to include in the contracts.

2. Identify suits against health care providers in your state that allege breach of implied or express warranty. Analyze the data obtained as to types of health care providers sued; specific allegations in the suits; types of damages sought by the plaintiffs; and how the suits were resolved (e.g., settlement, verdict).

3. Write a paper on a specific remedy for breach of a contract. Discuss the mechanisms of the remedy and what types of damages can be obtained in your state. Suggest options for a resolution of the situation sued for other than the remedy selected for the paper.

4. Compare and contrast living will statutes in at least four states for language concerning the witnessing of the document by health care providers. Analyze the legislative history of the statute for reasons why the language was decided upon during the legislative process. Either support or reject the rationale in the paper and present reasons for either position.

REFERENCES

1. W. Page Keeton. *Prosser and Keeton on the Law of Torts.* 5th Edition. St. Paul, Minn.: West Publishing Company, 1984, 657 (with 1988 pocket part), *citing DuBois v. Decker,* 29 N.E. 313 (1891); *McNevins v. Lowe,* 40 Ill. 209 (1866); *Napier v. Greenzweig,* 256 F. 196 (2nd Cir. 1919).
2. *Id.* at 655.
3. *Id.* at 656.
4. Henry Campbell Black. *Black's Law Dictionary.* 7th Edition. St. Paul, Minn.: West Group, 1999, 318.

5. John Calamari and Joseph Perillo. *The Law of Contracts.* 4th Edition. St. Paul, Minn.: West Publishing Company, 1998 (with updates).

6. Black, *supra* note 4, at 318–327.

7. Calamari and Perillo, *supra* note 5, at 641–647.

8. Example adopted from "Question 34," in Gordon Schaber and Claude Rohwer. *Contracts in a Nutshell.* 3rd Edition. St. Paul, Minn.: West Publishing Company, 1990, 433.

9. Calamari and Perillo, *supra* note 5, at 680.

10. *Id.* at 701.

11. 730 ILCS 5/5-5-5 (1990).

12. *Id.*

13. Calamari and Perillo, *supra* note 5, at 280.

14. 750 ILCS 30/5 (1980).

15. 710 ILCS 15/7 (1977).

16. Black, *supra* note 4, at 111.

17. Calamari and Perillo, *supra* note 5, at 30–31.

18. *Id.* at 71.

19. *Id.* at 80.

20. Black, *supra* note 4, at 300–303.

21. *Id.*

22. See, generally, Calamari and Perillo, *supra* note 5.

23. Calamari and Perillo, *supra* note 5, at 148–166. See also *Restatement (First) of Contracts,* Sections 230, 233, 236 (1932); *Restatement (Second) of Contracts,* Sections 201, 202, 203, 211 (1981, with updated supplements).

24. *Restatement (Second) of Contracts,* Section 205 (1981) (with updated supplements).

25. *Restatement (Second) of Contracts,* Section 205, Comment d (1981) (with updated supplements).

26. Calamari and Perillo, *supra* note 5, at 461; John Perillo, "Abuse of Rights: A Persuasive Legal Concept," 27 *Pacific Law Review* (1995), 37, 44–47. Bad faith allegations are also known as "abuse of rights" allegations.

27. Calamari and Perillo, *supra* note 5, at 461–468; *Tymshare v. Covell,* 727 F.2d 1145, 1150 n.3 (D.C. 1984).

28. Black, *supra* note 4, at 1139–1140.

29. *Id.*

30. Black, *supra* note 4, at 1422.

31. Calamari and Perillo, *supra* note 5, at 710–778.

32. *Id.* at 758.

33. *Id.* at 759–760.

34. Calamari and Perillo, *supra* note 5, at 796–799.

35. Black, *supra* note 4, at 182.

36. 619 A.2d 1201 (1997).

37. Theodore LeBlang, Eugene Basanta, Douglas Peters, Keith Fineberg, and Donald Kroll. *The Law of Medical Practice in Illinois.* 2nd Edition. St. Paul, Minn.: West Group, 1996, 669 (with 1998 cumulative supplements).

38. *Id.* at 669–672.

Reproductive and Family Concerns

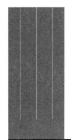

KEY PRINCIPLES

- Penumbra Doctrine
- Privacy
- Zones of Privacy
- *Parens Patriae* Doctrine
- Best-Interest-of-the-Individual Test
- Substituted Judgment Test

Although the right of privacy's beginnings were firmly planted in nonconstitutional ground—as a property right to be vindicated under a tort or contract theory—that viewpoint slowly changed. Privacy rights began to be rooted in several of the Bill of Rights' protections[1] and continued to further develop and change. In a 1928 U.S. Supreme Court wiretapping case, for example, Justice Brandeis in his dissenting opinion stated that the Fourth and Fifth Amendments provided a "right to be left alone."[2]

The First Amendment has also been cited as protecting privacy interests.[3] Also, the Fourteenth Amendment's Due Process and Equal Protection clauses respectively have also been cited as the basis for the privacy of personal decisions such as reproductive choice. Clearly these and other case law decisions have expanded the right of privacy from "interpersonal relationships to the level of individual choice."[4]

The expansion of the right of privacy is based on two constitutional doctrines—the penumbra doctrine and the zone of privacy doctrine. The penumbra doctrine, contained in Article I, Section 8(18) ("Necessary and Proper Clause") of the federal Constitution, states that when specific guarantees exist in the Bill of Rights, they contain additional protections containing implied rights, the exact extent of which is unclear.[5] The use of this doctrine with the right of privacy is important, since privacy is not specifically granted as a right in the U.S. Constitution. The right of privacy has been expanded by the courts in the penumbras of other clearly articulated constitutional rights, such as freedom of religion and association (First Amendment) and the protection against unreasonable searches and seizures (Fourth Amendment).

The zone of privacy is also an extension of the penumbra doctrine and expands clearly articulated rights to include the right of privacy. For example, the Ninth Amendment's statement that the rights listed in the Constitution "shall not be construed to deny or disparage others retained by the people" has been used to include the right of privacy in the Fifth and Fourteenth Amendments' protection of liberty.[6]

Like other rights, the right of privacy is not absolute. As a result, an individual's privacy interest must always be balanced with another's interest and with those of the government, whether local, state, or federal. The balancing of respective privacy rights is based on the *Parens Patriae* Doctrine, meaning "the parent of the country." This doctrine defines the state government as "sovereign"; that is, as a provider of protection to those unable to care for themselves, such as infants and legally disabled adults.[7] If necessary, the state can intervene by initiating a suit on behalf of the person who needs protecting, or becoming involved in a suit already in progress.

In either case, the state's purpose is to protect the individual or individuals involved because it has an interest in maintaining the well-being and productivity of its citizens. Even so, the state's concerns are not absolute, and they must be balanced with the individual's constitutional and

other rights. For example, on questions such as reproductive choice or custody of a minor child when a divorce occurs, the court always compares the state's interests and the individual rights of those involved before making a determination. That comparison must always conform to state and federal constitutional limitations on the ability of the government to unduly intervene in individual liberties.

To provide a consistent way in which respective rights can be carefully balanced, especially when one party cannot articulate his or her wishes, two tests are used in evaluating competing personal and state interests. One is the "best-interest-of-the-individual" test. In its pure form, it takes into account only the present welfare of the person and ignores societal, familial, or other secondary concerns that do not focus on what is best for the person at that time.[8]

. . . an individual's privacy interest must always be balanced with another's interest and with those of the government . . .

The second test, "substituted judgment," is based on the decision that the incompetent individual would make if he or she were able to do so. By its nature, this test requires clear, credible evidence of the individual's past preferences.[9] When such evidence is unreliable or unavailable, the use of this test is, in reality, the use of the "best interest" standard.[10]

Probably in no other area of the law is the balancing of such rights more delicate than in the exercise of such private decisions as procreation, choice of a mate, choice of living arrangement, family matters, and what treatment one will select or refuse.

SELECTED CONSIDERATIONS IN REPRODUCTIVE AND FAMILY AFFAIRS

Reproductive Choice

Sterilization

EUGENIC STERILIZATION. Eugenic sterilization—sterilizing those with certain "defects" to avoid

offspring in society who might inherit those defects—was a popular practice in the early 1890s. By 1917, 16 states had laws allowing compulsory sterilization of those who were found by the court to be insane, "feeble-minded," or moronic. Others with undesirable traits, including alcoholism, blindness, and deafness, were also included in these laws. By 1942, 32 states had enacted such laws.[11]

In a 1927 case, *Buck v. Bell*,[12] the U.S. Supreme Court upheld a Virginia law allowing the superintendent of a home for epileptics and the feeble-minded to sterilize inmates if it would be in the best interest of the inmate and society. However, in *Skinner v. Oklahoma*,[13] the U.S. Supreme Court held unconstitutional a law that allowed the state (under its Habitual Criminal Sterilization Act) to sterilize habitual criminals convicted of crimes involving moral turpitude. It is important to note that the Act was struck down because of the success of an equal protection argument—all criminals were not treated the same under the law—rather than because of outrage over the sterilization issue.

After the *Buck* and *Skinner* decisions, many states repealed their eugenic sterilization laws.[14]

INVOLUNTARY STERILIZATION. Involuntary sterilization laws exist in many states. The focus of these laws is not on the genetic impact of the offspring, but rather what is best for the individual having the child and the offspring. Many of these laws have been upheld by the courts under certain circumstances. Even so, they are subject to strict constitutional scrutiny, especially when the individual involved is not competent (that is, unable to give informed consent for the procedure).

Involuntary sterilization laws . . . are subject to strict constitutional scrutiny . . .

Involuntary sterilization most often arises with those who are mentally disabled or mentally retarded and whose sexual activity, or its potential, is of concern to family members, a guardian (if one has been appointed), or facility staff. Regardless of the circumstance, specific due process and other protections are afforded the individual unable to provide informed consent for this procedure.

Those protections include the right to a hearing, the right to counsel or a *guardian ad litem* (an attorney or other individual appointed by the court to represent the individual for the purposes of the hearing), the establishment of the need for the sterilization, and various medical and psychological examinations and opinions.[15]

VOLUNTARY STERILIZATION. The decision to terminate the ability to procreate can take place under various circumstances. When that decision occurs because children are not wanted, the choice is of a different character than when a disease or injury may necessitate removal of the reproductive organs. If the latter situation exists, it is probably not a voluntary choice in the sense that the removal of the reproductive organs is required for continued well-being. When the choice is truly voluntary, however, the most common method of sterilization is vasectomy for men and tubal ligation for women.

For competent adult men and women, the only legal prerequisite for voluntary sterilization is the provision of informed consent for the procedure. Most often, *written* informed consent is mandated, by either state or federal law. Spousal consent for sterilization is currently not universally required in the United States.[16] Although private hospitals or clinics can establish policies requiring spousal consent, public health care delivery systems cannot; doing so has been held to be a violation of the patient's right of privacy and therefore unconstitutional.[17]

Unmarried minors—those under 18 years of age—have several restrictions on the right to sterilization. Some states, such as Georgia and Connecticut, prohibit sterilization of unmarried minors. Others, like Colorado, allow it only when a parent or guardian also gives permission for the procedure. When the parent or guardian consents to sterilization but the minor objects, then a suit must be filed to provide the minor with certain protections and determine which decision will prevail.

Married minors, as well as minors emancipated in other ways, can consent to all medical treatments including sterilization. Therefore the only legal prerequisite for the married or otherwise emancipated minor in relation to sterilization would be the provision of informed consent.

NURSING IMPLICATIONS

The provision of care to one undergoing sterilization will vary depending on the circumstances surrounding that procedure. However, nurses who work in facilities for the developmentally disabled, those in home care, and those who provide nursing services for adult and minor women in ambulatory care and women's health centers will most probably be faced with patients who may undergo this procedure.

For the legally disabled patient or an unemancipated or unmarried minor, the nurse will be working with a guardian, other legally appointed consent giver, or the parent, especially in terms of explaining procedures, discussing nursing care, and relaying information from the physician concerning the patient's progress. Even so, it is important to include the patient in those discussions to ensure that the patient's dignity remains intact and that he or she is treated in a caring and humane way. For those patients who are able to make the decision themselves, the nurse will need to listen and clarify and obtain any additional information the patient may need to make an informed choice concerning the procedure.

The nurse will also need to be certain that the institution's or agency's policies concerning written consent are adhered to. Although it is clearly the physician's responsibility to go through the process of obtaining the informed consent of the patient, it is the nurse's responsibility to see that it has occurred. If, for example, the nurse in the operating room determines that the required written consent has not been obtained, the nurse must inform the surgeon and the nurse manager.

Furthermore, patients may request additional information from the nurse concerning the procedure. The nurse will need to ascertain what the patient had been told initially and, where possible, reinforce the information given by the physician. If necessary, the nurse may also need to contact the physician so that he or she can provide the additional details needed.

Any and all documentation that has taken place concerning the procedure should be a part of the medical record. Any communication to the physician, surgeon, or nursing administration concerning the patient and the procedure should be carefully and completely documented (see Documentation Reminder 11–1).

Last, if the nurse assesses that the patient may not be able to make an informed choice about the procedure, it is vital that the nurse share this information with the nurse manager and the physician, so that whatever evaluations are necessary concerning the patient's neurologic and psychiatric status can be carried out before the procedure is undertaken.

Birth Control Services and Information

The ability to obtain information concerning birth control is another fundamental issue for any individual, whether male or female, whether married or unmarried. Although one's religious beliefs may prohibit the use of birth control, the state or federal government cannot easily restrict an adult's access to birth control information, devices, and medications. The U.S. Supreme Court in 1965 and 1972 invalidated two respective state laws that restricted access to birth control devices.

In the 1965 case, *Griswold v. Connecticut*,[18] Connecticut's law made it a crime for married couples to use contraceptives and for anyone to counsel another to use them. The Court held that the right of (marital) privacy was one guaranteed by the Constitution's penumbras and zones of privacy of the First, Third, Fourth, Fifth, and Ninth Amendments. Furthermore, the Court suggested that privacy was also protected by the Fourteenth Amendment's Due Process Clause.

. . . reasonable constraints on a minor's access to [birth control] services and information . . . can occur.

In *Eisenstadt v. Baird*,[19] the Court struck down a Massachusetts law that prohibited unmarried couples from obtaining or using contraceptives. Based on an equal protection argument, the Court held that married or unmarried adults have the same right to obtain and use birth control devices.

Although restrictions on birth control services and information for adults are not constitutional, reasonable constraints on a minor's access to the same services and information, especially unemancipated and unmarried minors, can occur. Most often, access to birth control services and information is limited as a result of the state's requirement of parental consent for medical treatment of the minor. Some states, however, such as Illinois, provide a minor access to these services through a specific statute authorizing a physician or other

health care provider to provide services and information to the minor solely on the basis of his or her own consent.[20]

NURSING IMPLICATIONS

The nurse who works in a family planning or ambulatory care center where gynecologic services are offered will be the most directly involved in the provision of birth control services and information to clients. The information given must be clear, accurate, and understandable to the patient. Patient teaching concerning birth control is best done not only by direct discussion with the patient but also through evaluation of the patient's understanding of that information.

Nurse practitioners and nurses who are able to prescribe birth control medications in their particular state will need to do so only after careful and thorough assessment of the patient's physical status.

If the client is a minor, the nurse will need to be familiar with state law concerning consent and whether the minor needs parental consent for birth control information and devices. This need may depend on where the nurse is working. For example, a nurse who works in a public school clinic will most probably need to obtain the consent of the parent for any birth control services to the minor school child, even when state law might otherwise allow the minor himself or herself to consent. The requirement of parental consent is more a public relations issue and an attempt to avoid constitutional arguments; that is, the government might be seen to in some way sanction sexual activity or attempt to control the ability of minors to procreate.

Abortion

Abortion, the termination of pregnancy before the fetus reaches the stage of viability, can be spontaneous or induced, therapeutic or nontherapeutic.[21] Spontaneous abortions or miscarriages occur for many medical reasons, often without apparent cause.[22] Induced abortions, in contrast, are intentionally carried out for many reasons also, including the need to save the life of the mother. Although all of these situations raise controversial legal, ethical, and moral dilemmas, the focus of the development of the law has been on elective abortions that avoid a live birth.[23]

Abortion was a common form of birth control in England and America and was not considered a crime if it occurred before quickening.[24] However, after Connecticut passed the first law criminalizing abortion after quickening in 1821, other states followed. By 1900, abortion was illegal in all U.S. jurisdictions, and individuals who performed them were prosecuted as criminals.[25] In addition, medical licensing acts in most states allowed disciplinary proceedings against physicians who participated in illegal abortions.[26]

In the late 1960s and early 1970s, many of the antiabortion laws were amended to allow an abortion when there was a threat to the mother (either physical or mental), when the pregnancy was due to incest or rape, or when fetal congenital anomalies were diagnosed. It was not until 1973, however, that the U.S. Supreme Court held that the right of a woman to obtain an abortion was included in the right of privacy (Key Case 11–1).

Challenges to the *Roe* and *Doe* decisions were almost immediate. They centered not only on the holdings of the decisions but also on who should finance abortions when the mother could not do so herself or through private health insurance. The latter clearly became an access to abortion issue, for many poor women were effectively unable to have an abortion if they could not pay for the procedure.

Prerequisite procedures to obtain an abortion were also challenged, including procedural challenges involving a minor's access to abortion services. Table 11–1 summarizes several of the court challenges (p. 188).

Table 11–1 indicates a clear trend of retreat from the initial "strict scrutiny" test articulated in *Roe* and *Doe*. The *Rust* decision was particularly troubling to many health care providers, not only because it denied many poor women the right to counseling and abortion services, but also because of the restraints placed on the provider's right of free speech to counsel clients concerning what they determined to be sound medical advice. The regulations upheld by the court in *Rust* were dubbed "gag rules."

Because the regulations were so troublesome, the Department of Health and Human Services amended the rules to allow physicians to discuss abortion if based on "medical conditions." Nurses, counselors, and social workers, however, were still able to provide information on abortion to patients.[34] The U.S. Court of Appeals held that the revised gag rule was adopted in violation of the department's required procedure for changing its rules.[35] It was not until President Clinton rescinded the gag rule during his first week in office, however, that family planning clinics were able to provide medical advice and counseling concerning abortion without fear of violating the rule.

In 1992, the U.S. Supreme Court decided the most recent case concerning abortion rights. In *Planned Parenthood of Southeastern Pennsylvania v. Casey*,[36] the Court agreed to review a Pennsylvania law that (1) required physicians to tell women seeking an abortion about fetal development and alternatives to abortion, (2) had a 24-hour waiting period after the information was received, (3) required notifying the spouse of the intent to have an abortion, (4) mandated unemancipated minors to obtain consent from a parent or the court before obtaining an abortion, and (5) required physicians to keep detailed records on all abortions performed, with the records being subject to public disclosure.[37] The information to be maintained included the age and weight of the fetus and information about the female's past pregnancies or abortions.[38]

The Third Circuit Court of Appeals upheld all aspects of the Pennsylvania law except the spousal notification requirement. In doing so, it opined that based on the *Webster* and *Hodgson* decisions, the "strict scrutiny" test was no longer embraced by the majority of the Supreme Court justices. Rather, it continued, a lesser test—whether the law creates an "undue burden" on a woman's right to an abortion—was the appropriate standard.[39] Both sides appealed the Court of Appeals decision, asking for clarification on the law.

The U.S. Supreme Court upheld all of the Pennsylvania law's provisions except spousal notification as permissible ways in which a state's interest in the protection of fetal life and its preference for childbirth over abortion could be enforced.[40] The Court rejected the trimester approach established in *Roe*. In its place, the Court stated it would use the "undue burden" test in evaluating whether a state abortion law restricting abortion would be upheld or overturned. *Undue burden* is defined as whether a law restricting abortion has a purpose or effect of creating a substantial barrier to a woman's right to obtain an abortion.[41]

Although the *Casey* decision did not explicitly overrule *Roe v. Wade*, it effectively changed *Roe's* protections by placing limits—either real or potential—on a woman's choice concerning abortion.

One such limit that has received recent attention is what has been called "late-term abortion"

Plaintiff alleges criminal statute a violation of her due process rights under the Fourteenth Amendment

Court holds statute is vague and violates Ninth and Fourteenth Amendment rights

Fourteenth Amendment does protect personal liberty, which includes fundamental right of privacy to determine whether to terminate pregnancy

Court balances rights of mother with those of fetus

State does have interests, however, and court sets up trimester framework and state's ability to intervene in abortion decision within framework.

FACTS: A Texas criminal statute made it a crime to "procure" or "attempt" an abortion, except to save the life of the mother. Plaintiff, a single, pregnant female, wanted her abortion to be performed by a competent physician under acceptable medical conditions. She did not have the money to seek the abortion in another state, nor did she qualify for any of the exceptions in the Texas statute.

She filed suit, alleging that the statute was unconstitutional because it violated due process rights guaranteed under the Fourteenth Amendment of the U.S. Constitution.

DISTRICT COURT DECISION: The three-judge court held that the statute was vague and overly infringed on plaintiff's Ninth and Fourteenth Amendment Rights. A direct appeal to the U.S. Supreme Court was taken.

U.S. SUPREME COURT DECISION: The Court held that, under the Fourteenth Amendment's protection of personal liberty, which includes a fundamental right of privacy, a woman has a right to determine whether or not to terminate a pregnancy. In balancing the mother's right with that of the fetus, the Court held that (1) the fetus is not a person and thus not protected by the Constitution; (2) exempting only life-threatening situations from criminal liability does not consider other interests the female may have in terminating the pregnancy; and (3) although the decision to terminate a pregnancy is protected by the Constitution, the state *does* have legitimate interests in the general welfare of pregnant women, the unborn child, and the decision-making process after a certain point in time. Therefore, the Court held that during the first trimester of pregnancy, the decision to have an abortion is one between the mother and her physician. During the second trimester, the state may regulate the decision if the regulation is reasonably related to the state's interest in the health of the mother. During the last trimester, when the viability of the fetus is a legitimate state interest, the state may regulate and/or prohibit abortion, except when necessary to save the life of the mother.

ANALYSIS: The *Roe* decision was a landmark one and has been the subject of much controversy. In its companion case, *Doe v. Bolton,* the Court declared unconstitutional certain preabortion requirements in Georgia—state residency, approval by a hospital committee, and the procedure taking place only in a hospital approved by the Joint Commission on Accreditation of Healthcare Organizations (JCAHO). Although the two cases firmly rooted the right of a woman to make a choice about an abortion with limited governmental intervention, their respective parameters were tested by subsequent cases at both the federal and state levels (see discussion below).

It is also important to note that the *Roe* decision is an example of the use of the "strict scrutiny" test. Only when a "compelling state interest" exists can governmental intrusion into a "fundamental" right occur. As with many other constitutional rights, the right of privacy is not absolute. The Court's role here was to determine when the government can assert its interests and how an individual's rights may be narrowed.

TABLE 11–1

Court Cases After *Roe*

CASE NAME (YEAR)	CHALLENGE(S)	U.S. SUPREME COURT DECISION
Harris v. McRae (1980)[28]	Medicaid funding for abortions	No
Akron v. Akron Center for Reproductive Health, Inc. (1983)[29]	Restrictions on access: 24-hour waiting period, parental consent for unmarried minors, hospital procedure only for abortions after first trimester, detailed informed consent with MD's statement	Strikes down restrictions
Webster v. Reproductive Health Services (1989)[30]	Missouri statute stating life begins at conception; informed consent and information on abortions to patient; if pregnancy 20 or more weeks, MD must do tests to determine viability of fetus; and prohibition of abortions at public facilities unless pregnancy life threatening	Upholds restrictions with caveat that law's statement on life starting at conception cannot deny abortion rights; Court also discusses *Roe* as "rigid," "unsound," "unworkable"
Hodgson v. Minnesota (1990)[31] and *Ohio v. Akron Center for Reproductive Health* (1990)[32]	Parental notification for minors seeking abortion and provisions for court hearing to bypass parental notification to determine if minor capable of making decision	Upholds notification of *one* parent as constitutional and bypass provisions constitutionally permissible
Rust v. Sullivan (1991)[33]	Title X (funding for public and private nonprofit agencies providing family planning services) regulations interpreted by secretary of HHS to mean: no counseling about abortion, no referral for abortion, referral for "appropriate" prenatal services only, no "advocacy, promotion or encouragement" of abortion as method of family planning, and clear physical and organizational separation of facilities and staff from abortion services for those receiving Title X funds	Upholds regulations and finds they do not violate First or Fifth Amendment rights of patients or agencies

or "partial-birth abortion." Although the definition of either term is varied and confusing,[42] the debate centers on surgical procedures used to induce abortion during the second and third trimesters.[43] On both the federal and state level, laws proposed or passed make it a crime to use intact dilation and extraction (D & X) for late-term abortions.[44]

The debate over using D & X for late-term abortion includes maternal considerations, abortion mortality and morbidity, and the intrusion of the government—whether state or federal—into medical decision making, among other things.[45] Participants in the debate include physicians, anti-abortionists, the American Medical Society, and legal and other scholars who characterize the laws as "vague," "elastic," and an "undue burden" on a woman's right to abortion.[46]

On June 28, 2000, the U.S. Supreme Court, in *Stenberg v. Carhart* (99-830), held that Nebraska's statute criminalizing the performance of partial birth abortion(s) violated the federal Constitution as the Court interpreted it in the *Roe* and *Casey*

cases. In its opinion, the Court said the law also prohibited the "most common" method of abortions in the second trimester (the D & E procedure), thus placing an "undue burden" on a woman's right to "make an abortion decision." The Court also held the statute unconstitutional because there was no provision for a woman to obtain an abortion when needed to protect the female's health. The Court's 5–4 decision affects up to 30 similar state laws that had already banned the procedure, including Illinois, Ohio, and Wisconsin.[47]

. . . *the Casey decision did not explicitly overrule* Roe v. Wade *[but] it effectively changed* Roe's *protections by placing limits . . . on a woman's choice concerning abortion.*

ETHICS CONNECTION 11–1

Abortion has generated passionate human responses, including violence against staff of abortion clinics. Cogent moral positions have been developed both to support and refute the morality of abortion policies and practices. "Pro-life" supporters, on one hand, contend that a fetus is a person. Thus, they oppose abortion as the deliberate taking of a human life without the consent of the person whose life is at stake (the fetus). The "pro-life" argument is grounded in several moral principles, including but not limited to nonmaleficence, beneficence, respect for life, and the autonomy of the fetus. "Pro-choice" proponents, on the other hand, invoke the argument that a woman has the right to her own body and that she is not obligated to provide even temporary biological support for the fetus. This argument is grounded in the moral principle of respect for autonomy of the mother.

The distinction about when human life or personhood begins once was central to the debate about the morality of abortion but has been very difficult to establish. The quest to identify when a fetus could be considered a person was important for those who sought to support abortion early in the gestational period. More recently, moral arguments have been developed to both support and refute the practice of abortion, regardless of a fetus's claim to personhood. From the "pro-life" perspective, if a fetus has all the genetic attributes of being human, then theoretically the fetus is a person and thus entitled to human rights, especially the right to life. Abortion, thus, is the unjustified taking of a human life, or murder. Those who support the "pro-choice" argument contend that no human being has the right to depend upon the bodily processes of another person against that person's will. This argument is used particularly to justify abortion following rape or incest.

Ethical issues of abortion have become more complex as the practices of abortion and public policy related to abortion have changed. In addition, the question of fathers' and/or grandparents' moral rights in abortion decisions is part of the ethics conversation regarding abortion. Changes in abortion practices include the extension of the maximum gestation period at which abortion is legally permissible. Another change is the development of reproductive technologies that make it possible for multiple fetuses to compete with one another for sustenance during pregnancy. Technology has led to selectively aborting some fetuses in the interest of supporting life for others.[1] In addition, the technology that has led to *in utero* diagnosis and treatment of congenital anomalies also has created opportunities for parents to choose whether or not to abort the anatomically or physiologically imperfect fetuses.

Understanding the issues and taking a position on abortion is more than a theoretical exercise for practicing nurses, however. Because they are called upon to assist or attend during abortions and may, themselves, be faced with personal decisions about abortion, nurses must clearly understand their own values and beliefs. Those who cannot morally participate in abortions have the moral right, through conscience clauses, to refuse to participate. It is important that nurses know the extent of their legal rights and understand institutional policies related to attending or refusing to attend during abortion and invoking a conscience clause.

Some nurses are faced with deciding whether or not to care for women who choose to have abortions. All nurses, however, must address their values regarding this issue so that they can be active in developing public policy related to abortion. The course of public policy development has been contentious, fragmented, and delayed. Nurses and other health care professionals have a moral obligation to society to work toward developing or amending national policy so that it more fully reflects prevailing social moral values and those of the profession.[1] This is a daunting but important task in a pluralistic society and in a profession that reflects that plurality. (Refer to Chapter 3 for further discussion regarding the relationships between ethics and law in a pluralistic society.)

---

[1]Although abortion issues frequently are approached from the perspective of supporting parents' abortion decisions, there are times when health care professionals and ethicists advocate abortion and families refuse, choosing to carry the pregnancy to term. Issues of assisted reproduction, such as in the case of the McCaughey septuplets, offer a counterpoint to the usual abortion debate. When, upon ultrasound testing during a pregnancy facilitated by human chorionic gonadotropin (HCG), Bobbi McCaughey was found to be carrying seven fetuses, several options were presented, all of which would have meant reducing the total number of fetuses, by either selective abortion or other technologies. The McCaugheys rejected these options and Bobbi McCaughey gave birth to septuplets. Many ethical issues still surround this widely publicized decision and the social concerns that it raises. On a lighter note that nevertheless illustrates the McCaughey case as one that has broader social implications than those of individual or family autonomy, the city administrator commented, "They say it takes a village to raise children. We just didn't know it would be our village." See Arlene Judith Klotzko, "Medical Miracle or Medical Mischief?: The Saga of the McCaughey Septuplets," 23(5), *Hastings Center Report* (May-June 1998), 3–7.

NURSING IMPLICATIONS

The decision to have an abortion under almost any circumstance is difficult. Therefore, the nurse working with a patient who is faced with this choice needs to be especially sensitive to the patient's emotional stress during the time she is deciding what she will do. The provision of support, active listening, and information as needed will be very helpful to the patient during this process of decision making.

The nurse can reinforce the patient's right in seeking the treatment to terminate pregnancy consistent with the state law. For the adult patient, this right includes the fact that the decision can be made without notifying any other person, including a spouse. It also includes the right of the patient to seek whatever medical information is necessary from the physician to fully understand the implications of her decision.

If working with minors, the nurse will need to comply with state law concerning the rights of the minor to seek information about an abortion. If the minor patient has decided to have an abortion, the nurse will need to focus particularly on the need for parental notification or consent and any waiting period that is required before the abortion can occur. This will require up-to-date understanding of the law in the state in which the nurse practices. Although not always possible or desired, a careful discussion of seeking support and guidance from a parent can be explored with the minor.

Last, but by no means least, the nurse must explore his or her own feelings concerning abortion. This is important for the nurse so that personal values are clarified and owned.[48] Doing so also allows for the provision of care to the patient without infringing on her legal rights in relation to the procedure.

If, however, the nurse has determined not to provide care to a patient seeking abortion information or services, it is possible under many state laws (New York and Illinois, for example) not to participate in those services. The state statutes are often based on abortion being contrary to the health care provider's religious beliefs. An employer is prohibited by the statutes from retaliating against the nurse who raises this issue in the employment setting.

DOCUMENTATION REMINDER 11–1
Reproductive Choice

- Patient questions/comments/concerns
- Required forms—consent, notification of parent (if required for minor) and others—executed and in medical record
- Any and all patient teaching concerning procedure, follow-up care, discharge instructions
- Refusal of any part of procedure, follow-up care, discharge instructions
- Contact(s) with physician and others concerning care, nursing interventions, and patient response(s)

Reproductive Innovations
Artificial Insemination

Artificial insemination is the oldest reproductive technology. The process of artificially inseminating a female occurs by introducing viable sperm into the vagina, cervical canal, or uterus by artificial means.[49] Two processes exist—AIH (homologous insemination), which utilizes the sperm of the female's spouse, and AID or DI (donor insemination), which utilizes semen from a donor.[50]

Artificial insemination is the oldest reproductive technology . . .

AIH insemination is the less legally problematic of the two. Even so, clear concerns must be acknowledged. First and foremost, the procedure must be done in accordance with whatever statute may exist in the state. When a statute exists, a physician is usually the health care provider required to perform the procedure. Furthermore, the written informed consent of the couple is required. It is important that no guarantee of a full-term pregnancy or live birth be given to the couple.[51]

AID insemination, in contrast, is fraught with legal issues. This is particularly so in relation to consent issues and the support of the child. Clearly, the written informed consent of the woman to be artificially inseminated is mandatory. If the woman is not married, this requirement is not unusually problematic. Problems may arise in relation to the donor, however, especially if a state does not have a law concerning the legitimacy of the child and the donor's responsibilities, if any, after its birth. Some states have passed statutes specifying that a child from AID is legitimate, and the donor is not responsible for supporting the child because he is not considered the father. In those states that have not yet passed such statutes, issues of consent from the donor and support of the child will continue to exist.

If the woman is married and a decision is made to undergo AID without the consent of the husband, a legal battle may also occur. The husband may challenge his obligation to provide care and support of the offspring of the AID insemination to which he did not agree. If, in contrast, that husband has consented to the procedure, most state statutes clearly indicate that the child is the legitimate offspring of the couple who consented to the procedure, thus decreasing challenges of support obligations by the husband.

The utilization of donor sperm adds the requirement for the physician and the sperm bank, if one is used, to screen the donor for infectious diseases (including AIDS and hepatitis), Rh factor incompatibility, and inheritable diseases.[52]

In addition, facilities that "obtain, collect, process, furnish, distribute, or store" semen or tissue for use in humans must, by state law, register with the state's department of public health.[53]

Recently, AIH donation has received much attention surrounding the use of sperm from a deceased husband.[54] Most often, sperm is taken from an artificially sustained husband who is brain-dead.[55] However, other situations in which this method of AIH has occurred includes cadavers and frozen sperm willed to the surviving female in a relationship.[56] These situations raise many legal and ethical issues, including lineage questions, rights of inheritance, and a new husband's financial support of the child conceived in this manner prior to his marriage to the child's mother.[57]

NURSING IMPLICATIONS

Because physicians have been identified as the health care providers who are to conduct the process of artificial insemination, the nurse will not be directly involved in the actual process. Even so, the nurse may participate by doing an initial physical assessment of the woman who is to undergo the procedure and obtaining other preliminary information from her or the couple. Furthermore, the nurse may provide some information to the female or couple concerning the procedure prior to the physician's doing so.

In addition, the nurse who works in any physician's office or clinic providing artificial insemination services will need to be certain that all paperwork required for either procedure is in the patient's record (see Documentation Reminder 11–2). Furthermore, maintaining the privacy and confidentiality of the medical record, including the donor's identity in AID inseminations, is absolutely essential. Releases should be done only after written informed consent is obtained; records should be stored carefully and only certain staff granted access to them; and advice from legal counsel should be obtained whenever a subpoena is received for an individual record.

A nurse involved in the storage or handling of any semen must exercise care and caution. For example, policies and procedures should be developed and adhered to concerning receipt of semen from the donor; proper identification and storage of the sperm; and any treatment of the sperm (for example, centrifuge) prior to its use.[58] The development of policies and procedures should be based on guidelines established by such organizations as the American Association of Tissue Banks, the American Society for Reproductive Health, the Food and Drug Administration, and the Centers for Disease Control.[59]

Artificial insemination may be anxiety provoking and frightening to the patient, her husband, or significant other. The nurse's ability to provide support and care during the process can be invaluable to those undergoing this reproductive technique.

In Vitro *Fertilization*

Also a procedure of artificial insemination, *in vitro* fertilization (IVF) involves removing an ovum from the woman, fertilizing it *in vitro,* and then placing the fertilized egg into the uterus.[60] The procedure may take place with homologous or donor insemination. The birth of the first living child conceived as a result of this method occurred in 1978.[61] Since then, variations of the initial method have developed, including gamete intrafallopian transfer (GIFT), and zygote intrafallopian transfer (ZIFT).[62]

Many of the family, legal, and other concerns with this method of reproduction are similar to those discussed in the section on artificial insemination. However, an additional concern arises with

IVF regardless of the method used. That concern is what is to be done with an ovum or ova not implanted until a future date or not used for implantation at all.

[In vitro fertilization] may take place with homologous or donor insemination.

The storage of ova not used immediately raises concerns as to proper storage, labeling, length of ability to survive storage techniques (usually cryo-preservation), and ownership. For example, in a 1983 case, a California couple were both killed in a plane crash in South America after the successful fertilization of two ova in Australia, which were frozen and stored there. After the couple's deaths an Australian committee recommended that the embryos be destroyed, but the legislature passed a law suggesting the ova be implanted in another woman and if a child were born as a result, the child should be adopted. The California court, however, ruled that the children would not inherit from the deceased parents.[63]

In a 1989 divorce proceeding, the ownership of a divorcing couple's seven frozen embryos was disputed.[64] Initially the zygotes were awarded to Mrs. Davis so that she could utilize them for implantation. The ex-husband appealed the decision, arguing that the state could not force him to become a father. The Tennessee appeals court agreed with him, holding that the state could not force either one of them to use the embryos to be parents. Forcing the ex-husband to become a father against his will would violate his "constitutionally protected right not to beget a child where no pregnancy has taken place." The court awarded both joint custody of the embryos.[65]

On June 1, 1992, the Tennessee Supreme Court upheld the appeals court decision. In doing so, it held that when a divorcing couple is not able to agree on what is to be done with frozen embryos, the individual who does not want to be a parent should prevail, unless the party favoring parenthood has no other way of becoming a parent.[66] Furthermore, the Tennessee Supreme Court opinion clearly struck down the concept that the embryos were children; in other words, life does not

begin at conception.[67] Last, the court held that the clinic storing the embryos was "free to follow its normal procedures in dealing with the unused 'pre-embryos' [the court's term] as long as that procedure is not in conflict with this opinion."[68] The embryos were destroyed in 1993.[69]

The case, decided before the Pennsylvania abortion case, seems to favor parental rights over those of potential children. In addition, although both of the divorcing couple's viewpoints were considered, a balancing test was used to determine which position would prevail.[70]

Recent cases involving IVF issues provide additional decisions but no clear trends. For example, in *Kass v. Kass*,[71] a New York court required that frozen fertilized eggs be donated for research in accordance with the terms of the agreement executed by the former husband and wife.[72]

Haunting legal—and ethical—questions remain concerning what is to be done with fertilized zygotes. For example, how long can embryos be cryopreserved and still be used for implantation?[73] If not used for implantation, should they be destroyed? In what manner? Whose consent must be obtained to destroy them? Assuming their viability, can they be utilized by someone wanting to be a "surrogate mother"? Is the destruction of the fertilized cells covered in some way by state abortion statutes prohibiting destruction and experimentation with a fetus? And, as pro-life proponents suggest, do embryos need to be protected from destruction?[74]

Negligent destruction of the embryos creates additional concerns for health care providers. In a 1978 case, a university, hospital, and physician were found liable for the intentional destruction of a couple's cultured cells.[75] The plaintiffs sued under a theory of intentional infliction of emotional distress.

NURSING IMPLICATIONS

Many of the nursing implications discussed in the section on artificial insemination are applicable to this reproductive technique. Additionally, the nurse must keep up to date about existing state laws and the destruction of zygotes not used for implantation. The nurse will need to include in the written consent form all information concerning the use or destruction of cells not used for implantation. If the nurse assists the physician in the procedure, providing nonnegligent care before, during, and after the procedure is essential.

Surrogate Motherhood

Surrogate motherhood is an arrangement whereby one woman (the "surrogate") conceives and bears a child under an agreement to surrender the child to another person or persons, who must then adopt the child as their own.[76] Several variations of this arrangement exist. In one, an infertile couple agree to use the husband's sperm to artificially inseminate a woman who agrees to carry the child to term and then give up all parental rights. In another, an infertile couple use their respective ovum and sperm, fertilizing them in vitro and then having them implanted in a surrogate who carries the child to term and then gives up all parental rights.

Regardless of the method used, the agreement for this arrangement is regulated by state law. Some states, such as Arizona and Louisiana, have passed specific legislation concerning surrogacy. Those that have not passed specific laws utilize existing state laws dealing with adoption (for example, the illegality of selling babies or acting as an "intermediary" or "broker" in the process). Thus, where surrogate motherhood is not prohibited, the arrangement with the surrogate may include the payment of medical and living expenses but not a fee for her consent to give up the child for adoption.[77]

When a surrogate mothering arrangement goes well, there is little controversy. However, when the surrogate mother decides not to give up the child at birth, a whole myriad of legal issues arises, including the respective rights of all involved in the arrangement.[78]

NURSING IMPLICATIONS

The nurse's involvement with this type of reproductive technique most probably will be only in the provision of care to the surrogate mother, whether during regular prenatal checkups, delivery, or the postpartum period. Accurate and complete documentation concerning the care given will, of course, be necessary.

The nurse should not attempt to obtain information about the surrogacy relationship or participate in the decision concerning custody after the birth of the child. If, however, the surrogate mother initiates a discussion about her role, or expresses concerns about it, the nurse should provide whatever support is possible. Any concerns, as well as any interventions initiated by the nurse, should be documented in the medical record.

Although the nurse may be well-intended, trying to connect those interested in being a surrogate mother with couples who are looking for someone to act in that role, it is best not to do so. This prohibition is applicable not only to the nurse as employee but also outside of the employment setting. Involvement of this nature may clearly violate state laws concerning surrogacy or adoption or both.

Nurses who work in labor and delivery services must be certain to discharge a newborn pursuant to the policy in effect in that institution. If an infant is released to the wrong party or agency, the nurse and institution will most certainly face a lawsuit. When a nurse is unclear to whom the infant should be released, contacting the nurse manager is essential.

DOCUMENTATION REMINDER 11–2
Reproductive Innovations

- Patient questions/comments/concerns
- Consent forms complete and executed
- Coding of donor-identifying information to maintain confidentiality and privacy
- Any and all patient/family teaching concerning procedure, discharge instructions, follow-up care
- Complete donor sperm or ovum screening, results, and the like in chart, and information shared with female patient
- MD certification requirements mandated by state laws complete
- Storage of sperm, ovum, or zygotes and procedure documented
- Sperm, ovum, or zygote disposal recorded
- Refusal of any part of procedure, follow-up care, or discharge instructions

---

Genetic Counseling and Screening

Genetic counseling includes both the preconception determination of heritable disease and the prenatal diagnosis of fetal disease or abnormality.[79] Preconception counseling attempts to estimate the probability of recurrence of an identified genetic defect and aids prospective parents in deciding on a course of action.[80] If the female is already pregnant, specific diagnostic tests may be ordered, including amniocentesis, ultrasound, maternal blood tests, and chorionic villus sampling.[81]

Clearly the timing of genetic screening is crucial. As soon as it is determined that there is a potential for a particular heritable disease or a fetal disease or abnormality, a referral to a geneticist must be made. This is particularly important for the nurse-midwife who determines that a particular client may not be expected to have a normal pregnancy or delivery.

If the prospective parents decide not to have children based on the information the geneticist provides them, there is little else that can be done for the couple. They may consider adopting a child or children, however. If a fetal disease or abnormality is discovered, the care of the female during the pregnancy, should she decide to carry the fetus to term, must be carefully orchestrated.

NURSING IMPLICATIONS

The nurse working in a genetic counseling facility may take on any number of roles. For example, if an ultrasound examination is ordered, the nurse may function as an educator or coordinator of services.[82] If amniocentesis is required, the nurse may assist the physician. Any role requires that the nurse provide support to the female during the procedure, provide whatever patient teaching is necessary and consistent with the nursing role, monitor the patient's condition before, during, and after the procedure, and document the care given. If the nurse handles any specimens taken during the diagnostic test, careful labeling, management, and storage are also essential.

Alternative Family Structures

Adoption

Adoption has no historical basis in the common law and therefore is governed entirely by state statute.[83] The process involves termination of the legal relationship (and its rights and duties) between natural parents and their child and conferring the relationship upon adoptive parents and the child. The purpose of adoption is to promote the welfare of the child, especially when parents have died, or cannot, or do not, properly care for their child.

Adoption has no historical basis in the common law and therefore is governed entirely by state statute.

The specifics of the adoption process are varied, because each state has its own particular law governing adoption. Even so, some common elements can be identified. Adoption can occur through an agency or through private placement. Consent for the adoption must be given by the natural parents—both the mother *and* father—unless there has been a determination of "unfitness" of the parents or a judicial termination of parental rights has already occurred (e.g., in the case of proven child abuse). The buying and selling of babies is considered illegal.

Adoption records used to be sealed once the adoption was complete, and the records could not be opened unless "good cause" was shown. It is now more common for states to allow limited release of certain information in the adoption records if certain conditions are met. For example, some states allow the adopted person, or his or her representative, access to the birth certificate information and information identifying the birth parents.[84] Other states provide this type of information through the establishment of "mutual consent voluntary registries" whereby the adoptive and biological parents share identities and other information.[85]

In addition, because the need for medical information about the adoptee may be vital for treatment decisions, some states require medical information to be disclosed to the adoptive parents at the time of adoption while others allow access to this information under certain conditions.[86]

Because an adoption is a result of state law that terminates rights and creates new ones, certain constitutional requirements must be followed. To begin with, due process protections are afforded all parties. Thus, the biological parent(s) and the child to be adopted must be given notice of the pending adoption, and the father must be given the right to consent to, or contest, the adoption. In addition, any involuntary termination of the biological parents' rights cannot occur unless the decision is supported by "clear and convincing" evidence.

The adoption itself takes place in open court, with specific orders entered into the court record so that other documentation, such as the birth certificate, can reflect the adoptive parent(s) as the natural parent(s).

ETHICS CONNECTION 11–2

Although efforts have begun, nursing has been slow to address critical issues of professional and social values related to genetics. The international project, of which the Human Genome Project of the U. S. Department of Energy is a part, is an effort to understand "the sequences of genes that code the body's building blocks."[1,2] Newer understandings and better treatments of disease and disability were intended to emerge. For disability rights advocates as well as conceptions of nursing that view disease as part of human health patterns,[3] there is a hubris associated with the assumptions that disease and disability are inherently onerous. Some disability advocates conclude that this effort diminishes the worth of humans with disabilities or diseases and contributes to the widespread societal disregard for disabled persons, despite the Americans with Disabilities Act. There are, of course, counterarguments to this position. In an effort to carefully examine and present a balanced view of the nature and scope of the issues regarding genetic testing and disability, the Hastings Center published a special supplement.[4] This supplement contains reflections that are important for nurses to consider as they examine their own and the profession's moral values regarding genetic testing and its consequences, especially for nurses who participate in genetic counseling. In concluding the supplement the authors note that

> if prospective parents carefully ask themselves the hard questions about what they want and will appreciate in a future child, then they and any future children they raise have a better chance for fulfillment and for mutual, rewarding family life. And if genetics professionals (including nurses) learn more about what raising disabled children can mean, rethink their approach to parents, and help those parents better imagine what a child's disability might mean for their family, then some progress will be made in honoring the disability rights movement's central message that our society must be able to value people and lives of different sorts. Only as we take that message seriously can we be confident that our parental decisions will improve familial and communal life.

White[5] discusses the possibilities and challenges associated with an interpretive ethic for genetic decision making. This dialogical model is grounded in human relationships and, thus, is consonant with covenantal relationships and the ethic of care (see Chapter 3). In the dialogical model, genetics counselors hold a social rather than an individualistic view of autonomy and assist clients to explore and understand both the individual and social nature of the issues they are considering. Although counselors who use this approach serve as "gatekeepers to genetic services," they are not coercive and consider themselves bound to accept the choice of the client, regardless of whether it coincides with the counselor's own viewpoints. The effort is to help the client make as fully informed a decision as is possible. From this genetic counseling perspective, informed consent is considered to be a process rather than a single event. The plethora of genetic diagnostic and treatment possibilities increases daily. The ethical dialogue about genetic testing and the moral responsibilities of genetic counselors is developing and not yet fully formulated.

Nursing, health care, and society face many more ethical issues concerned with reproductive technology than can be adequately represented here. Currently, issues of the moral limits of technologically assisted reproduction such as the ultimate disposition of unused ova, stored sperm, and unimplanted embryos,[6] whether from live or dead donors, must be systematically, carefully, and responsibly addressed. At their center, these issues and others surrounding the beginning of life connect with end-of-life issues. Both are grounded in the broader individual, communal, and social discourse about the meaning and limits of human life, well-being, and mortality.

---

[1]The Hastings Center, Special Supplement: "The Disability Rights Critique of Prenatal Genetic Testing," 29(5) *Hastings Center Report* (September/October 1999), S1–S18.

[2]See Chapter 3 for additional information about the Human Genome Project and ethics.

[3]Margaret A. Newman. *Health as Expanding Consciousness*. 2nd Edition. New York: National League for Nursing Press, 1994 (Pub. No. 14-2626).

[4]The Hastings Center, *supra* note 1.

[5]Mary Terrell White, "Making Responsible Decisions: An Interpretive Ethic for Genetic Decisionmaking," 29(1) *Hastings Center Report* (January/February 1999), 14–21.

[6]John A. Robertson, "Meaning What You Sign," 28(4) *Hastings Center Report* (July/August 1998), 22–23.

Adoptive children enjoy all of the privileges of naturally born children, including the right of inheritance and recognition of the adoption in any state in which the family lives.

The Divorced Family

The process of divorce dissolves a marriage relationship.[87] As a result, the legal relationship between the former husband and wife is terminated, and therefore most, if not all, duties and obligations between the two are also terminated. If any duties or obligations survive the divorce, such as the payment of rehabilitative maintenance to the female or the continued payment of the mortgage on the home of the former couple, they would be included in the divorce decree.

If children were born during the marital relationship, their care, custody, and control would also be spelled out in the divorce decree. Although divorce terminates the duties and rights of the husband and wife, it does not terminate *parental* rights and responsibilities toward the children of that marriage. Rather, a divorce requires that the parental obligations be spelled out carefully, including child support payments, consent for and payment for medical care of the children, and custody arrangements.

Only when decisions concerning the custody of the children cannot be made by the divorcing couple does the court intervene to resolve the dispute. When confronted with custody battles, the court uses a "best-interest-of-the-child" test to make its determination; that is, the best placement for the child is based on such factors as the child's age, health, and desires (if ascertainable).

As with adoption decrees, a custody decree is valid in all other states because of the passage of the Uniform Child Custody Jurisdiction Act.[88]

Single-Parent Families

Single-parent families, once unusual, are common in today's society. Single-parent families can occur when there is a loss of a parent due to divorce, the death of one parent, or adoption by a single female or male.

Although at one time children born out of wedlock were considered illegitimate, today, children of single-parent families, whatever the cause, are legally no different from those of two-parent families. Specifically, they cannot be adopted without the consent of both biological parents, are entitled to full inheritance rights from both parents (when paternity is proven, if needed), and must be supported by the biological father (when paternity is proven, if needed).

Blended Families

The living arrangements possible for families in today's society are almost endless. A widowed man with children may marry a divorced woman with children, or a single mother may decide to live with another individual, or a divorced mother with one child may marry a previously unmarried man. The "blending" of these individuals into a family redefines the traditional notion of the "nuclear" or "primary" family of years past and adds new meaning to the term *stepfamily*.

Regardless of the manner in which the family comes together, traditional legal relationships remain unchanged. For example, unless any of the children in the aforementioned families are adopted by the respective spouse or live-in member, those spouses or live-in individuals have no legal obligation, rights, or duties in relation to the children. A subsequent marriage to another does not terminate the parental rights of the divorced couple. Likewise, marrying someone with children does not confer parental rights on the new spouse. Therefore, consent issues, custody concerns, and support obligations remain the duties, rights, and obligations of the biological parents until their rights are severed.

NURSING IMPLICATIONS

A nurse will most probably provide nursing care to at least one person in an alternative family structure.

A nurse will most probably provide nursing care to at least one person in an alternative family structure.

When confronted with a patient who is pregnant but who would like to give the baby up for adoption, it is best that the nurse who is working in the community help the patient contact a reputable private or public adoption agency. It is very important that the nurse not accept money or other items of value for referring the expectant mother to a prospective adopting couple.

If the nurse is providing care to an adopted child, the adoptive parents have full parental rights and can therefore be involved in the patient's care and must be consulted for their consent to the care of their child. If the adoption has not yet been finalized, but the couple has custody of the child during the pendency of the adoption procedure, they usually are given the right to consent to treatment of the child. The nurse may want to verify that fact with the couple before treatment is given.

The nurse working with a child who is experiencing the divorce of his or her parents will need to be sensitive to the emotional trauma the minor is going through. Once the divorce is final, it will be important to ascertain the parent who has been given the right to consent for medical treatment. Joint custody may have been agreed to or decided by the court. If that is the case, then the nurse must be certain that both parents give consent to the treatment needed by their child.

The nurse working with children in a blended family will need to assess who is the natural parent in that constellation. Generally only the natural parent can consent to or refuse treatment.

In addition to consent to treatment issues, the nurse, whether a school nurse or a nurse working in acute care, must be certain to release a child to the adult identified as being legally able to take possession of that minor. For example, the mother of a sick child may not be able to pick up the child from school. If, however, she contacts the school nurse and, consistent with the school's policy, she gives permission for her daughter to be picked up by her husband (who is not the child's father), then the school nurse can release the child to the designated person. The school nurse should document that permission in the child's school record.

SPECIAL CONSIDERATIONS IN REPRODUCTIVE AND FAMILY CONCERNS

Refusal of Treatment by Pregnant Woman

The right of the competent adult to refuse treatment, even life-sustaining treatment, has been firmly established as a protection under the Fourteenth Amendment's right of liberty (freedom from unwanted medical care) and privacy. That right becomes somewhat troublesome, however, when the competent adult is pregnant. No controlling decision declaring the fetus a person and therefore entitled to constitutional protections has been handed down by the U.S. Supreme Court. Even so, when the pregnant woman declines treatment, many legal issues arise in relation to the refusal's effect on the fetus.

Pregnant women have refused blood tests, diagnostic screening procedures, cesarean sections, and most often, blood transfusions.[89] To date, the cases dealing with this issue have been split; that is, some courts have ordered that the refused treatment should be given (cesarean section[90]) while others have upheld the right of refusal (blood transfusion[91]).

However, in a 1990 case, *In re A.C.*,[92] the District of Columbia Court of Appeals held that when a terminally ill pregnant mother is near death, the question whether or not a cesarean section will be done to possibly save the life of the fetus is to be decided by the pregnant woman. If the patient cannot make that decision because of incompetency or some other reason, then the substituted judgment test must be used to make the decision.[93]

The *A.C.* case notwithstanding, in view of the *Casey* decision discussed earlier in this chapter, arguments concerning the role of women in selecting medical treatment when pregnant may well be moot. The *Casey* Court held that a state's "legitimate" interest in "fetal life" exists "throughout pregnancy."[94] Indeed, the "balancing of fetal rights" with those of the mother insofar as consent to treatment is concerned is appearing in subsequent cases, albeit with varying results. In *In re Doe*,[95] the Illinois Appellate Court upheld a woman's decision not to have a cesarean section. Her decision, based on "her abiding faith in God's healing powers," was challenged by the state's attorney's petition to have the fetus declared a ward of the state.[96] The lower court refused to order the woman to have the recommended operation. An appeal was filed by the state and the public guardian, arguing that the interests of the fetus should have been balanced with those of the mother during the lower court hearing.[97] The appeals court rejected this approach and affirmed the lower court's decision.

In *In re Fetus Brown*,[98] the Illinois Appellate Court *did* utilize the "balancing test" in deciding whether a pregnant woman should be forced to undergo a blood transfusion. The competent woman, who was a Jehovah's Witness, refused the transfusion. The state again attempted to use the balancing test, but altered it by saying that the "balance" should occur between the state's interest in the fetus and the mother's interest.[99] The appeals court utilized this form of the test, but ruled that because a blood transfusion was a "substantial invasion" of the mother's bodily integrity, it could not be forced upon the mother.[100] The court did clearly state, however, that in certain circumstances—when treatment was "trivial"—another result might be appropriate. The court also suggested that the mother's interest outweighing the state's interest in the fetus is not certain in every instance.[101]

If future decisions follow *Casey* and the Illinois court's balancing rationale, restrictions on a pregnant woman's choices concerning treatment or nontreatment may well be considered subservient to treatment options that serve the fetus's well-being. Doing so may well create a burdensome adversarial relationship between the state, the fetus, and the pregnant female.[102]

High-Risk Maternal Conduct during Pregnancy

The well-being of both the mother and the fetus during pregnancy is a concern of health care providers. It is also a concern to the state, especially when the mother's conduct may create a risk to the well-being or very survival of the fetus. A well-known example of the type of conduct that places the fetus at risk is the use of alcohol and drugs. Other types of behavior, such as heavy smoking and lack of prenatal care, have also been identified.

A state's interest in a pregnant woman's high-risk behavior has been demonstrated in two ways, both involving the criminal law. In a 1999 case, a Wisconsin appellate court ruled that a woman who drank alcohol during her ninth month of pregnancy could not be charged with attempted murder of her fetus.[103] Despite the attempt by many states to charge high-risk maternal conduct as criminal causes of action, few are successful. Twenty-one other states have prohibited criminal prosecution of pregnant women whose behavior may cause harm to the fetus.[104]

A second approach to halt high-risk maternal behavior has been the use of the state's child abuse statutes. This approach has not been consistently successful. However, in some states including Colorado and South Carolina, child abuse laws have been used to successfully prosecute pregnant women when their behavior creates a risk to the well-being of the fetus.[105] In the case involving Cornelia Whitner, the South Carolina Supreme Court ruled that the child neglect prosecution against Ms. Whitner was proper.[106] The attorney general of South Carolina essentially argued that the fetus was a person who needed protection from its mother, who used crack cocaine during her pregnancy.[107] This decision is the only state ruling

that declares a fetus a person, thus entitling it to all protections afforded other persons, even when the person whom the fetus needs protection from is its own mother.[108] The U.S. Supreme Court refused to review the decision in the Whitner matter.

It may be that in the future, again in view of the *Casey* decision, additional steps may be taken by the state when pregnant women engage in behavior that endangers the fetus. For example, under the Fourteenth Amendment guarantee of privacy, could a state order a woman (or a man, for that matter) *not* to procreate when prior conduct has resulted in a finding of child abuse or neglect? In three cases, in California, Kansas, and Illinois,[109] the courts have held that a prohibition of procreation as a condition of parole was an impermissible intrusion on the right of privacy.

Use of Aborted Fetal Tissue for Transplantation or Research

The use of fetal remains for transplantation or research is a subject of great controversy, legally, ethically, and morally. The controversy stems mainly from the manner in which fetal tissue becomes available—through abortions.[110] Although using fetal tissue resulting from a spontaneous abortion or one induced to save the life of the mother may be less problematic to some, the use of an abortus from an elective abortion triggers objections from many individuals. Furthermore, the argument continues, using fetal tissue for experimentation and research, however noble, humane, and helpful that use may be, encourages abortion.[111]

The use of fetal tissue for research and transplantation is not new. It has occurred for some time pursuant to Department of Health and Human Services regulations, passed initially in 1975, and state laws such as the Uniform Anatomical Gift Act (UAGA), passed by all of the states between 1969 and 1973.[112] However, in March of 1988 during the Reagan administration, the assistant secretary declared a "temporary moratorium" on federally funded research that uses fetal tissue from induced (elective) abortions.[113]

Congress attempted to lift the ban on at least two occasions but was unsuccessful. President Bush established a tissue bank for fetal tissue resulting from miscarriages, stillbirths, or ectopic pregnancies in May of 1992, but critics stated that doing so was not enough. Such tissues are not easily available or suitable for transplant in many circumstances.[114]

On January 22, 1993 (2 days after he took office), President Bill Clinton directed his newly appointed secretary of Health and Human Services to lift the ban placed on federal funding for human fetal tissue transplantation research.[115]

Current regulations applicable to fetal tissue transplantation research define when the death of a fetus occurs,[116] prohibit those using the fetal tissue from deciding the "timing, method and procedures used to terminate the pregnancy,"[117] and prohibit the use of any inducements to influence the pregnant woman's decision to terminate her pregnancy.[118]

It is certain that the debate over the use of fetal tissue for research and transplantation will continue.

It is certain that the debate over the use of fetal tissue for research and transplantation will continue. Those who support fetal tissue use state that it holds promise for those with Parkinson's and Alzheimer's diseases, diabetes, and spinal cord injuries. Opponents, however, continue to argue that support of fetal tissue use supports only "a demand for tissues from unborn babies."[119]

Fetal Research

Fetal research is defined in three ways by the federal government: *in utero, ex utero,* or directed toward pregnant women.[120] The regulations mandate limitations on any of those types of research: (1) preliminary studies on animals and nonpregnant subjects must take place before experimentation occurs on pregnant human subjects; (2) nontherapeutic research can pose no more than a minimal risk to the fetus; (3) no inducements may be made to terminate a pregnancy; (4) abortion procedures may pose no more than minimal risk to the pregnant woman; and (5) researchers cannot take part in any decision concerning the timing or method of abortion or the viability of the fetus when the pregnancy terminates.[121]

In addition to these requirements, specific regulations require that when research is done *in utero,* the informed consent of both the mother and father be obtained, the research pose minimal risk to the fetus and serve the fetus's health needs, and the information obtained not be available in other ways.[122]

If a nonviable, *ex-utero* fetus is utilized for research, federal regulations specifically require that vital functions will not be artificially maintained; the research will not terminate heartbeat or respiration; and the information gained through the procedure is not obtainable in another manner.[123]

Freedom of Access to Clinic Entrances Act of 1994

Because abortion and reproductive health services are so controversial, many instances of violence have accompanied these issues. The violence has taken many forms, including the murder of those who perform abortion services[124] and blocking access to clinics providing abortion and other reproductive health care. In an attempt to prevent further violence from occurring, Congress passed the Freedom of Access to Clinic Entrances Act (Public Law 103-259).[125]

The Act provides civil and criminal remedies against those who block, assault, or commit other violent or threatening acts against women, their families, or health care providers at a facility providing reproductive services. The Act does permit peaceful picketing or other peaceful demonstrations protected by the First Amendment at such facilities.[126]

Cloning Human Beings

On July 5, 1996, Scottish scientist Ian Wilmut and his colleagues at the Roslin Institute successfully cloned a sheep. Wilmut used the technique of transplanting the genetic material of an adult sheep into an egg from which the nucleus had been removed.[127] The resulting sheep, named Dolly, was unique in that she contained genetic material of only one parent. Dolly was, in short, a "delayed genetic twin of a single adult sheep."[128]

Dolly's birth created legal, ethical, and moral controversy. President Clinton issued a ban on federal funding for attempts to clone human beings using this technique.[129] Questions were raised concerning the propriety of human cloning (e.g., is it ever acceptable?), the religious perspectives of cloning, and its potential for abuse.[130] Although

ETHICS CONNECTION 11–3

Cloning is a technology that is relevant to nurses as professionals and, more importantly, to nurses as human beings. Cloning is part of a genetic scientific revolution that "may both profoundly influence our beliefs and dramatically change how society functions."[1] Because much of the early research in reproductive technology was conducted in agriculture schools, the studies proceeded without regulation or monitoring by governmental agencies concerned with human health and welfare or oversight by institutional review boards (IRBs). Thus, the technological capability of recreating human life outstripped the capacity of ethicists and theologians to discern the nature and extent of related ethical concerns. The possibility of cloning human beings challenges contemporary ethics, particularly theological ethics, as perhaps few other scientific revolutions have done. In discussing cloning and genetic engineering, Cohen raises some intriguing and powerful questions for ethical consideration, including "Will designing our offspring someday be as easy and common as 'cut and paste' on a word processor? Are we on the cusp of an evolutionary advance toward being an 'autocreative species'?"[2] Ethicists who are examining issues of genetic engineering and cloning recognize that religious views are critically important dimensions to be considered. Cloning presents challenges for Jewish,[3,4] Christian,[5] and Western thought.[6,7] The moral conversation about cloning is ongoing and unresolved.

---

[1]Jonathan R. Cohen, "In God's Garden: Creation and Cloning in Jewish Thought," 29(4) *Hastings Center Report* (July/August 1999), 7–13.

[2]*Id.*

[3]Azriel Rosenfield, "Judaism and Gene Design," in *Jewish Bioethics,* Fred Rosner and J. David Bleich, Editors. New York: Hebrew Publishing, 1979, 401–408.

[4]Fred Rosner, "Genetic Engineering and Judaism," in *Jewish Bioethics,* Fred Rosner and J. David Bleich, Editors. New York: Hebrew Publishing, 1979, 409–420.

[5]Ronald Cole-Turner, Editor. *Human Cloning: Religious Responses.* Louisville, Ky.: Westminster John Knox Press, 1997.

[6]National Bioethics Advisory Commission. *Cloning Human Beings: Report and Recommendations of the National Bioethics Advisory Commission.* Rockville, Md.: Author, 1997.

[7]*Ethics and Theology: A Continuation of the National Discussion on Human Cloning.* Hearing Before the Subcommittee on Public Health and Safety of the Senate Committee on Labor and Human Resources of the 105th Congress, 1997.

far from reaching a consensus on the answers to these and other questions surrounding cloning, the 1997 report of the Rockville, Maryland–based National Bioethics Advisory Commission, *Cloning Human Beings,* has initiated an open debate that may begin to resolve some of the many questions raised about cloning human beings.

NURSING IMPLICATIONS

The nurse working with a patient in a situation in which any one of the special considerations arises will need to be certain that any informed consent or refusal documents are executed and in the patient's record. If a nurse or nurse-midwife provides prenatal care to a pregnant woman whose behavior is high risk, the nurse must adequately inform the patient of the ramifications of that behavior through patient teaching. Proper documentation in the chart is essential. Furthermore, if the nurse practices in a state where such conduct is considered child abuse or neglect under the state's statute, he or she is required to report that conduct to the state agency enforcing the law.

It is important to remember that in any of the situations mentioned, the medical record may be utilized in court, whether in a civil suit alleging negligence, a divorce action concerning the "best interests" of an embryo or child, or a criminal action alleging neglect or abuse on the part of a parent. Therefore, accurate, complete documentation is essential. If the nurse is subpoenaed to testify in court concerning the matter at issue, adequate preparation for that testimony is essential.

SUMMARY OF PRINCIPLES AND APPLICATIONS

Perhaps in no other area of the law are changes seen as rapidly and as frequently as in family and reproductive concerns. Furthermore, new and different legal, ethical, and moral dilemmas that follow these changes will need to be resolved.

For example, the birth of a child to a woman well past menopause as a result of *in vitro* fertilization brings into question the traditional reproductive period for women that existed prior to this birth. The ability of a mother to become the "surrogate mother" for her daughter and son-in-law by *in vitro* fertilization when the daughter cannot become pregnant also raises questions about established, traditional roles.

Moreover, the potential for abuse of reproductive innovations may well be a sign of things to come. The conviction of a physician utilizing his own sperm for *in vitro* transplantation of his patients without their consent is indeed troubling conduct on the physician's part.

There is constant concern over research involving the *ex-utero* reimplantation of a human embryo. Should such research be federally funded? Which embryos should be used for research? Will this technique be abused? The answers to these and other questions surrounding human embryo research will not be easily obtained.[131]

It is certain that additional developments will continue to occur in the area of reproductive health and the family. The nurse practicing in this area will need to continually update his or her knowledge base of legal developments *and* practice changes, especially as the effects of the *Casey* decision become clear. The nurse will need to be ever vigilant concerning the ethical and moral issues raised by advances in family and reproductive care. This is important not only in relation to the provision of care to patients but also for the nurse's own level of comfort with innovations in this interesting area of nursing practice.

Thus, the nurse will need to:

- Continually update practice skills and knowledge base in this area of nursing care

- Explore his or her own thoughts and feelings concerning family and reproductive issues

- Carefully consider the constitutional protections of the right of privacy for all patients when providing care

- Remember that no right is absolute and that, in some instances, a right may be limited by the government if that limitation can pass the applicable constitutional test

- Understand the two basic tests for decision making when an individual cannot make decisions for himself or herself—the "substituted judgment" and "best-interest-of-the-person" tests

- Remember that, currently, the U.S. Supreme Court has not ruled that a fetus or an embryo is considered a person under the law

- Remember that informed consent for reproductive innovations is necessary, and in some instances requires the biological father also to give his informed consent

- Remember that access to abortion and other reproductive health services is protected by federal law

- Understand that sterilization procedures are carefully scrutinized by the courts, and the procedure must conform with constitutional principles

- Document completely and accurately in this area of nursing practice

- Voice an inability to participate in any procedure that is offensive to religious beliefs, including abortion, and share those concerns with nurse managers and administration so that the nurse is not required to care for the patient

- Refrain from taking the role of "baby broker" in any private or agency adoption

- Conduct or participate in research in this area consistent with federal and state regulations

- Ensure that consent for treatment for minors is obtained from the proper person (e.g., parent, not stepparent)

TOPICS FOR FURTHER INQUIRY

1. Compare and contrast laws from selected states that govern involuntary sterilization to determine what protections are provided individuals who may be subject to involuntary sterilization.

2. Draft a model bill supporting or rejecting the right of a minor to obtain birth control services without parental consent.

3. Develop an interview guide for use with individuals who live in alternative family structures to measure experienced legal difficulties, if any, due to those alternative structures (e.g., discrimination, difficulty in obtaining loans).

4. Analyze selected cases reported in your state dealing with women who exhibited high-risk behaviors during pregnancy and what punishment, sanctions, or other limitations were imposed on the women by the court.

REFERENCES

1. Ralph Chandler, Richard Enslen, and Peter Renstrom. *Constitutional Law Deskbook: Individual Rights.* 2nd Edition. St. Paul, Minn.: West Group, 1987, 500 (with cumulative supplement issued May 1999).
2. *Olmstead v. United States,* 277 U.S. 438 (1928).
3. Chandler, Enslen, and Renstrom, *supra* note 1, at 498.
4. *Id.* at 501.
5. Henry Campbell Black. *Black's Law Dictionary.* 7th Edition. St. Paul, Minn.: West Group, 1999, 1155.
6. Chandler, Enslen, and Renstrom, *supra* note 1, at 499–500, *citing* Justice Goldberg in *Griswold v. Connecticut,* 381 U.S. 479 (1965).
7. Black, *supra* note 5, at 1137.
8. Alan Meisel, "Decisionmaking Standards for Incompetent Patients," in *The Right to Die.* Volume I. 2nd Edition.

New York: John Wiley & Sons, 1995, 351–352 (with 1999 cumulative supplement).

9. *Id.* at 349–351.

10. *Id.*

11. Theodore LeBlang, Eugene Basanta, and Robert Kane. *The Law of Medical Malpractice in Illinois.* Volume 2. 2nd Edition. St. Paul, Minn.: West Group, 549 (with 1998 supplement) (citations omitted).

12. 274 U.S. 200 (1927).

13. 316 U.S. 535 (1942).

14. LeBlang, Basanta, and Kane, *supra* note 11, at 550.

15. *Id.*

16. Robert D. Miller. *Problems in Health Care Law.* 7th Edition. Gaithersburg, Md: Aspen Publishers, 1996, 490.

17. *Id.*

18. 381 U.S. 479 (1965).

19. 405 U.S. 438 (1972).

20. 325 ILCS 10/1 (1993).

21. Miller, *supra* note 16, at 495.

22. *Id.*

23. Black, *supra* note 5, at 5–6.

24. Miller, *supra* note 16, at 495.

25. Jacquelyn Kay Hall. *Nursing Law and Ethics.* Philadelphia, Penn.: W. B. Saunders Company, 1996, 389.

26. See, generally, B. J. George, Jr., "The Evolving Law of Abortion," 23 *Case Western Reserve Law Review* (1972), 715–720.

27. 410 U.S. 113 (1973).

28. 448 U.S. 297 (1980).

29. 462 U.S. 416 (1983).

30. 429 U.S. 490 (1989).

31. 497 U.S. 417 (1990).

32. 497 U.S. 502 (1990).

33. 500 U.S. 173 (1991).

34. George Pozgar. *Legal Aspects of Health Care Administration.* 7th Edition. Gaithersburg, Md.: Aspen Publishers, 1999, 353.

35. *Id.*

36. 112 S. Ct. 2791 (1992).

37. Richard Carelli, "Court Hearing Abortion Case; Activists Say Rights Jeopardized," 138(76) *Chicago Daily Law Bulletin* (April 17, 1992), 1.

38. Henry J. Reske, "Is This the End of *Roe*? The Court Revisits Abortion," 78 *ABA Journal* (May 1992), 65.

39. *Id.*

40. Pozgar, *supra* note 34, at 353–354.

41. 112 S. Ct. 2791, 2820 (1992).

42. See "The Law, the AMA, and Partial-Birth Abortion," 282(1) *JAMA* (1999), 23–27 (letters section).

43. Janet Epner, Harry Jonas, and Daniel Seckinger, "Late-Term Abortion," 280(8) *JAMA* (1998), 724.

44. *Id.* Judy Peres, "The High Cost of Ambiguity in Abortion Laws," *Chicago Tribune,* May 31, 1998, Section 2, 1, 4.

45. "The Law, the AMA, and Partial-Birth Abortion," *supra* note 42; M. LeRoy Sprang and Mark Neerhof, "Rationale for Banning Abortions Late in Pregnancy," 280(8) *JAMA* (1998), 744–750.

46. See, as examples, David Grimes, "The Continuing Need for Late Abortions," 280(8) *JAMA* (1998), 747–750; John Gibeaut, "Strategic Adjustments: Abortion Opponents Focusing on Protection of the 'Partially Born,'" 4(3) *ABA Journal* (1999), 26–27.

47. Jan Crawford, "Late-term abortion ban voided," *Chicago Tribune,* June 29, 2000, Section 1, 1,22; *Stenberg v. Carhart,* Legal Information Institute, Supreme Court Collection, located at http://supct.law.cornell.edu/supct/htm199-830.ZS.html, accessed July 10, 2000.

48. See, generally, Chapter 3.

49. LeBlang, Basanta, and Kane, *supra* note 11, at 532.

50. Pozgar, *supra* note 34, at 358.

51. LeBlang, Basanta, and Kane, *supra* note 11, at 534.

52. *Id.* at 535–536.

53. *Id.*

54. See, for example, "Dead Man's Sperm Results in Birth: Delivery of Baby Girl Is First of Its Kind in the U.S.," *Chicago Tribune,* March 27, 1999, Section 1, 8.

55. LeBlang, Basanta, and Kane, *supra* note 11, at 534.

56. *Hecht v. Superior Court,* 16 Cal. App. 836, 20 Cal. Rptr. 275 (1993), *review denied,* Cal. LEXIS 4768 (September 2, 1993).

57. LeBlang, Basanta, and Kane, *supra* note 11, at 534.

58. See, as examples, American Fertility Society (now the American Society for Reproductive Medicine), *Guidelines for Gamete Donation,* 59 *Fertility and Society* (1993), 1S (Supplement); American Medical Association, Council on Ethical and Judicial Affairs, *Code of Medical Ethics: Current Opinions with Annotations,* No. 2.05 (1996).

59. *Id.* See also, Guidelines of the Center for Disease Control and Prevention; can be accessed at http://www.cdc.gov/. The Association of Women's Health, Obstetric and Neonatal Nurses (AWHONN) Resource Web Page can be accessed at http://www/awhon.org/resources/index.html.

60. LeBlang, Basanta, and Kane, *supra* note 11, at 536.

61. "Information Versus Choice in Infertility Treatment," 353(9168) *Lancet* (1999), 1895.

62. LeBlang, Basanta, and Kane, *supra* note 11, at 536.

63. *New York Times,* June 23, 1984, 9; October 24, 1994, 9; December 5, 1987, 11.

64. *Davis v. Davis,* No. F-14496, 1989 WL 140495 (Tenn. Cir. 1989).

65. *Davis v. Davis,* 1990 Tenn App. LEXIS 642 (September 3, 1990).

66. *Davis v. Davis,* 842 S.W.2d 588 (1992), *cert. denied,* 113 S. Ct. 1259 (1993).

67. *Id.*

68. *Id.*

69. *Palm Beach Florida Post,* June 16, 1993, 6A.

70. *CBS Nightly News,* June 1, 1992.

71. 696 N.E.2d 174 (1998).

72. Judy Peres, "Embryo Consent Forms' Validity Upheld," *Chicago Tribune,* May 8, 1998, Section 1, 3.

73. In Phoenix, Arizona, for example, a clinic storing cryopreserved sperm and embryos was closing, and notices went out to the general public that if they had embryos or sperm stored with the clinic, they must contact the clinic immediately. The notice went on to say that all unclaimed specimens would be destroyed as of a certain date. Matt Kelly, "Closure Opens Clinic to Dilemma on Embryos," *Chicago Tribune,* July 13, 1999, Section 1, 4. Because many of the cryopreserved specimens date back to the 1980s, they have no chance of surviving if implanted in a womb.

74. See, for example, "Groups Want to Save Frozen Embryos," *Chicago Tribune,* June 3, 1992, Section 1, 10.

75. *Del Zio v. Presbyterian Hospital,* 74 Civ. 3588 (S.D.N.Y. April 12, 1978).

76. LeBlang, Basanta, and Kane, *supra* note 11, at 540–541.

77. *Id.* at 541–542.

78. Because state laws vary, or are nonexistent, in such situations, several authors have proposed a model statute concerning surrogate parenthood. LeBlang, Basanta, and Kane, *supra* note 11, *citing* Mannus, "The Proposed Model Surrogate Parenthood Act: A Legislative Response to the Challenges of Reproductive Technology," 29 *University of Michigan Journal of Law Reform* 671 (1996).

79. LeBlang, Basanta, and Kane, *supra* note 11, at 551.

80. *Id.* For interesting articles on new issues emerging in the area of genetic testing, see Council on Ethical and Judicial Affairs, American Medical Association, "Multiplex Genetic Testing," 4(28) *Hastings Center Report* (1998), 15–21; "The Disability Rights Critique of Prenatal Genetic Testing: Reflections and Recommendations," 29(5) *Hastings Center Report* (1999), S-1 to S-25 (Supplement); Ronald M. Green, "Parental Autonomy and the Obligation Not to Harm One's Child," 25(1) *Journal of Law, Medicine & Ethics* (1997), 5–15.

81. Carolyn Harris, Carolyn Curtis, and Pamela Copeland, "Informed Consent," in *Liability Issues in Perinatal Nursing.* Donna Miller Rosant and Rebecca F. Cady, Editors. Philadelphia, Penn.: Lippincott, 1999, 190–195 (in conjunction with the Association of Women's Health, Obstetric and Neonatal Nurses [AWHONN]).

82. See, generally, *id.*

83. Black, *supra* note 5, at 50.

84. William Roach and the Aspen Health Law Center and Compliance Center. *Medical Records and the Law.* 3rd Edition. Gaithersburg, Md.: Aspen Publishers, 1998, 179–181.

85. *Id., citing* Illinois and Oklahoma as examples.

86. *Id.*

87. Black, *supra* note 5, at 494.

88. *Id.* The Act, its variations, and annotations concerning jurisdictions that have adopted it can be found in *Uniform Laws Annotated,* Master Edition, Volume 9, Pt. i (1988) (with updates).

89. Alan Meisel. *The Right to Die.* Volume I. 2nd Edition. New York: John Wiley & Sons, 1995, 645–646 (with 1999 cumulative supplement).

90. *In re Ayesha Madyren,* 114 *Daily Washington Law Report* 2233 (D.C. Superior Court, July 26, 1986).

91. *Mercy Hospital, Inc. v. Jackson,* 489 A.2d 1130 (1985), *vacated and remanded as moot,* 510 A.2d 562 (Md. App. 1986).

92. 573 A.2d 1235 (D.C. App. 1990) (en banc).

93. *Id.* at 1235.

94. See 112 S. Ct. 2791 (1992).

95. 632 N.E.2d 326 (1994).

96. *Id.* at 327.

97. Meisel, *supra* note 89, at 650.

98. 689 N.E.2d 397 (1997).

99. Meisel, *supra* note 89, at 651.

100. 689 N.E.2d 405.

101. Meisel, *supra* note 89, at 451, *citing* 689 N.E.2d 405.

102. See, generally, Wendy Chavin, Vicki Brietbart, and Paul H. Wise, "Finding Common Ground: Necessity of an Integrated Agenda for Women's and Children's Health," 22(3) *Journal of Law, Medicine & Ethics* (1994), 262–269.

103. Judy Peres, "A Setback for Fetal Rights in Wisconsin Alcohol Case: Pregnant Woman Who Drank Too Much Can't Be Prosecuted," *Chicago Tribune,* May 27, 1999, Section 1, 3. The female, Dorothy Zimmerman, was charged under Wisconsin's "born alive" law, which allows a person to be charged with murder if harm to the pregnant woman occurs and the fetus is subsequently born alive and then dies. The appellate court held that the legislative intent of the law was not to cover this type of case, but was for situations in which a third party injures the pregnant female and in so doing also injures and causes the death of the fetus. Ms. Zimmerman's daughter is now living with a foster family and is healthy.

104. *Id.* For an interesting commentary on the issue of maternal-fetal concerns in these and other situations, see Deborah Honstra, "A Realistic Approach to Maternal-Fetal Conflict," 28(5) *Hastings Center Report* (September-October 1998), 7–12.

105. *Id.*

106. *Id.*

107. *Id.*

108. *Id.*

109. See *People v. Pointer,* 199 Cal. Rptr. 357 (Cal. App. 1 Dist. 1984); *State v. Mosburg,* 768 P.2d 313 (Kan. App. 1989); "No Pregnancy Sentence Voided," 142(4) *Chicago Daily Law Bulletin* (January 5, 1996).

110. LeBlang, Basanta, and Kane, *supra* note 11, at 632.

111. *Id.*

112. Miller, *supra* note 16, at 340.

113. LeBlang, Basanta, and Kane, *supra* note 11, at 632–633.

114. *Id.*

115. LeBlang, Basanta, and Kane, *supra* note 11, at 632, *citing* Allred, "Fetal Tissue Transplants: A Primer with a Look Forward," 28(6) *Journal of Health and Hospital Law* (1995), 193.

116. 45 C.F.R. Section 46.203(f) (1991).

117. 45 C.F.R. Section 46.206 (a)(3).

118. 45 C.F.R. Section 46.206 (b).

119. Joan Beck, "Promising Fetal Tissue Research a Hostage to Politics," *Chicago Tribune,* June 1, 1992, Section 1, 13, quoting Rep. Barbara F. Vucanovich (R-Nev.).

120. LeBlang, Basanta, and Kane, *supra* note 11, at 673, *citing* 42 C.F.R. Section 46.201 *et seq.*

121. *Id., citing* 45 C.F.R. Section 42.206.

122. *Id.* at 673–674, *citing* 45 C.F.R. Section 46.207, 45 C.F.R. Section 46.207(b), 45 C.F.R. Section 46.209(d).

123. *Id.,* 674, *citing* 45 C.F.R. Section 46.209(a), 45 C.F.R. Section 46.209(b), and 45 C.F.R. Section 46.209(d).

124. See, for example, "Vermont Anti-Abortion Activist Sought for Information in Killing," *Chicago Tribune,* November 5, 1998, Section 1, 25 (in killing of Dr. Barnett Slepian on October 23, 1998 near Buffalo, N.Y.). The Internet has also been used to target physicians who do abortions. In one highly publicized case, several physicians and Planned Parenthood sued a group of antiabortion organizations who were publishing information about them on the World Wide Web. The site showed "dripping blood" and doctors murdered had lines drawn through their names in an attempt to "one day hold them (the doctors and Planned Parenthood) on trial for crimes against hu-

manity." Julie Robner, "Doctors Sue Internet Anti-Abortionists," 353(9149) *Lancet* (January 23, 1999), 303.

125. 108 Stat. 694 (1994).

126. 108 Stat. 696 (1994).

127. Executive Summary from "Cloning Human Beings: The Report and Recommendations of the National Bioethics Advisory Commission," 27(5) *Hastings Center Report* (October 1997), 7.

128. *Id.*

129. *Id.* Shortly after the announcement of Dolly's birth, a Chicago scientist, Richard Seed, proposed setting up clinics to clone babies for infertile couples in the United States. "Cloning Babies for Infertile Couples?" *Mayo Clinic Health Oasis* article, February 5, 1998, available on the World Wide Web at http://www.mayhealth.org/mayo/9802/htm/clone.htm, accessed November 11, 1999.

130. See, as examples, James Childress, "The Challenges of Public Ethics," 27(5) *Hastings Center Report* (October 1997), 9–11; Susan M. Wolf, "Ban Cloning? Why NBAC is Wrong," 27(5) *Hastings Center Report* (October 1997), 12–15; Daniel Callahan, "Cloning: The Work Not Done," 27(5) *Hastings Center Report* (October 1997), 18–20.

131. Symposium: "What Research? Which Embryos?" 25(1) *Hastings Center Report* (January-February 1995), 36–46.

Informed Consent and Refusal of Treatment

12

KEY PRINCIPLES

- Decision-making Capacity
- Patient Self-Determination Act
- Advance Directive
- Surrogate Decision Maker/Proxy Decision Maker
- Ethics Committee
- Informed Consent
- Informed Refusal

The legal doctrine of consent, informed consent, and refusal of treatment has been influenced by many disciplines, including ethics, moral philosophy, the behavioral sciences, and, of course, the law.[1] Legally, obtaining permission for treatment was initially derived from the common law and was the result of establishing its parameters and exceptions.[2] Furthermore, the early decisions were almost exclusively derived from the physician-patient relationship, as opposed to research, transplantation, and other clinical situations.[3]

The early decisions provided guidance for the health care provider, including the nurse, in terms of compliance with the doctrine of consent. Specifically, if the doctrine's parameters were not complied with, liability for assault and battery could occur. Although several earlier cases illustrated liability when consent was not obtained from a patient for treatment, the best-known case, *Schloendorff v. Society of New York Hospitals*,[4] clearly established this right. Justice Cardozo, in establishing the right of "self-determination," said:

> Every human being of adult years and sound mind has a right to determine what will be done with his own body; and a surgeon who performs an operation without his patient's consent commits an assault, for which he is liable in damages.

This is true, except in cases of emergency where the patient is unconscious, and where it is necessary to operate before consent can be obtained.[5]

The common law protection of the right of giving consent was later augmented by other cases that specifically required that the patient give *informed* consent for treatment; that is, the health care provider had a duty to provide certain information to the patient before consent was obtained.[6] If the duty was breached, then liability under a negligence theory could also be alleged by the patient.

The best known of the *informed* consent cases, *Salgo v. Leland Stanford Jr. University Board of Trustees,*[7] held that a physician had a duty to disclose "any facts necessary to form the basis of an intelligent consent by the patient to proposed treatment."[8]

Every human being of adult years and sound mind has a right to determine what will be done with his own body . . .

In addition to the common law protections that developed in relation to consent and informed consent, statutory mandates evolved. Constitutional protections concerning informed consent and refusal of treatment, based on privacy, liberty, and religious freedom (First Amendment), were applied to various treatment situations, including the right to refuse life-sustaining treatment. The latter has evolved as the "right to die."

INFORMED CONSENT

A patient's right of informed consent includes knowing and understanding what health care treatment is being undertaken. Obtaining informed consent is also important for the health care provider, for without it, he or she may be subject to a lawsuit alleging assault, battery, negligence, or a combination of these causes of action. Understanding the concept of informed consent, then, is important to both protect the patient's right to supply informed consent and avoid, insofar as is possible, suits against health care providers

for allegedly not obtaining the patient's authorization.

Types of Consent

Generally there are two types of consent: express and implied. Express consent is manifested by an oral declaration concerning a particular treatment ("yes") or by a written document (a consent form) that the patient signs. In health care, the written consent form is most often used, especially in hospitals, ambulatory surgery centers, and clinics.

It is important to note that except in certain situations (e.g., research), written consent for health care is not a requirement. Rather, it helps the patient understand what it is he or she is consenting to.

A written document indicating consent for treatment is a more reliable piece of evidence to prove that consent was obtained if a suit is filed alleging it was not. However, the use of consent forms cannot prevent the patient from taking legal action altogether. A patient can still challenge a health care situation in which a consent form was used to obtain consent. Nor can forms take the place of going through the *process* of obtaining informed consent from the patient. Obtaining informed consent is not just having a patient sign a consent form. Rather, it is the sharing of information whereby a dialogue takes place between the health care provider and the patient.

Implied consent is consent that is given by an individual's conduct rather than verbally or in writing. For example, when a nurse tells a patient that he or she is going to take the patient's blood pressure and the patient extends the arm, implied consent is given for that procedure. Likewise, when an individual stands in line, extends the arm and receives a vaccination without protest,[9] implied consent occurs.

Implied consent has also been found by the courts (1) when a true emergency exists and the individual cannot provide consent orally or in writing, (2) during a surgical procedure when additional surgery is indicated, so long as it is not substantially divergent from that originally consented to (the "extension doctrine"), and (3) when a patient continues to take treatments without objecting to them.

If an individual does object to the health care in any way, implied consent no longer exists. For example, if a patient in an emergency department refuses further treatment after being revived from an unconscious state, then no implied consent for treatment can be used to continue treatment. Also, as with oral consent, implied consent often raises difficulties in health care situations, one of which is proof of the reason for initiating treatment without the patient's express consent.

Elements of Consent

For consent to be valid, certain requisites need to be met. The first is decision-making capacity. Decision-making capacity is an essential element of giving informed consent or refusing treatment. Without it, consent or refusal is invalid.[10] It is defined as the "ability to appreciate the nature, extent or probable consequences of the [health care provider's] conduct to which consent is given."[11]

In the early development of the theory of informed consent and refusal this capacity was almost always called competency, and when not present, incompetency. However, the use of those terms led to much confusion for several reasons.

First, several definitions of incompetency exist. A person may be declared incompetent by a court (*de jure* incompetency) or an individual may be unable to function as a result, for example, of advanced Alzheimer's disease. Even though not declared incompetent by a court, the person may be regarded as incompetent (*de facto* incompetency).

Second, someone who has been declared incompetent by a court may not always lack the capacity to consent to treatment. Similarly, an individual with a progressive disease that eventually impairs cognitive ability is not always unable to consent in the early stages of the disease's progression.

Third, in many situations, an individual's "incompetency" is situational or transitional; that is, it is temporary. Clinically managing the environment with consistency in surroundings and personnel or appropriately using medication and adequate hydration and food reduces cognitive impairment.

Because of the confusion in the meaning and use of the terms *incompetency* and *competency,* the Presidential Commission for the Study of Ethical Problems in Medicine and Biomedical and Behavioral Research suggested that the use of the term *decision-making capacity* or *incapacity* be used to describe decision-making ability in treatment situations.[12]

Generally the adult is presumed to have decision-making capacity. Therefore, someone who is mentally ill, elderly, "confused," mentally retarded, or involuntarily committed to a psychiatric facility for treatment does not, by law, automatically lose decision-making capacity. Rather, a determination must be made as to the *effect,* if any, of the illness or condition on the ability to decide about treatment or nontreatment.[13]

Generally the adult is presumed to have decision-making capacity.

If clinical evidence demonstrates that decision-making capacity is compromised because of an illness or condition, then resort to the courts for an adjudication of the *legal disability* (current term for "incompetency" in many states) and the appointment of a guardian is necessary. Or, in those states that have adopted them, surrogate decision-making procedures can be followed to allow another to provide informed consent or refusal for the patient's treatment.

Some individuals are, by statute, presumed to lack decision-making capacity. For example, minors are not able to provide consent or refuse treatment. Instead, the parent(s) or legal guardian is given the ability to consent to and refuse treatment. However, there are exceptions to this general principle.

A second requisite for valid consent is that the individual must give consent voluntarily, that is, freely, without duress, coercion, or undue influence.[14] Although each case would be evaluated individually and include such factors as age of the patient, relationship between the patient and the health care provider, and the patient's mental capacity,[15] physically forcing a patient to provide consent, or restricting his or her liberty until a form is signed, might invalidate the consent.

A third factor necessary for valid consent is that it not be obtained under fraudulent circumstances. For example, asking a patient to sign what is described as a release of medical records that, in fact, is a consent form for a particular procedure would invalidate the consent.

Whether consent is given orally or in writing, the information given to the patient must be in a language that the patient can understand. This requirement is composed of two elements. First, the use of "medicalese" should be kept at a minimum, as it stands as one of the "greatest impediments" to patient understanding.[16] Second, the information shared must be in the patient's native language. Discussing the ramifications of a particular procedure in English with a patient who speaks and understands only Russian is of little help in obtaining consent or informed consent.

Last, but by no means least, valid consent requires that the patient have knowledge and understanding about the proposed medical regimen. Whether or not this element of consent has been met is likely the most problematic for health care providers and patients alike. Some studies indicate that despite adequate and accurate information given to patients about their proposed medical care, few truly understand what they consented to.[17] Thus there is a duty to ascertain whether the patient truly knows and understands what will be done. This can be evaluated without much difficulty. For example, simply asking if the patient has any questions, leaving adequate time for the patient to ponder information received and to make a decision, and providing written instructions concerning the treatment can clarify and assist in meeting this requisite of valid consent.

Knowledge and understanding become the foundation for a patient giving *informed* consent for treatment. Although all of the elements are vital for informed choice to be present, without adequate information concerning the proposed regimen and an understanding of it, no informed consent can occur.

Obtaining Informed Consent and Necessary Elements

Generally speaking, the physician is the one who has the duty to obtain the informed consent of the patient for medical care and treatment.[18] Hospitals and other health care delivery systems have not been held to share this duty, although in recent years, some court decisions have indicated that hospitals do have a duty to ensure that staff physicians obtain the informed consent of patients before providing treatment.[19] Other independent health care providers, such as nurse anesthetists or surgeons, are responsible for obtaining

informed consent for their particular procedures. When providing nursing care, the nurse would be the appropriate provider to obtain informed consent for that *nursing* care.

The elements of informed consent have been established by courts across the country when faced with deciding whether or not physicians gave patients adequate information concerning particular treatments. Although each particular situation may require more or less information, generally speaking the physician is to provide the following information to a patient:

1. The patient's diagnosis and name of the treatment, procedure, or medication
2. An explanation of the treatment, procedure, medication, and intended purpose
3. The hoped-for benefits of the proposed regimen (with no guarantees as to outcome)
4. The material risks, if any, of the treatment, procedure, or medication
5. Alternative treatments, if any
6. The prognosis if the recommended care, procedure, or medication is refused.[20]

The Therapeutic Privilege Doctrine

Although these elements are excellent guidelines to follow when obtaining informed consent from a patient, it is important to note that the law does not require this information to be given in each and every circumstance. Rather, it has developed the doctrine of therapeutic privilege that "suspends the duty to disclose if disclosure would be harmful to the patient."[21]

However, the privilege not to disclose certain information to the patient was narrowly drawn in the *Canterbury v. Spence* case.[22] The basis of the therapeutic privilege, according to the court, is not to influence the patient to undertake a medical regimen the physician thinks necessary by withholding information. Rather, its purpose is to allow the physician latitude of judgment when the information shared with the patient might be so detrimental to the patient that it is medically "unfeasible". . . or "contraindicated."[23]

A patient injured by the failure to share information can sue the health care provider for that injury under the concept of negligence. In determining whether the physician breached his or her duty of providing the elements necessary for the patient to give informed consent, two standards currently exist. One is the "professional standard";

that is, determining what other physicians in the same or similar circumstances would have revealed. This approach would require the use of an expert witness to establish the standard of care.

The second standard, the "reasonable patient" standard, looks at what "material information" the patient needed in the particular situation.[24] No expert testimony is needed to establish this standard because its focus is on the patient, not the physician. However, an expert witness—a physician—may be necessary if there is a question whether information concerning risks and alternatives to treatment should have been given to the patient.[25]

Other Exceptions to the Informed Consent Requirement

In some health care situations the law waives the need to obtain consent. In these cases, the state may have an interest in providing treatment to a particular individual.[26] Thus, neither the individual's right to give informed consent, nor the state's right to provide treatment, is absolute. As with many other circumstances, these rights must be balanced. In relation to informed consent, the nature of the exception *and* the facts and circumstances of the specific situation must be evaluated.[27]

TRUE EMERGENCY. One exception that has been established, for instance, is the case of a true emergency. In a true emergency, the life or the well-being of the individual is threatened and consent cannot be obtained, or if sought, might result in undue delay in treatment. In such a situation, the health care provider is able to provide necessary care. Some legal commentators have also found the ability to provide care in such circumstances because consent for treatment is implied, as discussed above.

For this exception to apply, however, there can be no patient directions to the contrary (for example, an oral declaration of refusal or an advance directive refusing care). Furthermore, it is the patient's *condition* that serves as the touchstone of the emergent need for care. Also, the exception is not a blanket one. For example, based on the patient's condition, *some* information can be provided to allow the patient to consent to the treatment, even if less information is given than if the patient's condition allowed fuller disclosure.

PATIENT WAIVER. Patient waiver of the right of giving informed consent is another exception recognized by the law. For various reasons, not all patients want to be given information concerning treatment. When the patient expresses a desire not to be informed, that right should be honored. However, it is important to note that simply because an individual chooses not to be informed about treatment, it in no way affects his or her right to *decide* about the medical regimen recommended, unless that right is waived as well.[28]

LACK OF DECISION-MAKING CAPACITY. The last exception is made when decision-making capacity does not exist. Although a health care provider may not be required to discuss treatment information with a patient who lacks decision-making capacity, he or she must share the information with a surrogate or proxy decision maker or a guardian. Thus, it is an "exception" only insofar as it means that the information is not shared with the patient but rather is shared with another who is legally recognized to provide or refuse authorization for treatment.

Documentation of Informed Consent

The documentation of the patient's informed consent to treatment in the medical record is important. Documentation guidelines exist in institutional policies, Joint Commission on the Accreditation of Health Care Organizations (JCAHO) accreditation standards, and state licensing laws for health care delivery systems.

The manner most often used to denote informed consent is the consent form. As was discussed earlier, its use should be "adjunctive" only; that is, as a supplement to the dialogue required between the patient and the health care provider in obtaining informed consent.[29] Most institutions and health care delivery systems develop their own specific forms for use in the facility. Their contents are based on applicable guidelines, including federal and state case and statutory law.

Three types of consent forms have been identified: blanket, battery, and treatment specific. Blanket forms, defined as a form that arguably gives a health care provider unbridled authority and discretion to provide whatever treatment is decided upon by the provider, are not recommended for specific treatments.[30] They can be used to cover situations in which general consent will suffice; for example, on admission to a facility and for *routine* care and procedures (e.g., blood pressure,

initial laboratory tests, and assignment of health insurance benefits to the institution).

Consent forms that protect health care providers against allegations of battery include information specific to a particular procedure or treatment. They are different from treatment-specific forms, however, in that the latter include *very* detailed information concerning the medical care recommended.[31] For example, when one is conducting research or experimental treatment, the consent form may contain more information than one used for more conventional treatment.

The use of written consent forms to document permission for treatment cannot avoid all legal problems. The patient can challenge the way in which his or her consent was obtained, what information was shared concerning the recommended treatment, or other aspects of the *process* of obtaining informed consent. Challenges can also be raised about the form itself. For instance, a patient may ask a court to render void any clauses that waive the patient's rights to sue or that limit damages if the patient is injured ("exculpatory clauses").

The use of written consent forms to document permission for treatment cannot avoid all legal problems.

Once informed consent is given and the form signed, the consent is valid unless or until it is retracted by the patient or a change in condition renders the informed consent invalid. Thus, generally speaking, there is no specific time limitation after which the consent of the patient is no longer valid.

Some institutions or agencies have adopted their own policies concerning this issue. For example, consent that is more than 20 days old may not be valid. However, a more reasonable approach is to consider each situation on a case-by-case basis that takes into account the patient's condition, the treatment consented to, and, of course, how long ago the consent was obtained.

Informed Consent for Adults and Minors

Adults are presumed to possess decision-making capacity, and therefore anyone 18 years

---

ETHICS CONNECTION 12–1

The doctrine of informed consent is an example of coextensive relationship between ethics and law (see Chapter 3). Grounded in self-determination, informed consent is a legal and ethical expression of the moral principle of respect for autonomy. In health care, informed consent holds that adults have moral and legal rights to freely determine whether to accept or refuse treatment. The elements of informed consent are addressed in this chapter. Most institutions have specific policies about informed consent protocols. Informed consent, in a less litigious era, was taken lightly in some institutions or by some providers. It now is recognized as a very important practice. In most institutions today, nurses are supported when they report that a consent form has not been signed or that a patient has reversed his or her decision. Employers and risk managers generally recognize that by calling attention to questions about the consent, the nurse is protecting not only the patient but also the institution. Nurses, particularly those who work nights, should be aware of the institutional policy on informed consent and how to report any problems or issues of informed consent. If necessary, treatments, including surgery, are postponed until the issues of informed consent are resolved.

Nurses play a critically important role in the consent process. Apart from checking that a consent form has been signed prior to treatment, particularly for surgery or other invasive treatments, nurses usually are able to assess the extent to which the patient understands the treatment. Frequently, it is the nurse to whom the patient will disclose reservations or lack of understanding about the treatment. When nurses determine that patients do not understand the treatments, are unwilling to accept the risks of the treatment, or have changed their minds about the treatment, they have a moral obligation to see that the treatment is not carried out until there is further discussion with the patient, even if the consent form previously had been signed.

---

of age or older is able to provide his or her own consent. Thus, unless decision-making capacity does not exist, informed consent must be obtained from the adult patient. When a decision cannot be made by the patient, legal mechanisms exist for another to be consulted and provide informed consent.

Minors—those under 18 years of age—generally are seen as lacking decision-making capacity. As a result, the parent(s) or the legal guardian of the minor provide informed consent for the minor patient. However, most states have passed laws that allow a minor to provide informed consent for treatment in certain circumstances. Although the laws may vary, the following minors may be able to provide their own consent to treatment:

- Married minors
- Pregnant minors (for themselves and the fetus. However, once the fetus is born, the minor mother usually retains the right to provide consent for the minor child but not herself *unless* she fits into one of the other exceptions)
- Minors over a specified age—for example, 12 years of age—for sexually transmitted diseases, HIV testing, AIDS treatment, and drug and alcohol treatment
- Emancipated and mature minors (usually specifically defined by state law)
- Minors seeking birth control services
- Minors seeking outpatient psychiatric services or inpatient voluntary admissions to a psychiatric facility (the latter often requires *notification*—not consent—of the parents)

The exceptions to obtaining informed consent presented earlier in the chapter also apply to the minor patient. Thus, if an emergency exists or a waiver occurs, for example, then obtaining informed consent is not required.

NURSING IMPLICATIONS

Regardless of the setting, the nurse who works with patients will be involved in some way with obtaining informed consent. As a staff nurse in a home health care agency, hospital, or ambulatory care setting, the nurse will need to be certain to obtain consent for any nursing care directly provided the patient. This most often will be on an informal basis; for example, telling the patient that a nursing procedure is going to be done, if agreeable to the patient. It may be more formalized, however, if the nurse is doing discharge planning or teaching. In either case, making sure the patient agrees with the care will be important. Documentation of that agreement is also important.

Likewise, advanced nurse practitioners, such as nurse anesthetists, nurse practitioners, and nurse-midwives, will need to obtain written informed consent from their clients concerning the care they will be delivering. Independent nurse practitioners can clearly be sued for not obtaining the informed consent of their patients.

In addition to obtaining permission for nursing care, the nurse may be involved in the process of obtaining informed consent for medical procedures by *witnessing* the patient's signature on the consent form in some way after the physician has completed the informed consent *process*. This role is different from obtaining consent, for the nurse is either obtaining the patient's signature (where the nurse becomes a witness to the signing only) or observing the patient sign the form in the presence of the physician.[32] There is no legal requirement that the witness be a nurse or, in fact, that a witness be used at all.[33] The use of a witness is a good risk-management tool, however, and the role can be performed by *any* competent adult, including in most instances a family member.[34]

Regardless of the nurse's role in the informed consent process, certain guidelines are critical to keep in mind. The patient should never be coerced, threatened, or hurried when his or her signature is sought. If the patient raises questions concerning the procedure or treatment, the nurse must evaluate whether the patient is truly informed about that regimen. If there is any doubt, the nurse must ask the patient not to sign the form and must contact the physician or independent nurse practitioner so that the patient receives whatever additional clarification or information is needed. The nurse must also notify his or her nurse manager.

If the nurse questions the patient's decision-making capacity, notification of the physician or advanced nurse practitioner and nurse manager is vital so that an appropriate evaluation of the patient's ability to provide informed consent can occur. Likewise, if a change in the patient's condition takes place after informed consent has been obtained—an increase or decrease in blood pressure prior to surgery, for example—the appropriate health care provider and nurse manager must be informed.

If English is not the primary language of the patient or parent whose consent is needed, an interpreter will be necessary. When using an interpreter, the nurse or other health care provider is *not* certifying that the interpreter provided the information correctly. Rather, the health care provider is simply indicating that the duty to provide information in a language the patient understands was met. Again, *any* individual, including a minor family member, can fulfill this role.

Although information concerning the patient's age should be clear long before informed consent for treatment is obtained, the nurse may need to validate the patient's age in order that consent is obtained from the proper person. If the patient is a minor, any exceptions that might allow the minor to provide consent should be ascertained. If the minor's parents are divorced, it will be important to obtain informed consent from the parent awarded that right during the divorce.

Last, but not least, the nurse must be actively involved in developing and updating agency or institutional policies and procedures concerning informed consent and the nurse's role in the process. Clear policies and procedures that delineate the nurse's role can be helpful in ensuring their consistent application and can be helpful in resolving controversies that may arise in practice.

DOCUMENTATION REMINDER 12–1
Informed Consent

- If nurse present when process of informed consent was carried out, who was present (by name), condition of patient, questions asked by patient, and the like

- Signed consent form (done pursuant to policy) included in patient record

- Communication with physician, advanced nurse practitioner and/or nurse manager as to time, discussion, instructions, and changes of orders, patient response

- Presence of interpreter by name, address, time, others present in medical record and on consent form

- Any exceptions to the need for informed consent (detailed as to circumstance, attempts to obtain consent, knowing waiver)

- If consent withdrawn by patient, notification of appropriate health care provider, time called, patient statement, individuals present, other actions taken

---

INFORMED REFUSAL

The right of informed refusal of treatment is analogous to informed consent to treatment.[35] A refusal of treatment can take place at the initiation of treatment, or it can occur at any time after treatment is begun. Furthermore, a refusal is valid even after informed consent has been given.

In some instances, the right to refuse treatment may result in a compromise of the individual's overall health and well-being. In other circumstances, the refusal may result in the death of the patient who refuses medical intervention. The latter, known as the "right to die," is the ultimate outcome of the right to refuse treatment.

The right of informed refusal of treatment is analogous to informed consent to treatment.

Types of Refusal

There can be two types of refusal of treatment. One is, of course, an express refusal. Either through an oral declaration or written document, the patient articulates what he or she does not want done when medical care is contemplated. Most often, in health care settings a written form to document refusal is used. This may take the form of an advance directive or a refusal of treatment form developed by the institution that substantiates the refusal and becomes a part of the patient's medical record.

Refusal of treatment may also be implied; that is, the patient's conduct indicates unwillingness to undergo medical intervention. For example, if a nurse in the emergency department tells a patient that the physician has ordered an injection and asks the patient to extend the arm for the shot, and the patient holds the arms tightly to the body instead, the patient has refused that treatment. Likewise, if attempt is made to give oral medication, and the patient refuses to open his or her mouth, a refusal of that medication has occurred.

Elements of Refusal

The refusal of treatment requires that the patient possess decision-making capacity; the refusal must be voluntary, uncoerced, and not made under fraudulent circumstances; and the patient must refuse treatment with knowledge and understanding of the refusal.

Obtaining Informed Refusal and Necessary Elements

The obligation to obtain informed refusal of treatment rests with the independent health care provider who is providing care to the patient. Thus, for medical issues, the physician would be responsible for ensuring that the refusal of the patient is obtained and is informed. A nurse who functions in an advanced role would also be the responsible health care provider to procure this information.

A health care institution's potential liability in refusal of care situations is somewhat different than for informed consent situations. When a patient does refuse care, the institution is obligated to make sure that no institution staff perform the refused treatment.[36] Furthermore, along with the health care provider, the facility is obligated to continue to provide "the best medical care possible" within the parameters of the patient's refusal.[37] In other words, informed refusal does not imply consent to "mistreatment."[38]

The elements of informed refusal are, in essence, the same as those required when the patient gives informed consent to treatment. In other words, the patient must be given all information necessary under the circumstances, including treatment options, risks, benefits, and the prognosis if the treatment is not undertaken.[39] The reason for refusal is immaterial. So long as the patient has decision-making capacity, the refusal must be honored.[40]

Exceptions to Honoring Informed Refusal by Patient

Although the right of informed refusal of health care has been articulated in a long line of cases, including the *Cruzan v. Harmon* decision[41] that was affirmed in the U.S. Supreme Court case *Cruzan v. Director*,[42] the right is not absolute. Special populations and circumstances require exceptions to the general principle that informed refusal must be honored. Those populations and circumstances will be discussed later in this chapter.

Documentation of Informed Refusal

When a patient refuses treatment, the informed refusal must be documented in the medical record. If the refusal is in a form other than an advance directive, then specific documentation must be done pursuant to the facility's policies and procedures.

Most health care delivery systems use an informed refusal form when a patient orally refuses to undergo treatment. The patient would be asked to sign the form, fashioned in a manner similar to informed consent forms, in the presence of a witness or witnesses. Areas that might be included in the form would be (1) an explanation of what treatment, surgery, or medication was recommended and refused, (2) the hoped-for benefits had the treatment been undertaken, (3) the ramifications of the refusal, and specifically the prognosis, and (4) any alternative treatment that was recommended and refused.

In addition, the institution may include a waiver of the right to sue the institution and the health care provider and/or a hold-harmless clause in the event the patient experiences injury or death due to the refusal of treatment. The validity of such clauses is questionable. In most instances, such clauses are not upheld by the courts because they are against public policy. This position is based on the fact that the patient does not have the same ability to bargain with the institution in such situations and therefore may feel there is no choice but to sign such an agreement.[43]

An example of a situation in which a form is often used to document refusal of care is when a patient decides to leave the institution against medical advice (AMA). When used, the form should include the fact that the patient was informed of the risks and consequences of leaving without continued treatment; who, if anyone, the patient left with; and the fact that the patient can return for treatment if he or she changes his or her mind.[44]

Informed Refusal for Adults and Minors

Informed refusal of treatment is given by the adult with decision-making capacity. When decision-making capacity is absent, the use of an advance directive, if one exists, is acceptable, or a legally recognized substitute/proxy decision maker can make the decision.

In situations in which minors are able to give informed consent to treatment, they are also usually given the right to provide informed refusal of treatment. When the minor does not possess that ability, it is the parent(s) or legal guardian who have the legal right to decide whether or not treatment will be refused.

However, the right to refuse treatment is not absolute, for either the adult or the minor patient. The limitations on the right to refuse treatment will be discussed later in this chapter.

NURSING IMPLICATIONS

Many of the same implications discussed under informed consent are applicable to the nurse when a patient refuses treatment. Those implications include not coercing an individual into refusing treatment, clarifying any concern over a patient's ability to provide informed refusal, and participating in the development of policies and procedures governing refusal of treatment.

One of the most important things for the nurse working with a patient who refuses treatment is to make certain that the request is honored. Generally speaking, a refusal should alert the nurse not to initiate care, to contact the physician and nurse manager, and to document the refusal in the record. The nurse should not hold the patient down physically or otherwise force or coerce the individual to accept treatment. Unless there is a true emergency or a situation in which treatment is necessary because of a danger posed by patients to themselves or others (e.g., when a psychiatric patient is acting out by hitting others or self-mutilating), coercion or force could result in allegations of false imprisonment, battery, and a violation of the patient's constitutional rights.

If an adult patient announces an intent to leave the facility against medical advice (AMA), he or she should be requested to stay until the physician has the opportunity to speak with the patient. If the patient refuses to wait, then an against-medical-advice form should be offered to the patient for signing. If the patient refuses to sign the form, however, the nurse should let the patient leave and document the incident in the patient's medical record. Notification of appropriate staff and the physician is also vital.

When a parent or a guardian refuses treatment for the minor child or ward, the physician and others in the facility must be notified according to institutional policies and procedures. The refusal may trigger mandatory reporting requirements (e.g., if the refusal results in the neglect of the minor). If so, the nurse will need to comply with those requirements and document his or her actions in the minor patient's medical record.

If required by institutional policy, an incident report should also be filed by the nurse and sent to the designated individuals in the facility.

The refusal of treatment may raise controversial issues for the nurse, especially if the refusal results in the death of the individual. Nursing staff should feel free to discuss these thoughts and feelings with other staff and nursing administration to obtain support and clarification of the potential conflict of values the refusal may raise.

DOCUMENTATION REMINDER 12–2
Informed Refusal

- If nurse present when treatment refused, who was present (by name), condition of patient, statement(s) made by patient
- Signed refusal form by patient, included as part of patient medical record and discussed in nursing notes
- If patient leaves against medical advice, complete and concise entry in nursing note concerning refusal and other information contained on form (e.g., time left, with whom left, risks and consequences of no further treatment, who will be notified)
- Incident report documentation should completely and accurately include the same information as the nursing note

---

LEGAL MECHANISMS FOR CONSENT OR REFUSAL OF TREATMENT WHEN PATIENT LACKS DECISION-MAKING CAPACITY

When an adult patient or a minor who is legally able to provide consent or refusal of treatment is unable to personally express treatment decisions, the law has provided several mechanisms for voicing the individual's choices. Many times the approach used is the advance directive. Three examples of advance directives most often seen are the living will, the durable power of attorney for health care,[45] and the "medical directive."

An advance directive is a written statement that directs health care providers concerning consent or refusal of treatment when the individual patient does not possess decision-making capacity. As such, it is an anticipatory rather than contemporaneous document.[46]

Advance directives are not cumulative and are not the exclusive manner in which an individual may direct decisions concerning treatment.

Rather, they are but one way for the patient to express treatment choices in the event he or she cannot do so personally. They provide guidance for health care providers when decisions must be made and the patient cannot be consulted.[47] When the directive provides for the appointment of a surrogate decision maker or a proxy decision maker, health care providers have the opportunity to work with that individual to provide care consistent with the patient's wishes.

An advance directive is a written statement that directs health care providers concerning consent or refusal of treatment when the individual patient does not possess decision-making capacity.

Living wills and durable powers of attorney are most often created by state statutes and are called natural death acts, medical treatment decisions acts, and substituted consent acts, for example. The statutes vary from state to state. Even so, an advance directive may instruct (state care to be carried out, withdrawn, or withheld), may appoint a surrogate/proxy decision maker, or do both.[48]

If an advance directive does not exist, then a second mechanism may be the use of a surrogate/proxy decision maker. Established by state law, this mechanism may be specific to a particular situation, such as donating organs or body parts for transplantation or refusing life-sustaining treatment, or may be of a more general nature in *any* health care situations in which the principal lacks decision-making capacity.

A third manner in which decisions for another may be made is through the state guardianship laws that have been in existence in most states for some time.

None of these mechanisms is exempt from challenges by family members or others who may not agree with an individual's choice or who may believe the decision concerning medical care was not freely given. As a result, contests can arise even with an advance care document or with surrogate/proxy decision making. When they occur, a resort to the state probate court is the only way to resolve

any questions concerning such issues as free choice, the presence or absence of decision-making ability, and whose decision concerning a particular patient should be given weight in treatment decisions.

Advance Directives
Living Will

A living will is a document that establishes a written mechanism for an individual to specify wishes about withdrawing or forgoing life-sustaining treatment (treatment that only prolongs or delays the process of dying). Typically the individual must be an adult or an emancipated minor (as defined by state law) to execute a living will. In addition, the presence of a terminal condition, persistent vegetative state, or permanent unconsciousness must exist before any instructions in the will are given effect.[49] Currently, 47 states, the District of Columbia, and Guam have living will statutes.[50]

The instructions in a living will direct health care providers concerning types of treatments the individual does not want initiated, or wants withdrawn, when the patient's condition meets the requisite diagnosis. The diagnosis is certified to by at least one physician and documented in the patient's medical record. Orders are then written by the physician that are consistent with the patient's instructions. Specific treatments that can be withdrawn or withheld include, but are not necessarily limited to, surgery, blood transfusions, cardiopulmonary resuscitation, and artificial nutrition and hydration.

Living wills are required to be in writing and signed by the patient. The patient's signature must be either witnessed by specified individuals or notarized. Many states (e.g., Colorado, Hawaii, and West Virginia) exclude from being a witness any employee, including a nurse, of a facility where the declarant is receiving care. The form the living will is to take is frequently included in the state statute, and an individual should use that form for his or her own will. State statutes also include how a living will can be revoked after it is executed. Some examples include oral revocation, destroying the will, or amending it in writing.

Living will legislation most often provides immunity from civil and criminal suits and disciplinary actions by state licensing agencies for health care providers who in good faith and consistent with good medical and nursing practice abide by a patient's wishes in the document.

Durable Power of Attorney for Health Care

A durable power of attorney for health care is a written, signed, and witnessed document that appoints an individual ("agent") to make health care decisions when the patient (the "principal") cannot do so himself or herself. As such, it is different from the living will in that the instructions are communicated to the agent who as a proxy or surrogate decision maker works with the health care providers concerning the treatment decisions of the principal.

As with living wills, the person executing a durable power for health care decisions must be an adult or, in some instances, an emancipated minor. The agent or agents appointed (many statutes provide for successor agents to be listed in the event the first agent named cannot serve) can generally be anyone the principal selects; in other words, it does not have to be a family member, although it may be. However, there are some restrictions on who can serve as an agent. One restriction in many state statutes is the inability of a health care provider, including a nurse, to act as an agent when providing patient care to the principal.

The durable power of attorney for health care decisions is a much more flexible and broader-based document than the living will. To begin with, it often allows the agent to make all health care decisions, including consent to *and* refusal of treatment such as surgery, blood transfusions, dialysis, cardiopulmonary resuscitation, and artificial nutrition and hydration. Furthermore, it is not restricted to situations in which the principal is terminally ill but can be used for any treatment circumstance, such as elective or required surgery, in which decision-making capacity would not be present.

Health care durable power of attorney laws also provide for revocation, amendments, or alterations of the document. Similar to living will legislation, these statutes provide immunity from civil, criminal, and disciplinary actions for health care providers.

Currently, 50 states and the District of Columbia have health care power of attorney statutes.[51]

Table 12–1 summarizes some of the common provisions in both the living will and the durable power of attorney for health care.

Medical Directive

The medical directive is a non-statute-based advance directive suggested by its developers for use because it is designed as a "comprehensive" document; specifically, it can be used for various treatment and patient condition situations and also provides for the appointment of a proxy decision maker.[52]

TABLE 12–1

Selected Common Provisions in Living Will and Durable Power of Attorney for Health Care

LIVING WILL	DURABLE POWER OF ATTORNEY FOR HEALTH CARE
Directs health care professionals concerning withholding or withdrawing treatment	Appoints agent who makes decisions for individual concerning any treatment options (e.g., withholding treatment, initiating treatment)
Usually death must be imminent or within specified time	Usually, no requirement that person be dying or near death
Requires that patients be terminally ill or have an incurable illness or condition	No limitations on patient condition(s) in order for durable power to be effective
Patient must be unable to make own treatment decisions for document to be effective	Patient must be unable to make own treatment decisions for document to be effective
Requires document to be witnessed, with restrictions as to who can witness	Requires document to be witnessed, but with few, if any, restrictions on who can witness
Wide variety of treatments to be withdrawn or withheld possible, but may be restricted (e.g., no withdrawal of food and fluid)	Few, if any, restrictions on types of treatments that can be identified in document
May be revoked, amended, or otherwise changed	May be revoked, amended, or otherwise changed
Not considered support for suicide or assisted suicide	Not considered support for suicide or assisted suicide

Data from: Alan Meisel. *The Right to Die*. Volume 2. 2nd Edition. New York: John Wiley & Sons, 1995 (with 1999 cumulative supplement).

In states in which a particular form is not required or strongly suggested, the medical directive could be used as an instructive document as well as a mechanism to appoint a surrogate/proxy decision maker. Because it is not a state law, however, many of the protections afforded in advance directive legislation (e.g., immunity from suit and guidelines concerning witnesses and agents) may not be applicable when the medical directive is used. A portion of the Medical Directive is represented in Figure 12–1.

Surrogate/Proxy Decision Maker (Other Than a Guardian)

In health care situations, the surrogate or proxy decision maker is an individual who is an agent for the declarant or principal (the patient), representing and acting for the patient in making health

---

MY MEDICAL DIRECTIVE

This Medical Directive shall stand as a guide to my wishes regarding medical treatments in the event that illness should make me unable to communicate them directly. I make this Directive, being 18 years or more of age, of sound mind, and appreciating the consequences of my decisions.

SITUATION A

If I am in a coma or in a persistent vegetative state and, in the opinion of my physician and two consultants, have no known hope of regaining awareness and higher mental functions no matter what is done, then my goals and specific wishes—if medically reasonable—for this and any additional illness would be:

☐ prolong life; treat everything
☐ attempt to cure, but reevaluate often
☐ limit to less invasive and less burdensome interventions
☐ provide comfort care only
☐ other (please specify): _____

_____

Please check appropriate boxes:

	I want	I want treatment tried. If no clear improvement, stop.	I am undecided	I do not want
1. **Cardiopulmonary resuscitation** (chest compressions, drugs, electric shocks, and artificial breathing aimed at reviving a person who is on the point of dying).		Not applicable		
2. **Major surgery** (for example, removing the gallbladder or part of the colon).		Not applicable		
3. **Mechanical breathing** (respiration by machine, through a tube in the throat).				
4. **Dialysis** (cleaning the blood by machine or by fluid passed through the belly).				
5. **Blood transfusions or blood products.**		Not applicable		
6. **Artificial nutrition and hydration** (given through a tube in a vein or in the stomach).				
7. **Simple diagnostic tests** (for example, blood tests or x-rays).		Not applicable		
8. **Antibiotics** (drugs used to fight infection).		Not applicable		
9. **Pain medications, even if they dull consciousness and indirectly shorten my life.**		Not applicable		

FIGURE 12–1. Sample medical directive form (partial). From: Karla Kinderman. *Medicolegal Forms with Legal Analysis: Documenting Issues in the Patient-Physician Relationship.* Chicago, Ill: American Medical Association, 1999, 169. Copyright 1989, American Medical Association.

care decisions.[53] The surrogate decision maker can be designated either by a written document (e.g., advance directive) or by state statute.

If a written document has been executed by the principal or declarant, then the surrogate decision maker or proxy appointed in that document would make decisions in conformity with the patient's wishes and governing state law. If the person making health care decisions on behalf of another is doing so by statute, he or she must make decisions utilizing the "substituted-judgment test" (if other evidence exists concerning the patient's wishes) or the "best-interest-of-the-patient test."

The surrogate/proxy laws are often included in living will or durable power of attorney for health care decisions legislation, although Illinois has a separate statute for substituted decision making.[54] Surrogate/proxy laws that are separate from other statutes list individuals, in decending order of priority, who are able to make decisions for a person without decision-making capacity or an advance directive who fits the legislatively identified conditions (e.g., terminal illness or chronic vegetative state). Decision makers often include (in order of priority) a guardian of the person, spouse, adult children, adult parents, and adult siblings.

Immunity provisions for health care providers as well as ways to resolve a health care provider's objection to carrying out any decisions of the surrogate/proxy are also often included in this type of legislation. Moreover, provisions are included for disagreements among and between the listed individuals (e.g., petitioning for a guardianship); documentation requirements; and responsibilities of health care providers in identifying and following the directions of the surrogate/proxy decision maker.

It is important to contrast a guardian's role with that of a surrogate or proxy decision maker. Although a guardian is, technically, another who makes decisions on behalf of the ward (the person declared legally disabled), the guardian is appointed by the court after judicial determination of the nature and extent of the ward's disability. A surrogate or proxy decision maker is one who fills the role without appointment by a court.

Guardianship for Adults

Guardianship laws have existed for some time and are an example of the state's power to "act as a parent" (*parens patriae*) in protecting those who

---

ETHICS CONNECTION 12–2

Fulfilling the requirements of informed consent is complex, particularly with respect to the person's knowing and understanding the treatment and its consequences, both intended and unintended. There are some special considerations that relate to informed consent for surgery. Usually the surgeon discusses the surgery with the patient and obtains the consent. The nurse sometimes serves as witness to the signature. The anesthesiologist discusses the anesthetic and recovery process with the patient prior to surgery. What often is overlooked in these discussions, however, is the status of the patient's advance directive during surgery. It is the practice, if not the policy, of many institutions to suspend the advance directive and Do Not Resuscitate (DNR) orders during surgery. Although this may not be a legal practice, many surgeons and anesthesiologists are firm about needing to be free to attempt to reverse any adverse responses to the surgery or anesthesia. They contend that it is unacceptable to expect anesthesiologists, anesthetists, and/or surgeons to bear the moral burdens of being able to alter or suspend normal life processes through anesthesia or surgery while being constrained from reversing the effects of their own work. Often patients are not told that their advance directives will not be honored. Some institutions have developed consent policies that require surgeons and anesthesiologists to disclose that advance directives will be suspended during the perioperative period. Policies frequently state that for elective surgery this conversation be held prior to the patient's admission. Thus, patients who insist upon having their advance directives honored during surgery have the opportunity to discuss this with the surgeon. If the surgeons or anesthesiologists then refuse to proceed with the surgery, the patient can be assisted in finding a surgical team that will adhere to the advance directive.

Surgical consent forms usually include clauses about the administration of blood or blood products during the perioperative period. For patients who are Jehovah's Witnesses or members of other groups that prohibit receiving blood or blood products, it is important that they consider that clause before signing the consent form. Frequently, there is no problem about complying with the patient's refusal of whole blood, but some medications contain minute fractions of blood products that might inadvertently be administered. In some institutions, policies about specific clauses in consent forms are developed through consultation with community religious leaders regarding what treatments are acceptable or unacceptable to members of the respective religious groups that are served by the institution.

cannot make decisions for themselves because they lack decision-making ability. Prior to the enactment of advance directive legislation and in states in which surrogate/proxy decision making was not possible, the appointment of a guardian was one of the few, or only, legally recognized ways that health care decisions could be made for those who could not do so themselves. Guardianship is still used for treatment decisions today, although not as frequently, because of the advent of advance directive legislation and common law decisions developing alternate ways to establish decision-making abilities.

Although guardianship laws provide a useful and helpful mechanism for treatment decisions, the appointment of a guardian cannot be undertaken lightly. For example, when a guardian of the person is appointed, the individual (known as the ward) may lose other fundamental rights in addition to the ability to consent to treatment. If the patient's medical condition warrants it, the right to own property, vote, and obtain a divorce may also be removed from the ward.[55]

Many early state guardianship laws did not require the guardian to make decisions in accordance with the expressed desires of the ward.[56] Laws have been, in many instances, reformed, but even today a guardian is required to act in the best interests of the ward, which may or may not be consistent with the ward's desires.

As a result, in some states like Illinois, when an agent has been appointed pursuant to a durable power of attorney, a guardian has no power to make health care decisions unless the probate court enters an order to that effect. Other states have provisions in state medical treatment acts requiring a guardian to honor any declaration made by a ward pursuant to the act.

If a guardian is needed to make personal (in contrast to estate or financial) decisions for an individual, a "personal guardian" or "guardian of the person" is appointed. Generally the personal guardian has the responsibility to provide for the care, support, comfort, health, education, and maintenance of the ward. Additional powers may be specifically granted by the court, or limitations may be imposed on the guardian's powers, depending on state law. Some of the limitations may include the guardian's inability to admit a nonconsenting ward to a mental health facility for treatment as a voluntary patient or to consent to highly invasive medical treatment. The state's pro-

bate law usually provides that the guardian can seek permission for these procedures from the court after evidence is presented for the need to do so. If granted, an order is entered giving the guardian authority to act as requested.

In some instances, a minor may have a personal guardian who makes decisions concerning health care if parental rights have been limited or rescinded. The personal guardian of a minor is granted specific rights depending on the circumstances of the appointment. Although education and custody of the minor may be given to the personal guardian, he or she may not have permission to consent to medical care for the minor ward. In such an instance, the order granting guardianship must be consulted to determine the specific powers of the minor's personal guardian.

It is important to distinguish a guardian from a *guardian ad litem*. A *guardian ad litem* is appointed by the court during the course of a proceeding to protect the interests of the alleged disabled adult or minor.[57] The *guardian ad litem* has no control over the person or his or her estate. Rather, the *guardian ad litem* serves as the court's investigator, providing information to the court as to what is in the best interest of the alleged disabled adult or minor concerning the appointment of a guardian. Once a guardian is appointed, the *guardian ad litem*'s role may end. If there are other judicial proceedings concerning the ward, the *guardian ad litem*'s role may continue, especially when the guardian appointed by the court is unwilling or unable to make decisions concerning the ward's personal or financial matters.

Not all states provide for the appointment of *guardians ad litem* in guardianship proceedings. In addition, their roles vary considerably even when they are used.[58]

Patient Self-Determination Act (PSDA)

Because of the difficulty many people had in deciding about health care decisions, especially decisions about the termination of treatment, Congress passed the Patient Self-Determination Act.[59] It was passed as part of the federal Omnibus Budget Reconciliation Act (OBRA) of 1990. Effective December 1, 1991, the Patient Self-Determination Act requires hospitals, nursing homes, health maintenance organizations (HMOs), and home health care agencies receiving Medicare and Medicaid funds to (1) have written policies and procedures concerning adult patients and their ability to provide informed consent and refusal of treatment, and inform patients of those policies, (2) inform patients concerning their rights under state law, including the use of advance directives, to make decisions concerning treatment or nontreatment, (3) assess the existence of any advance directives and document the same in the patient's medical record, (4) not condition the provision of care or otherwise discriminate against the patient who does or does not have an advance directive, (5) comply with state law concerning advance directives, and (6) provide educational programs to facility staff and the community on the law and on advance directives.[60]

The assessment of whether or not an advance directive exists, or of the patient's preference to execute one, must occur at the time of admission if the facility is a hospital or skilled care facility. For an HMO or other prepaid health care program, the information must be gathered at the time the individual enrolls in the health care plan. For home health care agencies and hospice programs, the requirement is "in advance" of providing care and "at the time of initial receipt" of hospice care.[61]

An advance directive is defined by the Patient Self-Determination Act as a *written* instruction, like a living will or durable power of attorney for health care, recognized under state law and relating to the provision of care when the individual is incapacitated.[62]

Requirements of the Patient Self-Determination Act are enforced through the usual Medicare and Medicaid procedures by the secretary of Health and Human Services and the Health Care Financing Administration (HCFA). These procedures include on-site surveys, withdrawal of funding under the applicable program, and failure to renew a provider agreement.[63]

The requirements of the Act do not apply to providers of outpatient services. Nor does the Act require a patient to execute an advance directive. The content and format of the written information to be given to the adult patient concerning advance directives are not dictated by the Department of Health and Human Services or the Health Care Financing Administration.[64] Also, a health care provider is not required to carry out an advance directive if state law allows objection on the basis of his or her conscience.[65]

NURSING IMPLICATIONS

There is no doubt that a nurse will provide care to patients who have advance directives. In fact, the nurse may be the first person the patient discusses the advance directive with. Because the Patient Self-Determination Act requires a health care facility, nursing home, and home health care agency to determine whether the patient has an advance directive, that responsibility may be assigned to the nurse. The American Nurses Association (ANA) recommends that determining if an advance directive exists be a part of the nursing admission assessment.[66]

The American Nurses Association . . . recommends that determining if an advance directive exists be a part of the nursing admission assessment.

When opening a new case, the home health care nurse will need to ascertain whether an advance care document exists. The triage nurse in the emergency department will also need to do so.

Even if the responsibility for determining the existence of an advance directive is assigned to another health care provider or employee, it is the nurse's responsibility to ask about the advance directive when the patient is admitted to the unit or service. Because the advance directive must be made a part of the patient's medical record, the nurse should get the advance directive from the patient or family, place it in the record, document its existence in the nursing note or admission form, and notify the physician so that orders can be written consistent with the advance directive.

It is important for the nurse to remember that unless orders are given or written consistent with the advance directive, the nurse cannot institute care or withdraw or withhold care as directed by the patient. Although this prohibition may seem ethically contraindicated, legally the nurse cannot prescribe medications or treatments (unless able to do so by the state nurse practice act). Furthermore, advance directive laws require certification of any prerequisite patient condition by a physician or other designated health care provider (e.g., advanced practice nurse, physician's assistant). As a result, the nurse needs to obtain orders from the attending physician or other health care provider that complies with the state advance directive laws in relation to certification and documentation requirements. Once obtained, care should be provided consistent with those orders.

If a patient does not have an advance directive on admission and wishes to execute one, the nurse should document this request and notify the appropriate department in the facility pursuant to policy. The nurse needs to remember not to be a witness to a living will or durable power of attorney. If asked, the nurse should refuse to act as an agent for the patient under a durable power of attorney for health care. Also, the nurse should not condition care on the existence or nonexistence of an advance directive or coerce, intimidate, or force a patient to initiate one.

If an advance directive is revoked, altered, or amended by the patient, the physician and the nurse manager should be notified consistent with facility policy. Care must be provided without regard to the instructions in the directive until new medical orders are provided by the physician.

When no advance directive exists and use of a surrogate/proxy decision maker is necessary, the nurse should obtain information as to care decisions from the decision maker and the physician only. The identity of the surrogate/proxy decision maker needs to be clearly noted on the patient's chart.

If a guardian has been appointed for the patient, it is imperative that the *type* of guardian and *powers* be ascertained. This can be done best by asking for a copy of the order appointing the individual as guardian and making it a part of the patient's medical record. In addition, notifying the physician and nursing administration is necessary.

If the nurse practices in the neonatal intensive care unit or with pediatric clients, a guardian for the minor may be making treatment decisions. As with the guardian for an adult, the nurse must ensure that the minor's guardian is legally able to provide consent or refusal of treatment.

The nurse must be active in developing clear, concise policies and procedures concerning the nurse's role and advance directives. This can be accomplished through membership on the policy and procedure committee or by communicating issues and concerns to those who serve on the committee. Important components to include in institutional policy are (1) who is to be contacted when a document exists, (2) who is to be notified when a revocation occurs, (3) the nurse's role in providing care when a revocation takes place, (4) definition of terms used in the policy (e.g., *DNR,*

assisted ventilation, artificial food and hydration), (5) who is to verify the appropriate surrogate/proxy decision maker, and (6) documentation requirements.

The nurse should also be actively involved on the facility ethics committee. Ethics committees were initiated primarily as a result of the *In re Quinlan*[67] decision. In that case, the court, in holding that Karen Quinlan's father, who was her legal guardian, could remove her from the ventilator, stated that no criminal liability would occur so long as the hospital's ethics committee (really a *prognosis* committee at that point) reviewed and confirmed her prognosis.[68]

The functions of ethics committees vary. They include educating, contributing to the development of institutional or agency policies and procedures, supporting those who are involved in treatment decisions, providing a forum for airing treatment issues and resolving disputes, and providing a vehicle for analytic moral and legal inquiry.[69]

The American Nurses Association has published a position statement on ways in which nurses can consider ethical issues.[70] The statement suggests nurses actively participate in review processes, serve as a resource for individuals and groups exploring health care ethics, and develop programs for nurses requesting assistance in addressing ethical concerns in nursing practice. Nursing has an invaluable contribution to make in resolving difficulties arising from refusal situations, especially when a conflict among family surrogate decision makers or a difference of opinion among health care providers can obscure the intent of an advance directive's instructions.

Last, if the nurse is unable to carry out the instructions of a patient's advance directive or surrogate/proxy decision maker, he or she should notify nursing administration and be assigned to another patient, as has been previously discussed.

DOCUMENTATION REMINDER 12–3
Advance Directives

- If advance directive made out by patient, include document in medical record

- Notification of physician, nurse manager, and others concerning patient's advance directive

- Name of surrogate/proxy decision maker or guardian and if involved in decision making

- Orders provided by physician

- If care transferred to another staff nurse, to whom, when, and summary notation in nursing notes

- If present when revocation or alteration occurs, specifics of revocation (what patient said, who was present, when and manner of revocation)

- Guardianship court papers included in medical record

- If present when care withdrawn, document details clearly and concisely (when, who present, who terminated care, patient response)

- Document other patient care provided that is not limited or rejected by patient

SPECIAL CONSIDERATIONS

Consent/Refusal for Organ and Tissue Transplantation

Organ and tissue donation is a fairly common occurrence in health care today. With the many advances in medical science and the development of drugs to minimize or eliminate rejection, transplants of livers, kidneys, and hearts, for example, have been done with varying degrees of success.[71] Likewise, tissues such as bone marrow, skin, and corneas have also been transplanted.[72]

For the most part, cadavers are the primary source of donated organs.[73] Although consent or refusal for such a donation could occur orally or by a written document immediately before the patient dies, often the decision to donate is made long before the end of life. As a result, the donation of organs or tissues is often done through a uniform law that has been passed in all states, the Uniform Anatomical Gift Act (UAGA).[74]

The Uniform Anatomical Gift Act allows an adult "of sound mind and body" to donate all or part of his or her body as a gift that takes effect upon his or her death. The gift can be made formally (e.g., in a will) or through another written and signed document, such as a donor card that is included on some state driver's licenses or an advance directive. The signature of the donor can be certified by two witnesses. If no prior donation has occurred, the Act provides a list of individuals (in descending order of priority) who can consent to donation at the time of death.

Likewise, some states have passed other statutes granting the right of the individual and/or the family to donate specific organs or tissues, such as corneas, when death occurs.

When an organ or tissue donation is made by a living person to another, different legal and ethical problems arise. When the donor is an adult who possesses decision-making capacity, the main legal concern is that the donor has been fully informed of the procedure to be undertaken. When the donor is a minor or an adult who lacks decision-making abilities, however, the crucial question is whether or not the guardian, parent, or other surrogate decision maker has the authority to provide consent for the procedure.

Some courts across the country have allowed donations by substituted consent to occur, while other jurisdictions have not. Because every organ donation from an adult lacking decision-making ability or a minor is unique, the best option is to resort to the court for determination of the issue.[75]

The National Organ Transplant Act[76] was passed by Congress to provide for a Task Force on Organ Procurement and Transplantation to oversee and report on issues in this area, including equitable access to organs and insurance reimbursement for transplantations. The Act also established organ procurement organizations (OPOs), federally funded, nonprofit organizations established to coordinate organ donation and procurement in identified service areas.[77] The Act, like many state laws, also prohibits the sale of human organs "for valuable consideration."

In order to increase the number of organ transplants, in June of 1998 the Health Care Financing Administration (HCFA) adopted a rule requiring hospitals to notify the appropriate organ procurement organization (or a predesignated third party) of all patient deaths or imminent patient deaths.[78] Once notified, the organ procurement organization is then responsible for assessing the suitability of the potential organ donor.[79] If the potential organ donor is deemed suitable, family consent for the donation must be obtained by the organization or by someone trained by it.[80]

Continued advances can be expected in organ and tissue transplantation in the years ahead. For example, animal-to-human transplantations have already occurred. In the first instance, "Baby Fae" received the heart of a baboon at Loma Linda University Medical Center in 1984 and lived for 10 days. In 1992, the use of a baboon liver for an adult male recipient at the University of Pittsburgh Hospital made the headlines. In 1992, an AIDS

ETHICS CONNECTION 12–3

Nurses are central to participation in morally responsible procurement of donor organs for transplantation. Collectively, nurses provide care to both donors and recipients. As organ procurement and transplantation technology has improved, organ transplants have become more common than in the past. Whether or not the dying individual has indicated on a driver's license or in some other way that he or she has chosen to donate organs, families generally are asked, as well. Nurses and others who are designated to approach families and support them as their family member dies must be extremely sensitive to the possibility of unintentional coercion about organ donation during what is a very vulnerable time for families. The current critical shortage of organs has led to statutory changes in procurement through the regional procurement agencies that may have the unintended effect of subtle, unintended coercion for families to consent to organ donation. Issues in organ procurement and transplantation also have highlighted the need for new definitions of death. New technologies that make possible the transplantation of more visible body parts, such as hands, may require extension of the usual consent forms.[1]

Organ swapping[2] and increased commercialization of organ donation is another consequence of the current scarcity of organs. Although consent regulation has been in place for medically procured organs and their transplantation, consent processes for persons who sell their organs or parts thereof currently are not well regulated. Although legally prohibited in the United States, there is an increasing international market for organs to be purchased or obtained through other *quid pro quo* arrangements. The social justice of the emerging marketplace model of organ procurement and transplantation is in question. Donors typically are vulnerable people who need money desperately or indigenous people who do not fully comprehend the meaning of donating their organs. Attempts are being made to halt these commercial practices and to further protect donors by developing informed consent legislation and processes that include commercial organ procurement arrangements.[3]

Xenotransplantation, the transplantation of animal organs and other parts into humans, poses other ethical issues. Technology is rapidly making such transplantations possible, but critical questions about xenotransplantation need to be addressed further. There is a public health concern, as well, that through animal to human transplantation, diseases may be transmitted across species, particularly from animal to human. HIV/AIDS is an example of cross-species transmission.[4] In addition, advocates of animal rights are concerned about the ethical treatment of the animals that are prospective donors. Informed consent about xenotransplantation, when it becomes available for treatment, will be complex indeed. It will be very difficult to foresee all the benefits and burdens of this and other emerging technologies.

---

[1]Arthur L. Caplan. "In Brief: Wearing Your Organ Transplant on Your Sleeve." 29(2) *Hastings Center Report* (March/April 1999), 52.

[2]Jerry Menikoff, "Organ Swapping," 29(6) *Hastings Center Report* (November/December 1999), 28–33.

[3]Dorothy Nelkin and Lori Andrews, "Homo Economicus," 28(5) *Hastings Center Report* (September/October 1999), 30–39.

[4]Lori P. Knowles, "Xenotransplantation: Full Speed Ahead, Slow Down," 29(4) *Hastings Center Report* (July/August 1999), 47; Mark J. Hanson and Lilly-Marlene Russow, "A Xenotransplantation Protocol," 29(6) *Hastings Center Report* (November/December 1999), 25–25.

---

patient received a bone marrow transplant from a baboon.[81] As a result, in 1996 the U.S. Public Health Service (USPHS) issued guidelines for cross-species transplantation, termed xenotransplantation.[82] The guidelines acknowledge the shortage of human organs for transplantation and provide procedures to minimize the risks possible when cross-species transplantation occur. Among other procedures, the guidelines identify the following areas of concern: (1) hospital infection control practices to reduce the transmission of infectious agents, (2) creation of a central database for safety data important for public health investigations, and (3) clinical protocol and the informed consent vital to public health concerns about infections with such transplants.[83]

These and other developments to come raise new and different ethical and legal implications for nursing and other health care professionals.

Consent/Refusal for Human Subject Research

Nursing research is defined as the conduct of systematic studies to generate new knowledge or confirm existing knowledge.[84] Generally speaking, however, there are two types of health care research—therapeutic and nontherapeutic.[85] Therapeutic research is aimed toward aiding all humans, including the individual undergoing the care or treatment. In contrast, in nontherapeutic research, treatment is carried out on individuals who have no medical need for the treatment.[86] For either type of research with humans as subjects, the law has established clear guidelines that must be followed to avoid, insofar as possible, abuse and misuse of the research process.

The first standards established to regulate research were the Code of Ethics in Medical Research,[87] promulgated by the Nuremberg Tribunal after World War II to avoid a duplication of the "research" done by Nazis in their concentration camps. This and subsequent codes, both national and international, led to the establishment of research guidelines by professional organizations as well as state and federal governments.

Current guidelines covering research are governed by several federal laws and regulations. For example, the Department of Health and Human Resources (HHS) requires that all research supported by it must comply with federal regulations for the protection of human subjects.[88] Among other things, the HHS regulations require the establishment of an institutional review board (IRB) through which all proposed research must be approved before support from HHS is forthcoming.[89] Each institution seeking HHS approval must submit its assurance that it will comply with the promulgated HHS regulations before HHS will review submitted proposals.[90]

In addition to the HHS regulations, research involving investigational new drugs or devices must comply with regulations promulgated by the Food and Drug Administration.[91]

An IRB is required to ensure that human research subjects are protected by ensuring that (1) the risks to the subjects are minimized; (2) selection of subjects is done in an equitable manner; (3) legally informed consent is obtained and documented appropriately in the medical record; and (4) adequate safeguards are in place for the protection of subject safety, privacy, and freedom from duress or undue influence.[92] In short, two areas of importance stand out—analyzing risk/benefit to the subject and obtaining informed consent.[93]

IRBs and research on human subjects have been subject to close scrutiny in recent years.[94] Lack of accountability for research involving human subjects, failure to obtain proper informed consent, and lack of oversight of institutional research are just a few of the concerns identified.[95]

For informed consent from human subjects to be consistent with federal requirements, the following information should be provided:

- Knowledge that the study involves research
- Any reasonably foreseeable risks or discomforts
- Procedures that will be followed
- How long the research will be provided
- Purposes of the research
- Reasonably expected benefits from the research
- Alternative treatments, if any
- Confidentiality of research records in relation to the subject's identity
- When more than a minimal risk is involved, whether compensation and additional medical treatment are available and where further information can be obtained
- Identity of person to contact for additional questions concerning the research, the subject's rights, and if an injury occurs
- Statement that participation in the research is voluntary, and refusal to participate or withdrawal from study can occur without retaliation[96]

Depending on the type of research project, these minimum requirements for informed consent may be supplemented by additional requirements, including circumstances under which the individual subject's participation in the study may be terminated by the researcher without the participant's consent.[97]

The federal regulations, as well as ethical codes established by professional associations and most health care delivery systems, require the individual's informed consent to be in writing.[98]

Further federal guidelines have also been promulgated for research with special populations. For example, minors are afforded specific protections that include obtaining the minor's consent, where possible, in addition to that of *both* parents (except in certain situations).[99]

When research involves prisoners, the rules categorize research that is permissible. Permissible topics include the study of health problems affecting prisoners as a class (e.g., hepatitis, chemical use) so long as consultation with medical and ethical experts occurs.[100] An institutional review board must determine if the research proposal conforms with requirements already discussed for informed consent.[101]

Research participants who are mentally ill, especially those who are institutionalized, may not be able to exercise free choice in the same manner that noninstitutionalized individuals do. Although decision-making capacity is retained upon admission to a psychiatric facility, continued hospitalization may weaken the individual's ability to make decisions freely. Therefore, strict compliance with federal and state guidelines concerning informed consent and research, and the use of an institutional review board to oversee the study, are vital.[102]

Consent/Refusal for HIV Testing

Obtaining informed consent when testing persons for the human immunodeficiency virus (HIV) is important not only because of the reasons already presented in this chapter, but also because of the possible stigma of the testing itself. For example, many persons tested for HIV experience difficulty in obtaining health or life insurance.[103] As a result, many states have enacted informed consent requirements for HIV testing.

Although state statutes vary, most require that written, informed consent of the test subject be obtained before testing for HIV status. Particular information may include an explanation of the test procedure, policies concerning confidentiality of the test results, the requirement of counseling if the test is positive, and what a seropositive result means.

In some states, minors over a certain age can consent to their own HIV testing. For minors who are taken into temporary custody under the state's child abuse law, the state agency administering and enforcing the law may be given the power to consent to HIV testing so long as the consent conforms to the state HIV testing laws.

In some states, minors over a certain age can consent to their own HIV testing.

Informed consent for HIV testing is not required in all circumstances. When, for example, a health care worker is accidentally exposed to blood or body fluid, some states allow testing of the patient without his or her consent. Particular

ETHICS CONNECTION 12–4

Informed consent for clinical experimentation is another area of special concern to nurses. Because patients often turn to nurses to discuss the proposed experimental treatment and its benefits and burdens, the nurse may be in the conflicting position of wanting to support the physician in giving the experimental treatment while assuring that the consent is fully informed and freely given. In these situations, communication among the patient, nurse, and physician is critically important. Tabak[1] has developed a worksheet to help nurses resolve this dilemma of divided loyalties. In Tabak's model, the nurse's individual and personal moral values are included as part of the decision making, as is the *ANA Code for Nurses: With Interpretive Statements.*[2] Recent changes in federal legislation affect ethics of nursing research and of nurses who participate in interdisciplinary clinical trials. In addition to understanding the increased monitoring of institutional review boards[3] (see Chapter 3), nurses who receive federal support for their own research projects or who participate in federally funded research projects directed by others must be aware of recent changes in disclosure of data about human subjects. With increasing technology, including the National Institutes of Health Web site and database, a repository for information about clinical trials is accessible.[4, 5] This accessibility, coupled with a controversial change in federal reporting requirements that disclose some previously privileged information, provide the ability to make better informed decisions about health care treatments. This technology also creates the burden of increased risk of disclosure of confidential information. Informed consent for research needs to address the possibility of data being accessible via the Internet. In addition, for research that involves treatment protocols, third-party payers are becoming more reluctant to pay for experimental treatment. Consent should include a statement that the cost of the treatment may need to be borne by the research subject.

---

[1]Nili Tabak, "Informed Consent: The Nurse's Dilemma," 15(1) *Medicine and Law* (1996), 7–16.

[2]American Nurses Association. *Code for Nurses: With Interpretive Statements.* Kansas City, Missouri: Author, 1985.

[3]Rebecca Dresser, "Time for New Rules on Human Subjects Research?" 28(6) *Hastings Center Report* (November/December 1998), 23–24.

[4]Rebecca Dresser, "Surfing for Studies: Clinical Trials on the Internet," 29(6) *Hastings Center Report* (November/December 1999), 26–27.

[5]Joanne Silberner, "Federal Science Policy: Changing Battle Lines, New Fronts," 29(4) *Hastings Center Report* (July/August 1999), 6.

requirements must be met in these cases, including a physician determining that the individual's blood or bodily fluid "may be of a nature to transmit HIV" or obtaining a court order mandating the test.

Informed refusal of HIV testing is possible, although it is not an absolute right. For example, when a rape or another type of criminal sexual assault has allegedly occurred, in some states a victim can request that the offender be tested for HIV status.[104] If the state's attorney obtains a court order to compel testing, the accused can be tested over his or her objection.

Consent/Refusal and Law Enforcement

Nurses working in the emergency department (ED) of a health care facility, or staff nurses providing care for a patient under police guard, may be asked to perform procedures that are aimed at obtaining medical evidence to support a particular criminal charge against the individual. These procedures include drawing blood (for a blood alcohol or drug screen), removing stomach contents, performing physical examinations, and assisting with surgery (to remove a bullet or a swallowed object). Because they risk being charged with the commission of a crime, many, if not most, of the individuals refuse to consent to the requested procedure.

The refusal cannot be taken lightly by nursing staff, regardless of the circumstances under which the individual denies consent for treatment. Clear nursing implications exist when a refusal occurs, but it is important for the nurse to know that many states have implied consent statutes, especially in

---

ETHICS CONNECTION 12–5

Persons who are 18 and older are considered to be adults, and those younger than 18 are considered to be minors. Therefore, with several exceptions, the latter are unable to provide consent. Parents or guardians typically give or refuse consent for their minor children. This practice and policy poses problems in some situations, such as in Human Immunodeficiency Virus (HIV) testing. Informed, voluntary testing of all individuals who potentially are infected is an important strategy in controlling the spread of Acquired Immune Deficiency Syndrome (AIDS). A number of states, including Texas, have amended state laws so that minors can give consent for the diagnosis and treatment of infectious, contagious, or communicable diseases that are subject to mandatory reporting, including HIV and AIDS. Informed consent about the limits of confidentiality and privacy is a key issue in HIV testing. Part of the information that adolescents seek before signing consent is what their parents will be told. Many adolescents who are at risk for HIV/AIDS are not tested because they fear that information about the testing and its results will be disclosed to their parents or guardians. From the moral perspectives of autonomy and beneficence, it is important that minors know that in some states, the laws about confidentiality conflict with one another. In Texas, for example, statutes require written consent from minors before releasing test results. Other statutes permit parents to obtain information about actual treatment for sexually transmitted diseases with or without their children's consent.[1] Thus, confidentiality is protected for testing but not for treatment. This situation is complicated further by the responsibility to inform sexual partners when the minor's test results are positive and there is "knowledge of possible HIV transmission to a third party." Until such conflicting laws are changed, individual practitioners have discretion about the burdens and benefits of protecting the minor's privacy and confidentiality versus disclosing medical information to the parents and others who might have been infected. Individual practitioners must be very clear about the moral values underlying their decisions. Further, they have a public responsibility to work toward making the legislation clear and consistent with prevailing social and professional moral values.

The question of minors' ability to consent to their own health care in other aspects of their lives is called into question, as well. Eighteen is the age of consent in the United States; however, studies of human development show that adolescents aged 13 and older have the capacity to give informed consent.[3] In practice, parents often discuss prospective treatment, especially invasive treatment such as surgery, with their minor children and come to consensus about consenting. This becomes difficult, however, for children who are in foster care and for children whose parents are in the midst of divorce proceedings in which the custody of the children is contested.

[1] J. L. Richardson, "Legal Issues for Nurses: Minors and the Ability to Consent to HIV Testing," 70(4) *Texas Nursing* (April 1996), 12–13.

[2] *Id.*

[3] J. Shields and A. Johnson, "Collision between Law and Ethics: Consent for Treatment with Adolescents." *Bulletin of the American Academy of Psychiatry Law* (1992), 314.

relation to driving under the influence of chemical substances (DUI). In other words, by obtaining a driver's license, the individual provides implied consent to be tested for drugs or alcohol when suspected of being impaired when driving. When such a law exists, and the individual refuses to consent to a blood test, it is unlikely that an action for assault and battery against the nurse or health care facility would be successful if the sample is taken over his or her objection.

Obtaining a blood sample is not as invasive a procedure as, for example, surgery to remove a bullet lodged in the patient's abdomen. The more invasive the procedure refused, the more likely an action for assault or battery (or violation of the patient's constitutional rights if the facility is a public facility) would be successful. Even so, a good rule of thumb is for the nurse not to participate in any refused procedure. The police can obtain a search warrant or a court order if the alleged offender refuses the desired medical intervention. If either of those are obtained, the protection of the nurse and health care facility against suit is almost certain.

Consent/Refusal and the Psychiatric Patient

Individuals receiving mental health services are presumed to possess decision-making capacity, regardless of whether their admission to a mental health facility is a voluntary or involuntary one (commitment). In fact, this presumption is often codified in state mental health statutes. In any case, the recipient of mental health services retains the right to provide informed consent or refusal of treatment, including but not limited to electro-convulsive therapy, psychosurgery, dental and medical treatment, and medications. The only way in which this right can be limited in some way is through the appointment of a guardian or the use of advance directives.

Because of the far-reaching effects of some treatment methods in psychiatry, informed consent for treatment has been clearly defined in many state mental health statutes. For example, Illinois, Massachusetts, Michigan, and New York provide for informed consent by the psychiatric client.[105]

The psychiatric patient's right of refusal is not absolute. In addition to the traditional exceptions to the mandate of obtaining informed consent for treatment, some additional ones exist for the psychiatric patient. One exception involves medica-

tions, particularly psychotropic medications. The right of refusing medications has been firmly established. Many cases, however, have limited that right to situations in which the patient is not a danger to himself or to others as a result of that refusal, including *Rennie v. Klein*[106] (Thorazine and Prolixin) and *Rogers v. Orkin*[107] (several medications). These and other court challenges have been based on several legal theories, including the First Amendment (freedom of speech, freedom of association) and Fourteenth Amendment (privacy, due process) constitutional protections.

A second area in which refusal of treatment presents unique issues in psychiatry is when the individual refuses to be hospitalized for a psychiatric problem. Although this topic will be discussed at length in Chapter 17, it is necessary to point out here that a refusal of admission may not be honored if the individual fits the criteria in the state mental health code for an involuntary civil admission (commitment). In a far-reaching 1975 U.S. Supreme Court case, *O'Connor v. Donaldson*,[108] those criteria were defined as requiring a finding by the court that the individual is a danger to himself or others *as well as* being mentally ill. The decision was steadfastly based on the constitutional protections of liberty and due process guaranteed by the Fourteenth Amendment.

If a psychiatric client is determined to be in need of a guardian, the judicial procedure is separate from any other judicial determination. If a guardian is appointed, the guardian may be able to provide informed consent or refusal for treatment in the psychiatric ward consistent with provisions in the state mental health code. When the treatment contemplated is particularly invasive or experimental, many state statutes require the guardian to seek court approval before consent or refusal is given. For example, in Illinois, a court order must be obtained by the guardian for electroconvulsive therapy, psychosurgery, or other "highly invasive medical treatment."[109]

Other Parameters of Consent/Refusal

Other boundaries exist in relation to an individual consenting to or refusing treatment. Insofar as informed consent is concerned, four additional limitations on an individual's authority to consent to treatment have been identified. Those limitations include consent for (1) mayhem, (2) aiding suicide, (3) medical products and drugs prohibited by law, and (4) inappropriate treatment.[110]

Mayhem is defined as the intentional and knowing permanent disfigurement or dismemberment of a body part without justification.[111] In many states it is currently called aggravated assault or battery[112] and is a criminal violation. A patient's consent to perform a procedure that would result in disfigurement or dismemberment does not protect the individual whose actions resulted in the bodily injury. For example, in a 1961 case, a physician was convicted of aiding and abetting mayhem as a result of his anesthetizing a patient's finger (at the patient's request) so it could later be removed by the patient's brother.[113]

Inducing, aiding, or forcing another to commit suicide is a crime in many states; that is, murder.[114] This is so even if the individual does so at the request of the person and with his or her consent. Moreover, a conviction for murder may result even when the request is to end suffering experienced in a serious or terminal illness.[115] This particular issue will be discussed at length in Chapter 13.

If a medical device or drug has not been approved by the Food and Drug Administration and is used in patient care situations other than those approved for testing, the practitioner using the device or drug may face several legal problems. To begin with, if there is injury to the patient, he or she may be able to sue the health care provider under a negligence theory. In addition, the practitioner would most probably face disciplinary action by the state licensing agency, by the institution where he or she practices, and by various professional associations. Again, the consent of the patient to use untested or unapproved devices or drugs would not protect the health care professional from these legal challenges.

Similarly, a health care provider is bound by ethical *and* legal mandates to provide appropriate care. A patient's expressed request and permission for the provider to do something illegal or contrary to standards of good medical or nursing practice is no justification to do so. Penalties for carrying out inappropriate or illegal care can include a suit alleging malpractice, licensing and other disciplinary actions, and even criminal charges.

NURSING IMPLICATIONS

The special considerations in informed consent and refusal of treatment raise additional nursing ramifications. For example, when working with patients or their families where organ or tissue donation is a possibility, adherence to established policies and procedures concerning donation can be helpful to the nurse. The nurse may have a pivotal role in approaching the patient or family concerning their decision to donate an organ, especially when the nurse works in a health care facility with a transplant unit or where the nurse has been trained by the organ procurement organization in his or her geographic area.

Initially assessing whether the patient has executed some type of document like a donor card is also important because it may alleviate the need to determine this issue after death has occurred.

The nurse should be clear about the fact that procuring and selling body parts for donation is a crime in most states, unless done pursuant to established laws (e.g., the Uniform Anatomical Gift Act). If someone approaches the nurse concerning willingness to donate an organ or informs the nurse that a source is available, referral to an attorney, an organ procurement agency, or other advisor who can aid the person in donating the organ legally is best.

Whatever the legal status of payment for organs or bodily tissue will ultimately be,[116] ethical dilemmas surrounding payment for organs will exist. One proposal, for example, provided a death benefit payment of $1,000 to a family who consented to the donation of a deceased family member's organ(s).[117] The nurse must actively ensure that organ and tissue donations are carried out with dignity and respect for the donor and donee.[118]

The nurse must actively ensure that organ and tissue donations are carried out with dignity and respect for the donor and donee.

A nurse may be involved in research in a number of roles. If a participant in a clinical study, the nurse must be certain that the patient is fully informed concerning the research and that the written consent is present in the medical record. If questions are raised by the patient, the nurse can help the patient obtain whatever additional information is needed.[119] If the nurse researcher is the principal investigator, he or she will need to ensure that the patient's informed consent is obtained consistent with all applicable laws and the institution's institutional review board.[120]

Recent changes in informed consent requirements regulated by federal agencies require that the nurse researcher be clear about when informed consent is necessary and when it may be waived. The Department of Health and Human Services' waiver applies to a small class of research activities involving human subjects when emergency medical intervention is needed but informed consent cannot be obtained and no surrogate decision maker is available to represent them.[121] Called the Emergency Research Consent Waiver, it can apply to any specific situation only where the institutional review board has approved both the research and the waiver of informed consent.[122]

The Food and Drug Administration also announced similar changes in its informed consent requirements for emergency treatment research activities involving an investigational new drug application or an investigative device exemption.[123]

The nurse researcher will also need to be clear about his or her own feelings concerning the emergency consent waiver. Although many supporters believe that the waiver will help those seeking treatment in emergency departments to have improved care, critics view the new regulations as a threat to patient rights and well-being.[124]

HIV testing requires that written, informed consent be obtained and in the medical record before testing occurs, unless an exception exists. If an exception excuses the requirement of obtaining informed consent, the nurse should carefully and completely document the facts surrounding that exception in the medical record.

If a patient is accompanied by a law enforcement officer and refuses care, the nurse should consult established policy and procedure in the facility concerning his or her role. Contacting the nurse manager is always a wise option if the nurse is unclear about what to do in the situation. If the patient consents to whatever treatment request the officer makes, the use of a facility consent form that specifically covers consent for a procedure at the request of a law enforcement officer is a good risk management approach. The form would become a part of the patient record as would any other consent form signed by a patient.

Psychiatric clients must be treated like all other clients in relation to informed consent and refusal of treatment; that is, they are able to grant or refuse permission for treatment. If an exception arises in which the decision cannot be honored (e.g., the patient is a danger to himself), then appropriate medical or nursing intervention should occur and those actions should be documented. This requires a thorough knowledge of the state mental health code's provisions on consent and refusal of treatment.

Many of the special considerations in informed consent/refusal require the nurse to exercise common sense. Yet, because the legal issues are unique, the nurse should seek guidance from his or her nurse manager and facility policies and procedures when necessary.

ETHICS CONNECTION 12-6

The practices and ethics of obtaining informed consent are changing as decision making becomes more focused on the family and the community. In the past, informed consent often was seen as an event, such as with therapy or cancer treatment protocols that an individual had the right to consent to or refuse. More recently, consent sometimes is considered to be a process of consent as individuals think about consequences of their decision over a longer period of time, whenever possible. They may, for example, choose to begin long-range treatments, such as a series of reconstructive surgeries, with the understanding that if the treatment becomes too burdensome, it will be discontinued, if possible. Knowing and understanding the full impact of any given treatment plan is very difficult, if not impossible, until one actually begins to experience the treatment and its outcomes.

Newer models of family and communal decision making are being developed that have potential to influence the moral foundations and practical processes of obtaining informed consent. In these models, consent more commonly is seen as a communal process rather than simply an individual practice that is grounded in notions of individual autonomy. It is not solely the individual client who benefits from or experiences the burdens of treatment. Humans are frequently embedded in relationships; thus, promoting autonomy "can require that others support and encourage the patient in complex ways."[1]

---

[1]Gregory E. Kaebnick, "From the Editor," 29(5) *Hastings Center Report* (September/October 1999), 3–6.

The ethical dilemmas raised by these situations may be more difficult to resolve than the legal concerns. Seeking out support, identifying one's own thoughts and feelings about these issues, and consistently reviewing theories of ethical decision making and models of practice can help the nurse begin to formulate his or her own resolution to these complex patient care situations.

SUMMARY OF PRINCIPLES AND APPLICATIONS

The right of self-determination is an important one that should not be abridged by health care entities or health care providers. Whether founded upon constitutional underpinnings or couched in terms of power, autonomy, or respect, self-determination is important to those consumers of health care, whether voluntarily or involuntarily. The nurse plays an essential role in aiding the patient to provide or withhold consent to treatment. Moreover, the nurse is a patient advocate. As such, he or she must protect the patient when the ability to provide continuing input into medical and nursing treatment is questioned or threatened. The nurse can fulfill those roles by:

- Being knowledgeable about state and federal informed consent and informed refusal laws

- Recognizing that the right of informed consent/refusal is based on many legal theories, including the constitutional rights of privacy, due process, liberty, and freedom of religion

- Protecting the patient's rights under the Patient Self-Determination Act

- Understanding the various advance directives, their use, and the nurse's roles concerning them

- Volunteering to serve on the facility's ethics committee

- Documenting carefully, accurately, and completely in the medical record information concerning informed consent and refusal

- Understanding substituted consent/refusal mechanisms, especially with minors, guardians, and others

- Remembering that adults enjoy a presumption of possessing decision-making capacity

- Remembering that some minors can provide their own consent/refusal for treatment

- Remembering that living wills, durable powers of attorney, and medical directives are examples of advance directives

- Differentiating among a guardian of the person, a guardian of the estate, and a *guardian ad litem*

- Remembering that special circumstances in informed consent/refusal present additional nursing implications

- Keeping in mind that the rights of informed consent and refusal of treatment are not absolute

- Identifying the many ethical dilemmas raised in informed consent/refusal situations

TOPICS FOR FURTHER INQUIRY

1. Develop a study to compare the right of minors to consent to or refuse medical treatment in at least three states by reviewing all of the respective state statutes covering this topic.

2. Review institutional policies on informed consent/refusal for treatment in at least three health care facilities and evaluate their conformity with the Patient Self-Determination Act.

3. Write a position paper on the sale of human organs and human tissues. Compare and contrast the legal issues inherent in the position taken with the ethical issues raised. Develop the nurse's role based upon the legal and ethical issues identified.

4. Compare the rights of nonpsychiatric patients to consent to or refuse treatment with those of psychiatric patients in at least two states and propose needed changes.

REFERENCES

1. Ruth Faden and Tom Beauchamp. *A History and Theory of Informed Consent.* New York: Oxford University Press, 1986, 23.
2. *Id.* at 25.
3. *Id.*
4. 105 N.E. 92 (1914).
5. *Id.* at 93.
6. Faden and Beauchamp, *supra* note 1, at 125.
7. 317 P.2d 170 (1957).
8. *Id.* at 181.
9. *O'Brian v. Cunard S.S. Co.*, 28 N.E. 266 (Mass. 1891).
10. *Restatement (Second) of Torts*, Section 892A (2)(a)(1977).
11. *Id.* at 892(a), Comment b.
12. President's Commission for the Study of Ethical Problems in Medicine and Biomedical and Behavioral Research. *Making Health Care Decisions: The Ethical and Legal Implications of Informed Consent in the Patient-Practitioner Relationship.* Washington, D.C.: U.S. Government Printing Office, 1982, 169–175; *Deciding to Forego Life-Sustaining Treatment.* Washington, D.C.: U.S. Government Printing Office, 1983, 119–126.

13. Alan Meisel. *The Right to Die.* Volume I. 2nd Edition. New York: John Wiley & Sons, 1995, 225 (with 1999 cumulative supplement).

14. *Id.* at 98–99.

15. *Restatement (Second) of Torts,* Section 892B(3)(1977).

16. Theodore LeBlang, W. Eugene Basanta, and Robert Kane. *The Law of Medical Practice in Illinois.* Volume I. 2nd Edition. St. Paul, Minn.: West Group, 1996, 778 (with regular updates) (citation omitted).

17. See, for example, Melina Gattellari, Philip Botow, and Martin Tattersal, "Informed Consent: What Did The Doctor Say?" 353(9165) *Lancet* (May 1999), 1713 (correspondence section).

18. LeBlang, Basanta, and Kane, *supra* note 16, at 777.

19. See, for example, *Tobias v. Winkler,* 509 N.E.2d 1050 (1987), *appeal denied,* 517 N.E.2d 1096 (1987); *Kus v. Sherman Hospital,* 644 N.E.2d 1214, *appeal denied,* 652 N.E.2d 343 (1995).

20. Meisel, *supra* note 13, at 95–96.

21. *Id.* at 107–108.

22. 464 F.2d 772 (Washington D.C. 1972).

23. *Id.* at 789.

24. Robert Miller. *Problems in Health Care Law.* 7th Edition. Gaithersburg, Md.: Aspen Publishers, 1996, 380 (citations omitted).

25. *Id.*

26. Meisel, *supra* note 13, at 103–104.

27. *Id.*

28. *Id.* at 108–109.

29. William Roach and the Aspen Health Law and Compliance Center. *Medical Records and the Law.* 3rd Edition. Gaithersburg, Md.: Aspen Publishers, 1998, 81–82.

30. Karla Kinderman. *Medicolegal Forms with Legal Analysis: Documenting Issues in the Patient-Physician Relationship.* Chicago, Ill.: American Medical Association, 1999, 111.

31. Miller, *supra* note 24, at 386–387.

32. Roach and the Aspen Center, *supra* note 29, at 78–81.

33. Even so, the nurse acting in this capacity must do so consistent with established policies. Roach and the Aspen Center, *supra* note 29, 62–86.

34. LeBlang, Basanta, and Kane, *supra* note 16, at 777.

35. See, generally, Meisel, *supra* note 13.

36. George J. Annas. *The Rights of Patients.* 2nd Edition. Totowa, N.J.: Humana Press, 1992, 98.

37. *Id.*

38. *Id.*

39. Meisel, *supra* note 13, at 149–150.

40. *Id.* at 151, *citing St. Mary's Hospital v. Ramsey,* 465 So. 2d 666 (Florida App. 1985) (refusal of a blood transfusion regardless whether the decision is based on fear of an adverse reaction, religion, hesitation to undergo the process, or cost); see also *Normal Hospital v. Munoz,* 564 N.E.2d 1017 (1991).

41. 760 S.W.2d 408 (Mo. 1988).

42. 110 S. Ct. 2841 (1990).

43. Annas, *supra* note 36, at 96.

44. Kinderman, *supra* note 30, at 33 (sample form).

45. Meisel, *supra* note 13, Volume 2, at 8–11.

46. *Id.* at 5.

47. *Id.* at 6–7.

48. Meisel, *supra* note 13, Volume 2, at 8–10.

49. Meisel, *supra* note 13, Volume 2, at 94–101.

50. *Id.* at 120.

51. *Id.* at 211–213.

52. Linda Emanuel, Michael Barry, John Stoeckle, Lucy Ettelson, and Ezekiel Emanuel, "Advance Directives for Medical Care—A Case for Greater Use," *New England Journal of Medicine* (March 28, 1991), 889. See also Kinderman, *supra* note 30, at 195–203.

53. Henry Campbell Black. *Black's Law Dictionary.* 7th Edition. St. Paul, Minn.: West Group, 1999, 1241.

54. *Id.* See 755 ILCS 40/1 *et seq.* (1998) (Health Care Surrogate Act). Other states that have similar statutes include Colorado, South Carolina, and West Virginia. Meisel, *supra* note 13, Volume 2, at 267.

55. See, for example, 755 ICLS 5/11a–17 (1991) (Illinois Guardians for Disabled Adults Act).

56. Annina M. Mitchell, "Involuntary Guardianship for Incompetents: A Strategy for Legal Services Advocates," 12 *Clearinghouse Review* 451, 460 (1978).

57. Henry Campbell Black. *Black's Law Dictionary.* 7th Edition. St. Paul, Minn.: West Group, 1999, 713.

58. See, generally, Meisel, *supra* note 13, Volume 1, 454–457.

59. Pub. L. No. 101-508 Sections 4206–4207; 4751–4752; Omnibus Budget Reconciliation Act of 1990, 42 U.S.C. Section 1395cc(f)(1) and 43 U.S.C. Section 1396a(a) (Supp. 1991).

60. *Id.*

61. *Id.* at Section 4206(a)(2), 42 U.S.C. Section 1395cc (f)(2) (A)–(E); Section 4751(a)(2), 43 U.S.C. 1396 a(w)(2) (A)–(E).

62. *Id.* at Section 4206 (3); Section 4751 (4).

63. Final Rule, 60 Fed. Reg. 33,262 (June 27, 1998).

64. *Id.* at 8196–8198.

65. *Id.* at 4206(c); 4751(a)(2); 42 U.S.C. Section 1396a(w)(3).

66. American Nurses Association. *Position Statement on Nursing and the Patient Self-Determination Act.* Washington, D.C.: Author, November 18, 1991.

67. 355 A.2d 647, *cert. denied sub nom. Garger v. New Jersey,* 429 U.S. 922 (1976), *modifying and remanding,* 348 A.2d 801 (1975).

68. *Id.* at 672.

69. Meisel, *supra* note 13, Vol. 1, 283–337.

70. American Nurses Association. *Mechanisms Through Which State Nurses Associations Consider Ethical and Human Rights Issues.* Washington, D.C.: Author, 1994; see also Margo Zink and Linda Titus, "Nursing Ethics Committees: Do We Need Them?" in *Current Issues in Nursing.* Joanne Comi McCloskey and Helen Kennedy Grace, Editors. 5th Edition. St. Louis, Mo.: Mosby, 1997, 640–646.

71. LeBlang, Basanta, and Kane, *supra* note 16, Volume 2, at 617.

72. *Id.*

73. *Id.* at 620.

74. *Uniform Laws Annotated, Master Edition.* Volume 8A, 63 (1993 & 1994 supplement).

75. LeBlang, Basanta, and Kane, *supra* note 16, Volume 2, at 620.

76. Pub. L. No. 98-507, 42 U.S.C. Section 273 *et seq.* (1984).

77. LeBlang, Basanta, and Kane, *supra* note 16, Volume 2, at 628–629.

78. *Id. citing* 62 Fed. Reg. 33,856 (June 22, 1998).

79. *Id.*

80. *Id. citing* "HHS Issues Rule to Spur Organ Donation," *Modern Healthcare* (June 22, 1998), 16.

81. LeBlang, Basanta, and Kane, *supra* note 16, Volume 2, at 635.

82. 61 Fed. Reg. 49,920 (September 23, 1996).

83. 61 Fed. Reg. 49,922 (September 23, 1996).

84. Mary A. Belgen and Toni Tripp-Reimer, "Nursing Theory, Nursing Research, and Nursing Practice: Connected or Separate?" in *Current Issues in Nursing.* Joanne Comi McCloskey and Helen Kennedy Grace, Editors. 5th Edition. St. Louis, Mo.: Mosby, 1997, 68.

85. LeBlang, Basanta, and Kane, *supra* note 16, Volume 2, at 650.

86. *Id.* at 651.

87. *Trials of War Criminals Before the Nuremberg Military Tribunals Under Control Council Law No. 10* (1949).

88. Miller, *supra* note 24, at 388.

89. *Id.*

90. *Id.*

91. *Id.* at 389.

92. LeBlang, Basanta, and Kane, *supra* note 16, Volume 2, at 661.

93. *Id.*

94. See, as examples, "Federal Regulators Impose Research Restrictions," 3(6) *UIC Alumni Magazine* (1999), 7; Jonathan Moreno, Arthur Caplan, Paul Wolpe, and the Members of the Project on Informed Consent, Human Research Ethics Group, "Updating Protections for Human Subjects Involved in Research," 280(22) *JAMA* (1998), 1951–1958; Daniel Greenberg, "When Institutional Review Boards Fail the System," 353 (9166) *Lancet* (1999), 1773.

95. See generally references in footnote 94; LeBlang, Basanta, and Kane, *supra* note 16, Volume 2, at 660–661.

96. 45 C.F.R. Section 46.116(a) (1985).

97. *Id.*

98. 45 C.F.R. Section 46.117(b) (1985); LeBlang, Basanta, and Kane, *supra* note 16, Volume 2, at 660.

99. 45 C.F.R. Section 46.404 (1985).

100. 45 C.F.R. Section 46.306 (1985).

101. 45 C.F.R. Section 46.305 (1985).

102. See, for example, Joan Stephenson, "Probing Informed Consent in Schizophrenia Research," 281(24) *JAMA* (1999), 2273–2274.

103. Mark Scherzer, "Insurance," in *AIDS Law Today: A New Guide for the Public.* Harlon L. Dalton, Scott Burris, Judith Miller, and the Yale AIDS Project, Editors. New Haven, Ct.: Yale University Press, 1993.

104. 720 ICLS 5/12-18(e) (1991) (Illinois). See also David McColgin and Elizabeth Hey, "Criminal Law," in *AIDS and the Law.* 3rd Edition. New York: John Wiley & Sons, 1997, 259–345 (with regular updates).

105. Robert Levy and Lenard Rubenstein. *The Rights of People with Mental Disabilities.* Carbondale, Ill.: Southern Illinois University Press, 1996, 102–151.

106. 462 F. Supp. 1131 (N.J. 1978); 476 F. Supp. 1294 (D. N.J. 1979).

107. 478 F. Supp. 1342 (D. Mass. 1979); 634 F. 2d 650 (1st Cir. 1980).

108. 422 U.S. 563 (1975).

109. 405 ICLS 5/2-110 (1979); Levy and Rubenstein, *supra* note 105, at 137–139.

110. Miller, *supra* note 24, at 406.

111. *Id.*

112. Black, *supra* note 57, at 993.

113. *State v. Bass,* 120 S.E.2d 580 (1961).

114. Wayne R. LaFave and Austin W. Scott, Jr. *Criminal Law.* 2nd Edition. St. Paul, Minn.: West Group, 1986, 650 (with 1999 update).

115. *Id.*

116. For an interesting case holding that the sale of chemicals in a man's blood without his knowledge or consent was permissible because a patient does not own his tissue, see *Moore v. Regents of the University of California,* 793 P.2d 479 (Cal. 1990). The court did hold that a clinician must inform a patient that his tissue could be used for research, but opined that to give a patient a property right to his tissue would "destroy the economic incentive to conduct important medical research." *Id.* at 495.

117. T. G. Peters, "Life or Death: The Issue of Payment in Cadaveric Organ Donation," 265 *JAMA* (March 13, 1991), 1302–1305.

118. See, for example, Dorothy Neldin and Lori Andrews, "Homo Economicus: The Commercialization of Body Tissue in the Age of Biotechnology," 28(5) *Hastings Center Report* (1998), 30–39.

119. Nancy J. Brent, "Legal Issues in Research: Informed Consent," 22(3) *Journal of Neuroscience Nursing* (June 1990), 190.

120. *Id.*

121. LeBlang, Basanta, and Kane, *supra* note 16, Volume 2, at 664, *citing* 61 Fed. Reg. 61,531 (October 2, 1996).

122. *Id.*

123. *Id., citing* 61 Fed. Reg. 51,498 (October 2, 1996).

124. *Id.* (citations omitted).

Issues in Death and Dying

KEY PRINCIPLES

- Life-Sustaining Procedures/Death-Delaying Procedures
- Suicide
- Assisted Suicide
- Euthanasia/Mercy Killing
- Death
- Decision-making Standards for Withdrawing or Withholding Treatment
- Lack of Decision-making Capacity

In Chapter 12, the concepts of informed consent and refusal of treatment were analyzed. Refusal of treatment may ultimately result in an individual's death, and the right to refuse treatment clearly includes the "right to die." The right to refuse life-sustaining treatment is not a new concept; rather, it is a by-product of the law of informed decision making limited by the restrictions of the criminal law.[1]

Although refusal of treatment that leads to one's death is not a novel concept, its acceptance has been fraught with controversy. The controversy has centered on the legal, ethical, and moral issues involved in the refusal of treatment; types of treatment refused; whether the patient refusing treatment was "terminally ill"; whether the patient possessed decision-making capacity; and, of course, health care professionals' obligations to provide treatment and concomitant liability issues if treatment was withheld or withdrawn.

Although all of the above factors are important, one author has identified the central problems in refusing treatment as the legitimacy of *forgoing* or *administering* treatment and the procedures used for those decisions.[2]

The previous chapter focused on the procedures for making treatment decisions. This chapter will center on the right to refuse life-sustaining treatment, including its legal development, specific cases involving that right, and special considerations that arise when an individual exercises his or her right to die.

HISTORICAL DEVELOPMENT OF THE RIGHT TO DIE

Adults

The right to refuse life-sustaining treatment is a relatively new right. Life-sustaining (or death-delaying) treatments or procedures sustain, restore, or supplant a necessary function of an individual patient's life.[3] They primarily serve to prolong the moment of death; if they were not utilized, death would be imminent.[4] The determination concerning the procedures' or treatments' effect on the life of the patient is certified by the attending and consulting physician in the patient's medical record. Examples of life-sustaining treatment may include ventilator support, artificial nutrition and hydration, hemodialysis, surgery, the administration of medications, cardiopulmonary resuscitation, and blood transfusions.

The right to refuse life-sustaining treatment is a relatively new right.

The first reported case concerning this issue, *In re Quinlan,* was decided in 1976. The right has been shaped, reshaped, expanded, and clarified since the *Quinlan* decision. Various individuals have refused life-sustaining treatment, including patients, family members, guardians, and other substitute/proxy decision makers. Moreover, refusal has found roots in many legal theories.

Many of the early cases, including *Quinlan,* were based on a constitutional right of personal privacy; that is, the ability to have control over what is done with one's body. The reader will recall that this rationale also formed the basis for reproductive rights discussed in Chapter 11. It was not until the U.S. Supreme Court decision in *Cruzan v. Director* in 1990, however, that the right was firmly couched in constitutional language.

It was not until the U.S. Supreme Court decision in Cruzan v. Director in 1990, however, that the right [to refuse treatment] was firmly couched in constitutional language.

A second legal theory supporting the right to refuse life-sustaining treatment was a common-law one. Its character was phrased in many ways, including the right to be free from unwanted bodily intrusions; the right to self-determination; and the right of bodily integrity.[5] Remedies for individuals who were not granted this right included suing for assault and battery, lack of in-

formed consent/refusal, and, of course, the intentional tort of invasion of privacy.

Other support for the right to die utilized state or federal legislation and concomitant regulations. For example, living wills were often successfully utilized in the early cases to support an individual's right to refuse life-sustaining treatment. However, some were not easily resolved because of the presence of advance directive legislation. For example, in one Illinois case, *In re Estate of (Dorothy) Longeway,*[6] the Illinois Living Will Act's definition of terminal illness was used to determine if artificial food and fluid could be removed at the request of the guardian (the patient's daughter). Although Ms. Longeway had never executed a living will, the Illinois Supreme Court held that the guardian had a right to refuse the treatment, but only if the patient's condition met the Living Will Act's definition of terminal illness as well as other conditions set forth by the court.

Sustaining challenges by citing other state or federal legislation or policies and regulations of the particular health care facility was another viable legal theory. For example, in *In re (Beverly) Requena*[7] and *Elbaum v. Grace Plaza of Great Neck,*[8] the respective institutional policies of not honoring a patient's refusal of life-sustaining treatment had to yield to the exercise of the rights of these two patients. In *Requena,* the institution did not inform the patient of the policy until after she had been hospitalized there for 15 months, and her deteriorating condition due to Lou Gehrig's disease (amyotrophic lateral sclerosis) resulted in her request not to institute administration of artificial food and fluid. Likewise, in *Elbaum* the nursing home failed to inform the family that it would not honor a refusal of artificial feedings and antibiotic therapy until after it was requested by the family (when subarachnoid bleeding resulted in Mrs. Elbaum's persistent vegetative state with no hope of recovery).

Last, it is important to note that another constitutional argument has been raised to support a right to refuse life-sustaining treatment—freedom of religion guaranteed by the First Amendment. Many of these cases were brought by Jehovah's Witnesses in an attempt to support their religious belief against blood transfusions. Generally the early cases mandated that the transfusions be given, especially if they were seen as life-saving and the patient was not terminally ill. That trend changed, however.

The change may be due in part to medical treatment advances that eliminate the need to seek court intervention. The use of autotransfusion (when possible) and the development of synthetic blood substitutes has begun to change the need for transfusing the blood of another. For example, perfluorocarbons (Fluosol-DA) and Perfluoro-cytlbromide (PFOB) showed promise when first used.[9] In 1984, Fluosol-DA was used in place of blood for a Jehovah's Witness who needed surgery for a trochanteric pressure sore.[10] Used not as a total blood replacement but rather as a transporter of oxygen and carbon dioxide, it allowed the surgery and outcome to be successful.[11] Recent developments include the use of hemoglobin solutions to create an artificial blood substitute. In fact, some published reports specify that a blood substitute may be near completion.[12]

In addition, the change may also have been due to heightened emphasis on sustaining a treatment decision based on an individual's religious beliefs. For example, in *In re Osborne,*[13] the court denied a hospital's motion for a court order to override a 34-year-old competent patient's refusal of a blood transfusion for internal bleeding. The court held that the patient's religious beliefs as a Jehovah's Witness and his interest in autonomy prevailed over any interest in preserving life and its sanctity.

Minors

Although reported cases testing the right of parents to make treatment decisions did not appear until the late 1800s,[14] parents since then have been testing and clarifying their rights in this regard. Clearly the legal issues involved in withdrawing and refusing life-sustaining treatment for a minor are somewhat more complex than those raised with adult individuals. The difficulty most probably stems from the fact that a minor, particularly if newborn or very young, has never possessed decision-making capacity. As a result, it is impossible to determine what the minor would want in a particular situation.

Decision making for such a minor is arguably no different than for an adult who has *never* possessed decision-making abilities (due to severe brain injury or retardation since birth, for example). Even so, the emotional issues involved in making treatment decisions for minors have raised additional legal concerns for health care providers. For example, specific legal protections are afforded

neonates born with congenital anomalies when refusing or withholding treatment is contemplated. This situation, as well as others affecting treatment decisions for minors, will be discussed in the Special Considerations section.

. . . the emotional issues involved in making treatment decisions for minors have raised additional legal concerns for health care providers.

Despite some of the unique issues raised in refusing or withholding life-sustaining treatment for minors, the difficulties in determining what to do in a particular treatment situation are conceptually similar to those for adults.[15] Essentially, the courts and federal regulatory laws concerning treatment and minors have taken a prognostic approach.[16] That is, if treatment is futile, it is not ordered. However, it should be noted that the cases cannot be cited for the proposition that only where treatment is futile will the courts uphold a refusal. Rather, as one author has suggested, this result is more reasonably related to the fact that the cases brought before the courts simply involve situations in which the minor is terminally ill.[17]

The reader will remember from Chapter 12 that parents are the natural guardians and provide informed consent or refusal of treatment for the child. As a result, most often court cases concerning treatment decisions for minors involve surrogate/proxy decision making. The parents of minors, exercising their constitutional rights to privacy in family affairs,[18] religious freedom under the First Amendment,[19] and state statutes applicable to treatment decisions and children (e.g., Rhode Island, Arizona, and Minnesota), have tested these rights in state and federal courts, especially as they relate to life-sustaining treatments. See Table 13–2 for a summarization of some of these cases.

Despite the ability of the parents to make treatment decisions, the right is not absolute. Rather, it has been balanced with various countervailing state interests. The four state interests used by a court in evaluating a parent's right (or for that matter, any person's right) to refuse treatment include the preservation of life, prevention of suicide, protection of innocent third parties, and protection of the ethical integrity of health care professionals.[20] Moreover, parents exercising a treatment decision for a minor must also do so utilizing certain standards. Those standards include the best interest or substituted judgment standards.[21] The best interest (of the patient) standard has been also described as the "objective approach" to decision making concerning treatment or nontreatment choices, because an "objective" evaluation as to what is "best" for the patient is made. In contrast, the substituted judgment standard has been looked at as a "subjective approach," meaning that a choice is based upon what the patient or minor would have wanted if he or she could make the choice personally. Which guideline is used for a minor will depend upon the minor's age. For example, a young infant (seen as incompetent by the law) would never have explained his or her wishes to the parents. As a result, the best interest standard might be the most appropriate one to use. In contrast, an older minor who expressed treatment preferences to the parents may be better served by the use of the substituted judgment test.[22]

These tests are often supplemented with others: whether the regimen in question (1) is a burden or a benefit to the patient; (2) will cause indignity, will relieve suffering, is intrusive, or has additional material risks; and (3) will affect the patient's quality of life.[23]

Some cases involving minors also tested refusal of treatment by the minor himself or herself rather than the parents. These cases arose under varied circumstances. For example, in one 1941 case,[24] a 15-year-old won the ability to consent to a donation of skin to another who needed it for a skin graft operation. Other cases have involved situations in which, for example, the minor's wishes were different from those of the parents. At times the cases involved life-sustaining treatment, while in others the treatment at issue was not strictly life sustaining.

Several Key Cases involve the refusal of treatment for minors. In addition, in the Special Considerations section, additional cases concerning refusal of treatment for minors will be discussed in which allegations of child abuse or neglect (or other charges) are brought against the parents. A brief analysis of the law in relation to treatment decisions for newborns born with disabilities will also be highlighted. These types of cases raise unique and difficult legal issues.

KEY CASES INVOLVING ADULTS

Although all of the court cases in which individuals asserted their right to refuse treatment, either in their own behalf or through another, are important, two cases will be presented as key ones. The *Quinlan* and *Cruzan* cases are, literally, landmark decisions in relation to refusing life-sustaining treatment. *Quinlan* was the first to raise the country's awareness of the issue and initiated a plethora of subsequent cases. *Cruzan* was the first case decided by the U.S. Supreme Court concerning the right to die and under what circumstances this choice would be honored. In both cases, the individuals involved—Karen Quinlan and Nancy Cruzan—had lost their decision-making ability. Guardians—family members in both instances—exercised the right on behalf of their respective daughters. (See Key Case 13–1.)

Karen Quinlan's father did exercise his power as guardian and had his daughter removed from ventilator support. She continued to breathe on her own and was transferred to Morris View Nursing Home in New Jersey. The home had no respirator, so placing her back on respiratory support was not an issue. Its ethics committee (functioning in one author's viewpoint as a *true* ethics panel) confirmed the decision, in accordance with the court ruling, that she would not be resuscitated.[29]

Karen Quinlan survived for 10 years, sustained by nasogastric feedings and antibiotics. She died at the age of 31 from acute respiratory failure following pneumonia.[30]

It was not until 14 years after the *Quinlan* case was decided that the U.S. Supreme Court rendered its opinion in the *Cruzan* case. During that interim, many courts were confronting the right to refuse life-sustaining treatment with varying outcomes. Table 13–1 summarizes some of those court decisions. (See Key Case 13–2, p. 245.)

Ironically, after the Supreme Court decision, another hearing to present "new evidence" of Nancy Cruzan's treatment wishes was held before the same trial (probate) court that originally heard her case.[34] The state of Missouri did not contest the petition, and the court granted the coguardians' request to withdraw the feeding tube. Nancy Cruzan died on December 26, 1990, 11 days after the court granted permission to withdraw the gastrostomy tube.[35]

Text continued on page 246

KEY CASE 13–1   In re Karen Quinlan (1976)[25]

A 21-year-old patient on ventilator after respiratory arrests

A diagnosis of persistent vegetative state (PVS) is made

Father petitions court to be appointed guardian to give permission to remove daughter from ventilator

Court denies father's petition for guardianship and denies power to remove Karen from ventilator

Supreme Court of New Jersey grants father's requests

FACTS: Karen Quinlan, a 21-year-old, suffered two respiratory arrests at a party after reportedly ingesting drugs and alcohol. She was given mouth-to-mouth resuscitation by friends and was taken to a New Jersey hospital. She arrived unresponsive and unconscious and was placed on a respirator and a nasogastric feeding tube was inserted. After receiving treatment and continued monitoring, it was determined that she was in a PVS and would not be able to survive without the respirator. After a careful and difficult period of decision making, the family believed it best that Karen be removed from the respirator. Her physicians, however, refused to do so, stating that the removal would not conform to medical standards, practices, and traditions, especially because Karen was not brain dead and because the ventilator was not seen as "extraordinary," but rather "ordinary," treatment. The father then filed a petition in court asking that he be appointed the guardian of his daughter and that he be given the express power to provide consent to have Karen removed from the ventilator.

INITIAL COURT DECISION: The Chancery judge denied the father's petition to be appointed as a personal guardian for Karen. Rather, a *guardian ad litem* was appointed for Karen and the father was granted guardianship over her financial affairs. Furthermore, the power to remove Karen from the respirator was also denied. Mr. Quinlan appealed the decision to the Appeals Court and also asked for specific injunctive and declaratory relief.

APPELLATE COURT DECISION: The Appeals Court granted certification for the case to go directly to the New Jersey Supreme Court and did not hear the case.

NEW JERSEY SUPREME COURT DECISION: At this stage in the proceedings, a number of other parties had been added to the case because of the far-reaching impact the decision would have. The physicians, the hospital, and the prosecutor of the county where Karen lived were enjoined (through an injunction) from interfering with carrying out any court decision to allow removal if it was granted and from prosecuting anyone for a violation of the criminal laws, respectively. In addition, the attorney general of New Jersey was joined in the case because of his obligation to represent the state in its interest in the preservation of life.

The New Jersey Supreme Court granted Joseph Quinlan's requests. Specifically, it held that (1) Mr. Quinlan would be appointed the personal and estate guardian of his daughter; (2) full power was granted Mr. Quinlan to make treatment decisions; (3) if the physicians agree that no hope of recovery exists for Karen, with the concurrence of the guardian and the family, she could be removed from the respirator; (4) an "ethics committee" or similar institutional body should affirm the decision to remove the ventilator; and (5) if all of the guidelines were met, no civil or criminal liability would be possible against the hospital, guardian, or physicians. The court also

Key case continued on following page

KEY CASE 13-1	In re Karen Quinlan (1976)[25] *Continued*

held that its decision should not be interpreted as meaning that other treatment situations needed to obtain judicial review before implementing treatment choices.

ANALYSIS: The *Quinlan* court based its decision on the constitutional right to privacy, both federal and state, and cited many U.S. Supreme Court cases that supported that right. Furthermore, the court clearly upheld the power of a guardian to exercise that right on behalf of a ward. Also far-reaching was the court's analysis of the ventilator as "extraordinary" treatment *in this situation;* that is, it was not curative or restorative but served only to forcibly "sustain" cardiorespiratory functions of an "irreversibly doomed patient." This ordinary/ extraordinary treatment distinction was used for subsequent cases for several years after *Quinlan,* albeit unsatisfactorily, especially in view of the advancement of medical technology that has made the "extraordinary" ordinary. Because the distinction has been described as hazy (the *Quinlan* court itself used this term), it is rarely used today. When it is, it is often called the benefit/burden approach. The benefit/burden approach, however, has been supplemented by the best interest test and others.[26]

The *Quinlan* court also illustrated the use of the balancing test required when the interest of a state and an individual compete. Although the court clearly acknowledged New Jersey's interests in preserving life and ensuring that physicians practice medicine according to their best judgment without interference from others, the court held that those state interests did not outweigh Karen Quinlan's right to be free from unwanted treatment. The court's support of ethics committees also had far-reaching consequences. The input that was required by the court was more of a "prognosis" confirmation than anything else, for the committee was to evaluate if Karen Quinlan's diagnosed condition would ever reverse itself.[27] Even so, ethics committees slowly began to develop and have flourished since 1980.[28]

Last, the court's holding that no criminal or civil liability would result from the decision to remove Karen from the respirator was vitally important in giving some early guidance on culpability issues for health care facilities and practitioners. Despite this guidance, subsequent cases tested the liability waters in relation to such decisions.

TABLE 13-1

Selected Court Decisions after *Quinlan* and before *Cruzan* Concerning Right to Refuse Life-Sustaining Treatment

CASE NAME/YEAR/STATE	DIAGNOSIS	TREATMENT(S) AT ISSUE	GUARDIAN, FAMILY, OTHER	DECISION	STANDARD(S) USED	COMMENTS
Superintendent of Belchertown State School v. Saikewicz (1977) (Massachusetts)[1]	Leukemia	O (Chemotherapy)	GAL	Ct. upheld no treatment	C (Privacy) S	Ct. held state's interests must give way to privacy; patient 67-yr.-old profoundly retarded male; treatment futile
Tune v. Walter Reed Army Medical Hospital (1985) (District of Columbia)[2]	Malignancy of pericardium; question of lung tumor	V (Removal)	Pt.	Ct. upheld removal	Q	First Fed. Ct. ruling on patient's right in military hospital to refuse life-sustaining treatment
Matter of Conroy (1985) (New Jersey)[3]	Arteriosclerotic heart disease; hypertension; diabetes; gangrenous leg	ANTH (Nasogastric tube)	GF (Nephew) and GAL appointed by court	Ct. upheld right to remove life-sustaining treatment from nursing home residents expected to die within 1 yr. even with treatment, using 3 tests (1) subjective; (2) limited objective; (3) pure-objective. Ct. also set up specific court procedures and documentation requirements before removing/withholding treatment	B & B (self-determination) CL B S	84-year-old nursing home resident; Ms. Conroy died during court battle; decision narrow in that only applied to nursing home residents; court supported use of living wills as a way for patient to express treatment wishes; feeding tube similar to other artificial sustaining measures

Table continued on following page

TABLE 13–1

Selected Court Decisions after *Quinlan* and before *Cruzan* Concerning Right to Refuse Life-Sustaining Treatment *Continued*

CASE NAME/YEAR/STATE	DIAGNOSIS	TREATMENT(S) AT ISSUE	GUARDIAN, FAMILY, OTHER	DECISION	STANDARD(S) USED	COMMENTS
Brophy v. New England Sinai Hospital (1986) (Massachusetts)[4]	Brain aneurysm; PVS	ANTH (Gastrostomy tube)	GF (wife)	Ct. upheld removal of G-tube	C (Privacy) S CL (Privacy)	Ct. held state's interests must give way to privacy rights even though pt. not terminally ill; no legal distinction between withholding/ withdrawing treatment; unwanted, painless feeding tube can be "intrusive" and "extraordinary"
Delio v. Westchester County Medical Center (1987) (New York)[5]	PVS after cardiac arrest	ANTH (Gastrostomy and jejunostomy tube)	CF (wife) and GAL appointed by court	Ct. upheld removal	CL (Self-determination)	First NY case to support withdrawal, especially with young (33), nonterminal patient; ct. held no legal distinction between withholding and withdrawing treatment
Matter of Farrell (1987) (New Jersey)[6]	Amyotrophic lateral sclerosis (Lou Gehrig's disease)	V	GF (husband) and GAL appointed by court for children	Ct. upheld removal with guidelines: pt. is competent and two nonattending MDs confirm decision-making ability and that informed consent/ refusal has occurred	CL (Privacy) C (Privacy)	Ms. Farrell died during ct. battle; first case dealing with removal of treatment *at home*; gave support to family (not courts) to make decisions; reemphasized no civil or criminal liability for "good faith actions" in removing/withdrawing treatment; two other cases, *In re Jones* and *In re Peter,* also decided on same day with essentially same outcomes

Case	Condition	Treatment	Decision-maker	Holding	Basis	Comments
Rasmussen v. Fleming (1987) (Arizona)[7]	Progressive neurological disorder (Multiple Sclerosis?); PVS or chronic vegetative state (CVS)	Do-not-resuscitate and do-not-hospitalize (DNR and DNH orders)	G and GAL approved by court	Ct. upheld ability of guardian to refuse treatment	SJ B CL (Bodily Integrity) C Q B & B	Ms. Rasmussen died during court battle; initial concern about nasogastric tube mooted when patient able to swallow, so case went forward on other medical treatment issues; one of first court decisions to hold no material difference between irreversible coma and PVS; ct. also emphasized when agreement exists as to course of treatment, no need for court intervention
Gray v. Romeo (1988) (Federal District Court, Rhode Island)[8]	Cerebral hemorrhage; PVS	ANTH (Gastrostomy tube) and further life support	G (Husband) and GAL appointed by court	Ct. upheld right of guardian to refuse treatment	C (Privacy) SJ	First federal decision (1) dealing with refusal of life-sustaining treatment (nonmilitary hospital); (2) based on federal constitutional right to privacy; (3) brought under Section 1983 because hospital refused to honor request and was state facility; (4) held state's interests must give way to individual choice, especially when family agrees

Table continued on following page

TABLE 13-1

Selected Court Decisions after *Quinlan* and before *Cruzan* Concerning Right to Refuse Life-Sustaining Treatment *Continued*

V = Ventilator
ANTH = Artificial nutrition, hydration
M = Medication
CPR = Cardiopulmonary resuscitation
O = Other
CF = Family member
C = Conservator
PT = Patient with diminished capacity
GAL = *Guardian ad litem*
G = Guardian
GF = Guardian/family member
LW = Living will
DPAHC = Durable Power of Attorney for Health Care
S = Statute
CL = Common law
SJ = Substituted judgment
B&B = Benefits/burden
Q = Quality of life
B = Best interest
C = Constitutional basis
IS = Interpretation of statute

[1]370 N.E.2d 417 (Mass. 1977)
[2]602 F. Supp. 1452 (D.D.C. 1985)
[3]457 A.2d 1232 (N.J. Super. Ch. 1983), *rev'd*, 464 A.2d 303 (N.J. Sup. A.D. 1983), *cert. granted*, 470 A.2d 418 (N.J. 1983), *rev'd*, 486 A.2d 1209 (N.J. 1985)
[4]497 N.E.2d 626 (Mass. 1986)
[5]510 N.Y.S.2d 415 (N.J. Sup. 1986), *rev'd*, 516 N.Y.S.2d 677 (N.Y. A.D. 2 Dept. 1987)
[6]529 A.2d 404 (N.J. 1987), *aff'g* 514 A.2d 1342 (N.J. Super. Ct. Ch. Div. 1986)
[7]741 P.2d 674 (Ariz. 1987)
[8]697 F. Supp. 580 (D.R.I. 1988), 709 F. Supp. 325 (1989)

| **KEY CASE 13-2** | Cruzan v. Director, Missouri Department of Health (1990)[31] |

Nancy Cruzan suffers cardiopulmonary arrest after a car accident

Cardiopulmonary functions restored, but coma occurs

Diagnosis made of persistent vegetative state

Gastrostomy tube inserted

Parents ask that food and fluid via tube be terminated, but hospital refuses

Parents, as coguardians, file a petition asking for authority to remove gastrostomy tube

Trial court grants permission to coguardians to remove gastrostomy tube

Decision is appealed to Missouri Supreme Court

Missouri Supreme Court reverses trial court decision

The Cruzans appeal the decision to the United States Supreme Court

FACTS: On January 11, 1983, Nancy Cruzan apparently lost control of her car. It overturned, and she was thrown into a ditch. When the paramedics arrived, she had no heart beat and was not breathing. Those functions were restored at the accident scene, and she was taken to the hospital in an unconscious state. The physicians at the hospital estimated she had not had cardiopulmonary functions for at least 12 to 14 minutes and diagnosed "probable cerebral contusions" compounded by the anoxia. Nancy remained in a coma for 3 weeks, when her condition was diagnosed as persistent vegetative state. Even though she could take some food and fluid orally, consent was given by her then-husband to implant a gastrostomy tube. When her condition did not improve and it became clear that it would never do so, Nancy's parents asked the hospital to terminate the artificial food and hydration. There was no doubt that the withdrawal of food and fluid would result in her death. The hospital refused to do so without a court order. The parents, appointed coguardians of their daughter in 1984, filed a petition in 1988 asking for the power to authorize the removal of the feeding and hydration tube.

TRIAL COURT DECISION: The state court granted the parents as coguardians the power to provide consent to withdraw the gastrostomy tube. It based its decision on the Missouri and federal Constitutions' protection of the right to refuse "death-delaying procedures." In addition, the court held that Nancy Cruzan had expressed her wishes not to be kept alive unless she could "live at least halfway normally." The conversation with a friend suggested to the court that her present condition was one in which Nancy herself would not want artificial feedings and hydration to continue.

The decision was appealed to the Missouri Supreme Court by the state and the *guardian ad litem.*

MISSOURI SUPREME COURT DECISION: In reversing the trial court, the Supreme Court of Missouri (1) recognized the right to refuse treatment that was supported by the common-law doctrine of informed consent, but was not certain that it applied in this case because of Ms. Cruzan's inability to speak for herself; (2) declined to read a broad right of privacy to refuse treatment in all circumstances into either the Missouri or federal Constitution; (3) read the Missouri Living Will statute as favoring the preservation of life, and therefore Ms. Cruzan's statement concerning her life and death were "unreliable" for determining her intent to have medical treatment withdrawn; (4) held that the coguardians could not exercise substituted judgment on behalf of their daughter because no "clear and convincing" evidence existed nor had a living will been executed by Nancy; and (5) believed that issues bearing on life and death are better addressed by a legislative body than by the courts. The Cruzans appealed the decision to the U.S. Supreme Court, which granted *certiorari* to consider the issue whether Nancy Cruzan had a right under the federal Constitution to mandate removal of life-sustaining treatment "under these circumstances."

Key case continued on following page

KEY CASE 13–2	Cruzan v. Director, Missouri Department of Health (1990)[31] *Continued*

The U.S. Supreme Court affirms the Missouri Supreme Court decision

U.S. SUPREME COURT DECISION: The U.S. Supreme Court affirmed the Missouri Supreme Court's decision. It held that (1) Missouri's requirement of "clear and convincing evidence" was not forbidden under the federal Constitution; (2) a person has a *liberty* interest in refusing unwanted medical treatment, but that right must be balanced with the state's interest in preserving life, especially when a surrogate decision maker is giving permission to withdraw food and fluid that will result in the person's death; (3) no clear and convincing evidence existed concerning Ms. Cruzan's wishes to withdraw food and fluid; and (4) because there was no such evidence, the state was not required to honor the wishes of the parents.

ANALYSIS: The *Cruzan* decision has been scrutinized carefully since its publication.[32] Although other cases may test the guidelines set forth in *Cruzan,* some consensus exists as to what guidelines were established. They are: (1) because the right to refuse treatment for a competent adult was supported by a "liberty" interest rather than a right of "privacy," a state must show only a rationally related interest (e.g., preservation of or protection of life) to place restrictions on the right; (2) the "right to die" is not a fundamental right but an "interest"; (3) states would most probably have to abide by a health care surrogate's decision to terminate/withdraw treatment for another when that person expressed that in an advance directive; (4) a feeding tube is one of many life-sustaining treatments that an individual may refuse; and (5) those who lack decision-making capacity and who have not expressed wishes concerning life-sustaining treatment with the clarity required by a state need protection from potential abuse and the "loss of life involuntarily" when others assert that right on their behalf.[33]

Two Post-*Cruzan* Cases

Two interesting post-*Cruzan* cases bear mentioning because both of them raised additional issues the *Cruzan* court had only set the stage for.

In the case *In the Matter of Sue Ann Lawrance,*[36] the Indiana Supreme Court upheld the right of Ms. Lawrance's parents to consent to the removal of artificial food and fluid from their 42-year-old daughter, who had been injured in an accident at the age of 9 years that left her mentally retarded. A second injury resulted in another craniotomy, a diagnosis of persistent vegetative state, and no hope of recovery. Despite Sue Ann Lawrance's death due to natural causes during the appeal of the case to the Indiana Supreme Court, both sides desired to have a ruling on the issues presented by her situation.

In upholding the parents' treatment decision to withdraw food and fluid, the court cited Indiana's Health Care Consent Act (HCCA) that specifically spelled out the procedures for a competent patient or an incompetent patient's family member to follow. In addition, the court continued, the removal of food and fluid was permissible under the Act.[37]

The court also held that a court proceeding was not required for situations similar to this case in which the Indiana Health Care Consent Act's procedures were met; specifically, that the family was authorized and willing to make a treatment decision, and the family and physician concurred in the decision.

The *Lawrance* case is noteworthy for several reasons. To begin with, it was the first case to be decided after *Cruzan* concerning a person in a persistent vegetative condition and in a state with no prior case law on the right to die.[38] Yet, the Indiana court never mentioned the *Cruzan* decision in its opinion. Moreover, the case dealt with surrogate/proxy decision making allowed by a state statute rather than through the use of an advance directive. Also, contrary to the *Cruzan* Court's opinion, the *Lawrance* decision may well stand for the axiom that others can make such choices without meeting a "substituted judgment" rationale.[39] There is no doubt that Sue Ann Lawrance's parents had no other "good-faith" guidance for their decision but what might be called the "best interest" of their never-competent daughter.

It is also important to point out how hauntingly similar the *Lawrance* decision was to the *Quinlan* opinion: (1) both dealt with individuals in a persistent vegetative state; (2) neither New Jersey nor Indiana had any prior case law interpreting state law or statutes in relation to the removal or withdrawal of medical treatment; (3) both cases involved parents asserting rights on behalf of their daughter, albeit in different roles (guardian vs. surrogate decision makers by statute); (4) both courts resoundingly held that with consensus among those who are legally involved in the decision-making process, no resort to the courts is necessary; (5) each court ruled that ventilator support and artificial fluid and nutrition respectively were "medical treatments" that could be refused or withdrawn; and (6) both courts held that no liability would result for those involved in the decision and the carrying out of that decision if the respective guidelines set forth in the opinions were followed. Perhaps these similarities simply support the opinion that the *Lawrance* court reaffirmed most of the post-*Quinlan* decisions and that the *Cruzan* decision was a clear departure from earlier decisions.[40]

A second case, *In re Busalacchi*,[41] illustrates other potential ramifications of the *Cruzan* decision. Because *Cruzan* supports the ability of the respective states to set their own standards concerning the removal of death-delaying medical treatment, a "patchwork" effect may occur. Thus, one state may authorize those decisions in a manner quite different and perhaps less restrictive than a neighboring state.

In the *Busalacchi* case, also decided in Missouri, the father of Christine Busalacchi was appointed guardian of his daughter, who had suffered severe head injuries as the result of a car accident. A persistent vegetative state was diagnosed and a gastrostomy tube implanted. After it was clear that rehabilitation was not possible, a recommendation was made that Christine be placed in a skilled nursing facility. The father was unable to get her admitted to any in Missouri or California, and then began to look at other states, including Minnesota.

When admission to a Minnesota home seemed likely, the rehabilitation agency changed Christine's diagnosis to one less serious than persistent vegetative state and filed a petition for a temporary restraining order (TRO) and a permanent injunction prohibiting Mr. Busalacchi from removing Christine from the state, alleging that he was doing so to remove the gastrostomy tube. The trial court denied the state's motion for a permanent injunction and dissolved the temporary restraining order.

The decision was appealed to the Missouri Court of Appeals, which reversed the lower court decision and remanded the case to that court. The court opined that the issue to be decided was not whether the feeding tube should be removed, but rather whether the guardian was acting in the ward's best interest by removing her to another jurisdiction where allegedly the feeding tube could be removed more easily than in Missouri.[42] Furthermore, the court held that the state had the burden of proving that Christine Busalacchi's needs were being adequately met in Missouri. If the state met its burden, then the guardian must prove that a move to another state was in her best interests.

The decision of the Missouri Court of Appeals was appealed to the Missouri Supreme Court, then sent back to the lower court for additional information on Ms. Busalacchi's diagnosis of persistent vegetative state. The lower court, after reconsidering the evidence, upheld the decision to transfer, but that decision was also appealed by the state of Missouri. Several days later, the Supreme Court of Missouri dismissed the case on the motion of the state. In an interesting twist, a "right to life" advocate then filed a petition requesting a temporary restraining order, which was granted by a St. Louis court.[43]

Christine Busalacchi died on March 7, 1993, after her feeding tube was removed, almost 6 years after the accident that left her in a persistent vegetative state.[44]

These and other cases will continue to test the parameters of the *Cruzan* decision. What standard will be applied when others make removal/withholding decisions? Will an advance directive be required? If an advance directive is required in a particular state, will it suffice as "evidence" of an individual's specific treatment preferences? Will a surrogate/proxy decision-making statute withstand legal challenge?

Despite the less-than-clear parameters of *Cruzan*, it can be said with certainty that there is legal support for the right to die, although the nature of that right may be called by other names (e.g., right to refuse treatment). Even so, *Cruzan* appears to have raised more questions than it answered. The decision also seems to clearly underscore the fact that the law has not progressed as far as many would like to believe it has in resolving issues surrounding the withholding or withdrawing of medical treatment that results in death.

Despite the less-than-clear parameters of Cruzan, *it can be said with certainty that there is legal support for the right to die . . .*

NURSING IMPLICATIONS

There is no doubt that nurses providing health care in almost any delivery system will work with a patient who is dying. In many of those situations, the issue of withdrawing or removing medical treatment will arise. To provide competent, compassionate, and caring nursing care, the nurse must be clear about his or her personal feelings concerning dying, death, and withholding or withdrawing treatment. The nurse can utilize many resources to help clarify those feelings, including ethics texts and chapters, professional organization position statements, professional journal articles, and formal and informal support groups.[45]

Whatever the nurse's feelings, they must not interfere with a patient's decision concerning treatment. The nurse can, and should, exercise the right not to participate in whatever treatment or nontreatment he or she objects to. Notifying the nurse manager and asking for another assignment is certainly permissible both legally and ethically.

If the nurse decides to care for the individual from whom treatment is withdrawn or withheld, it is important to do so by continuing whatever treatment is *not* refused. Furthermore, the comfort of the patient and any relief of pain, if it exists, is vital. The American Nurses Association's 1991 *Position Statement* on this topic fully supports the need for the proper management of pain in the dying patient and the utilization of full and effective doses of pain medication consistent with the patient's wishes, even at the expense of the patient's life.[46]

The nurse should also take advantage of the institution's ethics committee, grand rounds, or other vehicles to resolve complex care situations in which treatment is withheld or refused. One study indicated that registered nurses are not likely to utilize ethics committees as a first option when dealing with clinical ethical issues.[47] Many reasons for this are proposed. One troubling analysis is that the structure of the nursing hierarchy in a facility may not provide an easy mechanism for a nurse to freely bring patient care concerns to a nonnursing arena.[48] If that commentary is correct, nurse managers must establish a mechanism that helps nursing staff obtain input and guidance from ethics forums for complex patient care situations. Concomitantly, all nursing staff should take advantage of the opportunity to seek guidance and input from multidisciplinary bodies in complex care situations. In addition to participation in an institutional ethics committee, nurses should also explore the option of establishing and participating in a *nursing* ethics committee.

Nurses will also need to be knowledgeable about state legislative developments and case law concerning refusal of life-sustaining treatment. Participating in legislative hearings, writing legislators, and educating the public are examples of how nurses can be proactive and possibly aid in the development of law in this area.

Last, but by no means least, the nurse must push for clear policies and procedures to be developed and implemented in the institution or agency concerning refusal of life-sustaining treatment. Those policies should include the patient's right to refuse treatment and any limitations on that right; the documentation of refusal; pain control; definitions of terms (such as cardiopulmonary resuscitation); management of patient comfort; and the nurse's role in the care of the patient whose treatment has been withdrawn or withheld according to his or her wishes.

DOCUMENTATION REMINDER 13–1
Refusal/Withdrawal of Treatment

- Accurate, complete description of actual withdrawal of treatment (e.g., who present, time, patient response)
- Results of continued care/monitoring of patient
- Consistent notations as to patient condition
- Patient comments, complaints
- Notification of other health care providers when condition changes or additional orders needed
- Family presence, requests, concerns

KEY CASES INVOLVING MINORS

Many of the well-known cases involving minors and the refusal of life-sustaining treatment center around criminal charges or termination of parental rights proceedings brought against the parents. However, many other cases have been decided when those types of allegations are not the issue. Rather, the issues involved are similar to those decided by cases with adult individuals; that is, establishing the legal parameters of the family's or the minor's right to refuse life-sustaining treatment. (See Key Cases 13–3 and 13–4, pp. 250–251.)

Subsequent decisions involving minors, especially after *Quinlan* and *Cruzan*, have shaped the right of the minor or the minor's parents to make decisions concerning withholding or withdrawing life-sustaining treatment. Some of those decisions are summarized in Table 13–2 (pp. 252–253).

The treatment issues surrounding the removal of life-sustaining treatment with minors will continue to be molded and shaped by additional court decisions. Support of a mature minor's choice to refuse life-sustaining treatment may continue to be the touchstone of those decisions. They may

also continue to underscore the family's authority to assert the right on behalf of a minor child. It will take a U.S. Supreme Court decision, however, to begin to resolve the multifarious legal issues with more certainty.

NURSING IMPLICATIONS

Many of the nursing implications discussed in the section on cases involving adults and the removal or withholding of life-sustaining treatment are applicable here. What is unique about working with minors, however, is clearly the parents' role when treatment issues need to be decided. The nurse must be cognizant of the fact that the parents are experiencing a great deal of emotional distress. As a result, they will need emotional support, clarification of information concerning the treatment issues germane to their child's situation, and time to make whatever decisions are made.

In addition, whether the minor is 7 years old or 17, young family members and friends of the patient may also be present in the hospital setting. A knowledge of child and adolescent behavior and their reactions to death and dying will help the nurse interact with them as they struggle to understand what is happening to their family member or friend.

If the nurse is able to obtain membership on an ethics committee or institutional review committee (IRC), he or she can be a valuable contributing member.

If the nurse is able to obtain membership on an ethics committee or institutional review committee (IRC), he or she can be a valuable contributing member. In fact, nursing membership is recommended.[55] If, however, that option is not open to the nurse, membership on a *nursing* ethics or institutional review committee is a consideration. This type of forum provides many benefits to nursing staff, not the least of which is a resource group in which ethical issues can be shared and analyzed and a model for decision making adopted.[56]

Text continued on page 254

In re L.H.R. (1984)[49]

A 15-day-old newborn suffers medical problem

Diagnosis made of persistent vegetative state and newborn placed on respirator

Parents and others file petition to remove ventilator support

Trial court grants relief and suggests appeal to state supreme court

Georgia Supreme Court upholds trial court decision

FACTS: Fifteen days after a normal birth, a medical problem (unspecified) left L.H.R. in a persistent vegetative state with an "absence of cognitive function." There was no hope of recovery. The infant had been placed on a respirator shortly after the medical crisis arose. The physician and the parents agreed that the respirator should be withdrawn. The hospital's Infant Care Review Committee (ICRC) agreed with that decision. After obtaining an agreement with the Georgia attorney general and the local district attorney, the parents, physician, and hospital filed a declaratory judgment action in the local state court seeking authorization to withdraw the ventilator.

TRIAL COURT DECISION: The De Kalb County Superior Court granted the relief requested by the petitioners. It also ordered the attorney general to file an appeal to the Georgia Supreme Court so that guidelines would be established for future cases.

GEORGIA SUPREME COURT DECISION: The Georgia Supreme Court upheld the decision of the trial court and set specific guidelines for both adults and minors in a persistent vegetative state with no chance of recovery and set guidelines for removal of ventilator. They were (1) the termination of treatment in the situation can be authorized by family or a legal guardian; (2) the diagnosis and prognosis must be made by the treating physician and two other physicians who agree; (3) no prior court approval is needed nor does the decision need to be reviewed or affirmed by a hospital committee.

ANALYSIS: The court's decision was based on the constitutional right of privacy to refuse treatment when a "terminal" condition exists. In addition, the court supported this right regardless of whether the patient lost decision-making capacity or was young. Furthermore, the court's decision clearly underscores the fact that it is the family or legal guardian who are the most appropriate persons to make the decision. The holding was the first to diminish the role of ethics or infant care review (ICR) committees in decisions concerning the withdrawal or withholding of life-sustaining treatment. This was a curious development, especially in view of the growth of institutional ethics bodies during the period in which *L.H.R.* was decided (see Special Considerations section). It is also important to note that there was no disagreement in this case concerning the diagnosis or recommended course of treatment. Had L.H.R.'s condition not been terminal or if no consensus had been reached by the physician, parents, and legal community, the progress and the outcome of this case might have been very different indeed.

In re Chad Eric Swan (1990)[50]

A 17-year-old is in a car accident that leaves him in a persistent vegetative state

Gastrostomy tube inserted

FACTS: Seventeen-year-old Chad Swan was in a car accident that left him in a persistent vegetative state without ever regaining consciousness. A gastrostomy tube was inserted. Because there was no hope of recovery, his parents and older brother agreed that the feeding tube should be removed. They decided to file a petition for declaratory judgment, asking that no civil or criminal liability would

Petition filed by parents asking for gastrostomy tube to be withdrawn

Complications arise with gastrostomy tube

Gastrostomy tube "closes" and infection occurs

Neither gastrostomy tube nor nasogastric tube can be inserted

Central venous line inserted pending court decision

Trial court orders central venous line to be removed, but stays order until appeal taken

Appellate court unanimously upholds trial court decision

be incurred by the family, the physician, or the medical center if the feeding tube were removed. The petition was supported by affidavits from Chad's brother and mother that Chad told them he would not want to be kept alive by artificial means. Shortly after the petition was filed, an infection was discovered around the entry point of the feeding tube. A consultation with a gastrointestinal specialist determined that Chad's body had "rejected" the tube and the tube and opening were sealed. As a result, no food or hydration could be administered. Further complicating the matter was the fact that until the infection cleared, no reinsertion could take place. And, because of Chad's severe facial injuries sustained in the accident, a nasogastric tube was not feasible. The physician suggested that another tube not be inserted. The family agreed with this decision.

Prior to the hearing on the declaratory judgment petition, the medical center asked for directions while awaiting a hearing on the petition. The court ordered a central venous line be inserted to provide Chad with fluid until a decision was made.

TRIAL COURT DECISION: With all interested parties but the district attorney supporting the petition, the court entered an order allowing the central venous line to be removed. The court further opined that this kind of decision was best made by the parents in conjunction with the physician. The district attorney and the *guardian ad litem* asked that the line be continued until an appeal was taken. Because the court was concerned that Chad could die before the appeal was completed, it stayed the order removing the line until the appeals court rendered its decision.

APPELLATE COURT DECISION: In a unanimous decision, the appeals court upheld the lower court's decision. Chad's age was only "one factor" in determining if he had "clearly and convincingly" stated his treatment preferences. The court held a minor has that capacity when he or she has the ability of the average person to understand and weigh risks and benefits. In Chad's case, he had discussed treatment choices on two separate occasions, one time 8 days before the accident. In both instances, he clearly indicated his preference not to be kept alive if there was no hope for recovery. The court also held it made no difference that the gastrostomy tube was "rejected," thus making the issue "reinsertion" rather than "withdrawal." Citing another Maine case, *In re Gardner,*[51] the court said that the distinction did not decrease *Gardner's* binding authority.

ANALYSIS: This case is a noteworthy one in supporting the removal of life-sustaining treatment, and specifically food and fluid, for a minor. By citing the *Gardner* case, which dealt with a 22-year-old adult's expressed wishes concerning treatment, the *Swan* court gave credence to an oral advance directive by a minor.[52] Furthermore, by stating that Chad Swan's oral advance directives were "clear and convincing," the substituted judgment test often used when a surrogate/proxy decision maker is involved was seemingly not important. It is ironic to note that during one of the two conversations that Chad Swan had concerning his treatment preferences, he referred to the *Gardner* case. Swan was talking with his mother about the case because of its wide publicity and also because Joseph Gardner was the stepgrandson of a close friend of Chad's grandmother.[53] Then 16 years old, he told his mother that he could not understand why they would not let Gardner die. After discussing Gardner's condition (persistent vegetative state), Swan stated: "If I can't be myself . . . no way . . . let me go to sleep."[54]

TABLE 13-2

Selected Court Decisions after *Quinlan* Concerning Right to Refuse Life-Sustaining Treatment Involving Minors

CASE NAME/ YEAR/STATE	DIAGNOSIS	TREATMENT(S) AT ISSUE	GUARDIAN, FAMILY, OTHER	DECISION	STANDARD(S) USED	COMMENTS
In re Guardianship of Barry (1984) (Florida)[1]	PVS	V; O (all life-sustaining)	CF	Ct. upholds right of parents to reject treatment	SJ	Ct. decision similar to *In re L.H.R.*, in text; minor was an infant
Newmark v. Williams (1991) (Delaware)[2]	Burkitt's lymphoma	O (Chemotherapy)	CF (parents)	Ct. upheld no treatment	B B&B	Parents refused treatment based on religious grounds; child was 3 years old; court clearly stated treatment very risky, invasive, and painful; no neglect on parents' part for refusing treatment
Rosebush v. Oakland County Prosecutor (1992) (Michigan)[3]	PVS	V	CF (parents)	Ct. upheld removal of life support	S	Minor was 16 years old; when $10\frac{1}{2}$, she made oral statement about her treatment wishes; when parents tried to remove daughter from state rehabilitation center to hospital, prosecutor attempted to stop transfer

Case	Condition	Treatment	Parties	Holding	Basis	Notes
In the Matter of Baby K (1994) (Virginia)[4]	Anencephaly, but with functioning brain stem; minor permanently unconscious	V; CPR; O	GAL and S (federal and state); hospital requested interpretation of laws if it did not ventilate without mother's consent	Ct. upholds mother's right to require ventilation; holds hospital would violate one specific federal law if treatment not given	IS	Although district ct. held not treating Baby K would violate Section 504 of the Rehabilitation Act, the Americans with Disabilities Act, the Child Abuse Act, and the Emergency Medical Treatment and Active Labor Act, appeals court held that because it found a violation of the EMTALA, it would not rule on others; raises question again as to futility of care concerns, as in *Wanglie*

V = Ventilator
ANTH = Artificial nutrition, hydration
M = Medication
CPR = Cardiopulmonary resuscitation
O = Other
CF = Family member
C = Conservator
PT = Patient with diminished capacity
GAL = *Guardian ad litem*
G = Guardian
GF = Guardian/family member
LW = Living will
DPAHC = Durable Power of Attorney for Health Care
S = Statute
CL = Common law
SJ = Substituted judgment
B&B = Benefits/burden
Q = Quality of life
B = Best interest
C = Constitutional basis
IS = Interpretation of statute

[1] 445 So. 2d 365 (Fla. Dist. Ct. App. 1984)
[2] 588 A.2d 1108 (Del. 1991)
[3] 491 N.W.2d 6331 (Mich. Ct. App. 1992)
[4] 832 F. Supp. 1022 (E.D. Va. 1993), *aff'd.*, 16 F.3d 590 (4th Cir. 1994), *cert. denied*, 115 S. Ct. 91 (1994)

SPECIAL CONSIDERATIONS

Defining Death

Originally, death was defined medically and by the common law as the cessation of spontaneous function of the cardiac and respiratory system ("heart death"), using accepted medical criteria when making such a determination.[57] As advances in medical technology occurred, however, this definition was difficult to adhere to because these systems could be maintained for long periods by such devices as the ventilator and other life-sustaining medical equipment. As a result, an alternative definition was proposed. That definition was the brain death standard: that is, death occurs when all vital functions of the brain, brain stem, and spinal reflexes are irreversibly nonexistent, again determined by accepted medical standards.[58]

The brain death standard was initially used for donor-donee situations and, in fact, had been incorporated into the Uniform Anatomical Gift Act (UAGA) discussed in Chapter 12. The criteria proposed to determine if brain death occurred were developed by the Harvard Medical School's Ad Hoc Committee to Examine the Definition of Death, chaired by Dr. Henry K. Beecher.[59] Briefly, the initial criteria to determine if an "irreversible coma" was present were (1) absence of reflexes; (2) no spontaneous respirations or muscular movements; and (3) no response to normally painful stimuli.[60] These clinical signs were to be confirmed by a flat EEG (two readings at least 24 hours apart), computerized tomography (CAT scan), and other diagnostic measures. Furthermore, ensuring that no drug intoxication or hypothermia was present was also important.[61]

These guidelines were expanded upon by various groups, including the President's Commission for the Study of Ethical Problems in Medicine and Biomedical and Behavioral Research.[62] In 1980, the Harvard criteria were adopted into the Uniform Determination of Death Act (UDDA),[63] along with the common-law "heart death" standard.[64] Thirty states and the District of Columbia have adopted the Uniform Determination of Death Act (e.g., Colorado, Delaware, Idaho, Maryland, Pennsylvania, and Nevada). However, all 50 states and the District of Columbia have adopted brain death as a legal definition of death, whether by case law, amendments to current statutes, or regulatory means.[65]

If brain death is diagnosed in an individual, there is no legal duty to provide continuing treatment because that person is clinically dead. Therefore, treatment can be discontinued without criminal or civil liability. In fact, continuing to treat a dead individual can be a basis for liability if the surrogate/proxy decision maker does not consent to additional treatment.[66]

Despite its wide use, the brain death standard has not been universally accepted. Its critics question whether the concept is "theoretically coherent and internally consistent."[67] Others express a concern that it is "confused in practice," citing a 1989 study indicating that only 35% of nurses and physicians who were most likely to be involved in organ procurement for transplantation correctly knew the legal and medical criteria for death determinations.[68] These and other critics suggest a return to the former cardiorespiratory standard.[69]

Proponents of maintaining the brain death standard also abound. Interestingly, the proponents believe that, among other uses, the brain death standard is invaluable in organ transplantation situations.[70] In fact, some authors describe organ transplantation as "the engine driving the brain death train" because the brain death standard has not been a prerequisite for the termination of life-sustaining treatment during the past 20 years.[71] Yet, with multiorgan procurement, brain death *is* the required standard of death.[72]

The controversy is far from resolution. Even so, it is necessary, at least according to one author, that variations on the determinations of when an individual is dead and when life-sustaining treatment can be removed are difficult for society to accept. What is more acceptable is a "legally codifiable consensus" on defining death and leaving to personal choice and individual freedom decisions concerning when life-sustaining treatment may be withdrawn or withheld.[73]

Brain death is different from a persistent vegetative state in which substantial losses of function in the cerebral cortex occur but autonomous functions continue because there is no damage to the brain stem. Although a diagnosis of brain death does not ensure the absence of legal issues when treatment is withheld or terminated, a diagnosis of persistent vegetative state raises very different legal, and other, issues.[74] In fact, cases challenging the right to refuse life-sustaining treatment, including the two key cases in this chapter and many of those in Tables 13–1 and 13–2, involved individuals in a persistent vegetative state.

Refusal of Cardiopulmonary Resuscitation

The type of life-sustaining treatment refused or withdrawn has been as controversial, both legally and ethically, as the right to refuse treatment. The specific types of treatments focused on have, of course, changed. For example, the early cases involved ventilator support. Later cases involved artificial nutrition and hydration. One particular treatment that needs specific discussion is the refusal or withholding of cardiopulmonary resuscitation (CPR). It was one of the first specific treatments tested in the judicial system after the *Quinlan* case.

The type of life-sustaining treatment refused or withdrawn has been as controversial, both legally and ethically, as the right to refuse treatment.

The historical development of CPR has a great deal to do with its course in the right to refuse life-sustaining treatment. It has long been used; one of the earliest accounts appears in the Old Testament.[75] It was not until the 1960s, however, that research demonstrated that circulation could be maintained by external cardiac massage.[76] External cardiac massage was adopted quickly in hospitals and over the next 15 years became a routine procedure.[77] In fact, it was used for virtually *every* patient who experienced cardiopulmonary arrest.

It became clear to both the medical community and the consumer of health care that perhaps CPR was not indicated for every patient. However, there was concern about the liability of not initiating CPR. As a result, many "slow codes," "no codes," and removable purple dots on charts were used formally and informally when a discussion was made not to initiate CPR with certain patients.

In 1974, the National Conference on Standards for CPR and Emergency Cardiac Care stated that (1) the purpose of CPR is to prevent unexpected death; (2) it is not indicated in certain situations,

such as terminal irreversible illness; and (3) when CPR is not indicated, it should be noted in the patient's medical record (progress notes and order sheet).[78] After that statement, many institutions developed policies and began to utilize do-not-resuscitate (DNR) orders. It was not until a 1978 Massachusetts case, however, that the legal status of do-not-resuscitate orders was clarified. (See Key Case 13–5, p. 256.)

Since *Dinnerstein*, do-not-resuscitate orders have had a circuitous development. Even though they were somewhat legitimized after the court opinion, the liability concerns associated with such orders continued to abound. This was not helped when, for example, in 1982 a criminal investigation was initiated against a hospital in Queens because of reported do-not-resuscitate orders being written for elderly, incompetent patients.[80]

Despite these concerns, most hospitals and other health care delivery systems began to develop policies to cover do-not-resucitate orders and essentially treat them as any other medical order. For example, the policies require that (1) the order is written in the patient's medical record like other medical orders; (2) the order is reviewed and/or renewed on a specific basis; (3) a telephone do-not-resuscitate order is valid only under limited circumstances and must be witnessed by two registered nurses and documented as such in the patient's record; (4) if no do-not-resuscitate order exists, a patient must be resuscitated; (5) the patient or the legally recognized decision maker must be informed and provide consent for the treatment; and (6) do-not-resuscitate and CPR must be clearly defined so that other treatment not refused can be continued.[81]

Several states, including New York, Georgia, and Montana were so concerned about liability and do-not-resuscitate orders that the state legislatures passed specific acts or authorized state agencies to promulgate rules and regulations to deal with such orders.[82] Many other states followed suit, with "do-not-resuscitate legislation" passed by state legislatures as "freestanding" statutes or provisions in other state legislation, such as advance directive laws.[83]

The development of clear do-not-resuscitate policies in health care facilities, and perhaps a decrease in some of the liability concerns, was augmented by the Joint Commission on Accreditation of Health Care Organizations (JCAHO) re-

KEY CASE 13–5	In re Shirley Dinnerstein (1978)[79]

A 67-year-old woman with Alzheimer's disease suffers stroke

FACTS: Shirley Dinnerstein was a 67-year-old woman in whom Alzheimer's disease had been diagnosed in 1975, although she may have had the disease as early as 1972. She had been placed in a nursing home in 1975 when her family could no longer care for her at home. Her condition at that time was considered to be similar to a persistent vegetative state. In 1978, Ms. Dinnerstein suffered a massive stroke that left her paralyzed on the left side. A nasogastric tube and catheter were inserted by the hospital to which she was admitted after the stroke. The physician's opinion was that Ms. Dinnerstein would never recover and that her condition was terminal, although a prediction as to the length of her life could not be made. What was clear, however, was that if she suffered a cardiopulmonary arrest, she would die Thus, the physician's opinion was that she should not be resuscitated should an arrest occur. The patient's son (a physician) and daughter agreed with the physician. The hospital, physician, and family filed a declaratory judgment action in the probate court asking the court to guide them in making this type of decision (that is, writing a do-not-resuscitate order) or, if need be, authorize such a medical order.

Nasogastric tube and catheter inserted

Physician suggests do-not-resuscitate order be written, for condition would never improve

Family and others file case asking for guidance with do-not-resuscitate order

Trial court sends case to Appeals court

TRIAL COURT DECISION: The trial court did not make a decision in the case. Rather, it appointed a temporary guardian to protect Ms. Dinnerstein's interests, appointed a *guardian ad litem* (who opposed the do-not-resuscitate order), and made an extensive factual report for the Appeals Court to consider.

Appeals court remands case to trial court for an order granting the do-not-resuscitate order to be written by M.D.

APPEALS COURT DECISION: The appellate court remanded the case to the trial court for an order granting the relief requested. Specifically, the court held that the law would clearly allow a course of medical treatment that included a do-not-resuscitate order. In addition, the court opined that when there is full agreement by all those involved, no court order is necessary prior to the initiation of such medical treatment. Only if there is disagreement, or a physician's decision to initiate a do-not-resuscitate order is inconsistent with acceptable medical practice, should a court order be sought.

ANALYSIS: The *Dinnerstein* decision was a far-reaching one, for it clarified an earlier Massachusetts decision, *Saikewicz* (see Table 13-1). There had been some speculation after that decision that a court order would be necessary for any withholding or removal of life-sustaining treatment. The *Dinnerstein* court specifically held that "life-sustaining treatment" meant medical care in which a temporary or permanent cure would result. In both cases, the medical regimen to be withheld or withdrawn was not curative. Thus, court orders were not needed. The case again supports the right of a patient without decision-making capacity to decide against treatment, albeit through another, whether that other be a court, guardian, and/or family member.

quirement in 1988 that all hospitals seeking to be accredited have policies on resuscitation.[84]

A continuing issue with do-not-resuscitate orders is ironic in view of the solid development of the right of the patient to have input into treatment decisions. Although not yet definitively litigated, the propriety of a physician writing a do-not-resuscitate order without informed consent from the patient or surrogate/proxy decision maker, or writing one when no consent has occurred, is of constant concern, both legally and ethically.[85]

When Treatment Decisions Conflict with Medical Treatment Recommendations

The right to refuse treatment is not absolute and may need to be balanced against other interests, including the maintenance of the ethical integrity of the health care profession. Situations raising a threat to the ethical integrity of medicine or nursing are manifold. However, two general categories in which those situations arise can be identified: first, when treatment is refused that a physician or nurse believes should be provided, and second, when treatment is seen as necessary by the patient or family but is not medically indicated, or additional treatment is seen as "futile" by the health care provider.

The right to refuse treatment is not absolute and may need to be balanced against other interests, including the maintenance of the ethical integrity of the health care profession.

The first category applies to almost all of the cases dealing with the right to refuse life-sustaining treatment, including but not limited to *Saikewicz, Brophy,* and *Gray* (see Table 13–1). Generally the case decisions have clearly held that the state's interest, if it exists, must give way to the right of the patient to refuse life-sustaining treatment.

In the second category were some reported cases in which surrogate/proxy decision makers refused to allow the termination of life-sustaining treatment with brain-dead patients.[86] In 1991, an-

other case received attention. That case decided the propriety of continuing ventilator support at the insistence of a surrogate/proxy decision maker when it was not medically recommended. (See Key Case 13–6, p. 258.)

Helga Wanglie was kept on the ventilator in accordance with the court order. She died 4 days after the decision.[94]

Unfortunately, the *Wanglie* case provided little guidance in future cases dealing with the issue of futile or medically unnecessary treatment, most probably due to the varying fact situations of subsequent cases. In most instances, these cases have been decided only at the trial level; few have reached the state appellate courts.[95] Those cases include *Gilgunn v. Massachusetts General Hospital*[96] (whether treating physicians violated patient's daughter's right to be free from emotional distress because physicians unilaterally terminated treatment of her mother); and *Rideout v. Hershey Medical Center*[97] (whether parents of two-year-old could sustain certain causes of action, e.g., negligent and intentional infliction of emotional distress, against the hospital and treating physicians for the death of their daughter after extubating her without parents' consent and presence at daughter's bedside).

Hospice Care

The purpose of hospice care is to provide services to the terminally ill and their families that is focused upon palliation of pain and control of other symptoms.[98] An interdisciplinary team provides medical, nursing, psychological, and other support. The emphasis is on quality of life for as long as it lasts.[99]

Hospice care originated in Canada and England. Its acceptance in the United States was controversial. Hospice care has now gained recognition as an alternative to hospital care for the terminally ill. It is cost effective and provides needed services for many patients, including the elderly with cancer and those suffering from AIDS.[100]

One of the goals of hospice care—pain management—can be a disputatious issue when adequate amounts of medication are not provided to the patient or are unavailable to nursing staff to administer. In August of 1991, charges were brought against six hospice nurses (the "Hospice Six") of the Hospice of St. Peter's Hospital in Montana. Specifically, the Montana Department of Commerce, Professional and Occupational Licens-

In re Helga Wanglie (1991)[87]

An 86-year-old breaks hip

FACTS: Helga Wanglie broke her hip at the age of 86 years when she slipped on a rug in her home. After successful repair of the hip fracture, she was sent to a nursing home. She was readmitted to the hospital that repaired her hip after she developed respiratory failure due to emphysema. She was placed on a respirator. Several attempts to wean her from the respirator were unsuccessful. She was then transferred to another medical facility that specialized in the care of ventilator-dependent patients.[88]

In nursing home, Mrs. Wanglie develops respiratory failure and is placed on ventilator

Additional attempts at weaning occurred, one of which resulted in cardiopulmonary arrest. She was resuscitated and admitted to another hospital. Because of severe and irreversible brain damage due to the arrest, a persistent vegetative state and hopeless condition were diagnosed. The facility ethics committee and physicians recommended that the ventilator be removed and further life-sustaining treatment be withheld. The husband, as her guardian, and the family would not agree because Mrs. Wanglie would want treatment. She was then transferred back to the hospital where her hip had been repaired.[89]

Attempts to wean patient from ventilator result in cardiopulmonary arrest

Revival occurs, but diagnosis of persistent vegetative state made

The physicians there also recommended that the respirator should be removed, but the family and husband/guardian refused to agree. They did agree to a do-not-resuscitate order, however, because of the fact that recovery from an arrest would be unlikely. Despite the facility's ethics committee also recommending the withdrawal of the ventilator, the family would not waver from its decision. The basis for their position was an expressed desire by Mrs. Wanglie that her life not be prematurely "shortened or taken" if anything happened to her and she could not care for herself.[90]

M.D. recommends removal of ventilator
Husband, as guardian, and family will not consent to removal

Do-not-resuscitate status OK'd by husband

After many attempts to resolve the situation with the family, the hospital filed a petition seeking the replacement of Mr. Wanglie as the guardian of his wife.

Hospital files petition to replace Mr. Wanglie as guardian

TRIAL COURT DECISION: The probate court refused to replace Mr. Wanglie as guardian (conservator) of his wife, holding that he was "dedicated to promoting his wife's welfare" and was competent to continue in his role.[91]

Trial court denies hospital's request

ANALYSIS: The decision resulted in a flood of reactions. Some believed the decision was appropriate, especially in view of her wishes and the fact that the patient's private medical insurance would pay for the continued care.[92] Others discussed how a determination is made about "medically necessary" as opposed to "medically futile" treatment.[93]

The impact of the case will continue to be seen in future cases. The court clearly held that a competent family member is a more suitable surrogate/proxy decision maker than a stranger in the same role. In addition, the court's decision also stands for the principle that treatment decisions to withhold or withdraw treatment must be followed by health care practitioners. Mrs. Wanglie was not brain dead, a situation in which the appropriateness of continuing ventilator support would be highly questionable, to say the least. Rather, she was in a persistent vegetative state, and her guardian refused to give permission to have the ventilator removed.

ing Bureau challenged their conduct of keeping a "stash" of narcotics (including morphine) in a locked drawer for use when patients' conditions deteriorated, or when obtaining a new order or a change in medication was not possible (when the pharmacy was closed or the physician was not available).

After a hearing, the Montana Board of Nursing held that the six nurses committed unprofessional conduct by (1) altering and/or manipulating drug supplies, narcotics, or patients' records; (2) appropriating medications of patients; and (3) violating state or federal laws relative to drugs.[101] The board also held that the nurses (1) dispensed, or possessed with intent to dispense, morphine and other controlled substances without authority to do so; (2) did not keep records of the drugs received, dispensed, or possesed; (3) functioned as a medical doctor or pharmacist rather than as a nurse; (4) transferred controlled substances among and between patients contrary to federal and state laws on controlled substances; and (5) violated Montana criminal statutes regarding dangerous drugs.[102]

The board instituted probationary status on the licenses of the nurses for 3 to 5 years. The conditions of probation included barring the nurses from holding supervisory positions, making them obtain the board's approval before taking a new position, and making them submit quarterly reports to the board.[103]

After the board decision, only two of the nurses remained on staff at the hospice. Two others took a leave, one resigned, and another took a nonnursing position in the hospital.[104]

The nurses filed an appeal asking for judicial review of the board's final order. They alleged the board had rejected the hearing officer's recommendations and ordered different discipline, which was an abuse of its discretion. The court reversed the findings, conclusions of law, and final order of the board and adopted the hearing officer's recommendations. The board then appealed that decision. The Supreme Court of Montana upheld the hearing officer's findings, conclusion, and order. The hearing officer's findings and order were that (1) charges against the nurses for "unprofessional conduct" were not proven and should be dismissed; (2) letters of reprimand should be placed in the files of the nurses for 3 years; and (3) all charges against one nurse, Verna VanDuynhoven, should be dismissed.[105]

The case centered on the legalistics of the practice of nursing, dispensing vs. administering medications, and the role of the nurse (as opposed to the physician or pharmacist) in prescribing controlled substances. However, the "real issue" of the case was the social and medical ethic of how to let dying people die.[106]

Montana's living will statute did not authorize health care providers to "hasten death."[107] Because the hospice's living will form stated that medications "can and should" be administered to alleviate suffering, even though death could be hastened as a result, the nurses, according to the allegations of the attorney for the state agency, overstepped the legal limits of their practice.[108]

The goal of pain management in hospice care—indeed in health care generally—can also be thwarted by concerns of health care providers about criminal and other liability when the death of the patient is alleged to have been caused by large doses of pain medication.

The appropriate utilization of narcotics and sedatives to control pain and provide relief from suffering—palliative care—is a subject that has received little attention until recently.[109] Interestingly, some state courts have equated the right to be free of pain with the right to refuse medical treatment and have explicitly authorized the use of such medications.[110] In addition, other states have passed legislation, administrative rules, and/or guidelines authorizing physicians to prescribe adequate medications to treat "intractable pain," even when the death of the patient may be hastened.[111] Immunity from liability in these laws, administrative rules, and/or guidelines varies considerably, however, so concerns, including suspension or revocation of their licenses, still exist among health care providers.[112] In addition, the ethical issues raised by the use of adequate pain medication that may hasten the patient's death continue to be debated.[113]

When Withdrawal or Withholding of Medical Care for a Minor Results in Alleged Child Abuse or Neglect, Criminal Conduct, or Juvenile Proceedings

The cases dealing with this issue with newborns and minors can be categorized into two general classifications: minors with varying medical conditions and "seriously ill newborns" (a term coined by the President's Commission in its 1983 study), including those with congenital anomalies. The legal responses to these two categories have differed.

Minors with Varying Medical Conditions

In this group, allegations of criminal behavior or child abuse and neglect are brought against the parents. Charges result after a report is made to the state agency responsible for enforcing the state child abuse and neglect reporting statutes or when a petition is filed in the state juvenile court system.

When criminal conduct is alleged, the case is filed against the parents in the state criminal court. Specific causes of action when death of the minor occurs include involuntary manslaughter and murder.

Two cases alleging neglect in state juvenile court systems, one of the first such cases and one decided more recently, are presented as Key Cases. Selected other cases, including those involving criminal charges against the parents, are presented in Table 13–2. (See Key Case 13–7, p. 261.)

Ricky testified about his preferences for treatment in a hearing conducted pursuant to the Pennsylvania Supreme Court decision. It was clear he did not want the operation. The case worked its way up to the Pennsylvania Supreme Court again,[115] and the court upheld his wishes. (See Key Case 13–8, pp. 262–263.)

Seriously Ill Newborns, Including Those with Congenital Anomalies

When treatment decisions involve newborns with such conditions as prematurity and its concurrent developmental problems, spina bifida cystica, and anencephaly, the legal and ethical issues are volatile.[117] Two early examples of these situations illustrate the emotional nature of those decisions.

In 1970, a film produced by the Joseph P. Kennedy Foundation entitled *Who Should Survive?* depicted an actual case at Johns Hopkins University.[118] The parents of a 2-day-old infant with multiple anomalies, including Down's syndrome and duodenal atresia, asked that no surgical intervention take place, and the physicians agreed. The infant was given nothing by mouth and intravenous therapy was discontinued; 15 days later, the child died.

In 1973, a study done by two physicians at Yale–New Haven Hospital reported practices at that particular institution concerning treatment

decisions for newborns with birth defects.[119] In a 2½-year period of study in the special care nursery, 299 deaths occurred. Of those 299 deaths, 14% transpired because of a decision to withhold or withdraw treatment.[120] The conditions of the infants who died included spina bifida, trisomies, and multiple anomalies.[121]

It was not until 1982, however, that situations concerning the nontreatment of infants with congenital anomalies received national attention as they worked their way into the judicial system. Although a few earlier cases had been decided in other jurisdictions, including Florida and New York, one particular decision set the stage for far-reaching changes in federal and state law concerning newborns and treatment decisions. The case, *In re Treatment and Care of Infant Doe,* is discussed as Key Case 13–9 (p. 263).

Baby Doe died within 6 days of the decision of his parents to refuse treatment, surrounded by the legal frenzy to obtain treatment for him.

As a result of the Baby Doe case, the Reagan administration began to respond to the issue of withholding and withdrawing treatment from newborns with disabilities. The director of the Office of Civil Rights of the U.S. Department of Health and Human Services (DHHS), directed by President Reagan, issued a notice to 7,000 hospitals receiving federal funding.[125] The notice specifically stated:

> Under Section 504 (of the Rehabilitation Act of 1973) it is unlawful for a recipient of federal financial assistance to withhold from a handicapped infant nutritional sustenance or medical or surgical treatment to correct a life-threatening condition if (1) the withholding is based on the fact that the infant is handicapped; and (2) the handicap does not render the treatment or nutritional sustenance medically contradicted.[126]

Furthermore, the Department of Health and Human Services stated that Down's syndrome was a handicap covered under the Act and threatened to terminate financial assistance to any hospital that engaged in discriminatory conduct against handicapped newborns or "facilitated" such conduct by parents of handicapped newborns.

The initial notice was followed by an interim final rule.[127] Again citing Section 504 of the Rehabilitation Act, the Department of Health and Human Services required health care facilities to post

KEY CASE 13–7   In re Green (1972)[114]

Ricky Green's M.D. recommends a spinal fusion

Jehovah's Witness mother OK's surgery but refuses consent for blood transfusion

Hospital files petition to have 16-year-old declared "neglected child" and to have guardian appointed

Trial court denies request

Appeals court unanimously reverses decision

Pennsylvania Supreme Court reverses appeals court and remands case to trial court with specific guidelines

FACTS: Sixteen-year-old Ricky Green suffered two attacks of polio that resulted in obesity and paralytic scoliosis (94% curvature of the spine). As a result, he was wheelchair bound. His physicians recommended a "spinal fusion," which would require taking bone from his pelvis and placing it in his spine. Ricky's mother, a Jehovah's Witness, agreed to the operation provided that no blood transfusion occur. The orthopedic specialist informed Mrs. Green that the operation is "not without risk."

Because Mrs. Green would not consent to blood transfusions, the State Hospital for Crippled Children filed a petition to initiate juvenile proceedings to declare Ricky a "neglected child" under Pennsylvania's Juvenile Court Law. The hospital also asked for a guardian to be appointed for Ricky (Ricky lives with his mother, who is separated from his father).

TRIAL COURT DECISION: After an evidentiary hearing, the trial court dismissed the petition. The hospital filed an appeal.

APPEALS COURT DECISION: The appeals court unanimously reversed and remanded the case to the trial court for the appointment of a guardian. That decision was granted review by the Pennsylvania Supreme Court.

PENNSYLVANIA SUPREME COURT DECISION: The Pennsylvania Supreme Court reversed the appeals court decision and remanded the case to the trial court for additional proceedings. In so doing, the Supreme Court instructed the trial court to evaluate the following issues: (1) the charge of neglect is based on a religious belief; therefore, the exercise of religious freedom is an important constitutional right; (2) any state impingement of religious freedom must be justified; (3) the treatment in the case is not life sustaining; (4) Ricky's wishes must be determined; and (5) whose religious beliefs will prevail if there is a parent-child conflict concerning the treatment.

ANALYSIS: This case essentially stands for the principle that unless the life of a child is at stake, the state does not have an interest strong enough to override a parent's right to refuse treatment based on a religious belief. In addition, the case supported the now established trend of allowing input from the minor (especially the "mature minor") concerning treatment preferences. This is especially important when the child's religious preferences or beliefs may be different from those of the parent(s) and when the treatment is not lifesaving.

---

notices in a conspicuous place in pediatric wards, newborn nurseries, and special care units to alert staff that "discriminatory failure to feed and care for a handicapped infant" was prohibited by federal law.[128] In addition, a hotline number was listed with instructions for anyone with information concerning discrimination against a handicapped infant to report that conduct anonymously.[129] Last, the notice clearly stated that retaliation or intimidation of any person who did report conduct

KEY CASE 13–8	In re E.G., a Minor (1989)[116]

Jehovah's Witness mother and patient refuse blood transfusions

FACTS: E.G., 17 years old, contracted leukemia and required blood transfusions. Her mother and E.G., both Jehovah's Witnesses, refused the treatment based on their religious beliefs. All other treatment was consented to by E.G.'s mother.

Illinois files "neglect" petition Trial court holds 17-year-old a "neglected minor" and appoints guardian

TRIAL COURT DECISION: The trial court found E.G. to be medically neglected and appointed a guardian over the person to make medical decisions. The court stated that the appointment was in the child's best interest, despite describing her as a "mature 17-year-old." Even though E.G. was clear about her wishes and understood that death was "assured absent treatment," the court held that the state's interest in the preservation of life outweighed that of E.G. and her mother. The decision was appealed.

Appeals court vacates trial court order in part and modifies it in part

APPEALS COURT DECISION: The appeals court vacated the trial court order in part and modified it in part. Citing an Illinois case that upheld a Jehovah's Witness's First Amendment right to refuse transfusions, the court extended that right to "mature minors" based on the long line of U.S. Supreme Court decisions allowing minors to consent to abortions (without parental consent). That right, the court opined, was based on the constitutional right of privacy and that extended to the right to refuse medical treatment. Somewhat surprisingly, however, the court upheld the neglect finding against the mother.

The decision was appealed to the Illinois Supreme Court.

ILLINOIS SUPREME COURT DECISION: The Illinois Supreme Court made its decision despite E.G.'s turning 18 years old—the age of majority in Illinois—prior to its decision. In so doing, the court held that the issues in the case, although technically moot, were of "substantial public interest" and therefore should be decided. The court held that (1) a mature minor has a right to give consent or refusal for treatment; (2) the right is based not only on constitutional protections but state law as well; (3) state interests must be balanced against the rights afforded the mature minor; (4) if the treatment refused is life-threatening, the state's interest may be greater than the mature minor's; (5) the mother and E.G. agreed in this case, but when others—family, adult siblings, for example—disagree, their opposition to the mature minor's refusing treatment "would weigh heavily against the minor's right to refuse"; and (6) the neglect finding against the mother must be expunged.

Illinois Supreme Court upholds refusal

ANALYSIS: This case is an interesting one in supporting the common-law right of a minor to refuse treatment. Even though the court discussed many of the constitutional arguments for allowing the refusal of treatment by a minor, it declined to rule on the constitutional issue because it could rest its decision on other precedent. The decision's impact may not be as far-reaching as it seems upon a first reading, however. The Illinois Supreme Court points out in its opinion that if E.G. had refused the transfusions and her mother had consented to them, E.G.'s wishes may have had to give way to her mother's request. Perhaps, then, the right of the

KEY CASE 13–8 — In re E.G., a Minor (1989)[116] *Continued*

mature minor to refuse treatment in Illinois is conditioned on the parental support of that choice. Also, it is important to point out that although not a basis of the decision, the court relied on the abortion decisions granting a minor the right to seek those services without parental consent. Obviously the decision was reached prior to the U.S. Supreme Court decision in *Casey v. Planned Parenthood* discussed in Chapter 11. Whether that opinion will impact, directly or indirectly, on a minor's right to refuse medical treatment will remain to be seen.

KEY CASE 13–9 — In re Treatment and Care of Infant Doe (1982)[122]

Baby John Doe born with multiple anomalies

Parents refuse surgery and intravenous therapy discontinued

Hospital files petition to reverse parents' decision

Court upholds parents' decision

Appointed guardian ad litem does not appeal decision

"Neglected child" petition denied

Appeal to U.S. Supreme Court denied

FACTS: Baby John Doe was born with trisomy 21, a tracheoesophageal fistula, and esophageal atresia. The parents (the father was a teacher and had worked with Down's syndrome students "occasionally") believed that their son would not have "minimally acceptable quality of life" and that it was in his best interest, as well as in the best interests of the rest of the family (two other children) that surgical repair of the anomalies not take place. Since the infant could not be fed orally, intravenous therapy was discontinued. The hospital filed an emergency petition to override the parents' decision.

TRIAL COURT DECISION: After hearing testimony from several medical experts, including Baby Doe's pediatrician and a pediatric expert, the court held that the parents were fully informed of the treatment options available to their child and a decision concerning treatment in those circumstances was theirs to make. The court also appointed local child welfare authorities as a *guardian ad litem* in the event an appeal was to occur.

The *guardian ad litem* decided against an appeal.

JUVENILE COURT PETITION AND DECISION: The district attorney then petitioned the Indiana Juvenile Court asking for determination whether Baby Doe was a "neglected" child under Indiana law. The petition was denied.

Further attempts to have the case heard, including an appeal to the U.S. Supreme Court, were denied.

ANALYSIS: The case received nationwide publicity and was very controversial. According to one author, those responses are very curious, particularly because limited palliative therapy for seriously compromised handicapped infants was fairly common at the time.[123] The author also speculates that the controversial issue in the case was the presence of Down's syndrome, a handicap not particularly serious when compared with other congenital anomalies.[124]

was prohibited and that the noncare and nonfeeding of infants may also violate state civil and criminal law.

If any calls were received through the hotline, the Office of Civil Rights was prepared to initiate an immediate on-site investigation concerning the conduct. The investigators were nicknamed the "Baby Doe squads." They had the authority to question all health care providers and/or family members and had access to health care records and facilities.

The interim final rule was challenged by the American Academy of Pediatrics. The rule was invalidated 3 weeks after its effective date because of noncompliance with rulemaking requirements of the federal Administrative Procedure Act (APA).[130]

As a result of the invalidation of its rule, the Department of Health and Human Services proposed another rule and allowed for public comment under the Administrative Procedure Act. It elicited 17,000 responses.[131] The final rule, which was to take effect in February of 1984, contained the following provisions: (1) smaller notices similar to the earlier ones were to be posted, but not in public places; (2) the information reported would be kept confidential; (3) illustrative conditions requiring treatment were listed; (4) hospitals should establish Infant Care Review Committees (ICRCs); and (5) state child protective agencies receiving federal funds must establish procedures to receive and investigate allegations of medical neglect of newborns.[132]

Interestingly, the final rule was declared invalid by the U.S. Supreme Court in 1986 in *Bowen v. American Hospital Association*.[133] The Court declared the final rule was not authorized by Section 504 of the Rehabilitation Act and upheld the decisions of the lower federal courts as the case made its long, circuitous route to the Supreme Court. The Court was clear in its analysis of the Rehabilitation Act. It held that (1) when parents refuse treatment for their newborn, no discrimination by a health care facility takes place; (2) the final rule was not based on evidence that any facility had failed to report instances of discrimination under Section 504; and (3) the Department of Health and Human Services had no authority to require state agencies to investigate allegations of medical neglect.

Despite the Supreme Court's decision, the matter concerning treatment for newborns with handi-

caps had already been put to rest. During the legal course of *Bowen* and its "companion" cases in the lower federal courts, Congress passed the Child Abuse Amendments of 1984 (CAA),[134] altering the Child Abuse Prevention and Treatment and Adoption Reform Act originally passed in 1974.[135]

The Child Abuse Amendments, although controversial, were much more far reaching than a court decision testing the final interim rules would have been. Had a favorable decision for the Department of Health and Human Services been reached, compliance with the court order would have been required only of health care facilities receiving federal funds—Medicare specifically. The amendments, in contrast, required state child protective agencies receiving federal grants to (1) change the definition of child abuse and neglect to include the "withholding of medically indicated treatment"; and (2) establish programs in their systems to ensure that reports of medical neglect were investigated and, if appropriate, take necessary action.

Thus, those health care providers mandated to report child abuse and neglect under their respective state laws were required to report instances of "medical neglect" when "medically indicated treatment" was withheld, including nutrition, hydration, and medication. Several exceptions to the requirement of reporting include when (1) an infant is chronically and permanently comatose; or (2) treatment would only prolong dying, not correct an infant's life-threatening condition, and/or is futile; or (3) the treatment would be futile and may in fact be inhumane.[136]

It is difficult to evaluate the effects of the Child Abuse Amendments. Despite the attempt by the Reagan administration and Congress to prohibit the nonprovision of "medically indicated treatment" for newborns with congenital handicaps, the amendments have been cited in only one dissenting opinion (in which the judge criticizes a lower court's decision for ignoring the amendments when allowing the entry of a DNR order for an infant).[137] In other reported cases where the amendments were applicable, the court opinions did not even mention them.[138]

Euthanasia/Mercy Killing

In the United States, both of these terms mean mercifully putting to death people who suffer from painful, incurable, and distressing diseases.[139] The word *euthanasia*, meaning "good death" in Greek, is further defined in terms of active or passive and voluntary, involuntary, or nonvoluntary. It has also been contrasted with assisted suicide by focusing on the role of the health care provider. With assisted suicide, the health care provider only provides the means with which the patient ultimately acts "last" to end his or her life. In contrast, in euthanasia, the health care provider acts "last" by performing the act that results in the death of the patient.[140]

In the United States, [euthanasia and mercy killing] . . . mean mercifully putting to death people who suffer from painful, incurable, and distressing diseases.

The health care provider's actions would, of course, be seen as an example of active euthanasia. Moreover, it would most likely result in criminal liability for the health care provider. In addition to the potential legal ramifications, such conduct on the part of health care practitioners also raises complex ethical issues.[141] Nevertheless, attempts have been made by state legislatures and professional groups to pass legislation allowing for active euthanasia under certain limited circumstances. This development will be discussed in the Assisted Suicide section.

Passive euthanasia is, in fact, the "right to die" as it has been developed to date by the courts and legislative process.[142] However, it is still fraught with some confusion, mainly because of the inability of society to differentiate between the conduct of the health care provider in withholding or withdrawing specific treatment (acts of "commission" or "omission") and the underlying medical condition that ultimately causes the death of the patient.[143] Even so, most court decisions wrestling with this issue have held that it is the *underlying condition* that causes the death of the individual and not the withholding or withdrawing of the treatment, whether the treatment be artificial food and fluid[144] or other forms of medical care.[145]

Voluntary euthanasia usually denotes a situation in which the patient is actively involved in the decision to withdraw or withhold treatment by providing informed refusal of treatment, whether by an oral declaration or an advance directive. In contrast, involuntary euthanasia is defined as withholding or withdrawing treatment without the individual's informed consent to do so.[146] Nonvoluntary euthanasia takes place when the individual without decision-making capacity has not expressed his or her desires, and a decision is made without any real or presumed understanding of what the patient would have wanted.[147]

Suicide

Suicide is the deliberate termination of one's life by one's own hand.[148] Although suicide was a felony under the English law (forfeiture of the estate and burial in the highway as punishment), American jurisdictions no longer impose penalties for successful suicide.[149] However, attempted suicide is sometimes categorized as illegal or unlawful in some states. If so, the jurisdiction may require a psychiatric hospitalization for the individual. The rationale for this position is that the state has an interest in the preservation of life.

In relation to the refusal of life-sustaining treatment, the courts have been careful not to equate suicide with refusal of treatment.[150] The basis for not equating the two involves two theories: causation and intent. The causation approach rests upon the premise that it is the underlying condition, and not self-destruction, that causes the death.[151] Likewise, the intent theory is based on the fact that the individual intends only to forgo life-sustaining treatment—treatment that is seen as futile, painful, and/or burdensome—and does not intend death.[152] In fact, in one case, *Satz v. Perlmutter*,[153] which involved a competent patient suffering from Lou Gehrig's disease (amyotrophic lateral sclerosis), the court squarely rested its decision on both theories in upholding Mr. Perlmutter's request to be removed from the ventilator.

In relation to the refusal of life-sustaining treatment, the courts have been careful not to equate suicide with refusal of treatment.

In another important case, *Bouvia v. Superior Court (Glenchur)*,[154] the California Court of Appeals distinguished suicide from the patient's refusal to accept artificial food and hydration and forced spoon feeding as her resignation to accept an earlier death rather than accept forced feeding.[155] Ms. Bouvia was a patient whose disease—cerebral palsy—did not affect her decision-making capacity. The court upheld her refusal, stating that the right to terminate one's life is based on the right of privacy.[156] It is important to note that, unlike Mr. Perlmutter and many others involved in the right-to-die cases, she was not terminally ill.

Like courts that distinguish between suicide and the right to refuse life-sustaining treatment, most state legislatures have made this demarcation clear. Advance directive legislation in most states contains a provision clearly stating that the refusal of any treatment, including life-sustaining treatment, is not considered suicide. Furthermore, the legislation often contains a clear disclaimer that the state does not condone or support suicide.

Assisted Suicide

Assisted suicide is inducing, aiding, or forcing another to commit suicide.[157] In all American jurisdictions, if an individual forcibly or under conditions of duress causes another to kill himself or herself, a charge of murder would be brought against the individual.[158] Moreover, even if the deceased asked a person for help in achieving death for any reason, including a desire to end suffering from an illness or injury, a charge of murder would most probably be brought against that person.[159,160]

In the health care arena, if one accepts the premise that refusing life-sustaining treatment is not suicide, then it follows that if a health care provider adheres to a patient's oral or written request to refuse treatment or have certain treatment withdrawn, there can be no liability for assisted suicide, so long as the provider does not overstep the patient's requests. This conclusion was not initially clear, however, and many of the initial right-to-die cases focused on the liability issues for physicians, nurses, and health care institutions if care was withdrawn or withheld.[161] The result of the early decisions clearly articulated the principle that health care providers, institutions, and ethics committees would not be liable for assisting suicide.[162]

That principle was again affirmed in the *Bouvia* case discussed above. The court clearly held that a health care provider's presence (when a patient exercises his or her constitutional right of refusing life-sustaining treatment) is not the same as "affirmative assertive, proximate, direct conduct such as providing a gun, poison or . . . another instrumentality" that the person uses to "inflict injury upon himself."[163]

Most advance directive legislation also protects health care providers who "in good faith" abide by a patient's advance directive. The protection lies in immunity from criminal, civil, or disciplinary actions brought by others challenging the decision or actions of the health care practitioner or institution.

Health Care Provider–Assisted Suicide

In rare situations, the protection against liability for assisted suicide may not apply to actions of a health care provider. A health care provider may be liable for overstepping his or her role when a patient exercises the constitutional right to refuse life-sustaining treatment. This is especially so when the health care provider's conduct receives national attention.

The issue of health care provider–assisted suicide is not new, at least in the world arena. In the Netherlands and Germany, for example, suicide assisted by physicians is firmly planted in the respective countries' cultures.[164] It was not until recently, however, that this issue was openly dealt with in the United States.

> *It was not until recently, however, that [assisted suicide] was openly dealt with in the United States.*

Commentaries on the topic of assisted suicide existed prior to 1988.[165] It was not until 1988 that consistent media coverage began on the issue when the article "It's Over, Debbie"[166] appeared in the *Journal of the American Medical Association*. In March of 1990, another article, by Dr. Timothy Quill, openly discussed how he aided a young cancer patient to die by prescribing a lethal dose of barbiturates at her request, so she could take them and end her suffering.[167]

Health care provider–assisted suicide was catapulted into the national spotlight in the United States in 1990. Dr. Jack Kevorkian, a University of Michigan medical school graduate with a specialty in pathology, aided 54-year-old Janet Adkins achieve her death with his homemade "suicide machine." Suffering from Alzheimer's disease, she traveled to Royal Oak, Michigan, from her home in Portland, Oregon, with her husband and several friends to effectuate her death. Before she died, she reportedly wrote a suicide note stating that the decision was freely entered into because she did not want her disease to progress any further.[168]

After Ms. Adkins' death, Kevorkian, who became known as "Doctor Death," continued to help more than 130 people achieve death.[169] Despite continuing legal and ethical challenges to his conduct, including the summary revocation of his Michigan license to practice medicine, the suspension of his medical license in California, five unsuccessful criminal and civil trials or charges alleging a violation of Michigan's assisted suicide law and its common law, Kevorkian remained undaunted in his self-proclaimed quest to make health care provider–assisted suicide acceptable to society.[170]

On November 22, 1998, Kevorkian's quest began to end. Kevorkian videotaped himself giving a lethal injection to 52-year-old Thomas Youk, who suffered from Lou Gehrig's disease. Kevorkian then contacted CBS's *60 Minutes* and it showed the tape on national TV. On November 25, 1998, Michigan charged Kevorkian with first-degree murder, violating the assisted suicide law (a second law outlawing physician-assisted suicide went into effect in the fall of 1998), and the delivery of a controlled substance without a license in the death of Youk.[171]

Although the Michigan prosecutors dropped the assisted suicide charge as a "tactical" move to prevent Kevorkian from presenting evidence on the pain and suffering of Youk,[172] the first murder trial against him resulted in a conviction of second-degree murder and the delivery of a controlled substance without a license. Kevorkian represented himself in the trial. He was sentenced to 10 to 25 years in prison for the murder of Youk and 3 to 7 years for the delivery of a controlled substance.[173] The sentences are to run concurrently. Kevorkian must serve a minimum of 6 years, 8 months in prison before becoming eligible for parole.[174]

Kevorkian's conviction will certainly not end the debate surrounding health care provider–assisted suicide. Proponents and opponents alike staunchly try to ensure their viewpoints are adopted by society as a whole. In fact, while the Kevorkian drama was being played out, other developments—the U.S. Supreme Court decisions in *Washington v. Glucksberg*[175] and its companion case, *Vacco v. Quill*,[176] and the state of Oregon's residents voting to uphold its state's assisted suicide law—provided strength to both the support and opposition respectively to health care provider–assisted suicide.

Three states set the stage for determining the legality of legislative prohibition or support of physician-assisted suicide. Two of the states, Washington and New York, sought clarification of their respective state laws banning physician-assisted suicide. Both state statutes made it a crime to assist a person to commit suicide. In the third state, Oregon, the question of support of a state law *allowing* physician-assisted suicide was at issue.

The first physician-assisted suicide case was decided *en banc* by the Ninth Circuit Court of Appeals in *Compassion in Dying v. Washington State*.[177] Among other rulings, the court held that Washington's ban on assisted suicide was unconstitutional as applied to terminally ill, competent patients who ask physicians for help in ending their lives with dignity.[178] The court rested its decision on the constitutional liberty interest those patients have in determining the time and manner of their own death.[179] The court also held that some state regulation of assisted suicide might be constitutional, especially where state interests outweigh the exercise of the right (e.g., avoiding undue influence).

In New York State, the Second Circuit Court of Appeals held that a lower district court erred in upholding the New York law banning assisted suicide.[180] Prohibiting the right of physicians to assist mentally competent, terminally ill patients with death is unconstitutional according to the court.[181] The *Quill v. Vacco* decision was based upon the constitutional right of equal protection found in the Fourteenth Amendment and state and statutory law recognizing an individual's right to hasten one's own death.[182]

Both the *Washington* and *Vacco* cases were appealed to the U.S. Supreme Court. The Court agreed to hear both cases and rendered its decision in *Washington* and *Vacco* on the same day in separate opinions. Both opinions detail analyses of applicable prior decisions (e.g., *Cruzan* and *Casey*), suicide, and applicable constitutional principles. The Court essentially ruled that there was no constitutional right of assisted suicide, and held that states were free to decide how, if at all, physician/health care provider–assisted suicide would be regulated.[183] Both decisions initiated a plethora of discussions, commentaries, and arguments concerning the scope and ramifications of the decisions.[184]

Case law, like *Vacco* and *Washington*, certainly had an impact upon the second major area of development surrounding health care provider–assisted suicide—that of "voter initiatives" to legalize physician-assisted suicide.[185] Although such initiatives had begun in the early 1990s,[186] the state of Oregon's Death with Dignity Act[187] received a great deal of national attention, especially because Oregon is in the Ninth Circuit, whose Court of Appeals had a pivotal role in the *Washington* case.

The Death with Dignity Act allows physicians to *assist* death under very limited circumstances. As examples, a person seeking assisted suicide under the act must be an Oregon resident, over 18 years of age, "capable," and suffering from a terminal disease that will lead to death within 6 months.[188] The person must make several requests for the assistance—one written and two oral—by requesting medications to take himself or herself to end life.[189] The request for self-administered medications to end life must be an "informed" one.[190] In addition, a physician other than the one to whom a request for assistance is directed must confirm that the individual is voluntarily making the choice, has decision-making capacity, and is indeed terminally ill.[191] Waiting periods and the requirement of family notification are also included in the Act.[192]

The Death with Dignity Act did not go into effect initially. A case, *Lee v. Oregon*,[193] was filed in federal district court in Oregon seeking an injunction against the law going into effect because it violated, among other things, due process and equal protection guarantees under the U.S. Constitution. A preliminary injunction was granted by the federal district court but was reversed by the Ninth Circuit Court of Appeals,[194] The U.S. Supreme Court denied an appeal.[195]

During the pendency of the litigation surrounding the act, the Oregon legislature permitted the voters of Oregon to decide if they wanted to repeal the Act in 1997.[196] The repeal failed by a 60% to 40% margin, and in late 1997 the Act finally went into effect.[197]

The Act was amended in 1999, and those amendments are seen more as "clarifying" language in the original Act than adding additional substantive provisions.[198] Some of the amendments include adding factors which "demonstrate Oregon residence" (e.g., Oregon driver's license, registration to vote in Oregon), including pharmacists within the act's definition of *health care provider,* and expanding its immunity provisions.[199]

Although the law took effect, the Act was still subjected to legal challenges. One interesting challenge occurred on the federal level when the director of the U.S. Drug Enforcement Administration ruled that it would prosecute physicians or revoke their DEA registration if they prescribed narcotics for use in assisted suicide situations because it would violate the federal Controlled Substance Act for any physician, including Oregon physicians, to dispense controlled substances for that purpose.[200] Because the director had not issued this ruling in accordance with proper administrative procedures, Attorney General Janet Reno investigated the ruling and the purpose of the Controlled Substance Act (to prevent trafficking in illegal drugs and to prevent the abuse of legitimate drugs). She determined that the federal Controlled Substance Act did not support a ban on their use for an approved medical purpose.[201]

The legal and ethical debate over health practitioner–assisted suicide will continue, as perhaps it should, openly and analytically.[202] Despite the discomfort of such controversy, many believe it is better to deal with the issue openly rather than in a clandestine manner, which had been the case prior to 1988.

Death and Dying in Correctional Facilities

Individuals incarcerated in U.S. jails and prisons will reach 2 million by the end of the year 2000.[203] Regardless of the reasons for which they were incarcerated, inmates are not immune to health problems, including AIDS, mental illness, and tuberculosis.[204] Nor are they immune to the process of dying and end-of-life issues.[205]

End-of-life issues are more difficult to acknowledge and positively respond to in prison and jail settings, however, because of the systems' emphasis on "security and detention," the lack of

ETHICS CONNECTION 13–1

Although arguments in support of and against assisted suicide both cite the moral principle of autonomy as ethical rationale for their respective positions, Safranek argues that in both instances, an appeal to autonomy is flawed. He contends "The debate involving assisted suicide, like so many other social disputes, hinges on discrepant views of the good, rather than on autonomy or beneficence. Only by focusing on the conflicting views of the goods at stake—and abandoning or reformulating the argument for autonomy—will ethicists and legal scholars resolve this controversial issue.[1]

Despite disagreement about the morality of assisted suicide, the Oregon Death with Dignity Act[2] legally sanctioned physician-assisted suicide. Although many health care professionals, including nurses, physicians, and pharmacists, opposed the law, it was passed and organizations sought to develop guidelines for complying with the law. The law addressed only the role of physicians; it included no guidelines for nurses, pharmacists, or others. Therefore, the Oregon Nurses Association requested specific standards so that nurses would have some practice guidelines in order to avoid disciplinary action. One year following the effective date of the legislation, several reports of the response to the law were presented, including an article in the *New England Journal of Medicine*.[3] The Oregon Health Division (OHD) published a report that contends "assisted suicide is being carried out successfully under the state's Death with Dignity Act."[4] The report itself has been criticized for drawing conclusions from limited data and for its unfounded assertion that patients who requested physician-assisted suicide had been receiving adequate end-of-life care. An audiotaped interview made by a physician several days before his patient's death seems to refute the contention that adequate care was received. The patient, who was a woman in her mid-80s, had metastatic breast cancer and was in a hospice program. She did not seem to know, however, that she had the right to refuse unwanted treatments. She said, "I've seen people suffer, they give them artificial feeding and stuff, which is really not doing anything for them in the long run." The physician did not respond to this statement, but proceeded to ask her how she felt about the forthcoming assisted suicide.[5]

Proponents of assisted suicide tend to use autonomy-based arguments. Opponents of assisted suicide take the position that dying persons choose assisted suicide because they fear suffering, pain, abandonment, or being a burden for their families. If people had appropriate and adequate care during their dying, the argument goes, they probably would not choose physician-assisted suicide. The American Nurses Association opposes assisted suicide and has joined with several other organizations to influence assisted suicide legislation and policy.

Ethical distinctions are made between assisted suicide and pain management that may hasten death. It is permissible within the *Code for Nurses: With Interpretive Statements*[6] for nurses to administer medications intended to manage pain that also inhibit respirations. Pain management is a critically important end-of-life practice that is especially relevant for nurses. Nurses are skilled in pain management and know that it is considered morally reprehensible for nurses to allow dying patients to be in pain when such pain is avoidable, even at the cost of a hastened death. This process of pain management differs from assisted suicide, as does euthanasia.[7, 8]

[1]John P. Safranek, "Autonomy and Assisted Suicide: The Execution of Freedon," 28(4) *Hastings Center Report* (July/August 1998), 32–36.

[2]Joan Woolfrey, "What Happens Now? Oregon and Physician-Assisted Suicide," 28(3) *Hastings Center Report* (May/June 1998), 9–17.

[3]Arthur Eugene Chin, Katrina Hedberg, Grant K. Higginson, and David W. Fleming, "Legalized Physician-Assisted Suicide in Oregon—The First Year's Experience," 340 *New England Journal of Medicine* (1999), 577–583.

[4]Kathleen Foley and Herbert Hendin, "The Oregon Report: Don't Ask, Don't Tell," 29(3) *Hastings Center Report* (May/June 1999), 37–42.

[5]*Id.*

[6]American Nurses Association. *Code for Nurses: With Interpretive Statements.* Kansas City, Missouri: Author, 1985.

[7]Nicholas Dixon, "On the Difference between Physician-Assisted Suicide and Active Euthanasia," 28(5) *Hastings Center Report* (September/October 1998), 25–29.

[8]Hastings Center, "From the Editor," 28(5) *Hastings Center Report* (September/October 1998), 3–5.

public compassion for end-of-life care for inmates, lack of funds to provide adequate care and clinical resources, and the difficulty of providing discharge planning or medical leave for many in the prison population.[206]

Superimposed upon all of these conflicting issues is the constitutional requirement guaranteed by the Eighth Amendment and the Due Process Clause of the Fourteenth Amendment that a basic level of health care must be provided to all prisoners (discussed at length in Chapter 7). Although an important right, the parameters of its enforcement are limited because of the inmate's dependence on a correctional institution for that care.[207]

End-of-life concerns in correctional facilities is increasing in importance because of two main factors: the prevalence of HIV infection in prison populations and tougher sentencing laws requiring longer prison sentences.[208] Unfortunately, data concerning how terminally ill prisoners are treated in correctional facilities are difficult to obtain because most facilities do not keep complete data on the placement and care of terminally ill prisoners.[209]

Despite these and other difficulties in identifying, treating, and evaluating care given to terminally ill prisoners, "palliative care" to dying prisoners is occurring in the United States. A 1998 study by the National Institute of Corrections Information Center identified that 12 correctional agencies of the 53 surveyed established "formal" hospice programs in their respective facilities, 8 were developing formal programs, 12 were considering the establishment of "hospice care," and at least 9 other correctional facilities offered some form of palliative care "outside a formal hospice setting."[210] States in which formal hospice programs are available in state facilities or in U.S. Bureau of Prisons facilities include California, Colorado, Illinois, North Dakota, Louisiana, and Pennsylvania.[211]

All of the 12 formal hospice programs surveyed had passed specific policies and procedures to guide prison staff when working with the terminally ill prisoner. Admission procedures, special privileges, housing options, and do-not-resuscitate orders were most often included in the adopted policies and procedures.[212]

Pronouncement of Death

Traditionally death has been determined by the patient's physician or, in cases of a death occurring outside of a hospital situation or under suspicious circumstances, a coroner. Nurses have also begun to take over this task, albeit in some instances in limited circumstances.

Governed by state law, nurses in long-term care, a home health care agency, a hospice, and, in some instances, a hospital are given the authority to pronounce an individual dead, especially in situations when death is expected.[213] Even so, it is still usually required that the physician sign the

---

ETHICS CONNECTION 13–2

The role of nurses in correctional facilities has expanded in recent years, becoming a specialized area of practice. Nurses who are employed in correctional facilities realize that they have opportunities to provide health care to a traditionally underserved community. Ethical issues of caring for prisoners have not been extensively addressed. Health care usually is concerned with distributive justice, the allocation and distribution of health care resources. The criminal justice system focuses on compensatory and retributive justice. Although it is possible to argue for limits on services to prisoners because of the harm they purportedly have done to others, such arguments are not sustainable from the perspective of ethics of care and covenantal relationships. Proponents of providing care to imprisoned individuals argue that many people have been incarcerated because they did not have the financial resources for the same quality of defense that others have had. African-Americans, in particular, are disproportionately represented in urban correctional facilities.

In caring for individuals who are imprisoned, it is important for the nurse to differentiate his or her emotional responses from ethical positions. There may be emotional reasons why nurses cannot attend prisoners who are dying. From a moral perspective, however, dying prisoners are members of the inclusive covenant to which all humans belong and are to be afforded competent, humane care at the end of life. Schools of nursing are beginning to offer student clinical practicum experiences in correctional facilities so that students can learn how to provide care to persons whose liberty interests have been restricted by imprisonment.

---

death certificate.[214] New Jersey, Connecticut, New Hampshire, Massachusetts, Georgia, Hawaii, and Alaska have authorized nurses in long-term care to declare specific patients dead.

As this legal role continues to develop, it may become more commonplace, especially for nurses who function in more independent, advanced practice. For example, South Dakota specifically grants this power to nurse practitioners.

NURSING IMPLICATIONS

The nurse working with patients who are dying must take into account all of the legal and ethical ramifications associated with their care. For example, it is important that a do-not-resuscitate order

ETHICS CONNECTION 13-3

Dying is the one thing in life that is done alone. It is the common connection among all human beings. Yet, North American societal values typically deny human mortality, and health care practices treat disease and death as the enemy. It is morbidity and mortality rates that are counted, not caring, healing, and peaceful dying. Until recently, end-of-life issues focused on limiting treatment. In managed care systems, there has been a subtle shift away from limiting treatment toward patients' or family members' insisting on providing treatment that may be medically futile. Nurses are well positioned to work with clients and families to show them how to be present with their dying family member without resorting to invasive or futile treatments. Nurses currently are concerned with how to provide comfort care and be present for dying patients and their families when cure-oriented treatment has ceased. They are working to recover their skills of providing competent, compassionate care to those who are dying. There is a national interdisciplinary initiative to improve education of health care professionals regarding hospice and palliative care.

Respect for autonomy is one of the most important moral principles that concern nurses and their clients at the end of life. Several studies of preferences of nursing home residents about their end-of-life treatments revealed that although nearly a third had discussed their preferences with family members, only 12% had talked about their treatment preferences with their health care providers.[1,2] Regardless of the age of the dying person or whether the person is dying at home or in an institution, morally responsible nursing practice includes providing comfort and initiating discussions about what is important to the person who is dying and to his or her family. With the increased attention to spirituality in health care as a counterpoint to the domination of science and technology, supporting patients' religious practices and understanding their beliefs about suffering are important.[3,4]

[1]Anonymous, "Most Nursing Home Residents Prefer Life-sustaining Treatments, but Do Not Discuss This Topic with Caregivers," 193 *Research Activities* (May 1996), 5.

[2]Anonymous, "Nursing Home Residents and Their Families Often Have Little Input into End-of-Life Medical Decisions," 223 *Research Activities* (January/February 1999), 18–19.

[3]David B. McCurdy, "Religion and Spirituality in the Clinical Setting: Ethical Challenges and Opportunities," 32 *Insights* (Winter 1999), 2–10 (Ethics Newsletter of Mercy Health Systems of Chicago, Illinois.)

[4]Stan Van Hoof, "The Meaning of Suffering," 28(5) *Hastings Center Report* (September/October 1998), 13–19.

be obtained consistent with the institution or agency policy. Under no circumstances should a nurse accept and carry out a do-not-resuscitate order that is not consistent with policy. Rather, the nurse should inform the nurse manager of a request to do so inconsistent with the policy. Also, the nurse must be clear that, unless a contradictory order exists, the do-not-resuscitate patient must be given all other nursing care that is not refused. Studies have shown that nurses believe all other care can—and should—be provided; in fact, they do provide that care consistent with the patient's or surrogate/proxy decision maker's decisions.[215] Family members and others should be reassured by the nurse that other care will not be neglected for the do-not-resuscitate patient.

The nurse working with patients who are dying must take into account all of the legal and ethical ramifications associated with their care.

The nurse should be ever vigilant about ensuring that any decision to withhold or withdraw treatment is made with the patient's, or the legally recognized surrogate/proxy's, informed refusal. If the nurse determines that informed refusal has not been obtained, the nurse should contact the nurse manager. Furthermore, the situation may be one that needs to be brought before the institution's ethics committee or nursing ethics committee.

When patient care disagreements surrounding pain management arise, whether the nurse works in a hospice or an acute care setting, he or she should raise the disagreement through the established institutional avenues.[216] Under no circumstances should the nurse decide to "take matters into his or her own hands" and alter medication doses or orders or initiate the administration of new medications. In addition, the personal storage of medications, especially controlled substances, in violation of the agency or facility policy is not recommended.

The nurse working with minors has additional concerns, especially if the older or mature minor refuses treatment that has been consented to by the parent(s). The physician and nurse manager should be contacted immediately. Furthermore, if the minor's treatment wishes conflict with the parent's treatment decisions, the physician and nursing administration again must be notified.

The nurse may be subpoenaed to testify in court if a treatment situation involving a minor or other patient has not been resolved through other routes. The nurse should contact the risk management department of the facility and also seek legal advice (from the institution's attorney and/or his or her own attorney) before responding to the subpoena in any way.

If the nurse in the neonatal intensive care unit is faced with refusal of treatment because of the presence of a disability, and none of the exceptions discussed in the Federal Child Abuse Amendments apply, the nurse should seek legal advice concerning her responsibilities in that situation. At issue, of course, is whether the nurse would be required to report that situation under the state's child abuse laws. Another way of handling the situation would be to bring the issue before the institutional review committee or other ethics group, if possible.

Insofar as assisted suicide is concerned, the nurse would need to carefully evaluate his or her participation in an assisted suicide. A complete understanding of state criminal and civil law is vital, as are the ethical and professional issues assisted suicide raises.[217] It is important, however, that the nurse be active in raising the issue generally in nursing ethics committees, team meetings, and with other nurse colleagues to establish open channels of communication concerning the matter.[218] Keeping abreast of the latest legislative developments in his or her own state and other states is also important.

If the nurse works in Oregon, or a state in which assisted suicide is permitted through legislation, the nurse will need to comply strictly with the assisted suicide statute. For example, Oregon's law does not permit the physician to terminate a patient's life through lethal injection, mercy killing, or active euthanasia.[219] As a result, the physician—or any future health care provider to whom the Act applies, if it is amended—must ensure that the patient "remains in control of the decision, timing, and every aspect" of the self-administration of the medication prescribed for suicide.[220] Accurate and complete documentation in the individual's medical record consistent with any statutory mandates is absolutely vital to support the health care provider's actions and, at the same time, support the patient's decision.

Whether the nurse works in a state that has assisted suicide legislation or works where the issue has not yet been legislated, research and evaluation of the benefits and drawbacks of assisted suicide and the health care provider's role, including that of the nurse, will be necessary. For example, preliminary data about assisted suicide under the Oregon statute indicate that in the first year of its existence, 15 terminally ill people used it to end their lives.[221] Thirteen of the 15 individuals who took legal prescriptive medications were cancer patients, and the average age of those who took their lives was 60.[222] In addition, it appears that those who sought to end their lives under the Act did not suffer painful or lingering deaths. Moreover, those who used their right to assisted suicide did so because of their desire to exercise some control over the way they died rather than take an "easy way out" of financial difficulties or extreme pain.[223]

Despite these initial, favorable findings, additional data on health care provider–assisted suicide are needed. Other research and data arguably contradict the positive results under the Oregon statute.[224] Moreover, the effect upon health care providers who have a role in health care provider–assisted suicide must be carefully scrutinized.[225]

Nurses in correctional facilities must work within the system to establish end-of-life care for dying prisoners. The establishment of palliative care in such settings requires the nurse to be creative in using existing facilities or, if possible, in seeking new physical surroundings for hospice care. Educating and training all staff who will be working with the dying patient is necessary due to the "team approach" in the provision of such care.[226] Providing services to the families of dying prisoners, including counseling on death and dying issues, referrals to community resources, and assistance with funeral arrangements, is also essential.[227]

If the nurse practices in a state where he or she can pronounce patients dead, the nurse should do so consistent with the state law granting that authority. The notification of required individuals should also occur.

Last, but by no means least, nurses need to have systematic support as they work with patients like Nancy Cruzan, Baby Doe, and others who are struggling with the issues surrounding the dying process. Working with the dying is often very rewarding but it can also be emotionally overwhelming. Providing support for nurses who care for patients at the end of life cannot be overlooked.

DOCUMENTATION REMINDER 13–2
Special Considerations

- Document completely and accurately any and all medical orders for withdrawing or withholding treatment, including do-not-resuscitate orders, doing so consistent with facility policy

- If do-not-resuscitate order given inconsistent with facility policy, document who notified and file incident report

- Utilize proper forms when requesting any and all medical supplies, including medications and controlled substances

- If controlled substances or other medications not obtained from pharmacy, contact nursing administration and file incident report

- Any and all telephone or other requests for changes in medications

- Any and all orders given for changes in medications, especially controlled substances

- Any and all contacts, discussions, and the like with pharmacy, physician, nursing management

- Utilize required reporting forms when reporting child abuse/neglect pursuant to state law and when working in a state where assisted suicide legislation requires the use of specific forms

- Accurate and complete entry concerning mandated report; incidents with family or others concerning withdrawal or withholding of treatment; results of reporting; presentation before ethics committee

- Accurate and complete entry concerning pronouncement of death following state law mandates

---

SUMMARY OF PRINCIPLES
AND APPLICATIONS

The issues surrounding death and dying will probably never be fully resolved. Just as one particular issue is met with perhaps some "comfort," another begins to create discomfort, discord, and introspection. As uncomfortable as those feelings may be, health care and its practitioners, including nurses, cannot shy away from meeting the innumerable issues that will continue to be raised by the refusal of life-sustaining treatment. Credit should be given to those individuals who, in their role as patients, demanded that health care and society as a whole wrestle with those issues head on.

Nurses, then, can continue to grapple with issues in death and dying by:

- Understanding the various legal and clinical terms associated with death and dying, including brain death, suicide, and euthanasia

- Comparing and contrasting the many ethical and legal issues surrounding decisions to withhold or withdraw life-sustaining medical care

- Keeping abreast of the legislative and case law development concerning refusal of treatment

- Comparing and contrasting an adult's right to refuse life-sustaining treatment with that of a minor (or the parents of a minor)

- Carefully evaluating the differences, if any, between refusal of life-sustaining treatment and health care practitioner–assisted suicide

- Firmly identifying and articulating one's own values and beliefs concerning refusal of life-sustaining treatment

- Protecting those who cannot protect themselves—the disabled newborn, minor, or "incompetent" adult—when the need exists (lack of informed input into treatment decisions or conflict surrounding treatment decisions, for example) by notifying appropriate individuals and organizations

- Aiding patients and families in obtaining necessary information to make reasoned, informed decisions concerning medical treatment

- Complying with the law when a treatment situation requires it (mandatory reporting, testifying at a trial or hearing)

- Actively participating on institutional committees that explore issues in death and dying (institutional review, ethics, or nursing ethics committees)

- Testifying at hearings when legislative changes are proposed concerning the right to refuse life-sustaining treatment

- Understanding that the right to refuse life-sustaining treatment is not absolute but may be balanced against particular state interests

- Striving to keep open lines of communication between and among nursing and other medical colleagues, the family, and the patient

- Supporting, and participating in, research involving identified[228] or new issues surrounding the dying process[229]

TOPICS FOR FURTHER INQUIRY

1. Compare and contrast the nursing profession's positions on assisted suicide with those of other health care professions, including medicine and social work. Identify and analyze any similarities and differences. Suggest reasons for any similarities and differences, including an evaluation of the historical development of the profession and an evaluation of changes, if any, of the ethical principles upon which the positions are based.

2. Develop a model institutional policy for use in a particular health care delivery system concerning a nursing ethics committee. Include its purpose, composition, and how the committee will function, especially if another ethics committee already exists.

3. Research your state law on the reporting of abuse or neglect of minors involving the parents' refusal of treatment or the withdrawal of treatment that is considered lifesaving. Determine how many cases were successful, how many were dismissed, and how many went to a hearing or trial. Suggest ways in which the system for reporting such alleged situations can be improved or changed.

4. Develop a questionnaire interview tool to evaluate nurses' attitudes about refusal of life-sustaining treatment or assisted suicide. If possible, include a nurse or nurses who work in correctional facilities in the sample. Include questions such as how the nurse would react in a given situation and the basis for his or her actions; when the belief or beliefs about the topic were formed by the nurse; and how the nurse sees nursing roles in the topic under investigation. After the data are analyzed, present the findings at a nursing meeting or publish the results in a nursing journal.

REFERENCES

1. Alan Meisel. *The Right to Die*. Volume 1. 2nd Edition. New York: John Wiley & Sons, 1995, 16 (with 2000 cumulative supplement).
2. *Id.* at 5.
3. Henry Campbell Black. *Black's Law Dictionary*. 7th Edition. St. Paul, Minn.: West Group, 1999, 937.
4. *Id.*
5. Meisel, *supra* note 1, Volume 1 at 56–61.

6. 549 N.E.2d 292 (Ill. 1989).
7. 517 A.2d 886 (N.J. Super. 1986), *aff'd*, 517 A.2d 869 (N.J. Super. A.D. 1986).
8. 544 N.Y.S.2d 840 (N.Y. App. Div. 1989).
9. Theodore R. LeBlang, W. Eugene Basanta, and Robert Kane. *The Law of Medical Practice in Illinois*. Volume 2. 2nd Edition. St. Paul, Minn.: West Group, 1996, 638–639 (with 1998 supplement).
10. *Id., citing* Brown, "Fluosol-DA, a Perfluorochemical Oxygen-Transport Fluid for the Management of a Trochanteric Pressure Sore in a Jehovah's Witness," 12 *Annals of Plastic Surgery* (1984), 449.
11. *Id.*
12. *Id.* at 639 (citations omitted).
13. 294 A.2d 372 (D.C. App. 1972).
14. Meisel, *supra* note 1, Volume 2, at 285, *citing Heinemann's Appeal*, 96 Pa. 112 (1880). In this case, the father's custody of his children was terminated and the children given to the grandmother because he had refused to call a physician for needed medical care.
15. Meisel, *supra* note 1, Volume 2, at 290–291.
16. *Id.* at 292.
17. *Id.* at 290–291.
18. *Id.* at 283–284, *citing Wisconsin v. Yoder*, 406 U.S. 205 (1972); *Pierce v. Society of Sisters*, 268 U.S. 510 (1925); *Meyer v. Nebraska*, 262 U.S. 390 (1923).
19. *Wisconsin v. Yoder*, 406 U.S. 205 (1972).
20. Meisel, *supra* note 1, Volume 1, at 69.
21. *Id.*, Volume 2, 293–297.
22. See, for example, *In re Swan*, 569 A.2d 1202 (Me. 1990); *In re Beth*, 587 N.E.2d 1377 (Mass. 1992); Key Case 13–4.
23. Meisel, *supra* note 1, Volume 1, at 341–464. See also Thomas Hafemeister and Paula Hannaford. *Resolving Disputes Over Life-Sustaining Treatment: A Health Care Provider's Guide*. Williamsburg, Va.: National Center for State Courts, 1996.
24. *Bonner v. Moran*, 126 F.2d 121 (App. D.C. 1941).
25. 355 A.2d 647 (N.J. 1976), *cert. denied sub nom. Garger v. New Jersey*, 429 U.S. 922 (1976), *modifying and remanding*, 348 A.2d 801 (N.J. Sup. Ct. Ch. Div. 1975).
26. Meisel, *supra* note 1, Volume 1, at 343–347.
27. *In re Quinlan*, 355 A.2d 647, 671–672 (N.J. 1976).
28. Margo Zink and Linda Titus, "Nursing Ethics Committees: Do We Need Them?" in *Current Issues in Nursing*. Joanne Comi McClaskey and Helen Kennedy Grace, Editors. 5th Edition. St. Louis, Mo.: Mosby, 1997, 640.
29. Bowen Husford. *Bioethics Committees: The Health Care Provider's Guide*. Rockville, Md.: Aspen Publishers, 1986, 70.
30. *Id.* at 71.
31. 497 U.S. 261 (1990).
32. See, for example, "*Cruzan*: Clear and Convincing?" 20(5) *Hastings Center Report* (September/October 1990), 5–12 (a series of articles dealing with the decision); Alexander Capron, Guest Editor, "Medical Decision-Making and the 'Right-to-Die' After *Cruzan*," 19(1-2) *Law, Medicine & Health Care* (Spring, Summer 1991) (the entire edition includes reactions to the Supreme Court decision); Mila Ann Aroskar, "The Aftermath of the *Cruzan* Decision: Dying in a Twilight Zone," 38(6) *Nursing Outlook* (November/December 1990), 256–257; Mary Hansen, "Com-

parison of *Quinlan* and *Cruzan* Decisions," 23(4) *Nursing Management* (April 1992), 40–41.

33. James Bopp and Thomas Marzen, "*Cruzan:* Facing the Inevitable," 19(1-2) *Law, Medicine & Health Care* (Spring, Summer 1991), 37–51; Larry Gostin, "Life and Death Choices after *Cruzan*," *id.*, 9–12; William Colby, "Missouri Stands Alone," 20(5) *Hastings Center Report* (September/October 1990), 5–6; Charles Baron, "On Taking Substituted Judgment Seriously," *id.*, 7–8.

34. *Cruzan v. Mouton*, Estate No. CV 384-9P (Cir. Ct. Jasper County, Mo. December 14, 1990).

35. *New York Times*, December 27, 1990, A9 (National Edition).

36. 579 N.E.2d 32 (Ind. 1991).

37. *Id.* at 38–41.

38. *Id.* at 41 (footnote 8).

39. Meisel, *supra* note 1, Volume 1, at 393–394.

40. *Id.* at 41–49.

41. *In re Busalacchi*, No. 59582, 1991 WL 26851, 1991 Mo. App. LEXIS 315 (March 5, 1991), *reh'g and/or transfer denied* (Mo. App. March 26, 1991), *cause ordered transferred to* Mo. Sup. Ct. (Mo. Ct. App. April 15, 1991), *appealed and remanded sub nom. Busalacchi v. Busalacchi*, No. 73677, 1991 Mo. LEXIS 107 (October 16, 1991), *appeal dismissed*, No. 73677, 1993 WL 32356 (Mo. January 26, 1993).

42. Meisel, *supra* note 1, Volume 1, at 132, *citing In re Busalacchi*, No. 59582, slip. op. at 3 (Mo. Ct. App. March 5, 1991).

43. "Father Regains Control in Right-to-Die Case," *Chicago Tribune*, February 20, 1993, Section 1, at 2.

44. Meisel, *supra* note 1, Volume 1, at 134, *citing* "Comatose Woman, Focus of Court Battle, Dies," *New York Times*, March 8, 1993, at A7 (National Edition).

45. See, for example, American Association of Colleges of Nursing, *Competencies Necessary for Nurses to Provide High-Quality Care to Patients and Families During the Transition at the End of Life*, reprinted in Betty Rolling Ferrel, "Caring at the End of Life," 25(4) *Reflections* (1999), 31–37, at 36.

46. American Nurses Association. *Position Statement on Promotion of Comfort and Relief of Pain in Dying Patients*. Kansas City, Mo.: Author, September 5, 1991. See also the special projects and research on pain and end-of-life care done by Betty Rolling Ferrel, RN, PhD, FAAN, including the establishment of a Pain Resource Center, in *Reflections, supra* note 45. The Center's Website is located at http://mayday.coh.org. Also helpful on the many facets of pain management is the symposium edition "Legal and Regulatory Issues in Pain Management," 26(4) *Journal of Law, Medicine & Ethics* (1998).

47. Zink and Titus, *supra* note 28, at 641, *citing* Diane Hoffmann, "Does Legislating Hospital Ethics Committees Make a Difference? A Study of Hospital Ethics Committees in Maryland, the District of Columbia, and Virginia," 19(1-2) *Law, Medicine & Health Care* (Spring, Summer 1991), 118–119.

48. Hoffman, *id.*

49. 321 S.E.2d 716 (Ga. 1984).

50. 569 A.2d 1202 (Me. 1990).

51. 534 A.2d 947 (Me. 1987).

52. Meisel, *supra* note 1, Volume 2, at 39.

53. *In re Chad Eric Swan, supra* note 50, at 1205.

54. *Id.*

55. Meisel, *supra* note 1, Volume 1, at 297–298.

56. Zink and Titus, *supra* note 28.

57. Robert Miller. *Problems in Health Care Law*. 7th Edition. Gaithersburg, Md.: Aspen Publishers, 1996, 506–507.

58. *Taber's Cyclopedic Medical Dictionary*. 16th Edition. Philadelphia, Pa.: F. A. Davis, 1989, 457–458.

59. Ad Hoc Committee, "A Definition of Irreversible Coma," 205 *JAMA* 337 (1968).

60. *Id.*

61. *Id.*

62. President's Commission. *Defining Death: Medical, Legal and Ethical Issues in the Determination of Death*. Washington, D.C.: U.S. Government Printing Office, 1981.

63. 12 Uniform Laws Annotated (U.L.A.) 412 (Supp. 1994).

64. Meisel, *supra* note 1, Volume 1, at 625.

65. *Id.* at 625.

66. *Id.* at 631, *citing Strachan v. John F. Kennedy Memorial Hospital*, 538 A.2d 346 (N.J. 1988).

67. Robert Truog, "Is It Time to Abandon Brain Death?" 27(1) *Hasting Center Report* (1997), 29–37.

68. *Id.* at 31, *citing* Stuart Younger and others, "Brain Death and Organ Retrieval: A Cross Sectional Survey of Knowledge and Concepts Among Health Professionals," 261(13) *JAMA* (1989), 2205–2210.

69. *Id.* at 33.

70. James Bernat, "A Defense of the Whole-Brain Concept of Death," 28(2) *Hastings Center Report* (1998), 14–23.

71. *Id.* at 21–22.

72. *Id.*

73. *Id.* at 22.

74. For interesting commentaries on this issue, see, as examples, Richard Gillion, "Persistent Vegetative State, Withdrawal of Artificial Nutrition and Hydration, and the Patient's 'Best Interests,'" 24(2) *Journal of Medical Ethics* (1998), 75–81; Mark R. Tonelli, "Substituted Judgement in Medical Practice: Evidentiary Standards on a Sliding Scale," 25(1) *Journal of Law, Medicine & Ethics* (1997), 22–29; Albert Fenwick, "Applying Best Interests Standard to Persistent Vegetative State—A Principled Distortion?" 24(3) *Journal of Medical Ethics* (1998), 86–89; John Oldershaw, Jeff Atkinson, and Louis Boshes, "Persistent Vegetative State: Medical, Ethical, Religious, Economic and Legal Perspectives," 1(3) *DePaul Journal of Health Care Law* (1997), 494–536.

75. President's Commission for the Study of Ethical Problems in Medicine and Biomedical and Behavioral Research, "Resuscitation Decisions for Hospitalized Patients," in *Deciding to Forego Life-Sustaining Treatment: Ethical, Medical and Legal Issues in Treatment Decisions*. Washington, D.C.: U.S. Government Printing Office, 1983, 231, *citing* 2 Kings 4:31–37 (New English).

76. *Id.* at 233, *citing* W. B. Kouwenhoven, J. R. Jude, and G. G. Knickerbocker, "Closed-Chest Cardiac Massage," 173 *JAMA* 1064 (1960).

77. *Id.* at 234.

78. National Conference on Standards for Cardiopulmonary Resuscitation and Emergency Cardiac Care, "Standards for Cardiopulmonary Resuscitation (CPR) and Emergency Cardiac Care (ECC)," 227 *JAMA* 837, 864 (1974).

79. 380 N.E.2d 134 (Mass. App. 1978).

80. President's Commission, *Deciding to Forego Life-Sustaining Treatment, supra* note 75, at 238, *citing* David Margolick, "Hospital Is Investigated on Life Support Policy," *New York Times,* June 20, 1982 at A/34.

81. *Id.* at 248–252; see also William Roach and the Aspen Health Law and Compliance Center. *Medical Records and the Law.* 3rd Edition. Gaithersburg, Md.: Aspen Publishers, 1998, 171–174; American Nurses Association. *Position Paper on Nursing Care and Do Not Resuscitate Decisions.* Washington, D.C.: Author, 1992.

82. N.Y. Public Health Law Article, 29-B, Section 2960 *et seq.* (1988); Ga. Code Ann. Sections 31-39-1 to -9 (1991); Mont. Code Ann. Sections 50-10-101 to -106 (1991); Tenn. Code Ann. Section 68-11-224 (1990).

83. Meisel, *supra* note 1, Volume 1, at 559–560.

84. Joint Commission on Accreditation of Healthcare Organizations. *1996 Accreditation Manual for Hospitals.* 1996. RI 1.d, RI 1.2.5, 1.2.6.

85. Meisel, *supra* note 1, Volume 1, at 554–555.

86. Meisel, *supra* note 1, Volume 2, at 532–533, *citing Dority v. Superior Court,* 193 Cal. Rptr. 288 (1983); *Alvarado v. New York City Health and Hospitals Corp.,* 547 N.Y.S.2d 190 (1989), *vacated and dismissed sub nom. Alvarado v. City of New York,* 550 N.Y.S.2d 353 (1990).

87. No. PX-91-283 (4th Dist. Ct. Hennepin County, Minn. July 1, 1991).

88. Ronald E. Cranford, "Helga Wanglie's Ventilator," 21(4) *Hastings Center Report* (July-August 1991), 23.

89. *Id.*

90. *Id.*

91. *Wanglie, supra* note 87, slip. op. at 5 (finding of fact #4), *reprinted in* 2 Biolaw (August-September 1991), U:2161.

92. Felicia Ackerman, "The Significance of a Wish," 21(4) *Hastings Center Report* (July-August 1991), 27.

93. Daniel Callahan, "Medical Futility, Medical Necessity: The Problem without a Name," 21(4) *Hastings Center Report* (July-August 1991), 30–35.

94. *New York Times,* July 6, 1991, 8, col. 1 (National Edition).

95. Meisel, *supra* note 1, Volume 2, at 533.

96. No. SUCV92-4820 (Super. Ct. Suffolk County, Mass., April 21, 1995 *as reported in* Meisel, *supra* note 1, Volume 2, at 533).

97. 16 Fiduc. Rep. 2d 181 (C.P. Dauphin County, Pa. 1995, *as reported in* Meisel, *supra* note 1, Volume 2, at 533).

98. LeBlang, Basanta, and Kane, *supra* note 9, Volume 1, at 418. See also Jane Adler, "Care Packages," *Chicago Tribune,* April 25, 1999, Section 16, 5.

99. *Id.*

100. Anthony Kovner and Steven Jonas. *Health Care Delivery in the United States.* 6th Edition. New York: Springer Publishing Company, 1999, 221–222.

101. *In the Matter of the Proposed Disciplinary Treatment of the Licenses of Mary Brackman, RN, Mary Mouat, RN, Debbie Ruggles, RN, Ruth Sasser, RN, Verna VanDuynhoven, RN, and Lynn Zavalney, RN,* Docket Nos cc-90-68-RN, cc-90-66 RN, cc-90-69 RN, cc-90-70-RN, cc-90-71-RN, cc-90-67, RN. Finding of Facts, Conclusions of Law and Final Order, 20–24, June 28, 1992.

102. *Id.* at 24–31.

103. *Id.* at 34–37.

104. "Montana's Hospice Six Raise Issue of 'Compassion'" *AJN* (August 1991), 65, 71 (news section).

105. *Brackman v. Board of Nursing,* 820 P.2d 1314 (Mont. 1991); 851 P.2d 1055 (Mont. 1993), *rehearing denied,* May 20, 1993.

106. *AJN, supra* note 104, *citing The Independent Record,* a Montana newspaper.

107. *Id.* at 65, *citing* Steven Shapiro, attorney for the Montana Department of Commerce, Professional and Occupational Licensing Bureau.

108. *Id.*

109. Meisel, *supra* note 1, Volume 1, at 589, *citing* Institute of Medicine. *Approaching Death: Improving Care at the End of Life.* Marilyn J. Field and Christine K. Cassel, Editors. Washington, D.C.: National Academy Press, 1997.

110. Meisel, *supra* note 1, Volume 1, at 590. As examples, Georgia and Nevada courts have held that medications for the relief of pain for palliative care is acceptable.

111. *Id.* at 591. States passing "intractable pain" statutes include Florida, Nevada, Ohio, Tennessee, and Virginia.

112. Meisel, *supra* note 1, Volume 1, at 589–592. See also *Board of Nursing v. Merkley,* 940 P.2d 144 (Nev. 1997) (nurse's employment terminated and license suspended in connection with the administration of morphine for pain relief); Sandra H. Johnson, "Disciplinary Actions and Pain Relief: Analysis of the Pain Relief Act," 24(4) *Journal of Law, Medicine & Ethics* (1996), 319–327; Robyn Shapiro, "Health Care Providers' Liability Exposure for Inappropriate Pain Management," 24(4) *Journal of Law, Medicine & Ethics* (1996), 360–364; Ann Alpers, "Criminal Act or Palliative Care? Prosecutions Involving the Care of the Dying," 26(4) *Journal of Law, Medicine & Ethics* (1998), 308–331.

113. See, as examples, Ann Martino, "In Search of a New Ethic for Treating Patients with Chronic Pain: What Can Medical Boards Do?" 26(4) *Journal of Law, Medicine & Ethics* (1996), 332–349; Glen Johnson, "Commentary: A Personal View on Palliative and Hospice Care in Correctional Facilities," (27)3 *Journal of Law, Medicine, & Ethics* (1999), 238–239; Edmund Pellegrino, "Emerging Ethical Issues in Palliative Care," 279(19) *JAMA* (1998), 1521–1522; Kathleen Foley, "A 44-Year-Old Woman with Severe Pain at the End of Life," 281(20) *JAMA* (1999), 1937–1944.

114. 292 A.2d 387 (Pa. 1972).

115. 307 A.2d 279 (Pa. 1973).

116. 549 N.E.2d 322 (Ill. 1989), *aff'd and rev'g* 515 N.E.2d 286 (Ill. App. Ct. 1987).

117. See, for example, *In re Baby K,* 832 F. Supp. 1022 (E.D. Va. 1993), *aff'd,* 16 F.3d 590 (4th Circ. 1994), *cert. denied,* 115 S.Ct. 91 (1994); Ellen Flannery, "One Advocate's Viewpoint: Conflicts and Tensions in the Baby K Case," 23(1) *Journal of Law, Medicine, & Ethics* (1995), 7–12; Mark Crossley, "Infants with Anencephaly, the ADA, and the Child Abuse Amendments," 11(4) *Issues in Law and Medicine* (1996), 379–389.

118. Joseph P. Kennedy, Jr. Foundation, West Hartford, Conn., 1971.

119. Raymond Duff and A.G.M. Campbell, "Moral and Ethical Dilemmas in the Special Care Nursery," 289 *New England Journal of Medicine* (1973), 890.

120. *Id.*

121. *Id.*

122. No. GU 8204-00 (Ind. Cir. Ct. Monroe County April 12, 1982), *writ of mandamus dismissed, sub nom. State ex rel. Infant Doe v. Baker,* No. 482 S 140 (Ind. May 27, 1982), *cert. denied,* 464 U.S. 96 (1983).

123. Meisel, *supra* note 1, at 308.

124. *Id.* at 309.

125. "Discrimination against the Handicapped by Withholding Treatment or Nourishment: Notice of (sic) Health Care Providers," 47 Fed. Reg. 26,027 (1982).

126. *Id.*

127. "Non-Discrimination on the Basis of Handicap," 48 Fed. Reg. 9630 (March 7, 1983).

128. *Id.* at 9631.

129. *Id.* at 9631–9632.

130. *American Academy of Pediatrics v. Heckler,* 561 F. Supp. 395 (D.D.C. 1983).

131. Margaret M. Mahon, "The Nurse's Role in Treatment Decisionmaking for the Child with Disabilities," 6(3) *Issues in Law & Medicine* (Winter 1990), 247, 254, *citing* 48 Fed. Reg. 30,846 (1983).

132. "Procedures Relating to Health Care for Handicapped Infants," 45 C.F.R. Section 84.55 *et seq.* (1989).

133. *American Hospital Ass'n v. Heckler,* 585 F. Supp. 541 (S.D.N.Y.), *aff'd,* 794 F.2d 676 (2d Cir. 1984), *aff'd sub nom. Bowen v. American Hospital Association,* 476 U.S. 610 (1986).

134. Pub. L. No. 98-457, 98 Stat. 1749, 42 U.S.C. Sections 5101–5107 (October 4, 1984).

135. Pub. L. No. 93-247, 88 Stat. 4 (1974).

136. 42 U.S.C. Section 5102(3); 42 C.F.R. Section 1340.15(b)(2) (1985). See, generally, 42 C.F.R. Section 1340 *et seq.* (1985) for additional definitions, objectives, and interpretive guidelines.

137. Meisel, *supra* note 1, Volume 1, at 320, *citing C.A. v. Morgan,* 603 N.E.2d 1171 (Ill. App. Ct. 1992) (Judge McMorrow, dissenting).

138. *Id., citing Stolle v. Baylor College of Medicine,* 981 S.W.2d 709 (Tex. Ct. App. 1998); *Branom v. State,* 974 P.2d 335 (Wash. Ct. App. 1999).

139. Black, *supra* note 3, at 575.

140. *Id.*

141. See, for example, Daniel Callahan, "Terminating Life-Sustaining Treatment of the Demented," 25(6) *Hastings Center Report* (1995), 25–31; Nicholas Dixon, "On the Difference Between Physician-Assisted Suicide and Active Euthanasia," 28(5) *Hastings Center Report* (1998), 25–29.

142. Meisel, *supra* note 1, at 452, 472.

143. Meisel, *supra* note 1, Volume 2, at 452, 472.

144. See, for example, *In re Estate of Greenspan,* 558 N.E.2d 1194 (Ill. 1990), *on remand* No. 88P8726 (Ill. Cir. Ct. Cook County, October 3, 1990); *L.W. v. L.E. Phillips Career Dev. Ctr.,* 482 N.W.2d 60 (Wis. 1992).

145. *Barber v. Superior Court,* 195 Cal. Rptr. 484 (Ct. App. 1983).

146. Black, *supra* note 3, at 575.

147. Meisel, *supra* note 1, Volume 2, at 515.

148. Black, *supra* note 3, at 1447.

149. Wayne LaFave and Austin Scott. *Criminal Law.* 2nd Edition. St. Paul, Minn.: West Group, 1986, 649 (with 1999 updates).

150. See, for example, *In re Farrell,* 529 A.2d 404 (1987), *aff'g* 514 A.2d 1342 (N.J. Sup. Ct. Ch. Div 1986); *In re Conroy,* 457 A.2d 1232 (N.J. Sup. Ct. Ch. Div), *rev'd,* 464 A.2d 303 (N.J. App. Div. 1983) *rev'd* 486 A.2d 1209 (N.J. 1985); *McIver v. Krischer,* 697 So. 2d 97 (Fla. 1997); *Washington v. Glucksberg,* 117 S. Ct. 2258 (1997).

151. Meisel, *supra* note 1, Volume 2, *citing Gray v. Romeo,* 697 F. Supp. 580 (1988); *McKay v. Bergstedt,* 801 P.2d 617 (Nev. 1990); *People v. Kevorkian,* 527 N.W.2d 714 (1994).

152. See, for example, *Fosmire v. Nicoleau,* 551 N.E.2d 77, 82 (N.Y. 1990); *Thor v. Superior Court,* 885 P.2d 375, 386 (Cal. 1993).

153. 379 So. 2d 359 (Fla. 1980), *aff'g* 362 So. 2d 160 (Fla. Dist. Ct. App. 1978).

154. 225 Cal. Rptr. 297 (Ct. App. 1986), *review denied* (June 5, 1986).

155. 225 Cal. Rptr. 297.

156. *Id.*

157. LaFave and Scott, *supra* note 149, at 650.

158. *Id.*

159. *Id.* at 477–480.

160. *Id.* at 650.

161. See, as examples, *Satz v. Perlmutter, supra* note 153; *In re Eichner,* 423 N.Y.S.2d 580 (Sup. Ct. Nassau County 1979), *aff'd sub nom. Eichner v. Dillon,* 426 N.Y.S.2d 517 (App. Div. 1980), *modified sub nom. In re Storar,* 420 N.E.2d 64 (N.Y.), *cert. denied,* 454 U.S. 858 (1981); *In re Dinnerstein,* 380 N.E.2d 134 (Mass. App. Ct. 1978); other cases in Table 13-1.

162. Meisel, *supra* note 1, Volume 2, at 455–457.

163. Bouvia, *supra* note 154, at 297.

164. Margaret Battin, "Assisted Suicide: Can We Learn from Germany?" 22(2) *Hastings Center Report* (March-April 1992), 44–51; Maurice A. M. deWachter, "Euthanasia in the Netherlands," *id.,* 23–30; Ray Mosley, "Dutch Euthanasia Plan Lets Kids Make Choice," *Chicago Tribune,* August 26, 1999, Section 1, 1, 22.

165. See, for example, Derek Humphry. *Jean's Way.* Eugene, Ore.: Hemlock Society (1978); Brian Clark. *Whose Life Is It Anyway?* New York: Avon Books, 1980; Bonnie Steinbock, Editor. *Killing and Allowing to Die.* Englewood Cliffs, N.J.: Prentice-Hall, 1980; Christian Bernard. *Good Life, Good Death: A Doctor's Case for Euthanasia and Suicide.* 1981.

166. Anonymous, 259 *JAMA* 272 (1988).

167. Timothy Quill, "Death and Dignity: A Case of Individualized Decision-Making," 324 *New England Journal of Medicine* 691 (1991).

168. "Kevorkian Murder Charge Dropped but not Forgotten," *Hospital Ethics* (January/February 1991), 6.

169. "Kevorkian Fate Hangs on Definition of Murder," *Chicago Tribune,* March 22, 1999, Section 1, 5.

170. "Chronology of Dr. Jack Kevorkian's Life and Assisted Suicide Campaign," *Frontline: The Kevorkian Verdict,* 1–6, located at http://www.pbs.org. Accessed January 6, 2000.

171. "Kevorkian Fate Hangs on Definition of Murder," *supra* note 169.

172. "In Tactical Move, State Drops Kevorkian Assisted-Suicide Charge," *Chicago Tribune,* March 12, 1999, Section 1, 6.

173. Jim Kirk and Sue Ellen Christian, "Kevorkian Gets 10 to 25 Years for Murder," *Chicago Tribune,* April 14, 1999, Section 1, 1, 17; Sue Ellen Christian, "Kevorkian Con-

174. Kirk and Christian, *supra* note 173.

175. 521 U.S. 702 (1997).

176. 521 U.S. 793 (1997).

177. 73 F.3d 790 (9th Cir. 1996) (*en banc*), *rev'd sub nom. Washington v. Glucksberg*, 521 U.S. 702 (1997).

178. "Ninth Circuit Holds Unconstitutional Ban Against Physician-Assisted Suicide," 5(11) *BNA Health Law Reporter* (March 14, 1996), 369.

179. *Id.* Liberty interests, whether to be free from unwanted medical treatment or in choosing the manner and time of death, is found in the Fourteenth Amendment. See Key Case 13-2, *Cruzan v. Director, Missouri Department of Health,* in this chapter.

180. "Ninth Circuit Holds Unconstitutional Ban Against Physician-Assisted Suicide," *supra* note 178; *Quill v. Vacco,* 80 F.3d 716 (1996), *rev'd* 521 U.S. 793 (1997).

181. *Quill v. Vacco,* 80 F.3d 716, 718.

182. Meisel, *supra* note 1, Volume 2, at 503.

183. *Washington v. Glucksberg,* 521 U.S. 702 (1997); *Quill v. Vacco,* 521 U.S. 793 (1997); Meisel, *supra* note 1, Volume 2, 506–508.

184. See, as examples, Meisel, *supra* note 1, Volume 2, at 506–508; Michael Uhlmann, Editor. *Last Rights? Assisted Suicide and Euthanasia Debated.* Grand Rapids, Mich.: William B. Eerdmans Publishing Company, 1998 (with Ethics and Public Policy Center, Washington, D.C.); Tania Salem, "Physician-Assisted Suicide: Promoting Autonomy—or Medicalizing Suicide?" 29(3) *Hastings Center Report* (1999), 30–36; Mark Angell, "The Supreme Court and Physician-Assisted Suicide: The Ultimate Right," 336(4) *New England Journal of Medicine* (1997), 50; Renee Coleson, "The *Glucksberg* and *Quill* Amicus Curiae Briefs: Verbatim Arguments Opposing Assisted Suicide," 13(9) *Issues in Law and Medicine* (1997), 3–52.

185. Meisel, *supra* note 1, Volume 2, at 506.

186. *Id.* at 506–508. Some states in which unsuccessful attempts at legislation legalizing physician-assisted suicide occurred were New York and California.

187. Or. Rev. Stat. Sections 127.800–897 (1996), *implementation enjoined by Lee v. Oregon,* 891 F. Supp. 1429 (D. Or. 1995), *vacated and remanded,* 197 F.3d 1382 (9th Cir. 1997) (lack of federal jurisdiction), *cert. denied sub nom. Lee v. Harcleroad,* 118 S. Ct. 328 (1997).

188. The Task Force to Improve the Care of Terminally-Ill Oregonians. *The Oregon Death with Dignity Act: A Guidebook for Health Care Providers.* Portland, Or.: Author, 1998; Oregon Death with Dignity Act, *supra* note 187, Sections 1.01(1), 1.01(6), 1.01(12), 2.01, 3.18.

189. Death with Dignity Act, *supra* note 187, Sections 2.02(1)–(4), 3.06, 6.01(form); Task Force, *supra* note 188, 15–16.

190. Death with Dignity Act, *supra* note 187, Sections 3.01(2), 3.04.

191. *Id.*, Sections 3.02.

192. *Id.*, Sections 3.05, 3.08.

193. 891 F. Supp. 1429 (D. Or. 1995). The case was brought by two physicians, four "terminally ill or potentially terminal patients," a residential care facility, and individual operators of residential care facilities. Meisel, *supra* note 1, Volume 2, at 509. Interestingly, in its 1997 decision vacating and remanding the case to the federal district court,

194. 197 F.3d 1382 (9th Circuit 1997).

195. *Cert. denied sub nom. Lee v. Harcleroad,* 118 S. Ct. 328 (1997).

196. Meisel, *supra* note 1, at 509.

197. *Id.*

198. Meisel, *supra* note 1, *Cumulative Supplement 2000,* at 74.

199. *Id.* at 74–76.

200. Meisel, *supra* note 1, *Cumulative Supplement 2000,* at 53.

201. Bureau of National Affairs, "DEA Won't Sanction Oregon Physicians Who Participate in Lawful Assisted Suicides," 7(24) *BNA Health Law Reporter* (June 11, 1998), 958–959.

202. See, for example, Steven King, "The Role of the Psychiatrist in a Patient's Right to Die," 279(17) *JAMA* (1998), 1346 (letters to the editor section); Donald Hermann, "The Question Remains: Are There Terminally Ill Patients Who Have a Constitutional Right to Physician Assistance in Hastening the Dying Process?" 1(3) *DePaul Journal of Health Care Law* (1997), 445–494; Barbara Daly, Devon Berry, Joyce Fitzpatrick, Barbara Drew, and Kathleen Montgomery, "Assisted Suicide: Implications for Nurses and Nursing," 45(5) *Nursing Outlook* (1997), 209–214; Judith Kennedy Schwartz, "Assisted Dying and Nursing Practice," 31(4) *Image: Journal of Nursing Scholarship* (1999), 367–373; Linda Emanuel, "Facing Requests for Physician-Assisted Suicide: Toward a Practical and Principled Clinical Skill Set," 280(7) *JAMA* (1998), 643–647; Marilynn Larkin, "Psychologists Grapple with Patient Requests to Hasten Death," 353(9170) *Lancet* (1999), 2133.

203. Nancy B. Mahon, "Symposium Introduction: Death and Dying Behind Bars—Cross-Cutting Themes and Policy Imperatives," 27(3) *Journal of Law, Medicine, & Ethics* (1999), 213.

204. *Id.*; Sue Buckley, "Best Practices: How Jails Are Addressing Evolving Inmate Health Care Needs," *American Jails* (1998), 1; Ellen Brown, "Managed Health Care in Prisons: The Untold Story," 6(3) *Managed Health Care* (1996), 3–6; Michael Sniffin, "Jailing Mentally Ill Is Widespread," *Chicago Tribune,* July 12, 1999, Section 1, 4.

205. Mahon, *supra* note 203, at 213.

206. *Id.* at 213–214; Felicia Cohen, "The Ethics of End-of-Life Care for Prison Inmates," 27(3) *Journal of Law, Medicine, & Ethics* (1999), 252.

207. Cohen, *supra* note 206, at 252.

208. U.S. Department of Justice, National Institute of Corrections, "Hospice and Palliative Care in Prisons: Special Issues in Corrections," (1998), accessed March 13, 2000, at the National Institute of Corrections Information Center Web site: http://www.nicic.org, 1.

209. *Id.* at 2.

210. *Id.*

211. *Id.* at 2–4.

212. *Id.* at 5.

213. Miller, *supra* note 57, at 508.

214. *Id.*

215. See, for example, Karin Kirchoff, Vicki Spuhler, Ann Hutton, Beth Vaughan Cole, and Terry Clemmer, "Intensive Care Nurses' Experiences with End-Of-Life Care," 9(1)

American Journal of Critical Care (2000), 36–42; Roberta Kaplow, "Use of Nursing Resources and Comfort of Cancer Patients with and without Do-Not-Resuscitate Orders in the Intensive Care Unit," 9(2) *American Journal of Critical Care* (2000), 87–95. See also, American Nurses Association. *Position Statement on Nursing Care and Do-Not-Resuscitate Decisions.* Washington, D.C.: Author, 1992. This ANA position statement, and its other statements, can be accessed on the ANA Home Page at http:// www.nursingworld.org.

216. See, for example, American Nurses Association. *Position Statement on Promotion of Comfort and Relief of Pain in Dying Patients.* Washington, D.C.: Author, 1991.

217. See, for example, Deborah Lowe Volker, "Assisted Suicide and the Domain of Nursing Practice," 5(1) *Journal of Nursing Law* (1998), 39–50; Barbara Daly, Devon Berry, Barbara Drew, and Kathleen Montgomery, "Assisted Suicide: Implications for Nurses and Nursing," 45(5) *Nursing Outlook* (1997), 209–214; American Nurses Association. *Position Statement on Assisted Suicide.* Washington, D.C.: Author, 1994; American Nurses Association. *Position Statement on Active Euthanasia.* Washington, D.C.: Author, 1994; Nancy J. Brent, "The Home Healthcare Nurse and Assisted Suicide," 15(10) *Home Healthcare Nurse* (1997), 691–693; Chapter 3.

218. Daly, Berry, Drew, and Montgomery, *supra* note 217.

219. Oregon Death with Dignity Act, *supra* note 187; Task Force, *supra* note 188, 26; Kathy Kirk, "How Oregon's Death with Dignity Act Affects Practice," 98(8) *AJN* (1998), 54–55.

220. Kirk, *supra* note 219, at 55, *citing* Task Force, *supra* note 188.

221. "Suicide Law Painless, Oregon Says," *Chicago Tribune,* February 18, 1999, Section 1, 6.

222. *Id.*

223. *Id.*

224. "Euthanasia Frequently Goes Awry Study Says," *Chicago Tribune,* February 24, 2000, Section 1, 10; Kathleen Foley and Herbert Hendin, "The Oregon Report: Don't Ask, Don't Tell," 29(3) *Hastings Center Report* (1999), 37–42; "Doctors Often Act on Their Own, Study Finds," *Chicago Tribune,* August 12, 1998, Section 1, 9.

225. Ezekiel Emanual, Elizabeth Daniels, Diane Fairclough, and Brian Clarridge, "The Practice of Euthanasia and Physician-Assisted Suicide in the United States: Adherence to Proposed Safeguards and Effects on Physicians," 280(6) *JAMA* (1998), 507–513.

226. National Institute of Corrections, *supra* note 208, at 6; Glenn G. Johnson, "Commentary: A Personal View on Palliative and Hospice Care in Correctional Facilities," 27(3) *Journal of Law, Medicine, & Ethics* (1999), 238–239.

227. National Institute of Corrections, *supra* note 208, at 6.

228. Support of, and participation in, research in the area of death and dying must also include the critical evaluation of all research and the results obtained in terms of its study design, validation and reliability of instruments used, and the use of any anecdotal comments of those who participated in the study. See, for example, Colleen Scanlon, "Euthanasia and Nursing Practice: Right Question, Wrong Answer," 334(21) *New England Journal of Medicine* (1996), 1401–1042 (editorial).

229. For example, a relatively "new" issue surrounding the dying process is how the nondisclosure to the patient of his terminal status affects the nursing care of that person. Preliminary data reveals that nondisclosure can negatively influence nursing care because of the patient's lack of adequate and timely information concerning a terminal prognosis. Mary Ann Krisman-Scott, "An Historical Analysis of Disclosure of Terminal Status," 32(1) *Journal of Nursing Scholarship* (2000), 47–52.

Issues Related to Violence

Violence, abuse, neglect, and exploitation are widespread in the United States. Although homicide rates have declined to levels seen in the late 1960s, in 1998 the murder rate was 6.3 per 100,000 persons.[1] Aggravated assault totaled 61% of violent crimes in 1995.[2] Abuse, neglect, and/or exploitation of the elderly occurs at a rate of 1 to 2 million cases each year.[3]

"Intrafamilial violence" or "domestic violence" is also alarmingly prevalent and takes many forms. In 1995, for example, more than 1 million children nationwide experienced some type of abuse or neglect.[4] "Intimate partner abuse" (IPA) is seen in women who seek treatment in EDs at the rate of 2.7% to 3.1%.[5] Sadly, in 1996, approximately 1,800 domestic homicides were committed by "intimates" in the home; nearly three out of four murdered were women.[6]

Sexual abuse or exploitation, including criminal sexual assault and incest, is another common form of violent behavior. Sexual violence occurs within families and in extrafamilial relationships; no one is immune. Physical violence and sexual injury often occur together.[7]

Because nurses are involved in all aspects of health care and practice in all health care delivery settings, they can actively participate in reducing the continuing spiral of violence. Whether in the role of a school nurse, a home health care nurse, or a nurse psychotherapist, the nurse can play an important role in assessment, intervention, and prevention of violence.

The nurse's legal obligations include mandatory reporting of certain instances of violence. The nurse also needs to be aware of the potential for violence against patients by health care providers and violence and the potential for abuse against health care practitioners.

THE NURSE AS MANDATORY REPORTER

Both federal and state laws require certain individuals to report particular instances of violence, abuse, and/or neglect to governmental agencies. For example, the Federal Child Abuse Prevention and Treatment Act requires alleged instances of medical neglect to be reported to state agencies empowered to enforce child protective services.

Because health care practitioners, including nurses, are often in a unique position to identify and assess cases of violence against others, they are almost always included as *mandated reporters;* that is, when an identified instance of injury appears to be present and the result of abuse, neglect, or exploitation, the mandated reporter must report the situation to the proper authorities. Thus, mandatory reporting laws include two specific types: those for child abuse and neglect and those for injury to the elderly.

Because health care practitioners, including nurses, are often in a unique position to identify and assess cases of violence against others, they are almost always included as mandated reporters [in federal and state reporting laws].

Laws that mandate reporting specifically provide certain protections for the reporter. They include (1) not requiring "hard evidence" of the abuse or neglect in order to report, but rather a "good-faith belief" or a "reasonable suspicion" that the injury is the result of abuse or neglect; (2) immunity from civil and criminal liability and licensing actions for reporting "in good faith" or with a "reasonable suspicion" that the conduct required to be reported has occurred; (3) presumed "good faith" of the reporter so that good faith must be rebutted by anyone challenging it; (4) specifically nullifying any confidentiality, privacy, and privilege mandates the health care professional would otherwise be required to adhere to because of the health care provider-patient relationship; and (5) providing confidentiality to any report made under the particular law.

A health care provider who is a mandated reporter and does not fulfill his or her duties under the law faces various penalties. They include (1)

ETHICS CONNECTION 14–1

Prevention of injury and violence is a national health priority.[1] Patterns of violence in the United States have reached morally unconscionable proportions. There are many patterns of violence, including domestic violence, random violence, workplace violence, violence in schools, and violence against vulnerable populations, such as children, disabled elderly, mentally ill, and poor people.

Both official agencies and unofficial coalitions that are charged with developing and implementing strategic plans for prevention of violence have identified demographic patterns of violence. For example, men are more often the victims and the perpetrators of homicide than are women, and African-American males are seven times more likely than white people to be murdered.[2] Violence is not limited to crowded inner city neighborhoods, however. In recent years, episodes of violent tragedies in schools across the nation have become part of the national experience. Individualistic ethics is not particularly helpful in revealing the origins of violence nor in identifying morally responsible strategies to prevent tragedies. Ethics of community or communitarian ethics holds greater promise of exploring our collective accountability for violence prevention. The broader social discourse about violence, its origins, patterns, and prevention may help to inform society's ethical comportment regarding violence.

Violence is so prevalent in U.S. society that it is morally reprehensible to contribute to its power through using the language of violence. In the United States and other industrialized nations, residents are becoming desensitized to everyday expressions of violence. Media, including or perhaps especially news reports, portray violence; children's television programs and computer games often focus on "annihilating" invaders. In communicating with one another, we often use metaphors of violence, such as "If I only had a gun," "I could have killed" him or her, and so on. Health care, in particular, has adopted a language of violence. Metaphors for nursing therapies, medication management, and recovery processes often involve violent language. Disease is seen as an "enemy" to be "fought," clients "win" or "lose" their "battles" against "life-threatening" diseases, antibiotics "attack invading" microbes, and the like. As members of society as well as health care professionals, nurses can help to reduce the use of violent language through becoming more aware of its presence and thoughtful about its use. The *Code for Nurses: With Interpretive Statements*[3] obligates nurses to be involved in political action in support of nursing's social policy agenda, including prevention of violence. Weber[4] argues that this political action includes endorsement of political candidates who support nursing's health care goals and practices.

The ethics of violence can be discussed from a variety of ethical perspectives, including ethical theories, moral principles and covenantal relationships (see Chapter 3). Almost all moral principles are involved in ethics and violence, particularly nonmaleficence. From the perspective of covenantal relationships, violence violates basic human rights and, thus, addresses inclusive rather than special covenantal relationships. Inclusive covenantal conflicts have higher priority than do conflicts between special covenants.[5]

In a radically different approach to communal ethics, George Ellis, a cosmologist who supported antiapartheid efforts in South Africa, has developed an ethic of community service. This ethic is based, in part, on "Quaker tenets of confronting injustice through rational dialogue and advocating tolerance for those with different beliefs."[6] Through observations of human behavior, Ellis argues that a universal moral law does exist. "The foundation line of true ethical behavior, its main guiding principle valid across all times and cultures, is the degree of freedom from self-centeredness of thought and behavior, and willingness freely to give up one's own self-interest on behalf of others."[7] Ellis refers to this principle of community service ethics as "kenosis," meaning "self-emptying." Regardless of the ethical, philosophical, or theological approach to prevention of violence, it clearly is a moral obligation of nursing and nurses.

---

[1]Office of Disease Prevention and Health Promotion, U.S. Department of Health and Human Services. *Healthy People 2010.* Washington, D.C.: Author. See also Web site: http://health.gov/healthypeople/PrevAgenda/whatishp.htm

[2]*Id.*

[3]American Nurses Association. *Code for Nurses: With Interpretive Statements.* Kansas City, Missouri: Author, 1985.

[4]Eileen Weber, "Nursing's Ethical Mandate: Endorsing Candidates," 4(1) *Creative Nursing* (1998), 10–11.

[5]Joseph L. Allen. *Love & Conflict.* Lanham, Md.: University Press of America, 1995.

[6]W. Wayt Gibbs. "Profile: George F. R. Ellis: Thinking Globally, Acting Universally," 273(4) *Scientific American* (October 1995), 50–52.

[7]*Id.*

TABLE 14–1

Mandatory Reporting Statutes for Nurses Relating to Violence

CONDUCT/INJURY	WHERE REPORT MUST BE MADE
Child abuse and neglect	State child protective agency and/or police
Elder abuse and neglect	State department on aging and/or police
Suspicious or unnatural deaths	Medical examiner or coroner and/or police
Injuries due to lethal weapons (gun, knife)	Medical examiner or coroner and/or police
Injuries due to criminal conduct (criminal sexual assault, battery, assault)	Medical examiner or coroner and/or police

criminal prosecution (for a misdemeanor, for example); (2) proceedings under the applicable state licensing law for a violation of the particular licensing act (nursing or medical practice act in which a duty to report is included); and (3) proceedings to cancel any certifications granted by the state (a school nurse certificate, for example).[8]

Table 14–1 lists the more common mandatory reporting requirements for nurses and other health care providers in all health care delivery settings.

SETTINGS AND TYPES OF VIOLENCE

Regardless of the specific setting in which violence occurs, violence has a definition that transcends those sites. Violence is the unjust and unwarranted exercise of force, often physical (but also psychological) and accompanied by outrage, fury, or vehemence.[9] The use of violence is a deliberate act that can result in abuse, injury, or damage.[10]

Domestic/Intrafamilial Violence

The home is no stranger to violence. Domestic violence is insidiously brutal because it can go undetected for long periods, if not forever. Domestic violence is conduct of a family member or a member of a household toward another family or household member so that the result is physical, psychological, or developmental injury or damage. Domestic violence is a broad category. It typically encompasses abuse, neglect, and/or exploitation. A direct act of domestic violence occurs when a

spouse is physically beaten. A more indirect act of violence occurs when a spouse is psychologically terrorized by a partner. The nurse who observes belongings smashed and broken in a patient's home may be seeing evidence of violence.

In some types of domestic disorder, such as child abuse or neglect, the nurse can intervene more easily because of mandated reporting for health care providers. Thus, when a school nurse discovers unexplained bruises on a student's body or an emergency department (ED) physician is suspicious about an injury manifested by an infant, an evaluation of the injury and the family can begin when the reporting occurs.

Not all types of domestic violence, however, mandate reporting to governmental agencies. Spousal beating and, in some states, elder abuse in the home or community do not require reporting. Protection in these states can be sought only after consent of the victim is obtained or after the abused individual seeks aid using other judicial remedies.

One remedy is the protection afforded under a state's domestic violence law. Most laws broadly define violence covered under the act. Those instances include, for example, intimidation, interference with the personal liberty of another, and neglect (failure to provide food, medical care, and health and safety protections for a disabled or dependent individual).[11] In addition, they provide judicial relief (orders of protection) and police protection (e.g., arrest of offender, transportation of victim and family to a medical facility or shelter) to victims of domestic violence. Those covered under the state statutes include spouses, parents, adults with disabilities, family members, and household members.

The domestic violence statutes are civil and are not the only choice a person has to obtain relief from domestic terror. Other remedies that the victim can pursue, either alone or in combination with the laws governing domestic violence, include divorce (if applicable) and criminal actions. For example, the charge of aggravated criminal assault may be used, and victims may obtain a cease and desist or restraining order.

Child Abuse and Neglect

Abuse (mental or physical maltreatment)[12] or neglect (the failure or omission of proper attention to a person or thing, whether inadvertent, negligent, or willful),[13] can occur in any setting. The abuse or neglect of a minor—someone 17 years of age or younger—is no exception. Abuse or neglect often occurs in the home but can also occur in school, in a neighbor's home, or in a relative's residence. The most prevalent type of abuse or neglect against minors is physical; sexual abuse and emotional maltreatment are second and third.[14]

The most prevalent type of abuse or neglect against minors is physical; sexual abuse and emotional maltreatment are second and third.

Abuse can be evident in affirmative acts, such as striking an individual or verbally intimidating someone to force compliance. Abuse can also occur more indirectly when, for example, a child is not given the attention needed to become a healthy adult. Abuse can be sexual in nature as in intercourse and exhibitionism; incest may also occur.

Neglect also includes absence of care or attention in a particular situation.[15] When, for example, a minor child is not fed or is kept isolated and ignored in the home, psychological as well as physical neglect occurs.

As with abuse, neglect is specifically defined in child and elder abuse and neglect statutes passed by state legislatures.

All states and the District of Columbia have laws protecting abused and neglected minors,[16] through mandated reporting for specified individuals. Although the laws vary widely from state to state, all laws require that the reporter have a "good faith" or "reasonable belief" that abuse or neglect is occurring or has occurred. Specific definitions of abuse and neglect are also included in each state's law. Some definitions for abuse include physical injury (burns, internal abdominal injuries), psychological injury (scapegoating, repeated name calling), sexual abuse (including genital injuries), and cruel punishment. Neglect is often described as the deprivation of necessities, medical neglect, malnutrition, and even moral neglect (specifically in Arizona, Idaho, and Mississippi).[17]

Child abuse and neglect laws also contain unique provisions concerning the role of nurses and others when abuse or neglect is suspected. For example, statutes allow a physician or police officer to take a minor into temporary "protective" custody without the consent of the person caring for the child. This action can occur when returning the child to the person responsible for the child's welfare may, in the judgment of the physician or police, result in continued endangerment to the child's health or safety, and there is no time to obtain a court order for the temporary custody.[18]

When protective custody is possible, statutory provisions provide for the immediate care of the imperiled child. For example, notification to the child protective agency must occur; notification to the person responsible for the child's welfare must be undertaken; and the child must be placed in a foster or other home until a hearing on the parental or other person's custody issue is held.[19]

Child abuse and neglect statutes also give physicians and facilities authority to take photographic and radiographic films of the minor (if indicated) and to conduct other medical tests without parental consent if these measures will help confirm that abuse or neglect has occurred. Spiral fractures or a subdural hematoma evidenced by medical tests, for example, can help a health care provider decide about reporting the incident and/or taking the child into protective custody.

Nurses and other mandated reporters are usually informed in writing of the investigation done and the disposition of any case reported to the child protective agency. The records compiled by the state agency, including the identity of the reporter, are confidential, however, and can be disclosed only pursuant to the child abuse and neglect statute.

Nurses have been involved in child abuse cases with positive results. For example, in *State v. Gillard*,[20] an admitting nurse's testimony about a 7-year-old's statement to her concerning the child's injuries ("My Daddy did it. I was not kicked by a cow. My Mom was there but she just let him do it") helped convict the stepfather of felony child abuse. In *Commonwealth v. Garcia*,[21] a pediatric nurse who examined a 33-day-old child at the "well baby" program noticed the child's strange conditions. The infant's eyes were red and multiple bruises were present on the extremities and trunk. The eye condition was diagnosed as "subconjunctival hemorrhages," and X-rays and a CT scan showed 26 rib fractures, a skull fracture, two fractures of the left leg, and fractures of both clavicals.

The assessment, evaluation, and reporting of these and other injuries, as well as additional medical evidence gathered by the nurse and the clinic, resulted in a conviction of the parents for "wantonly and recklessly permitting another" to assault and batter the infant.[22] The parents had denied abusing the child, but the court held that there was sufficient circumstantial evidence to convict both of them.

Elder Abuse and Neglect

The problems of elder abuse and neglect are in their infancy.[23] Elder mistreatment has remained a hidden, shameful, and often ignored problem until very recently.[24] In addition, with an estimated 20% increase in the number of persons over 65 by the year 2020,[25] the problem can only continue to expand.

Because of reluctance on the part of the elderly to report it, the actual incidence of elder abuse and neglect is most probably underestimated and certainly not well documented.[26] This is so especially when abuse and neglect occur at the hands of family members or caretakers. Furthermore, health care providers often unintentionaly overlook elder abuse and neglect, explaining a fracture or loss of weight as expected consequences of the aging process (e.g., loss of balance, decrease in appetite). In other situations, health care providers, including home health care nurses, are reluctant to report elder abuse or neglect because of a lack of cooperation by the family, lack of cooperation by the patient, or doubt about whether the abuse or neglect really occurred.[27] Consequently, only one in eight instances of elder abuse and neglect are reported to elder protective services or other authorities.[28]

. . . health care providers often unintentionally overlook elder abuse and neglect, explaining a fracture or loss of weight as expected consequences of the aging process . . .

Laws protecting the elderly from abuse and neglect exist in almost every state. Unfortunately, the mistreatment of the elderly can occur in the community, including the home, or in health care facilities, including nursing homes or long-term care entities. Although anyone *could* report elder abuse or neglect to the state protective agency (a department on aging, for example), only 43 states have enacted some form of mandatory reporting of elder abuse or neglect.[29] Most often, these mandatory reporting statutes resemble child abuse and neglect laws. Unlike the child abuse and neglect legislation, however, many require reporting only when elder abuse or neglect occurs in health facilities.

For example, Illinois, Michigan, New Jersey, and California have mandatory reporting statutes for the mistreatment of the elderly in long-term care or nursing home facilities.[30] Definitions of abuse and neglect include physical or mental injury by other than accidental means, sexual abuse, and lack of adequate medical or personal care or maintenance. Mandatory reporters include nurses, nursing home administrators, and podiatrists.

Clearly, these statutes must also be read with other state and federal laws that protect the elderly in health care facilities. Illinois and New Mexico, for example, have criminal laws often making it a felony to abuse or neglect an elderly person in a long-term care facility.[31] State and federal laws also govern the use of chemical and physical restraints with elderly residents of health care facilities. A recent final interim rule promulgated by the Health Care Financing Administration (HCFA) and applicable to the Medicare and Medicaid programs, for example, affirmatively prohibits the misuse of medications and physical restraints in long-term care facilities. Guidelines for their appropriate use and the documentation of that use are also defined.[32]

While elderly residents in health care facilities are protected by states that have passed mandatory reporting laws, elderly individuals who live in their own homes, with their families, or in boarding homes may not be protected. Statistics reveal most of the abusers of elderly individuals in the community are relatives; 19.3% are spouses of elderly victims, 19.3% are children, and 8.6% grandchildren.[33]

Furthermore, the types of abuse and neglect that can occur in a domestic situation are much more elusive and insidious. Financial abuse (unusual checkbook activity, forcing the elder person to sign over property), improper medication administration, and environmental control (room or home not warm enough or cool enough, locking the elderly person in a room) are just a few examples.

Only a few states have passed mandatory reporting of elder abuse or neglect in the community. Alabama, California, Montana, and Florida are among them.[34] However, the laws vary widely in terms of their scope of coverage and in the actions mandated for required reporters.[35] Other states have passed protective laws for the elderly in the community, but they are voluntary "reporting statutes."[36]

In addition to the reporting laws concerning elder abuse or neglect, other state regulations protect the elderly in the community when no mandated reporting laws exist. For example, state criminal laws have been passed to punish the neglect of an elderly person or the financial exploitation of an aged citizen. The reporting of such conduct to the police can cut further abuse.[37]

In states in which no specific laws have been promulgated, use of already existing criminal laws, such as those prohibiting assault and battery, can also protect the elderly in the community. In fact, many states (including Florida, Louisiana, and Colorado) have made assault or battery against an elderly person an "aggravation" of the crime.[38] If convicted, the defendant can then be sentenced to additional prison time.

Abuse and Neglect of Disabled Individuals

Although a disability can be defined in many ways, for the purposes of this section of the chapter it is defined as an objectively measurable physical or mental condition of impairment which results in one's inability to function.[39] Disabilities include amputations, paralysis, mental retardation, and mental illness. Disability knows no specific age limitations. Estimates indicate that at least 43 million individuals in the United States have chronic, significant disabilities.[40]

The protection afforded the disabled against abuse and neglect is supported, in many instances, by other laws. For example, a disabled person in a nursing home has the same protections the elderly resident would have under the state's mandatory reporting of *any* abuse or neglect of a facility resident. A nursing home resident who does not receive proper and necessary care for a broken hip, for example, is experiencing criminal neglect. In

the same way, the abuse or neglect of a disabled minor would be reportable under the state child abuse and neglect law.

In addition, if an individual's disability requires hospitalization or institutionalization in a developmental disability or mental health facility, state codes regulating care, such as those in Illinois and Texas, include penalties for the abuse or neglect.[41]

When the disabled person lives in the community, however, less stringent reporting requirements apply. Both permissive and mandatory reporting statutes protect a disabled person who is abused, neglected, or exploited.[42] When not mandated to report instances of violence against the disabled, however, health care providers often face difficult choices concerning whether or not (1) the patient will consent to the reporting; (2) alternative living arrangements are possible; and (3) verification (insofar as possible) of the abuse, neglect, or exploitation can occur.

As with elder abuse and neglect in the community, a state's criminal code can be used to punish those who inflict abuse and neglect on the disabled. For example, "criminal neglect of an elderly or disabled person" makes it a felony to (among other things) endanger or cause to deteriorate a preexisting mental or physical condition of a disabled or elderly person. Such a law most often applies to "caregivers" in the community and broadly defines that role.[43]

Rape/Criminal Sexual Assault

At one time, rape was defined as the use of threat or violence to force a woman to engage in sexual activity against her will.[44] Now, to be more gender-neutral and reflect the unfortunate expansion of this type of violence among men and women alike, its name has changed. For example, in Illinois[45] rape is now called criminal sexual assault and abuse.

The definitions of force and sexual activity have also changed, although the changes vary from state to state. Common ones include (1) expanding to include specific acts that are gender-neutral, including "sexual penetration" and "sexual conduct"; (2) eliminating the need to prove consent for the conduct in question; (3) augmenting the definition of "force or threat of force" by the aggressor; and (4) abandoning the need to show evidence of the emission of semen to prove that sexual penetration took place.[46]

One of the early categories of sexual assault was that of statutory rape. It covered situations in which a young female of a specified age (e.g., 12 to 16) was involved in a sexual encounter with a male. The protection afforded the minor female was based on her inability to provide valid consent to sexual intercourse.[47] Currently, in those states with changed statutes, *any* minor under a specified age is a victim of sexual assault if the other requirements in the criminal statute are met.

Marital rape is a category of sexual violence against women, but surprisingly has only recently been made a crime. Oregon, Iowa, and the District of Columbia are among those with criminal statutes covering marital rape, while other states provide immunity from suit for husbands who force sexual activity on their wives. However, in some states in which a conviction is possible, it can be successful only if the husband and wife are not living together because of a court order or are legally separated.

Other states make a distinction between sexual assault between married couples and between nonmarried couples. Thus, if two people are not married but are living together, the woman cannot allege marital rape or sexual assault.

Sexual Abuse and Exploitation

Sexual abuse and exploitation (taking unjust advantage of another for one's own benefit or gain[48]) know no favorites. They can occur with adults, minors, the elderly, the disabled, within families, and outside families. In fact, their prevalence is so widespread that all mandatory reporting protective statutes include sexual abuse and exploitation. It is important to note that violence, abuse, neglect, and exploitation are not mutually exclusive. Any particular situation may result in all four types of conduct against an individual or individuals.

Sexual abuse and exploitation . . . know no favorites. They can occur with adults, minors, the elderly, the disabled, within families, and outside families.

Although common, sexual abuse and exploitation are sometimes difficult to identify because they can be manifested in many ways. Evidence may appear as a change in appetite in a minor child or as unexplained depression that a school nurse sees in an adolescent. More direct evidence might include a diagnosis of a sexually transmitted disease or genital/perineal trauma in a minor or in an elderly nursing home resident. A minor adolescent female may be sexually exploited if she is forced to provide sexual favors in return for a place to stay. Or an elderly female may be forced into giving a monthly Social Security check to the male boarding house owner who does not use it for the elderly boarder's living expenses in order to avoid sexual exploitation or abuse by the owner.

Perpetrators of sexual abuse and exploitation are as diverse as the forms this violence takes. Those who commit acts of sexual abuse and exploitation can be family members (spouses, parents, stepparents, siblings), caretakers, health care providers (facility staff, psychotherapists), teachers, clergy, strangers, pedophiles, males or females. When sexual abuse or exploitation is suspected, specific interventions must occur, and they will depend not only on the age of the suspected victim but also on the type of injury.

Because of the embarrassment, shame, fear, and stigma often felt by victims of sexual violence and exploitation, many states have enacted protective laws to minimize, insofar as possible, any unnecessary publicity. For example, mandatory reports concerning child abuse and neglect are considered confidential and can be released only under certain circumstances (to law enforcement officers or during a trial). In addition, if the suspected or documented victim is a child who receives treatment, all records are usually made confidential so that release occurs only in specified circumstances (to law enforcement agencies, for example).[49]

If an individual is a victim of a rape or criminal sexual assault and seeks counseling for that violence, in some states all communications between the victim and the "rape counseling staff" are confidential and cannot be released without the consent of the victim.[50] This prohibition includes release at the trial. If the latter is necessary, an *in camera* (in the judge's chambers) review is allowed to determine if the information should be released. If the information is needed in the case against the accused, the judge can order it to be released.[51]

In addition to concerns over confidentiality, victims of sexual abuse and exploitation are at risk for contracting sexually transmitted diseases, including AIDS. As a result, most state statutes requiring the mandatory reporting of child abuse contain provisions for testing the victim so that care and counseling can begin immediately if necessary.[52]

Adult victims can ask that the individual accused of rape or other criminal sexual assault be tested for HIV to effectuate the same results. This ability is usually provided under the state's criminal laws and also protects the subject being tested.[53]

NURSING IMPLICATIONS IN CASES OF ABUSE AND NEGLECT

Working with victims of abuse, neglect, and exploitation demands patience, empathy, and a thorough knowledge of the law. Because acts of violence can be inflicted on anyone, all nurses must be aware of the possibility of violent behavior with all patients.

Working with victims of abuse, neglect, and exploitation demands patience, empathy, and a thorough knowledge of the law.

Thus, policies and procedures concerning the nurse's role in abuse, neglect, or exploitation cases are essential. The guidelines must be specific for both adults and minors. The policies should include who is to be notified when suspected or documented abuse or neglect is present; documentation guidelines; and treatment issues and protocols.

Second, the nurse who encounters suspected or documented violence against a patient must follow state law and facility guidelines in reporting to the proper agency. Because the nurse is almost always identified as a mandatory reporter in statutes requiring compulsory reporting, there is no room for the nurse's discretion in reporting the incident. The only leeway the nurse has is whether or not the injuries are believed "in good faith" or "reasonably" to be the result of abuse, neglect, or exploitation. The nurse should also keep in mind

that many of the required reporting statutes prohibit anyone else in the facility or organization from hindering or obstructing a report.

The nurse can help intervene in violent behavior by obtaining as much information from the victim as possible. This will require good interpersonal communication skills, especially if the patient is young or is fearful of sharing information. A very young victim may not be able to discuss the incident directly, so careful listening to what is said—and not said—will be vital. In addition, particular methods—role-playing or storytelling—may help the minor share the incident.

Similarly, observing and noting any unusual behavior may indicate that abuse or neglect has occurred. For example, does the home health care nurse notice that the 10-year-old in the family seen for another health problem is suddenly truant from school? Does an elderly client being seen postoperatively suddenly seem lethargic and inattentive?

If the particular state in which the nurse practices protects the identity of victims of assault and abuse, the nurse should maintain that confidentiality by following the law's mandate. If a blood test of the victim is obtained, conforming with state statutes concerning confidentiality for HIV and AIDS is essential.

When the victim of violence is a child and protective custody is necessary, the nurse should be clear about the nurse's role in that situation. Most often it is the *physician* who is given the authority to place a child in protective custody. The nurse who is not authorized to perform this function can indirectly help with such an emergency by ensuring that the child does not leave the facility with the abuser. For example, the nurse may need to call security to help with the removal of the family or abuser or contact the facility administration about the problem.

If photographs are to be taken of the victim, especially a minor, the nurse should be clear about who is given the authority to do so. The nurse who is not granted that power can help as a witness by being present in the room with the victim or by fulfilling the mandate for reporting the situation to the proper agency.

The nurse in the community—whether as a visiting nurse, in home health care, or in a senior citizen center—must be attentive to abuse, neglect, and exploitation. If the state does not mandate reporting, the nurse can try to convince the elderly person to seek help through the state agencies set up to provide protection from the abuser. If persuasion does not work, providing support services for the abuser, including respite time, is another option.

Nurses may be involved in gathering evidence to document sexual abuse or neglect. Although this request can occur in any health care delivery setting, it will most often occur in the ED. Evidence often includes the results of a physical examination. The ED nurse should have an exhaustive orientation in the collection of evidence. Whether assisting in its collection, or collecting evidence personally, the nurse must exert great care to ensure that the evidence is collected properly and that any laboratory work, including a pregnancy and HIV test, is not overlooked. Any specimens taken, including vaginal aspiration, mouth and rectum swabs or foreign pubic hair, should be immediately and accurately labeled and sent to the laboratory for analysis. Of particular importance is the establishment of a "chain of custody" to ensure that the specimen is not lost, destroyed, or mishandled, making it inadmissible in a subsequent trial or other proceeding. Documentation Reminder 14–1 lists areas to remember when documenting violence.

DOCUMENTATION REMINDER 14–1
Violence

- Completion of all required forms for the reporting of abuse, neglect, exploitation (e.g., name and address, age of victim, type of injury, name and occupation of person who files report, actions taken)
- Condition of patient, who accompanied patient, quotes by patient, tests and care provided, who was notified, mandatory reporting completed
- Clothing, photographs, and so on, given to police, identity of officer by name, time, badge or star number, police station and district
- Patient refusal of treatment or consent to report incident (where applicable)
- Protective custody decisions, who was involved, who contacted, where minor taken (inpatient at facility or custody of state agency)
- Obtaining and handling of evidence
- Referrals to other social service agencies, including therapy for victim, home care or respite services, discussion in student care conference, legal services

- Informed consent for treatment and tests when obtained and given
- Discussion of problem with family, caregivers; their response, or actions taken
- Any follow-up care suggested or recommended, whether or not care was provided at time of discovery of abuse, neglect, or exploitation

---

The nurse must also promote awareness of sexual abuse, neglect, and exploitation for both colleagues and the public. For other nurses, continuing education or in-service programs can address these topics. These issues can also be included in nursing curriculums of all nursing education programs. Furthermore, exploring personally held values about women, aging, the disabled, and male-female relationships can help colleagues to clarify their feelings concerning violence against others.

Educating the public may be more difficult to achieve, but the prevention of violence, including sexual abuse and neglect, is a goal worth pursuing both formally and informally. The school nurse who meets with a student's parents and helping them identify better ways to cope with the stress caused by their school-age child may be preventing future violence.

The nursing association or school of nursing that sponsors a seminar on abuse and neglect may also serve the public. The participation of others who work with victims of violence—including social workers, mental health professionals, and those who have successfully overcome the problems of abuse and neglect—can be very effective.

The nurse should also be involved in legislative efforts on both the state and federal level to protect those who experience abuse, neglect, and exploitation.[54] Exercising the right to vote, especially for those who support protective laws, is essential. So too is attempting to influence the legislative process through testifying at public hearings on proposed legislative changes and fund-raising efforts. Without financial support or legislative appropriations for protective laws, new statutes become nothing but hollow victories.

The nurse who is involved in testifying at any judicial proceeding concerning abuse, neglect, or exploitation should seek counsel from the facility attorney and/or an attorney of the nurse's choice *before* responding to a subpoena or any other request to provide testimony. To protect the nurse during that process, it is imperative that representation continue throughout the proceeding. For example, the nurse may not be aware of the need to assert the confidentiality of the information requested or to request an *in camera* review of documents before they are released.

Obtaining adequate legal advice not only protects the patient but also shields the nurse against allegations of a breach of the patient's rights. For example, many state licensing laws prohibit a nurse from breaching nurse-patient confidentiality except in certain situations. Conformity with the technicalities of a nurse practice act or other state laws is critical for the nurse who must not only facilitate the patient's case but also meet personal and professional obligations.

Last, nurses and other health care providers must begin to routinely assess the presence of violence in all patients who present themselves for care within a health care setting. In a recent study of 131 women who were admitted to a nontrauma urban teaching hospital, 26% reported being in an abusive relationship at one time.[55] Interestingly, no respondents in the survey were asked about domestic violence by their treating health care providers.[56]

Another study indicated that 3,455 women who presented themselves to community hospital EDs had also experienced "intimate partner abuse" within the past year and at other points in their lifetimes.[57] Other studies indicate that women who are pregnant[58] and those seeking an abortion[59] are also at high risk for violence and abuse.

SPECIAL SITUATIONS INVOLVING VIOLENCE

Violence Against Patients and Residents by Health Care Providers

Violence by health care practitioners against patients in health care settings occurs in varying ways. Violence may take place when an overworked and overtired surgeon is unduly rough when removing a patient's postoperative stitches; abuse can happen when a nurse responds harshly to a patient who asks a seemingly innocent question. Abuse and neglect of vulnerable inpatients and residents of health care facilities—disabled, mentally retarded, and elderly persons—by health care providers occur frequently. The excuses offered for the maltreatment of patients and resident populations are numerous. They include over-

worked medical and nursing staff; vulnerable residents' inability to complain; frequent understaffing; large patient care assignments that result in staff frustration; and, in some instances, inadequate preparation of both professional and ancillary staff who work with the populations they care for.

> *The excuses offered for the maltreatment of patients and resident populations [by health care personnel] are numerous.*

Forms of Patient Abuse and Neglect

Maltreatment or injury to a patient is often obvious. In one case, a certified nurse assistant allegedly verbally harassed a nursing home resident and forcibly pulled her by her arm.[60] In another, a nurse assistant allegedly hit and rubbed soap in the eyes of a 70-year-old double amputee after the patient had soiled his bath water.[61] Misconduct by health care providers may, however, be more subtle. In one instance, a nurse assistant refused to provide a bedpan to a resident more than once per night so that the resident urinated in her bed and had to wait until morning to be bathed and have her bedding changed.[62] Also, abuse may occur when baths, shaving, and feeding are not carried out on a regular basis or are done in a substandard manner.[63] Forcibly providing medical care without consent, such as CPR or feeding tubes, is yet another subtle type of abuse.

Verbal abuse can occur when a patient is called a name or when belittling or derogatory remarks are made.[64] In one reported case involving an ED nurse, a patient with spinal meningitis whose behavior was difficult to control was called names and told to leave the hospital if he didn't like the way it was run.[65]

Abuse and neglect sometimes involve the misuse of methods of treatment. A patient may be subjected to medical procedures without required sedation or extubated too early. Medications or physical restraints may be used as punishment or as a convenience to the nursing staff. For example, a nurse in a long-term care facility may not have adequate staff to monitor residents who need observation. As a result, an unruly or fragile resident may be administered medication more frequently than necessary or be placed in a Posey belt or other restraint to reduce the need for frequent monitoring. In one reported case, a nurse's aide placed a wheelchair-bound resident in his room and moved his bed in front of the door so it only opened one third of the way to prevent the resident from "wandering."[66]

Neglect or exploitation by health care providers can also be obvious, as when a bedridden patient suffers from numerous infected bedsores. So too is severe weight loss in a resident who also complains of hunger and reduced portions at erratic mealtimes.[67] Unlawfully taking a patient's money, Social Security check, or other personal property is a form of exploitation that may go undetected for some time.

NURSING IMPLICATIONS IN CASES OF VIOLENCE BY HEALTH CARE PROVIDERS

Regardless of the type of violence and regardless of its being inflicted by a colleague or staff member, the nurse who knows of a problem must report it.[68] To whom the situation must be reported will depend on the type of health care facility.

In an acute care setting, the nurse should share concerns with the nurse manager and nurse executive. In addition, an occurrence report and any other required internal documents should be initiated. In a long-term care facility, the situation must also be reported to the appropriate state agency if mandatory reporting is required. Depending on the state law covering abuse in the community, the nurse may or may not be required to report the maltreatment of vulnerable community residents to identified authorities. If reporting is not mandatory, the nurse may work with the victim in obtaining consent to intervene in whatever manner is necessary to avoid further mistreatment.

When a patient or resident appears to have been abused or neglected, proper nursing and medical care must take place immediately. The nurse will need to notify the attending physician of the necessity for orders for diagnostic work and additional medical treatment.

The nurse who witnesses verbal or psychological abuse against a patient or resident should report the incident to the nurse manager and also initiate any required supporting facility or agency documents. Early intervention into inappropriate conduct by nursing and other staff is vital to help staff learn healthier ways of working with patients.

The nurse must also use medication and physical restraints judiciously and consistent with good nursing practice, institutional or agency policy, and state and federal law. If inadequate staffing is inhibiting the proper monitoring of patients, the nurse must inform nursing administration so that additional help can be obtained.

In addition, the nurse manager will need to carefully supervise and evaluate nursing staff and nurse assistants. If a performance problem arises in which residents are not treated properly, the employee must be informed and his or her conduct improved. If abuse or neglect occurs after the employee has been informed, the employee should be dealt with pursuant to facility guidelines for discipline, suspension, or termination.

Violence Against Health Care Providers

Perhaps the most common illustrations of violence against health care providers are injuries and maltreatment inflicted by patients against facility staff. Although no area of a facility or type of health care provider is immune from abuse or injury by patients, certain areas and practitioners have experienced greater incidence of injury than others.

Risks for Violence Against Nurses

The ED and mental health care units (including those providing substance abuse treatment and treatment for the developmentally disabled) are two areas with a high proportion of violence by patients. Increased violence in these areas may be due to many factors. For example, EDs function 24 hours a day, are unlocked, have minimal security, and are not physically designed for safety of staff (e.g., "panic buttons," bullet-resistant glass barriers).[69] Mental health care units and facilities are often understaffed and have inadequate security. Even so, they provide services to populations that, because of their emotional difficulties, may "act out" against facility staff.[70]

Violence experienced at the hands of patients can be physical or verbal. Kicking, beating, stabbing, and throwing objects are just a few samples of the physical violence that a patient may inflict. Verbal abuse or harassment may include name calling and shouting. Scores of studies indicate that verbal abuse by patients and by visitors make up the first and second most common sources of violence.[71]

A second type of abuse experienced by health care providers is inflicted by colleagues. Although a long-standing problem, such "horizontal violence" has only recently been documented.[72] It occurs against all types of health care providers, including nurses, medical students, social workers, respiratory therapists, and radiographers.[73] A study of nurse-physician relationships indicated that nurses are often subjected to temper tantrums, scapegoating, condescending attitudes, and public humiliation by physicians.[74] Likewise, physical abuse, including assault and battery, has also been imposed upon nurses by physicians.

Nurses have won several lawsuits against physicians who have inflicted violence against them. In one reported case, a nurse sued a physician for striking her on the forearm during provision of care to a patient who had a severe nosebleed.[75] Although the nurse experienced no physical injury, she won an award of $10,001 in punitive damages against the physician. In *Gordon v. Lewiston Hospital*,[76] a physician's statement to an emergency room nurse that "she should get off her ass," was a "wrench in the works," and "was obstructing patient care" resulted in the physician's suspension of his staff privileges. In upholding the suspension, the Commonwealth Court of Pennsylvania relied upon the fact that the hospital had warned Dr. Gordon that further "disruptive behavior" would result in his suspension.[77]

A study of nurse-physician relationships indicated that nurses are often subjected to temper tantrums, scapegoating, condescending attitudes, and public humiliation by physicians.

NURSING IMPLICATIONS IN CASES OF VIOLENCE AGAINST HEALTH CARE PROVIDERS

No nurse can stand by and let abuse occur without taking action. One most obvious response is to prevent the abuse, insofar as that is humanly possible. Therefore, nurses practicing in the ED and mental health units must be educated in the techniques and strategies to control abusive behavior, whether physical or verbal. These techniques and strategies include teamwork; careful assessment of prior violence by the patient, when possible; astute observation of current behavior; early intervention into potentially abusive situations (including, but not limited to, interpersonal approaches and medication); and adequate security and staff whenever abusive situations may arise.[78] In addition, nursing staff members must push for "architectural security" of the unit in which they practice,[79] including adequate room size, safety features (e.g., safety glass and alarm systems to call for help), and camera monitoring. Standing orders and written protocols for the use of medication and restraint, when clinically necessary, can also help the nurse when a decision must be made quickly to intervene in an explosive situation.

The nurse in the community must also be careful to avoid situations in which a patient may initiate violence. The nurse who is uncomfortable about seeing a patient alone should request that another nurse or agency staff member be present during the visit. The community nurse should always keep the agency informed of the planned route and should check in frequently with the agency.[80]

Although prevention is the best approach to avoiding violence in health care, it does not always work. Therefore the nurse who experiences violence by a patient should seek help and adequate protection, especially if the threat is physical. Obtaining help, retreating after isolating the violent patient, and protecting other patients and staff are all necessary.

Likewise, if a patient begins to seem out of control during a home visit, the nurse should attempt to calm the patient. If success does not occur quickly, however, the nurse should leave the situation and contact the agency, family, or other appropriate persons (e.g., police).

When a nurse is abused by another health care provider, the nurse should assertively request that the violence stop and not happen again. If that approach does not work, the nurse must report the incidents to the nurse manager and others in nursing administration. If appropriate intervention is not forthcoming, the nurse may need to report the circumstances to outside authorities, including the state licensing agency. In addition, the nurse should obtain legal advice about filing civil or criminal action against the abuser.

Last, but by no means least, the formal education of health care practitioners should include at least one ethics course so all students are "sensitized" to violence in health care. Including these issues can raise student awareness of the problem and offer a framework within which to resolve it. In turn, the graduate practitioner will be better able to treat others in a caring, rather than a violent, manner.

Violence in the School Setting

School violence is not what it used to be. At one time, if a child complained of being beaten up by older student bullies during recess, that was as bad as it got. Today, however, school violence runs the gamut of horror, including aggravated assault, stabbings, suicide, hate crimes, and shootings.[81] In fact, mass shootings in schools in Pearl, Mississippi; West Paducah, Kentucky; Jonesboro, Arkansas; Edinboro, Pennsylvania; and Littleton, Colorado, have resulted in the deaths of teachers and classmates.[82] Deaths on the property of a functioning public, private, or parochial elementary or secondary school (kindergarten through grade 12) totaled 268 in the years from 1992 to 2000.[83]

The reasons for violence in the school setting are varied. Some point to the atmosphere in the schools wherein students verbally harass classmates, place unacceptable graffiti in bathrooms identifying students by name, and sexually harass both male and female students.[84] Others indicate that having unclear rules or no rules concerning acceptable and unacceptable student conduct when not in class adds to the problem of setting realistic and fair limits in the school setting.[85] Still others see violence in school as due to the fact that the student who has witnessed violence or has been a victim of violence may act out against others due to feelings of anxiety, depression, or the need for self-protection.[86]

NURSING IMPLICATIONS

Regardless of the reasons for violence in the school setting, nurses have the potential to help identify, intervene, and prevent violence from occurring in schools. Perhaps no other group has this potential like school nurses. Because school nurses are visible, valuable members of the education team and are accessible to students, their interactions with the student body can begin the process of identifying a particular student who may be at risk for violent behavior. Referrals to appropriate community resources as well as on-site educational and support groups, anger management programs, and drug abuse prevention programs may help alleviate the need for intervention *after* violent behavior occurs. Working through parent associations and running parent skill training can increase parents' awareness of the potential for violence and how to constructively intervene before a tragedy occurs. Collaborating with other community groups and health care providers the parents and their student may be working with can hopefully provide a coordinated, consistent plan of support for the high-risk student.[87]

The psychiatric/mental health nurse, whether as a staff member in a psychiatric facility or as an advanced practice nurse, will need to assess all young and adolescent patients for the risk of violent behavior. Aiding patients to manage anger, improve self-control, and curb aggressive behavior are vital skills the psychiatric/mental health nurse must focus on in the established therapeutic relationship.[88] Also important is early intervention and competent management of existing emotional difficulties such as anxiety, depression, and identified psychiatric illnesses that might result in violent behavior.

Nurses who work in home health care are in a unique position to assess and evaluate children and adolescents in their home environment and the family's overall ability to handle problems and concerns in a nonviolent way. If, for example, an elderly and sick patient being seen by the home health care nurse is verbally abused and threatened by an adolescent grandson, the nurse can suggest other ways of working with the elderly patient. In addition, providing support to the grandson by listening to his concerns, suggesting other support options for him (increasing aide visits so that he can spend time with friends rather than always having to be home to care for the grandfather), and making appropriate referrals for additional help may keep the cycle of abuse from escalating. Adults in the family must also be supported. New ways of coping with the stress they are experiencing will need to be introduced by the home health care nurse whenever possible.

Pediatric nurses and pediatric nurse practitioners are also pivotal in assessing and intervening when they observe questionable behavior with their patient and/or the patient's family. Educating both the patient and his or her family about healthy ways to deal with violence, increasing positive, supervised recreation for children, and working legislatively to establish responsible gun ownership laws are all ways that can help decrease the chances of violence occurring.[90]

ETHICS CONNECTION 14–2

Violence in the workplace is a growing problem in the United States. Violence is the second leading cause of all on-the-job deaths and the leading cause of on-the-job deaths among women.[1] Nonfatal workplace violence also is a serious concern. Nurses often are victims of workplace violence. Inadequate staffing patterns purportedly contribute to increased violence in mental institutions. Emergency and trauma units are areas of especially high risk for violence against nurses and other health care employees. However, no area of health care is immune from violence. Violence against nurses is not limited to physical violence; verbal abuse is another common form of violence, particularly verbal abuse of nurses by physicians. This is intolerable and reportable. Violence of all forms is a breach of the moral principle of nonmaleficence. Violence in relationships of power imbalance also is an issue of social justice.

Nevertheless, few corporations, including health care institutions, are prepared to prevent violence in the workplace. Speer suggests that this apathy and lack of preparedness regarding violence in the workplace is a result of either denial or feelings of powerlessness to prevent such violence.

Arguing that most workplace violence is predictable and preventable, Speers proposes ways that companies can develop policies and practices to prevent violence and response teams to investigate and manage incidents that might lead to violence. In addition, Speer notes that domestic violence often is a precursor to workplace violence. Therefore, companies benefit from developing a responsible, compassionate plan of protecting employees who report that they are in abusive relationships. Speer reports that in a survey of corporate security and safety directors, 94% "ranked domestic violence as a high security problem."[2]

As with violence in general, ethical approaches related to workplace violence may be grounded in moral principles of nonmaleficence and beneficence, or in covenantal relationships. A profile of workplace mass murderers, however, reveals that there also are social justice issues associated with violence and its prevention. Speer's article includes a related article, "A Profile of Multicide" (mass murder) that is based on an interview with Deborah Schurman-Kauflin, an FBI-trained profiler of mass murderers. Schurman-Kauflin notes that mass murderers generally are people who have had psychosocial problems all their lives and typically are receiving psychiatric care. Developmental patterns of those who commit multicide have several commonalities. Many times, such individuals have experienced physical or emotional parental abandonment that leaves them unable to form attachments with other people. Potential mass murderers see less powerful humans and other creatures as objects; this detached view of living beings allows them to hurt smaller children and animals. They also have histories of property destruction, although they usually do not have criminal records. Because they see themselves as already dead, they are able to kill others and then kill themselves.[3] In a society that is committed to preventing violence, efforts need to start early if these repetitive patterns of isolation and abandonment are to be changed. Nursing can play a major role in assisting families, school systems, and other social institutions to obtain the skills, counseling, and other resources they need in order to prevent humans from feeling isolated and vulnerable.

Short-term prevention of workplace violence requires vigilance in identifying individuals who are at risk for committing violent acts. These individuals include not only full-time employees but also temporary employees, independent contractors, and anyone else who has a connection with the company. Schurman-Kauflin, in her appended article, further proposes a cluster of events that a company can watch for. She cautions that it generally is futile to attempt to dissuade a potential mass murderer from acting and warns employers and colleagues to take any threats of violence very seriously and to report them. "Creating a more humanizing workplace" is a very important practice in preventing violence. Sometimes corporate life dehumanizes or objectifies workers in the same way that the mass murderer objectifies his employer and colleagues. Through managing corporate actions, including layoffs, in a way that shows concern for those who work in a given institution, there is less likelihood of violence. Nurses in occupational health settings are well placed to work toward preventing workplace violence.

---

[1]Rebecca A. Speer, "Can Workplace Violence Be Prevented?" 60(8) *Occupational Hazards* (1998), 26–29.
[2]*Id.*
[3]*Id.*

ETHICS CONNECTION 14–3

Violence in the schools presents a growing concern in North America. Reports of a survey of youth violence conducted by the Josephson Institute of Ethics[1, 2] indicated that almost one-fourth of male high school students said that they had taken a weapon to school within the past year. Some 70% of the high school students said that they had struck another person in anger.

The loss through violence of so many children is a collective national and international tragedy. On a personal level, the loss is devastating to families, friends, and the wider community of all the children who have been killed or injured. Society readily acknowledges the grief of the families whose children have been killed. The grief and loss of families whose children actually or allegedly committed the violent acts that resulted in the deaths of others and themselves is less public. Although those acts never will be forgotten, there currently is a heightened concern for understanding the role of forgiveness in spiritual healing.[3]

A nurse, who is the mother of a 15-year-old daughter who was killed in a school shooting, recommends a broad range of individual, parental, and social action that nurses can initiate or support[4] and recommends additional reading on the subject of violence in schools.[5] This call for nurses to become more involved in social action clearly is consistent with the *Code for Nurses: With Interpretive Statements.*[6]

[1]American Public Health Association, "Survey Shows Propensity for Youth Violence," 29(6) *Nation's Health* (July 1999), 16–17.

[2]The Josephson Institute of Ethics is a nonprofit, nonpartisan organization that administers the Character Counts! Coalition. This coalition is an alliance of more than 300 national and regional groups working to help students develop trustworthiness, respect, responsibility, fairness, caring, and citizenship. See http://www.character-counts.org

[3]Avis Clendenen and Troy Martin. *The Forgiveness Exchange: To Forgive or Not to Forgive.* Unpublished Manuscript, 2000. *The Forgiveness Exchange* is a biblical, theological, and pastoral reflection. Dr. Avis Clendenen and Dr. Troy Martin are professors at Saint Xavier University, Chicago, Illinois. http://www.sxu.edu

[4]Sabrina Stenger, "Killed in School," 63(4) *RN* (April 2000), 36–38.

[5]See also C. R. DeBernardo and J. P. McGee, "Preventing the Classroom Avenger's Next Attack: Safeguarding against School Shootings," 4(2) *On the Move with School-Based Mental Health* (1999), 1.

[6]American Nurses Association. *Code for Nurses: With Interpretive Statements.* Kansas City, Missouri: Author, 1985.

SUMMARY OF PRINCIPLES AND APPLICATIONS

No one is immune from the effects of violence. It is global, threatening, and ubiquitous.[91] Violence has become a way of life, a common occurrence, in today's society. Acquiescence is not the answer, however, for the effects of violence are far reaching, permanent, and self-perpetuating. Research indicates, for example, that those who experienced abuse in childhood and as adults are prone to be abusers themselves, perhaps due to a fear of being victimized again.[92]

A recent study of abuse experienced by ED nurses accounted for compromised patient care, decreased morale, and "professional burnout."[93] These, together with other facts and figures, clearly support the need to intervene in the spiral of violence.

The nurse can play an active and important role in preventing violence in health care by:

- Attending continuing education programs and seminars on abuse, neglect, and exploitation

- Assessing the possibility of abuse, neglect, or exploitation with all patients

- Intervening consistent with legal and ethical duties when violence occurs against patients

- Educating patients and the public about the existence of abuse

- Protecting victims' confidentiality and privacy as mandated by law

- Testifying truthfully if called as a witness in any proceedings related to a patient who is the victim of violence

- Participating in the development of agency or facility policies and procedures dealing with patients who are victims of violence

- Reporting in good faith any concerns or beliefs that colleagues may be abusers of a patient or patients

- Eliminating abuse of staff by colleagues by reporting instances to appropriate agency or staff authorities

- Supervising staff carefully to intervene quickly in any staff-induced violence against patients

- Practicing nursing with an ever-vigilant eye toward personal safety when caring for potentially violent patients and/or families

- Documenting accurately and completely in any records concerned with instances of abuse, neglect, or exploitation

- Voting for elected officials who support laws deterring violence in the home, community, and health care

- Educating patients and their families about violence and self-protection, especially if mandatory reporting laws do not apply ·

- Encouraging state and federal legislatures to provide needed financial support for continued programs for victims of violence (e.g., therapy, shelters, health care)

- Acknowledging and positively working with one's own experiences as a victim of violence in order to stop its self-perpetuation

TOPICS FOR FURTHER INQUIRY

1. Design a study to determine if protective orders or other judicially developed mechanisms to prohibit violence against victims do, in fact, reduce or eliminate further injury.

2. Develop an interview tool to use with nurses and other health care providers (e.g., physicians, social workers, physical therapists) to identify respective experiences of violence by colleagues in health care settings.

3. Use an interview tool or questionnaire to evaluate how many nurses have been involved in reporting instances of child abuse and/or neglect to state agencies. Select particular practice areas (e.g., nursing, home health care nurses, nurses in child care clinics) and compare and contrast them.

4. Develop a model policy for reporting and intervening in violence against employees in your facility. Present it before the facility's policy and procedure committee for its feedback or ask the risk management committee or department to review it and make recommendations, if any, for changes.

REFERENCES

1. U.S. Department of Justice, Bureau of Justice Statistics. *Homicide Trends in the United States: Long Term Trends.* Available at: www.ojp.usdoj.gov/bjs. Accessed March 15, 2000.
2. U.S. Department of Justice, Federal Bureau of Investigation. *Uniform Crime Reporting Program Press Release.* October 13, 1996, 3, located at http://www.fbi.gov. Accessed March 31, 2000.
3. Seymour Moskowitz, "Saving Granny from the Wolf: Elder Abuse & Neglect—The Legal Framework," 31(77) *Connecticut Law Review* (1998), 85–86. See also Marshall Kapp. *Geriatrics and the Law: Understanding Patient Rights and Professional Responsibilities.* 3rd Edition. New York: Springer Publishing Company, 1999, 93.
4. National Center on Child Abuse and Neglect. *1977 Report,* cited in a review of *The Battered Child.* Mary Helfer, Ruth Kemp, and Richard Krugman, Editors. 5th Edition. Chicago, Ill.: University of Chicago Press, 1997. Review by Dr. Prasanna Nair, 280(5) *JAMA* (1998), 479–480.
5. Stephen Dearwater, Jeffrey Cohen, Jacquelyn Campbell, Gregory Nah, Nancy Glass, Elizabeth McLoughlin, and Betty Bekemeir, "Prevalence of Intimate Partner Abuse in Women Treated at Community Hospital Emergency Departments," 280(5) *JAMA* (1998), 433 (citations omitted).
6. Family Violence Prevention Fund. *Domestic Violence Is a Serious Widespread Social Problem in America: The Facts.* 1999, 1, located on the World Wide Web at the Fund's home page at http://www.fvpf.org. Accessed March 31, 2000.
7. Claire Burke Draucker and Christian Madesen, "Women Dwelling With Violence," 31(4) *Image: Journal of Nursing Scholarship* (1999), 328–329.
8. Robert Miller. *Problems in Health Care Law.* 7th Edition. Rockville, Md.: Aspen Publishers, 1996, 466; William Roach and the Aspen Health Law and Compliance Center. *Medical Records and the Law.* 3rd Edition. Gaithersburg, Md.: Aspen Publishers, 1998, 141.
9. Henry Campbell Black. *Black's Law Dictionary.* 7th Edition. St. Paul, Minn.: West Group, 1999, 1564.
10. *Id.*
11. See Illinois Domestic Act of 1986, 750 ICLS 60/101 *et seq.* (1986).
12. Black, *supra* note 9, at 10.
13. *Id.* at 1055.
14. National Clearinghouse on Child Abuse and Neglect Information. *In Fact . . . Answers to Frequently Asked Questions on Child Abuse and Neglect.* 1997 Statistics. Available at http://www.calib.com/nccanch. Accessed March 21, 2000, *citing* U.S. Department of Health and Human Services. *Child Maltreatment 1997: Reports from the States to the National Child Abuse and Neglect Data System.* Washington, D.C.: U.S. Government Printing Office, 1999.
15. Black, *supra* note 9, at 1055.
16. George D. Pozgar. *Legal Aspects of Health Care Administration.* 7th Edition. Gaithersburg, Md.: Aspen Publishers, 1999, 337.
17. *Id.* at 337.
18. See 325 ICLS 5/5 (1998); Ill. Admin. Code tit. 89, Section 300.120 (1991).
19. *Id.*
20. 936 S.W.2d 194 (Mo. 1999).
21. 713 N.E.2d 397 (Me. 1999).
22. *Id.* See also David Tammeleo, "Nurses Are Guardian Angels of Abused Children," 40(4) *Regan Report on Nursing Law* (1999), 4.
23. See, for example, Mark Lachs, Christianna Williams, Shelley O'Brien, Karl Pillermer, and Mary Charlson, "The Mortality of Elder Mistreatment," 280(5) *JAMA* (1998), 428.
24. Terry Fulmer, "Our Elderly—Harmed, Exploited, Abandoned," 25(3) *Reflections* (1999), 17.
25. *Id.* at 18.
26. Moskowitz, *supra* note 3, at 78–79.
27. Kapp, *supra* note 3, at 93–94.
28. Pozgar, *supra* note 16, at 339.
29. Molly Dickinson Velick, "Mandatory Reporting Statutes: A Necessary Yet Underutilized Response to Elder Abuse," 3 *Elder Law Journal* 190 (1995).

30. 210 ICLS 30/1 *et seq.* (1997) *as amended;* Michigan Compiled Laws Annotated, Section 400.11a (1993), *as amended;* New Jersey Statutes Annotated, Section 52: 27G-7.1 (West 1993) *as amended;* California Code, Section 15630 (West 1991), *as amended.*

31. 720 ICLS 5/12-19 (1991), *as amended* (Illinois); New Mexico Statutes Chapter 30 Article 47 Section 30-47-4 (1978), *as amended.*

32. 42 C.F.R. Section 482.13 (1999). See also, American Society for Healthcare Risk Management, "Health Care Financing Administration Imposes New Patients' Rights Conditions on Participation Requirements for Hospitals Effective August 2, 1999 (Final Interim Rule)," *ASHRM Member Alert* (July 20, 1999), 3; Chapter 19.

33. National Center on Elder Abuse, American Public Human Services Administration. *The National Elder Abuse Incidence Study: Final Report September 1998.* Washington, D.C.: Administration on Aging, U.S. Department of Health and Human Services, 1998. Available on the World Wide Web at http://www.aoa.dhhs.gov/abuse/report/. Accessed March 22, 2000.

34. Velick, *supra* note 29, at 190, *citing* Ala. Code Section 38-9-8 (Michie 1992 & Supp. 1994); Cal. Welf. & Inst. Code Sections 15-600 to 15-755 (West Supp. 1995); Mont. Code Ann. Section 52-3-811 (1993); Fla. Stat. ch 415.103 (West 1993).

35. See generally, Velick, *supra* note 29.

36. Velick, *supra* note 29, at 190. States which have passed voluntary reporting statutes governing elder abuse and neglect in noninstitutional settings include New Jersey, North Dakota, and Pennsylvania.

37. See generally, Robert Polisky, "Criminalizing Physical and Emotional Elder Abuse," 3 *Elder Law Journal* (1995), 377–382.

38. Florida Stat. Ann. Section 784.08 (West 1989), *as amended;* Louisiana Stat. Ann. Volume 9 Section 50.1 (West 1986), *as amended;* Colorado Revised Statutes Section 18-3-209 (1993).

39. Black, *supra* note 9, at 474.

40. Laura Rothstein. *Disabilities and the Law.* 2nd Edition. St. Paul, Minn.: West Group, 1997, 2 (with regular updates).

41. 405 ICLS 5/6-102 (1992), *as amended;* Texas [Human Resources] Code Annotated 48.036 (1990), *as amended.*

42. Illinois' Domestic Abuse of Disabled Adults Intervention Act, 20 ICLS 2435/15 *et seq.* (1997), (permissive reporting with consent of individual); Washington's Abuse of Children and Adult Dependent or Developmentally Disabled Act, Wash. Revised Code Annotated Section 26.44.010 *et seq.* (West 1993) (mandatory reporting).

43. 720 ICLS 5/12-21 (1997).

44. Susan Ross, Isabelle Pinzler, Deborah Ellis, and Kary Moss. *The Rights of Women: The Basic ACLU Guide to Women's Rights.* 3rd Edition. Carbondale, Ill.: Southern Illinois University Press, 1993, 221–222.

45. 720 ICLS 5/12-12 to 5/12-18 (1994), *as amended.*

46. *Id.*

47. NOW Legal Defense and Education Fund and Dr. Renee Chero-O'Leary. *The State-by-State Guide to Women's Legal Rights.* New York: McGraw-Hill, 1987, 81.

48. Black, *supra* note 9, at 600.

49. 325 ICLS 15/5 (1993), *as amended* (Illinois' Child Sexual Abuse Prevention Act).

50. See 735 ICLS 5/802.1-802.2 (1996).

51. *Id.*

52. See 325 ICLS 5/5 (1998), Abused and Neglected Child Reporting Act.

53. 720 ICLS 5/12-18 (1998) (Illinois).

54. In 1994, Congress passed the Violence Against Women Act, allowing women to civilly sue their attackers in federal court. In May, 2000, the U.S. Supreme Court invalidated the section of the Act that allowed victims of rape to civilly sue their attackers in federal court. In its 5–4 decision, the Court held that it is the states that have the power to govern such matters and not the federal government. Jan Crawford Greenburg, "High Court Ruling Further Clips Role of Congress," *Chicago Tribune,* May 16, 2000, Section 1, 1, 16. Prior to the May U.S. Supreme Court decision, many states, including Illinois, had proposed legislation to allow civil suits by rape victims.

55. Katherine C. McKenzie and others, "Prevalence of Domestic Violence in an Inpatient Female Population," 13 *Journal of General Internal Medicine* (1998), 277–279.

56. *Id.*

57. Dearwater and others, *supra* note 5.

58. Jacquelyn C. Campbell, "If I Can't Have You No One Can," 25(3) *Reflections* (1999), 8–12.

59. Susan Glander and others, "The Prevalence of Domestic Violence Among Women Seeking Abortion," 91 *Obstetrics & Gynecology* (1998), 1002–1006.

60. *Hearns v. Department of Consumer and Registration Affairs, D.C.,* 704 A.2d 1181 (1997).

61. *Ambassador Convalescent Center,* 83 Lab. Arb. (BNA) 44 (1984).

62. *IDAK Convalescent Center of Fall River (Crawford House),* 238 N.L.R.B. 410 (1978).

63. *Molden v. Mississippi State Department of Health,* 730 So. 2d 29 (1998).

64. See *Hall v. Bio-Medical Applications,* 671 F.2d 300 (8th Cir. 1982).

65. *Baptist Memorial Hospital v. Bowen,* 591 So. 2d 74 (Ala. 1991).

66. *Remmers v. DeBuono,* 660 N.Y.S.2d 159 (1997).

67. *State v. Serebin,* 350 N.W.2d 65 (Wis. 1984).

68. Failing to report instances of abuse can have serious implications. See *Wall v. Fairview Hospital,* 584 N.W.2d 395 (1998), in which a Minnesota psychiatric nurse's failure to report suspected patient abuse by the psychiatrist with whom she worked was at issue.

69. Pamela Levin, Jeanne Beauchamp Hewitt, and Susan Terry Misner, "Insights of Nurses about Assault in Hospital-Based Emergency Departments," 30(3) *Image: Journal of Nursing Scholarship* (1998), 253.

70. See, for example, "INA Zeller RN Seriously Injured in Workplace Assault: INA Demands Staffing and Security Improvements," 96(10) *Chart for Nurses* (1999), 1, 3 (the official publication of the Illinois Nurses Association).

71. Levin, Hewitt, and Misner, *supra* note 69, at 253–254 (citations omitted).

72. See, for example, Carrie Lybecker, "Violence Against Nurses a Silent Epidemic," 4(6) *Workplace Violence Prevention Reporter* (1998), 12 (available on the World Wide Web at http://www.nurseadvocate.org/silentepidemic.html); "Violence In Health Care Profession Enormous and Costly Problem," 4(5) *Workplace Violence Prevention Reporter*

(1998), 1–7; Barbara Mathews Blanton, Carrie Lybecker, and Nicole Marie Spring. *A Horizontal Violence Position Statement.* (1999). Available at http://www.nurseadvocate. org/hvstate.html. Accessed March 27, 2000.

73. See, for example, Kathryn Braun, Donna Christle, Duane Walker, and Gail Tiwank, "Verbal Abuse of Nurses and Non-Nurses," 22(3) *Nursing Management* (1991), 73–74.

74. *Id., citing* F. B. Friedmann, "A Nurse's Guide to the Care and Handling of MDs," *RN* (March 1982), 38–42.

75. *Peete v. Blackwell,* 504 So. 2d 222 (Ala. 1986), *rehearing denied,* March 20, 1987.

76. 714 A.2d 539 (Pa. 1998).

77. *Id.;* see also, David Tammelleo, "PA: Physician Verbally Abuses ER Nurse: Suspension of Staff Privileges Result," 39(4) *Regan Report on Nursing Law* (1998), 3.

78. See Emergency Nurses Association. *Violence in the Emergency Care Setting.* Des Plaines, Ill.: Author, 1997; U.S. Department of Labor, Occupational Safety and Health Administration. *Guidelines for Preventing Workplace Violence for Health Care and Social Service Workers.* Washington, D.C.: OSHA Publications, 1996 (OSHA Document #3148); Liza Little, "Risk Factors for Assaults on Nursing Staff: Childhood Abuse and Education Level," 29(12) *JONA* (1999), 22–29.

79. *Id.*

80. Barbara Youngberg, "Managing the Risk of Home Health Care," in *The Risk Manager's Desk Reference,* 2nd Edition. Barbara Youngberg, Editor. Rockville, Md.: Aspen Publishers, 1998, 382–383.

81. National School Safety Center. *In-House Report on School Associated Violent Deaths.* Westlake, Cal.: Author, 1999, 24. The report is available on the World Wide Web at http://www.nssc1.org. Accessed March 20, 2000.

82. *Id.;* see also, Lynne Lamberg, "Preventing School Violence: No Easy Answers," 280(5) *JAMA* (1998), 404–407.

83. National School Safety Center, *supra* note 81, at 25.

84. Lamberg, *supra* note 82, at 405 (citations omitted).

85. *Id.* (citations omitted). But see, Margaret Grahm Tebo, "Zero Tolerance, Zero Sense," 86 *ABA Journal* (2000), 40–46, 113, wherein the author discusses the drawbacks of establishing too-strict policies.

86. Lamberg, *supra* note 82, at 405 (citations omitted).

87. National Association of School Nurses. *Position Statement—Violence.* Scarborough, Me.: Author, 1995. The statement is available on the association's Web site at http://www.nasn/org. Accessed March 28, 2000.

88. See generally, Lamberg, *supra* note 82.

89. "Mental Illness and Violent Acts: Protecting the Patient and the Public," 280(5) *JAMA* (1998), 407–408 (Medical News & Perspectives section).

90. Jody Kurtt and Ginett Budreau, "Recent Changes and Current Issues in Pediatric Nursing," in *Current Issues in Nursing.* 5th Edition. Joan Comi McCloskey and Helen Kennedy Grace, Editors. St. Louis, Mo.: Mosby, 1997, 251-257. See also, Society of Pediatric Nurses. *Position Statement On Children, Violence and Resiliency,* 2000, 1–2, available on the World Wide Web at the society's home page at http://www.pednurse.org, accessed March 30, 2000; Society of Pediatric Nurses. *Action Plan for Prevention of Pediatric Firearm Injuries,* 1998, 1–2, on the society's home page (as above), accessed March 30, 2000.

91. Thomas Cole and Annette Flanagin, "Violence—Ubiquitous, Threatening and Preventable," 280(5) *JAMA* (1998), 648 (editorial).

92. Little, *supra* note 78; Lamberg, *supra* note 82.

93. Levin and others, *supra* note 69, at 253.

PART THREE

Legal and Ethical Concerns of Nurses in Diverse Roles and Settings

Licensure and Nursing Practice

15

Nurses, like other licensed professionals, are regulated by various state laws. One vitally important state law that directly affects the practice of nursing is the state nursing practice act. The ability of the state to govern nursing, other health care providers, and health care delivery systems is based in the state's constitution, which grants the state "police power" to ensure that its citizens' health, welfare, and safety are protected, and the federal Constitution's Tenth Amendment, which allows the respective states to establish and enforce any laws not prohibited or preempted by federal law.[1] Therefore, so long as the state laws are reasonable and further the overall objective of protecting its citizens, they stand as legitimate regulations of those individuals who seek to practice a profession or establish a health care entity.

Although the concept of state power is an important one, the ability of each state to regulate nursing and nursing practice has resulted in a wide variety of regulatory laws that are not consistent from state to state. The result is confusion among nurses and the public alike about scope of practice, educational issues, and specialties in nursing. Furthermore, this diversity has led to wide variations among state licensing boards or agencies regulating nursing practice, in terms of not only their structure but also their respective powers. For example, a 1985 study of boards of nursing conducted by the American Nurses Association's Center for Research cited five structure models for occupational licensing bodies.[2] They range from boards with complete autonomy (the ability to hire staff, discipline licensees, and set standards of practice, for example) to a "regulatory system" run by an agency director, commission, or council, in which the board or identified nursing group (e.g., a committee) functions as an advisory body to the agency head.[3]

Despite the multifarious laws governing nursing practice from state to state, any graduate nurse seeking licensure for the first time, or any licensed nurse, must be familiar with the agency or board administering the act, its rules and regulations, and his or her rights *and* responsibilities granted by the act. This chapter will provide such an overview that can form the basis for a more in-depth analysis of the nurse's own state practice act and state occupational licensing body (e.g., board of nursing or bureau of professional regulation).

NURSE PRACTICE ACTS

History

It is no secret that in the United States occupational licensure was first controlled by physicians. The American Medical Association, established in 1847, was very active in the political process, especially in relation to lobbying for state regulation of health care providers through licensure.[4] With the U.S. Supreme Court decision in 1888 that occupational licensure was within the legitimate "political power" of the state, the licensing of physicians was well established,[5] and physician licensure was rapidly adopted throughout the states.

> *It is no secret that in the United States occupational licensure was first controlled by physicians.*

This initial control over licensure by physicians clearly impacted on other health care professions later regulated by the states, including nursing. Because medicine was the first to define its practice, other professions had to be described by the states not only in very different terms but also by excluding any functions or responsibilities that were clearly included in the already established definition of medical practice.[6]

This impact can clearly be seen in the development of nursing practice acts across the country. In 1903 the North Carolina legislature passed the first registration act.[7] Other states soon followed North Carolina's example, and by 1923, all of the states then in existence had nurse practice acts. These were *permissive* acts, however, which meant that although one could register with the state agency or board to practice nursing, one did not *have* to do so. If an individual did not register with the state, that individual could continue to provide with.[8] In addition, and perhaps most telling, few if any nurses sat on the boards of nursing established by the acts. Rather, physicians composed the membership of the early boards.

In 1938, New York State passed the first *mandatory* nurse practice act. The New York legislation was remarkably different from the prior acts because it required individuals practicing nursing to be licensed to do so. Thus, no longer could an individual provide nursing care *or* use the initials "RN" after his or her name without being licensed. Moreover, the New York act included a definition of nursing practice and established a new nursing level, that of the licensed practical nurse. The licensed practical nurse role was also defined in terms of scope of practice and qualifications. Also, vitally important for the development of nursing as an autonomous profession controlled by *nurses* rather than *physicians,* registered nurses and licensed practical nurses began to compose the membership of nursing boards.

In 1938, New York State passed the first mandatory nurse practice act.

Around this time, an organization working toward licensure recognition of nursing and of the profession, the Nurses Associated Alumnae Organization of the United States and Canada, became the American Nurses Association. It continued to be active in supporting the regulation of nursing practice. In the early 1940s, a statement on provisions that should be included in nurse practice acts was prepared by the association.[9] In 1955, the association attempted to develop a "model definition" of professional nursing practice that unfortunately included a restrictive sentence stating that the practice of professional nursing "shall not be deemed to include any acts of diagnosis or prescription of therapeutic or corrective measures."[10] This language was necessary, so the thinking went, because mandatory acts needed to include a definition of nursing reflecting a distinction from medical practice that was already defined and carefully protected by the medical community.

The 1955 statement was followed in 1980 by another document, which was intended to serve as a policy guide for "nurses, state nursing associations, state boards of nursing, and state officials"

nursing care to patients but could not utilize the initials "RN" after his or her name. Furthermore, until the first *mandatory* act was passed, the permissive acts did not include any definition of the scope of nursing practice or had few prerequisites the individual seeking registration had to comply in amending nurse practice acts. The publication's purposes were to (1) reflect changes in the profession; (2) protect the public from unsafe practitioners; (3) ensure that the acts contained only those restrictions on licensure necessary to the regulation of safe practice; and (4) provide the minimal legal foundations in the acts for practice in the state, with control over the scope and definition of nursing practice remaining within the professional organization.[11]

Although the definition of professional nursing in this document did not include the restrictive language seen in the 1955 statement concerning what was the practice of nursing and what was to be reserved for physicians only, the 1955 language saw its way into many nursing practice acts, both before the 1980 position was adopted and afterward. In 1983, the American Nurses Association's own study indicated that nine states still had language similar or identical to the 1955 definition of nursing.[12]

Beginning in 1971, nurse practice acts were modified not only to provide a legal foundation for specialty areas of nursing practice, such as nurse practitioners, nurse-midwives, and nurse anesthetists, but also to eliminate the restrictive language established earlier. Again, New York became the first state, in 1972, to alter that restriction on practice.[13] In addition, terms like "nursing diagnosis," "expanded role," and "joint practice" (between nurses and physicians) were touchstones of this era.

The American Nurses Association also developed a new position statement (*Suggested State Legislation: Nurse Practice Act, Disciplinary Division Act and Prescriptive Authority Act*) concerning nurse practice acts, which reflected the many changes in nursing practice and health care delivery.[14] Insofar as the nursing practice acts are concerned, the document was important, not only for its support of advanced practice and its definitions of *delegation* and *supervision,* but also for its attention to boards of nursing. Boards, according to this publication, should be given clear powers and duties rather than simply inferring them.[15] Furthermore, the document clearly provided guidelines for the retention of responsibilities for boards that are not autonomous units, but rather function within a department or other state agency. They include (1) evaluating and approving requirements for licensure and renewal of that license; (2) disciplining professional nurses and licensed practical nurses who are not fit to practice, in accordance with due process principles; and (3) establishing and applying competency requirements to continue or reenter practice after a disciplinary action.[16]

In 1996, the American Nurses Association published its *ANA Model Practice Act.*[17] This model act was developed in order to "incorporate innovative approaches" to nursing practice acts that could withstand legal review and challenges.[18] Rather than develop the model on a particular state nurse practice act, the assocation drafted the model based on nursing needs identified in existing nurse practice acts and suggested language to focus upon anticompetitive barriers to practice.[19]

The 1996 model, among other provisions, specifically regulates licensed practical/vocational nurses, registered nurses, and advanced practice nurses. Board of nursing powers and responsibilities are also addressed and the model act expands the role of the board of nursing by granting the board the ability to issue advisory opinions on nursing practice, issue subpoenas, examine witnesses, and administer oaths. Language authorizing the board to address issues relating to the nursing profession's need and desire to develop limited liability and/or professional corporations was seen as an essential expanded power. The act also places the power to regulate prescriptive authority for nurses with the board of nursing.[20]

Current Status

Clearly, outside forces as well as state legislatures were responsible for molding nurse practice acts into various models. As a result, there is wide variation among state acts. Even with these variations, certain similarities exist, and consistency results more from concepts and principles of administrative law than from a consensus in nursing or the general public as to what should be included in these acts. Even so, nurse practice acts continue to be an important aspect of the regulation of nursing practice, nursing education, and the protection of the public from unsafe and unlicensed practice.

BOARDS OF NURSING OR OTHER REGULATORY UNITS

Composition and General Powers

The board of nursing or similar body is a creature of state law. The state nurse practice act con-

---

ETHICS CONNECTION 15–2

Although the American Nurses Association (ANA) code itself has not been revised since 1973, the *Interpretive Statements* were revised in 1985. The 1985 revisions specify the sequence of actions that nurses must take to comply with the safeguarding provisions of the *Code.* These *Interpretive Statements* are clear and unambiguous. When nurses first become aware that health care may be compromised by "inappropriate or questionable practice," they are morally required to express their concern to the person who is engaged in the inappropriate or questionable practice and to state the potential harm to the client. The nurse who identifies the potential harm also is responsible for documenting the inappropriate or unsafe comportment and reporting the behavior or practices through the process established by the health care institution.[1] When the practice is not ". . . corrected within the employment setting and continues to jeopardize the client's welfare and safety, the problem should be reported to other appropriate authorities."[2] Appropriate authorities include state professional organizations, state licensure regulatory agencies such as state boards of nursing, or other professional or "legally constituted bodies."

This final requirement to move beyond the walls of the institution has posed considerable difficulty to individual nurses in the past. Because most nurses are and were employees, the *Code's* moral obligation that nurses report their employers' failure to act in a morally responsible way created conflict and frequently resulted in damage to the reporting nurses' careers and loss of livelihood. It was this conflict between the ethical requirements of the *Code* to protect the client and nurses' loyalty to the institution that was so well illustrated in the 1986 report of the classic Yarling and McElmurry study.[3] Social, institutional, and regulatory (licensure) contexts are changing, however, and nurses in many areas are becoming more autonomous and are supported by either colleagues, their institutions, or the law when they comply with this provision of the *Code.*

---

[1]Institutions also are obligated to have "an established process for the reporting and handling of incompetent, unethical, or illegal practice within the employment setting," according to the American Nurses Association. Interpretive Statement 3.2, Acting on Questionable Practice. *Code for Nurses with Interpretive Statements.* Kansas City, Missouri: Author, 1985.

[2]American Nurses Association. *Code for Nurses with Interpretive Statements.* Kansas City, Missouri: Author, 1985. (Currently under revision. Revised *Code* anticipated in 2001).

[3]Rod Yarling and Beverly McElmurry, "The Moral Foundation of Nursing," 8(2) *Advances in Nursing Science* (1986), 63–73.

---

tains provisions concerning the board's or other unit's composition, power, and authority. Members of boards or committees are appointed in many ways. Some states mandate appointment by the state governor with professional organization participation.[21] Others require nomination from state nurses associations (e.g., state nursing and licensed practical nursing associations).[22]

Because the state legislature grants to the board of nursing or similar body certain powers clearly specified in the nurse practice act, the board can carry out only those powers or those that can reasonably flow from them. Thus, boards of nursing are considered to be of "limited jurisdiction." This limited jurisdiction may be further limited by the legislature. Common powers given to boards of nursing may include rulemaking, licensing, and the authority to conduct and participate in cases involving the discipline of nurses licensed under the act. Despite the wide variations

in power, these regulatory bodies are involved in administering and enforcing the state nurse practice act.

Disciplinary Process and Procedure
Grounds for Disciplinary Actions

The state nurse practice act section on discipline lists specific grounds upon which the board or regulatory unit can take disciplinary action against the nurse. Although variations exist, some common grounds to protect the public from unsafe or ineligible practitioners include:

- Violation of any provision of the nursing practice act
- Abuse of alcohol or other habit-forming drugs when the licensee has not requested or is not receiving treatment for drug addiction or abuse

- Falsification of patient records or failure to record essential information in the patient's record
- Unprofessional conduct likely to deceive, defraud, or harm the public
- Conviction of a felony or a crime involving moral turpitude, or pleading *nolo contendere* (no contest) to either
- Negligent or willful violation of nursing practice standards
- "Unlawful" acts, including practicing nursing without a license, fraudulently obtaining or furnishing any nursing license or diploma, or aiding and abetting another in such acts.[23]

Common powers given to boards of nursing may include rulemaking, licensing, and the authority to conduct and participate in cases involving the discipline of nurses licensed under the act.

Based on the common provisions of nurse practice acts, eight general categories of disciplinary actions can be taken against nurses. They are fraud and deceit; criminal activity; negligence, risk to clients, and physical and mental incapacity; violations of the nursing practice act or rules; disciplinary action by another board; incompetency; unethical conduct; and drug and/or alcohol use.[24]

Eight general categories of disciplinary actions can be taken against nurses.

FRAUD AND DECEIT. Although the specific conduct that might violate this general category can vary and can involve other violations, such as criminal activity or drug or alcohol abuse, many times the deceit and fraud can take place when the individual attempts to secure a nursing license and falsifies documents (e.g., fraudulent license or college transcript) in order to obtain licensure in a state.[25]

CRIMINAL ACTIVITY. Generally, two main provisions are included in most nurse practice acts concerning criminal activity: (1) conviction of a felony and (2) conviction of a crime involving "moral turpitude" or "gross immorality."

Although there are wide variations in the kinds of crimes that might be included under the latter two categories, generally they involve those that have dishonesty as a central element, such as theft, fraud, misrepresentation, and embezzlement.[26]

Felonies, on the other hand, are those violations enumerated in the federal or state criminal statutes, and because of their serious nature usually require more than 1 year in jail as punishment if convicted. Some examples include possession of a controlled substance, forgery, deception, and murder.

Regardless of the type of criminal activity that may be alleged against the nurse, criminal allegations raise additional implications. Specifically, the issue of self-incrimination must be carefully evaluated. The right against self-incrimination is based in the Fifth Amendment of the U.S. Constitution and similar state constitutional provisions. It protects an individual from being "compelled" to be a witness against himself or herself in a criminal case and requires the government to prove its case against the accused.

The right against self-incrimination applies in agency or board of nursing actions when the nurse or licensed practical nurse is accused of conduct that violates not only the nurse practice act but also state or federal criminal laws. If the conduct in question may violate state criminal law (e.g., diverting controlled substances from the employer or falsifying narcotics or medical records to cover the diversion), an admission by the nurse to investigators, either by an oral or written declaration or by any other act (and especially after being given a *Miranda* warning by those investigators), allows the state to bring criminal charges against the nurse. Of course, *any* admission, with or without a *Miranda* warning, can be used against the nurse in the disciplinary proceeding itself.

NEGLIGENCE, RISK TO CLIENTS, AND PHYSICAL OR MENTAL INCAPACITY. This overall category clearly reflects the board of nursing's concern about protecting the public from unsafe or incompetent practitioners. Although some states simply indicate "negligence" in the delivery of nursing care as a ground for discipline, many state statutes require "gross negligence" to occur, or require more than one incident to have taken place before taking action against the nurse. Likewise, the risks to clients that are grounds for actions against professional or licensed practical nurses are, most often, significant risks to the health, safety, or physical or mental well-being of the patient and may also include actual injury to the patient.

A nurse's physical or mental incapacity, whether due to disease or injury, must relate to the nurse's *current* ability to practice and deliver health care safely.[27] This is an important legal concept because it ensures that a board or other regulatory unit will not exceed its authority when evaluating conduct alleged to be in violation of the nurse practice act. If a nurse is unable to care for patients safely and competently because of any of the conditions in this category *at the time a complaint is filed,* and that inability is proven, then the nurse may not practice until and unless the disability is removed. To discipline a nurse when there is no *current* threat to the public's safety is to ignore constitutional and other protections afforded an individual in his or her due process and property rights.

VIOLATIONS OF THE NURSING PRACTICE ACT OR RULES. Almost all of the state nurse practice acts include language allowing discipline against a nurse for a violation of the act. Many acts also include any violation of the related administrative rules as valid grounds for taking action against the nurse or licensed practical nurse.[28]

Rules and regulations further define a particular statute by giving more details and guidelines concerning the administration and enforcement of the act. The administrative rules and regulations for nurse practice acts are as divergent as the acts themselves, but some areas of coverage include standards of conduct for professional and licensed practical nurses (e.g., Illinois and Wisconsin); definitions of terms used in the act (e.g., unprofessional conduct, negligence, and mental incompetency); and scope of practice statements, tasks allowed, and required collaboration in licensing specialty areas of practice (e.g., nurse-midwives or nurse practitioners).

With the establishment of the National Bank, the Healthcare Integrity and Practitioner Data Bank (HIPDB), and the National Council of State Boards of Nursing Disciplinary Data Bank established in 1981, tracking prior disciplinary actions against nurses will be easier for nursing boards.

DISCIPLINARY ACTION BY ANOTHER JURISDICTION. Prior to the Health Care Quality Improvement Act of 1986 and the Medicare and Medicaid Patient and Program Protection Act of 1987,[29] which require hospitals, licensing boards, professional associations, peer review committees, and insurers to report disciplinary actions to a national data bank, nurses and other health care providers could move from one state to another relatively easily without any tracking of prior disciplinary problems. As a result, states did not often file an action against a nurse or licensed practical nurse because of actions taken by another state unless that information was inadvertently discovered. However, with the establishment of the National Bank, the Healthcare Integrity and Practitioner Data Bank (HIPDB),[30] and the National Council of State Boards of Nursing Disciplinary Data Bank established in 1981,[31] tracking prior disciplinary actions against nurses will be easier for nursing boards. Thus, it is certain that this provision will continue to be included in nurse practice acts as a basis for disciplinary action against the nurse.

INCOMPETENCE. This general category as a basis for disciplinary action against nurses has not been specifically recommended by the American Nurses Association for inclusion in nurse practice acts.[32] Even so, this ground does appear, again in varying forms, in many acts. The various forms include mental disability that would interfere with safe patient care (many times phrased as an involuntary admission to a psychiatric facility); negligence; and failure to meet generally accepted standards of nursing practice.

UNETHICAL CONDUCT. Unethical conduct can include many types of behavior. Some nurse practice acts or their rules and regulations contain specific provisions concerning unethical behavior, including breach of nurse-patient confidentiality; refusal to care for someone of a certain race, creed, color, or national origin; fraud in obtaining reim-

ETHICS CONNECTION 15–3

From the perspective of covenantal relationships (see Chapter 3), nurses who observe reportable unsafe practice are faced with conflicts between and among several special covenants—with their colleagues and others in the work environment, with their employers, and with their profession. The accountability for safeguarding clients, however, is part of respecting human life and human rights. The primary conflict that nurses experience in safeguarding clients against harm from others, thus, is a conflict between special covenants and an inclusive covenant that preserves human well-being. Allen's presentation of covenantal conflict gives priority to inclusive covenants over special covenants.[1] The accountability to the client thus prevails over obligations either to institutions or to colleagues. Therefore, although it may be emotionally anguishing to report a colleague, it is morally indefensible to fail to report an individual who practices "incompetently, unethically, or unsafely."

---

[1]Joseph L. Allen. *Love and Conflict.* Lanham, Md.: University Press of America, 1995.

---

bursement; violation of the ethical code for nurses; and not maintaining competence in nursing practice.[33]

DRUG AND ALCOHOL USE. Impaired nursing practice is still a concern in the nursing profession.[34] The number of disciplinary actions against nurses utilizing this ground in nurse practice acts is disturbing and is on the rise. In one state alone, from November of 1997 through May of 1999,[35] there were at least 38 documented cases of disciplinary actions taken by the state board of nursing against nurses for drug and alcohol impairment or use that affected the nurse's practice. In addition to impairment or use, other problems that often concurrently arise with drug or alcohol use are diversion of an addicted-to drug (often controlled substances) from the employer, selling diverted drugs or drug paraphernalia (syringes, IV tubing) to others, and falsification of patient and other records.

Although it was once fairly common for state boards or other regulatory units to be punitive when nurses had an addiction problem, whatever the reason and however it manifested itself, they have shifted to acknowledging the addiction as an illness that requires treatment. Viewing addiction as an illness has not changed any board's responsibility to protect the public by removing the impaired nurse's license when needed, but it has resulted in a vision of treatment and rehabilitation for the impaired nurse so that continued recovery can be obtained and maintained. With the help of professional organizations such as the National Nurses' Society for Addictions, the Drug and Alcohol Nurses' Association, and the American Organization of Nurse Executives, treatment and educational programs, as well as input into legislative changes in nurse practice acts, have been established to help impaired nurses and, at the same time, protect the public from unsafe practitioners.

Two interesting results have taken place because of the efforts of these organizations. First, many nurse practice acts require certain nurses, such as nurse administrators or owners of nurse registries, to report impairment that affects the nurse's practice and diversion of controlled substances to the board of nursing or regulatory unit. Doing so creates many problems for the nurse who is reported. However, in an attempt to be more rehabilitative, some of the practice acts provide an exception to reporting when the nurse seeks treatment, is monitored by the facility, and stays employed there. The difficulties with this approach are varied. One is that many times, adequate treatment options are simply not available for the nurse in his or her community. A second problem lies in the act itself: If the nurse is fired, for example, for theft or forgery pursuant to the employer's disciplinary policy, the nurse must then be reported to the state agency because one of the key provisions of nonreporting—employment—cannot be met.

Second, developing alternative approaches to disciplinary actions against the nurse is perhaps more flexible and serves to protect the public *and* provide needed treatment and rehabilitation to the impaired nurse. The alternative approaches have been established in several states, including Florida and California. Other states have adopted varying forms of the community-based California model and the Florida approach, which allows the impaired nurse to enter an approved treatment facility, be shielded from disciplinary action so long as treatment is successful, and return to work with monitoring by the board.[36]

Because of the professional organizations' efforts, and because of better public understanding of the problem of addiction, several model acts have been proposed for state legislatures to follow in developing alternatives to disciplinary actions against nurses abusing drugs or alcohol.[37] Until *all* jurisdictions adopt such an approach to the impaired nurse, however, more traditional actions, including disciplinary actions, will continue against the nurse or licensed practical nurse whose chemical addiction affects his or her professional practice.[38]

Possible Actions of Board or Regulatory Agency

The ability of the board of nursing or regulatory agency to take action against the registered or licensed practical nurse rests with the statutory authority given the licensing authority by the state legislature. The American Nurses Association clearly supports the position that the licensing authority be given broad powers to discipline nurses. Those powers include denying an application for licensure; suspending or revoking a license or other authorization to practice; requiring a licensee to submit to treatment or therapy for initial,

continued, or renewed licensure; and administering a public or private reprimand.[39]

. . . the licensing authority [should] be given broad powers to discipline nurses. Those powers include denying an application for licensure; suspending or revoking a license or other authorization to practice; requiring a licensee to submit to treatment or therapy for initial, continued, or renewed licensure; and administering a public or private reprimand.

The regulatory agency or board is also usually given wide latitude in combining the possible actions. For example, when drug use is found to exist, the registered nurse's license may be placed on probation (e.g., periodic, random drug screens and employer reports to be submitted to the agency) in addition to requiring the nurse to successfully complete treatment for the drug problem.

If the registered or licensed practical nurse's license is suspended or revoked and the conditions specified in the case are met, the nurse may usually petition the board or regulatory agency for reinstatement of the license. The burden of proving that the reinstatement is warranted rests with the nurse. If that burden is met, then reinstatement can occur, with or without additional reporting to the licensing authority (e.g., additional employer reports). However, if the burden of proof is not met, the individual may be denied reinstatement of his or her license at that time.

Actions taken by the board or regulatory agency are often challenged by individuals seeking initial licensure when their application is denied;[40] by registered and licensed practical nurses when a revocation occurs;[41] and when the action is alleged to be a violation of certain due process rights of the licensee.[42] Unless the licensing authority's decision is beyond its scope of power, unconstitutional, or arbitrary, however, the decisions are not overturned by the reviewing court.

ETHICS CONNECTION 15–4

Frequently, other nurses shun nurses who report unsafe practices of their colleagues. Because the nurse who reports a colleague also protects that colleague's privacy whenever possible and respects the confidentiality required in such situations, other coworkers sometimes are unaware of the unsafe practices. Thus, both the nurse who reports a colleague and the nurse who is reported may experience social isolation in the work environment. The *Code of Ethics for Registered Nurses* of the Canadian Nurses Association clearly identifies the obligation of colleagues to respect one another, even while safeguarding clients: "Nurses support other nurses who act in good faith to protect clients from incompetent, unethical or unsafe care, and advocate work environments in which nurses are treated with respect when they intervene."[1] Nurses are morally required to support nurse colleagues who do, in good faith, report others for untoward practices.

---

[1]Canadian Nurses Association. *Code of Ethics for Registered Nurses,* Ottawa: Author, 1997.

KEY CASE 15–1	Rafferty v. Commonwealth of Pennsylvania and State Board of Nurse Examiners (1986)[43]

FACTS: Anne Marie Rafferty, a neurosurgical nurse in the ICU at Thomas Jefferson University Hospital, was to bathe a comatose patient who was on a respirator. She decided to disconnect the respirator during the bath to check for spontaneous respirations, because the patient began experiencing premature ventricular contractions (PVCs). After testing his breathing without the respirator (no spontaneous breathing occurred), she reconnected the ventilator. She resumed the bath, but noticed "significant changes" in the patient's blood pressure and PVCs. Nurse Rafferty did not call a code, despite being instructed to do so by several other ICU nurses who realized that the patient was experiencing cardiac arrest. The patient died. Ms. Rafferty was reported to the Pennsylvania Board of Nursing by the hospital and was charged with "willfully or repeatedly" violating several of the regulations of the Pennsylvania Nursing Act dealing with assessing human responses to nursing care, external cardiac resuscitation, and artificial respiration. The regulations also stated that the board could discipline a nurse when there were "willful or repeated" violations of the (nurse practice) act or regulations. There were never any allegations by the board that Ms. Rafferty caused the patient's death, nor were there any findings to that effect.

Pennsylvania Board revokes the license due to the nurse's conduct deviating from accepted standards of care

BOARD OF NURSING: After a hearing, the Pennsylvania Board of Nursing revoked Ms. Rafferty's license, because she violated several of the regulations of the Act, and her conduct deviated from accepted nursing practice. She appealed that decision to the Commonwealth Court of Pennsylvania.

The initial Court of Review reversed the board's decision due to insufficient evidence

COURT REVIEW OF FINDINGS: The initial court of review reversed the findings of the board, holding that there were no repeated violations, just the one incident; there was no evidence of any "willful" violation of the regulations; Ms. Rafferty's record prior to this incident was "unblemished"; and although Ms. Rafferty's conduct was in error and subject to "severe criticism," the board erred in finding substantial evidence on which to base the revocation. The board of nursing appealed the decision to the Pennsylvania Supreme Court.

The Pennsylvania Supreme Court reverses the initial review court decision, holding there was "ample evidence" in the record for its decision

PA. SUPREME COURT REVIEW OF FINDINGS: The Pennsylvania Supreme Court reversed the lower court decision and remanded the case to the Commonwealth Court of Pennsylvania. The Supreme Court held that the board was not required to prove specific intent when looking at "willful" conduct, because doing so would negate the board's charge of ensuring "safe nursing services for the citizens of the Commonwealth." The court also upheld the board's decisions that Ms. Rafferty's conduct in removing the patient from the respirator to check for spontaneous respirations rather than to do so by other means and the finding that her other conduct was "willful" were based upon ample evidence in the record.

KEY CASE 15–1	Rafferty v. Commonwealth of Pennsylvania and State Board of Nurse Examiners (1986)[43] *Continued*

The Pennsylvania Supreme Court also remands several issues to the Commonwealth Court for its decision

However, the court remanded several issues to the Commonwealth Court for its decision because they were raised during the appeal. They were whether or not the board regulations were constitutional; whether the presence of the hospital's attorney at the board hearing denied her a fair hearing; and whether the board's refusal to reopen the record for additional testimony of the treating physician was proper.

The Commonwealth Court holds that the decision stands because the issues it reviewed did not require a reversal of the board's decision

COURT DETERMINATION OF ISSUES ON REMAND: The Commonwealth Court affirmed the decision of the Pennsylvania Board of Nursing to revoke Ms. Rafferty's license, holding that the additional issues raised did not merit overturning that decision. In so doing, the court stated that (1) the rules were not vague as to *her* conduct (and therefore were constitutional); (2) the presence of the hospital attorney in no way prejudiced her or the board's decision; and (3) not reopening the record was proper since, according to Pennsylvania's Code of Procedure, there was no new evidence requiring the board to do so.

ANALYSIS: The *Rafferty* case is an example of how alleged due process rights violations are handled by the courts. Clearly, Ms. Rafferty was concerned with her rights to a fair hearing, a decision based on the evidence by an appropriate body, the opportunity to present and cross-examine witnesses, and, of course, judicial review. Although one may not agree about the ultimate outcome of this, or any other, case concerning licensing actions, it clearly illustrates that the process of review and the rights of the licensee are carefully protected.

Procedural and Substantive Due Process Rights of Licensees

The registered or licensed practical nurse possesses clear protections against any arbitrary and unfair actions by the state licensing authority. A nursing board or regulatory agency licensing nurses is a governmental agency and therefore must abide by both substantive *and* procedural due process principles. Procedural and substantive due process rights are based in the U.S. and respective state constitutions, as well as in the federal and state administrative procedure acts. The minimum protections afforded the nurse licensee are therefore fairly universal in practice acts and include:

- Notice of time and place of any proceeding
- A clear statement of the charge(s)
- Representation by counsel
- Cross-examination of adverse witnesses
- Presentation of own witnesses
- Hearing before a proper and authorized group that makes its decision in a fair manner based on the evidence presented
- Record/transcript of the proceedings
- Judicial review of the decision

> *A nursing board or regulatory agency licensing nurses is a governmental agency and therefore must abide by both substantive and procedural due process principles.*

Allegations of violations of these rights often serve as the basis for a challenge of the board or licensing authority's decisions concerning actions against the nurse, as seen in Key Case 15–1.

Burden of Proof and Evidence in Hearings

Any decision of a board of nursing or regulatory agency must be based on the facts introduced into evidence during the hearing. Generally the rules governing administrative hearings and evidence are not as rigid as when a civil or criminal hearing or trial takes place. Furthermore, because administrative hearings take place before a hearing officer who may or may not be a lawyer, the rules and regulations concerning evidence are relaxed somewhat. For example, in administrative hearings, hearsay (an out-of-court/hearing statement offered to support the truth of something at issue in the court or hearing) may be admitted into evidence more easily.

Although the more relaxed rules may be beneficial to the nurse who faces a disciplinary hearing, the inability to utilize the strict rules of evidence may also be harmful to the nurse. For example, if hearsay were allowed in a particular board hearing, and an *adverse* witness testified about something she said she heard another person say about the nurse whose license was at issue, and that other person could not be found to support or refute the statement, the licensee might not be able to defend herself as she more fully could if the rules of evidence were more strictly applied.

The burden of proof in administrative hearings varies from state to state and is based on statutory and case law. In addition, it may vary based on who initiates the hearing or proceeding. For example, in Illinois, if a nurse petitions the Department of Professional Regulation for reinstatement of his or her license after it has been suspended, the nurse must show, by a preponderance of the evidence, that the license should be reinstated.[44] If, however, the department initiates a disciplinary action against a professional or licensed practical nurse, the burden of proof the department must meet in proving the allegations is one of clear and convincing evidence.[45]

Although the clear and convincing evidence standard is a common one in administrative hearings, other evidentiary standards required for the board or regulatory agency to prove the allegations against the licensee include "substantial evidence," a preponderance of the evidence, a clear preponderance, and satisfactory proof.

When a board or regulatory agency does not meet its burden of proof, the nurse licensee can challenge the decision.[46]

Judicial Review of Board or Agency Decisions

The ability of the licensee to have a decision reviewed by the appropriate court is an important one, but it cannot be used unless the nurse meets certain prerequisites. As with many of the topics discussed thus far, judicial review varies from state to state, although it is clear that every nurse who decides to question a decision of a board or regulatory agency has the right to do so.

One of the usual requirements for judicial review is exhaustion of any and all remedies afforded for review of the administrative decision *within* the administrative agency or body itself. For example, if a nurse disagreed with a decision, a request for a rehearing before the same administrative officer or body might be required before any judicial review could occur.

When judicial review takes place, the reviewing court's role is dictated by state case and statutory law, including the state administrative procedure act. The reviewing court's main role is to ensure that the administrative hearing was a fair one and that the applicable law was interpreted and applied accurately. As a result, the reviewing court will most often uphold the decision of the board or regulatory agency unless one or more of the situations presented in Table 15–1 occur.

Judicial review of any administrative board decision must also be timely filed pursuant to state law. When the petition for judicial review is not timely filed, it will be dismissed.[52]

TABLE 15–1

Board or Agency Actions Not Upheld on Judicial Review

BOARD OR AGENCY	CASE EXAMPLES
Acted arbitrarily, capriciously, or in an unreasonable manner	*Scott v. Nebraska Board of Nursing*[47]
Abused its discretion	*State of Florida v. McTigue*[48]
Violated constitutionally protected right(s) of licensee	*Woods v. D.C. Nurses' Examining Board*[49]
Made an error of law	*Hoyte v. Board of Regents of the University of the State of New York*[50]
Based its decision on insufficient evidence	*Arkansas State Board of Nursing v. Long*[51]

When judicial review takes place, . . . the reviewing court's main role is to ensure that the administrative hearing was a fair one and that the applicable law was interpreted and applied accurately.

Challenges to Powers or Actions of Boards or Regulatory Agencies

Challenging board or agency decisions can take the form of a specific allegation by the nurse, or it may be a component of another objection to the regulatory agency's conduct (e.g., disciplinary action for "unprofessional conduct").

One type of specific challenge to the board or agency's filing of disciplinary actions against the nurse is when the agency has not done so in a timely manner. For example, in *Harper v. Louisiana State Board of Nursing,*[53] the board did not bring a complaint for more than 2 years after it was aware that Ms. Harper had "improperly handled" narcotics. In upholding the board's suspension of Ms. Harper's license, the court held that no specific time frames for bringing a case against a licensee were present in the Louisiana Nurse Practice Act and also held that because such cases do not become "stale," there is no need to file them within a certain time.

A different result would most probably occur, however, if a particular state nurse practice act *did* contain a specific period. Illinois' Nursing and Advanced Practice Nursing Act, for example, requires that any action against a registered nurse or licensed practical nurse must take place within 3 years from the commission of the conduct allegedly violating the Act or from a final conviction order.[54] This time limitation can be extended by 1 year when a professional negligence case, or a settlement of such a case, is pending against the licensee for the alleged conduct.[55]

A second challenge to board or agency power can rest on the jurisdiction of the entity to bring its complaint; that is, to its authority to exercise its powers. This challenge can take many forms, such as alleging that the board or agency exceeded its authority granted by the legislature in revoking a license because of intoxication while on duty;[56] alleging that the entity cannot take action against a *student* nurse who is not a "registered nurse" or a "licensee";[57] or alleging that no regulations existed to guide the board or agency in taking action against the nurse, as seen in Key Case 15–2.

Other Specific Duties

In addition to participating in disciplinary proceedings, a state board of nursing usually has additional responsibilities and duties delegated to it by the legislature. Common additional responsibilities of most boards or regulatory units include approval of educational programs, licensing powers, and rulemaking authority.[59]

Educational Responsibilities

The board of nursing or agency responsible for nursing practice in the state has, as one of its main goals, the setting of educational standards for nursing programs throughout the state, whether they be 2-, 3-, or 4-year basic programs, graduate programs, or continuing education and refresher courses. It is important to note that there is not total agreement on the actual powers to be given to state nursing boards in this role.[60]

The approval process for proposed nursing education programs can be quite involved and prolonged, but the procedure must be completed before any program can begin operating. The board or regulatory agency is usually given the ability to develop standards and rules for the curriculum, faculty, students, and facilities.

In addition to approving nursing education programs, many state boards of nursing are given the power to deny or withdraw approval after a hearing or other due process protections are afforded the program.

Licensing Powers

Regulatory units governing nursing practice have the ability to grant nursing licenses to those individuals who meet certain requirements so that those individuals can legally practice nursing.[61] The board or agency establishes the requirements through its statutory authority (the nurse practice act itself) as well as through developed standards, rules, and regulations. The requirements for initial licensure application usually include completion of or graduation from an approved nursing program; obtaining a passing score on the licensing

KEY CASE 15–2   Tuma v. Board of Nursing (1979)[58]

The Idaho Board of Nursing suspends Ms. Tuma's license for "unprofessional conduct"

The initial review court upholds the board's decision

The Idaho Supreme Court reverses the district court, holding that any disciplinary action must be done pursuant to notice of the misconduct to the licensee and pursuant to established rules and regulations

FACTS: Jolene Tuma was a registered nurse employed as a clinical instructor of nursing at the College of South Idaho. While performing those duties, she met a patient with myelogenous leukemia whose only hope of survival was chemotherapy. Ms. Tuma asked to administer the chemotherapy to the patient. During initiation of treatment, the patient brought up the subject of Laetrile and asked Ms. Tuma about it as an alternate form of therapy. After several discussions with Ms. Tuma about Laetrile, the patient withdrew her consent for the chemotherapy. A family member of the patient then contacted the doctor. The physician discontinued the chemotherapy, and the patient died about 2 weeks later. Although the death did not result from Ms. Tuma's actions "in any way," the physician reported her to the board of nursing for "interfering with the physician-patient relationship."

BOARD OF NURSING: After a hearing, Ms. Tuma was found to have engaged in "unprofessional conduct" under the Idaho Nursing Act and her license was suspended for 6 months.

COURT REVIEW OF FINDINGS: The District Court affirmed the 6-month suspension, and Ms. Tuma then appealed to the Supreme Court of Idaho on the grounds that her due process rights were violated. Specifically, Ms. Tuma alleged that the term *unprofessional conduct* was unconstitutionally vague and therefore did not give her notice that speaking with a patient about alternative treatment—Laetrile—would be a violation of the act.

IDAHO SUPREME COURT REVIEW OF FINDINGS: The Idaho Supreme Court reversed the district court's decision, holding that the board had not exercised its ability to expand the initial legislative definition of nursing prior to the *Tuma* case. Therefore it could not suspend the license of *this* person without a clear warning to Ms. Tuma that the conduct she engaged in—talking with a patient about alternative treatments—was "unprofessional conduct." Furthermore, the court held that in addition to giving adequate notice to Ms. Tuma of any prohibited conduct, developing specific rules and regulations was also necessary to guide the board in making judgments concerning any licensee who comes before it for alleged misconduct.

ANALYSIS: The *Tuma* case is an example of many of the points discussed throughout this chapter, including the importance of protecting the due process rights of nurses in disciplinary actions (notice and adequate hearing) and requiring clear, defined prohibitions of conduct when an adverse outcome—suspension or revocation of a license—may take place. The case also illustrates the interplay between the legislature and the entities it creates. It is not enough to be given the power to do something; rather, the agency, board, or other entity created must do so within the powers given *and* in a nonarbitrary manner.

examination; and proof of good character, age, and citizenship. If the applicant does not meet one or more of the requirements, the board or agency can, of course, deny the applicant the professional registered nurse license or the practical nurse license. Adverse decisions have been the subject of many cases by those denied a license. However, unless the unfavorable agency decision falls into one of the categories listed in Table 15–1, it will be upheld upon judicial review.

In addition to applications for *initial* licensure, the board or regulatory agency also has jurisdiction to make licensure decisions for those professional and licensed practical nurses who seek licensure in that state after holding a license in another state or foreign country. Although the manner in which the state grants an individual a license may vary, the four options available to the state agency are endorsement, reciprocity, waiver (or "grandfathering"), and examination.

Although the manner in which the state grants an individual a license may vary, the four options available to the state agency are endorsement, reciprocity, waiver (or "grandfathering"), and examination.

Endorsement and reciprocity differ. *Endorsement* refers to the process of granting a license after an evaluation of whether the individual already granted a license in another state, and *those* requirements, satisfy the requirements in the state where the application is pending. *Reciprocity,* on the other hand, is the process of granting a license when two states have exactly the same licensing requirements. This is a difficult standard to meet, given the wide variation in state nurse practice acts,[62] however, and therefore most, if not all, nurses receive a license in another state after initial licensure by way of endorsement.

Licensing powers of boards of nursing or regulatory agencies also may include the ability to grant temporary licenses, place a license on inactive status, and renew licenses during established renewal periods.[63] Clearly, these powers, when granted to the board, also include the ability to establish rules and regulations to carry out these responsibilities.

The licensing of foreign nurses in the United States continues to be the subject of much controversy and litigation. The debate has centered on qualifications and the need for the foreign nurse to be proficient in English. As a result of these concerns, most state nursing practice acts require a certificate by the Commission on Graduates of Foreign Nursing Schools (CGFNS) evidencing proficiency in English and satisfactory educational preparation before a license in that state will be issued.[64]

Rulemaking

The board of nursing or regulatory agency's ability to promulgate rules and regulations is usually found in the state's administrative procedure act and respective administrative law decisions. This aspect of board power is vital, for without the option of establishing rules and regulations to carry out the nursing practice act, the board or agency's power would indeed be a hollow one.

To promulgate rules, the governmental agency is required to adopt them in a constitutional manner; that is, with notice to the public, with a hearing for the purpose of allowing for public testimony in support of or against the proposed rules and regulations, and with publication of the final version of the adopted directives in the required reporter.[65]

As has been illustrated in this chapter, the rules and regulations adopted by the regulatory agency can be challenged but will withstand such a test unless the action taken, or the rule or regulation, is invalidated by the reviewing court.

Regulation of Advanced Practice

The ability of the state board of nursing or regulatory agency to regulate advanced nursing practice—the practice of clinical nurse specialists, nurse-midwives, nurse practitioners, and nurse anesthetists—has been the subject of much debate, not only within the nursing profession but also between the nursing profession and other professional groups.[66] The American Nurses Association has been involved in this debate, not only in supporting the ability of prepared nurses to practice in expanded roles but also in how specific nursing practice acts should be in regulating expanded roles.

Specifically, the American Nurses Association's position is that the state nurse practice act should give authority to the board or regulatory agency to "include advanced practice under the definition of nursing practice, thus allowing the BON to make professional distinctions in tasks (scope of practice) by levels of practice."[67] Certification, adopting rules for the practice of advanced nurse practitioners, and establishing categories of advanced nurse practitioners should rest with the professional associations, and doing so in a nurse practice act is seen as restricting "flexibility and expansiveness" of the practice of advanced and nonadvanced practitioners.[68] Even so, many state nurse practice acts establish categories of advanced practitioners, certify them, adopt rules for their practice, and/or define education and other qualifications for specialty practice.[69]

MULTISTATE LICENSURE

In 1995, the National Council of State Boards of Nursing initiated an inquiry into the possibility of and the need for multistate licensure, especially in view of the advent of telehealth and nursing's involvement in delivering nursing care services through this medium. In 1997, the council's Delegate Assembly ratified language for an interstate compact. The council then developed a Mutual Recognition Master Plan to implement the mutual recognition mode.[70] The final version of the Nurse Licensure Compact, which consists of 11 articles, was adopted on November 6, 1998.[71]

The council's compact is described as "an agreement between two or more states to coordinate activities associated with nurse licensure."[72] The end result of such a compact is to facilitate practice across state lines and, at the same time, help states protect the public's health and safety by ensuring competent nursing care; facilitate cooperation between states who are part of the compact; and promote compliance with the state laws governing the practice of nursing in each state which is a member of the compact, among other purposes.[73] Table 15–2 summarizes some of the provisions of the National Council's Nurse Licensure Compact.

There is no question that there is a need for an arrangement in which licensure and practice across state lines is made simpler. The Pew Health Professions Commission, for example, included such a recommendation in its 1998 report.[74] Yet,

---

TABLE 15–2

Selected Provisions of the National Council of State Boards of Nursing Nurse Licensure Compact

ESSENCE OF PROVISION	WHERE FOUND
• A state that adopts the Compact is called a "party state"	Article II j.
• "Nurse" defined as a registered nurse or licensed practical/vocational nurse	Article II i.
• Licensure issued in the "home state" of the nurse (the nurse's primary state of residence) is recognized by each party state as authorizing a multistate licensure privilege in each party state	Article II e.; Article III a.
• Compact establishes a Coordinated Licensure Information System (CLIS) that is to include information on licensure and disciplinary history of each state (reported by each party state) to help coordinate licensure and enforcement data	Article VII a.
• Disciplinary actions by boards of nursing against the registered nurse or licensed practical/vocational nurse can take place in any state which recognizes multistate licensure	Article V

Data from: National Council of State Boards of Nursing, "Nurse Licensure Compact," November 6, 1998 at http://www.ncsbn.org; National Council of State Boards of Nursing, "Nurse Licensure Compact: Setting the Record Straight," at http://www.ncsbn.org. Accessed April 4, 2000.

---

despite the identified need for a framework that would facilitate practice across state lines, there is little consensus as to what that framework should be.

The Nurse Licensure Compact has both supporters and critics. Some organizations that support its adoption include the American Association of Occupational Health Nurses (AAOHN)[75] and the Air and Transport Nurses Association.[76] Others, such as the American Nurses Association[77] and the National Association of Pediatric Nurse Associates & Practitioners, Inc. (NAPNAP),[78] are critical of the compact.

Despite the controversy surrounding the compact, as of March 2000, Arkansas, Iowa, and North Carolina have enacted the compact legislation. The state of Maryland's compact went into effect on July 1, 1999. Nebraska and South Dakota's state laws go into effect on January 1, 2001.[79]

The American Nurses Association has proposed three other models to facilitate practice across state lines that are not based upon a compact model. In contrast to an agreement model between states, all three ANA models suggest ways to provide for multistate licensure using the current licensure framework. The models are described by the ANA as rapid endorsement (when physically practicing across state boundaries), registration (practicing via Telehealth), and site of provider (practicing via Telehealth).[80]

Multistate licensure is still an evolving issue. It will take some time before it is clear whether one model excels over another and truly facilitates professional practice across state, or other, boundaries.[81] The nurse will need to keep abreast of all of the latest developments in the area of multistate practice. If the nurse is practicing in a state that has adopted the compact, he or she will need to conform with the compact when practicing physically or electronically in another state which has also adopted the compact. Continual evaluation of the compact and other models will be necessary in order to ensure the best solution for easing multistate licensure and, at the same time, continuing to provide quality nursing care to the public. Active participation in the nurse's professional organizations will be necessary to help those entities support and facilitate the best format for multistate licensure to thrive and be universally accepted.

TELEHEALTH AND NURSING PRACTICE

Telehealth has been defined in various ways due to its ever-changing and developing character. Even so, a clear definition is gleaned from how it operates: "the removal of time and distance barriers for the delivery of health care services and related health care activities through telecommunication technology."[82] Whether using the telephone,[83] computers, or videoconferencing, or transmitting data or images across other types of technological equipment, telemedicine has revolutionized health care delivery.[84]

There are many positive results due to the increased use of telecommunication in health care. Remote areas of the country—or the world, for that matter—have access to specialists and innovative medical procedures that they would not be able to take advantage of without telehealth. Consultations with health care providers and educational experiences for medical and nursing students no longer require face-to-face encounters. Triage decisions can be made without the need to have the patient come to the physician's or nurse practitioner's office.

Despite these positive effects, telehealth raises many legal and ethical concerns. Legally, one of the first issues focuses upon licensure. When a consultation or a triage decision is made across state or national lines, the question of practicing nursing or medicine without a license is immediately raised. Where should the health care provider be licensed? Is it acceptable for the health care provider *not* to be licensed in a state where the patient is physically located, as long as the practitioner is licensed in the state from which the information is provided? The regulatory issues surrounding telehealth are perhaps the most urgent ones that must be resolved. One solution is multistate licensure, discussed in the previous section of this chapter.[85] Another proposed resolution is a "limited telemedicine [telenursing] license" in each state in which a patient resides and receives services through telehealth procedures.[86] Interestingly, the Health Care Financing Administration (HCFA) of the Department of Health and Human Services has decided that for reimbursement purposes, when a teleconference consultation occurs, the state of practice is the site where the provider is located.[87] As a result, the patient, in essence, "travels" via telecommunication technologies to the site of the provider.[88] If one accepts this approach, perhaps multistate licensure is "unnecessary" because it is the patient who crosses state or national boundaries, not the provider.

A second concern in telehealth is the confidentiality and privacy of the health information sought and received with telecommunication technologies. Computerized medical records have been in use for some time, but concern surrounding their access, misuse, and interception is longstanding and ever present.[89] The same concerns are raised with other forms of telehealth, including videoconferencing and video consultations.[90]

A third legal concern centers on the issue of competencies in telehealth. The American Nurses Association has identified 11 competencies the registered nurse should demonstrate when using telehealth technologies in nursing.[91] They include establishing a therapeutic relationship with the client, ensuring clients are informed about their choices concerning the use of telehealth, and documenting and integrating into information systems the structure, process, and outcomes of telehealth events.[92] Along with other professional nursing organizations such as the American Academy of Ambulatory Care Nursing, the Home Health Nurses Association, and the National Association of Pediatric Nurse Associates and Practitioners, the association has also identified core principles related to clinical standards and the roles and responsibilities of health care professionals in the establishment of standards and guidelines in telehealth.[93] Standards and guidelines are essential in order to establish—and maintain—quality care using this medium.

The nurse who utilizes telehealth in whatever form will need to be sensitive to the fact that many of its applications have yet to be tested legally. As a result, a proactive, preventative approach to the liabilities that may be associated with its use is best.

Such an approach should include compliance with all agency policies and practices concerning confidentiality and privacy of teletronic information transmitted in telehealth and telenursing; a clearly defined informed consent policy for use with any telenursing should be established and followed (e.g., scope and purpose of the telenursing encounter, limits of the telenursing encounter)[94]; technological proficiency must be ensured through in-services, workshops, and continual updates, especially as changes in this area occur[95]; professional liability insurance for telenursing activities must be included in either the nurse's individual policy and/or the employer's insurance policy that covers the nurse employee[96]; and changes in tort law—especially professional negligence—will need to be reviewed regularly to determine if telehealth changes traditional liability principles (e.g., Is there a "duty" to provide telehealth? How may "reasonable care" be defined in this medium?).[97]

SUMMARY OF PRINCIPLES AND APPLICATIONS

Most nurses are familiar with liability principles related to professional negligence and attempt to practice their profession with those principles in mind. Equally important, however, is the value of the nursing license and potential liability the nurse faces if there is an alleged violation of the nursing practice act.

A registered nurse or licensed practical nurse possesses a "property right" in his or her license, meaning that the nurse has a legal claim to it.[98] The federal or state government cannot deprive an individual of life,

liberty, or property without due process of law.[99] Therefore the government cannot limit or take that right away unless clear due process protections are afforded the owner of the property right. When a nurse is accused of conduct that may jeopardize his or her license, fairness and justice must surround the proceedings to protect the nurse's clear "property right" in that license from being transgressed.

If there are allegations that the nurse has violated one or more of the act's provisions, and those allegations are proven, it is clear that the professional or licensed practical nurse will be disciplined in some way. Because the nurse's very livelihood is at stake when a disciplinary action is pending, the nurse should avoid, insofar as humanly possible, any potential violation of the state nurse practice act by:

- Understanding the history and purpose of nurse practice acts generally
- Knowing the state nurse practice act, and its rules and regulations, in the states in which she or he is licensed
- Obtaining legal counsel if an action by the state board of nursing or state regulatory agency is taken against the nurse
- Obtaining updates on cases decided by state courts and/or regulatory agencies concerning nursing practice and the nurse practice act
- Taking an active role in the professional associations of the nurse's choice, especially in relation to nursing practice issues
- Taking an active role in the legislative process, especially in relation to nursing practice issues, by writing legislators and providing testimony about pending bills or amendments to current statutory law
- Attending nursing board or committee meetings on a regular basis
- Considering applying for a position on the state board of nursing or committee and, if appointed, serving as a member of the board or committee, or suggesting names of nurse colleagues to serve on the nursing board or committee
- Keeping current on the developing issues in regulatory law, including multistate licensure and telehealth and nursing practice

TOPICS FOR FURTHER INQUIRY

1. Design a study to compare the following state practice acts in terms of similar provisions covering scope of

practice, delegation and supervision, promulgated rules and regulations, telehealth practice, and grounds for discipline: nursing practice act, pharmacy practice act, medical practice act, and social work practice act.

2. Interview a nurse or practical nurse who has been disciplined by the state regulatory agency for his or her impressions of the due process protections present during the process.

3. Obtain minutes of the meetings of the state nursing board or regulatory agency through the state Freedom of Information Act and analyze actions taken by the board or agency.

4. Interview a state legislator supportive of nursing practice and identify the various successes and failures experienced by the legislator in attempting to change the act through the legislative process. If possible, include attempted changes in relation to multistate licensure and/or telehealth.

REFERENCES

1. U.S.C.A. Const. Amend. 10: "The powers not delegated to the United States by the Constitution, nor prohibited by it to the States, are reserved to the States respectively, or to the people."

2. Clare LaBar. *Boards of Nursing: Composition, Member Qualifications and Statutory Authority.* Kansas City, Mo.: American Nurses Association Center for Research, 1985, 2, *citing* Council of State Governments. *Occupational Licensing: Centralizing State Licensing Functions.* Lexington, Ky.: Author, 1980, 1.

3. *Id.*

4. Bonnie Bullough, "Introduction—Nursing Practice Law," in *Nursing Issues and Nursing Strategies for the Eighties.* Bonnie Bullough, Vern Bullough, and Mary Claire Soukup, Editors. New York: Springer Publishing Company, 1983, 279; see also, Antoinette Inglis and Diane Kjervik, "Empowerment of Advanced Practice Nurses: Regulation Reform Needed to Increase Access tò Care," 21(2) *Journal of Law, Medicine, & Ethics* (1993), 197 (citations omitted).

5. Bonnie Bullough, *supra* note 4.

6. Inglis and Kjervik, *supra* note 4.

7. George Pozgar. *Legal Aspects of Health Care Administration.* 7th Edition. Gaithersburg, Md.: Aspen Publishers, 1999, 241.

8. *Id.*

9. American Nurses Association. *Suggestions for Major Provisions to be Included in a Nursing Practice Act.* Kansas City, Mo.: Author, 1943.

10. American Nurses Association. *Educational Preparation for Nurse Practitioners and Assistants to Nurses.* Kansas City, Mo.: Author, 1955.

11. American Nurses Association. *The Nursing Practice Act: Suggested State Legislation.* Kansas City, Mo.: Author, 1981.

12. Clare LaBar. *Statutory Definitions of Nursing Practice and Their Conformity to Certain ANA Principles.* Kansas City, Mo.: ANA, 1983, 51.

13. Pozgar, *supra* note 7, at 240.

14. American Nurses Association. *Suggested State Legislation: Nursing Practice Act, Nursing Disciplinary Diversion Act, and Prescriptive Authority Act.* Kansas City, Mo.: Author, 1990.

15. *Id.* at 13.

16. *Id.*

17. American Nurses Association. *Model Practice Act.* Washington, D.C.: American Nurses Publishing, 1996.

18. *Id.* at 5.

19. *Id.*

20. *Id.* at 10–16.

21. *Id.* at 40.

22. *Id.*

23. *Id.* at 49–50. See also National Council of State Boards of Nursing. *Model Practice Act.* Chicago, Ill.: Author, 1994, 29–33.

24. See, for example, Robert H. Gans, "Current Concepts in Dealing with Licensing Board Disciplinary Matters," in *1997 Wiley Medical Malpractice Update.* New York: John Wiley, 1997, 211–240; Ann Carruth and Donnie Booth, "Disciplinary Actions Against Nurses: Who Is at Risk?" 6(3) *Journal of Nursing Law* (1999), 55–62.

25. See, for example, *Nicholson v. Ambach,* 436 N.Y.S.2d 465, *appeal dismissed,* 446 N.Y.S.2d 1024 (1981). This ground can also be useful when an applicant for licensure cheats during the NCLEX exam. *Culpepper v. State of Arizona,* 930 P.2d 508 (1996).

26. See, generally, Wayne LaFave and Austin W. Scott. *Criminal Law.* 2nd Edition. St. Paul, Minn.: West Publishing Company, 1986 (with 1999 update); Chapter 9.

27. See, for example, *State Board of Nursing v. Crickenberger,* 757 P.2d 1167 (Colo. Ct. App. 1988).

28. ANA, *supra* note 17, at 49–50.

29. Pub. L. No. 99-660, 42 U.S.C.A. Section 11101 *et seq.* (1986); Pub. L. No. 100-93, U.S.C.A. Section 132-a-5 *et seq.* (1987).

30. For a brief discussion of the HIPDB, see Chapter 6.

31. For an interesting discussion of the current and proposed interplay between these three data banks, see the National Council of State Boards of Nursing's home page at http://www.ncsbn.org.

32. ANA, *supra* note 17, at 49–52.

33. *Id.* at 51.

34. Madeline Naegle and Ann Solari-Twadell, "Impaired Practice: Still an Issue," 10(2) *Journal of Addictions Nursing* (1998), 61–62 (editorial).

35. "Disciplinary Actions," *Pennsylvania State Board of Nursing* (Winter 1999–2000), 5–10. See also Alison Trinkoff and Carla Storr, "Substance Use Among Nurses: Differences Between Specialties," 10(2) *Journal of Addictions Nursing* (1998), 77–85.

36. For an interesting overview of "diversion programs" established by states, and research concerning Florida's Intervention Project, see Tonda Hughes, Linda Smith, and Marion Howard, "Florida's Intervention Project for Nurses: A Description of Recovering Nurses' Reentry to Practice," 19(2) *Journal of Addictions Nursing* (1998), 63–69.

37. American Nurses Society on Addictions. *Statement on Model Diversion Legislation for Chemically Impaired Nurses,* 1985. *Reprinted in* Tonda Hughes and Ann Solari-Twadell, "Responses to Chemical Impairment: Policy and Program

Initiatives," in *Addiction in the Nursing Profession: Approaches to Intervention and Recovery.* Mary Hack and Tonda Hughes, Editors. New York: Springer Publishing Company, 1989, 200–217; National Council of State Boards of Nursing. *Model Guidelines: A Nondisciplinary Alternative Program for Chemically Impaired Nurses.* Chicago, Ill.: Author, 1994.

38. As of 1998, 25 states have developed formal diversion programs. Hughes, Smith, and Howard, *supra* note 36, at 63.

39. ANA, *supra* note 17, at 52.

40. *Richardson v. Brunelle,* 398 A.2d 838 (1979).

41. *Mississippi Board of Nursing v. Hanson,* 703 So. 2d 239 (1997).

42. *Slagle v. Wyoming State Board of Nursing,* 954 P.2d 979 (1998).

43. 471 A.2d 1339 (Pa. Comm. 1984), *rev'd in part, remanded in part,* 499 A.2d 289 (1985), *on remand,* 505 A.2d 357 (1986).

44. 68 Illinois Administrative Code, Chapter I, Subchapter a, Part 110 (*Rules of Practice in Administrative Hearings*), Section 110. 190 (1983).

45. *Id.*

46. For an interesting recent case concerning which standard of proof should be used in a disciplinary action against a nurse who challenged the standard applied by the Vermont Board of Nursing, see *In re Smith,* 730 A.2d 605 (Vt. 1999).

47. 244 N.W.2d 683 (Neb. 1976).

48. 387 So. 2d 454 (Fla. 1980).

49. 436 A.2d 369 (D.C. App. 1981).

50. 304 N.Y.S.2d 693 (1969).

51. 651 S.W.2d 109 (Ark. 1983).

52. *Bowman v. Indiana State Board of Nursing,* 663 N.E.2d 1217 (1996).

53. 484 So. 2d 857 (La. App. 1986).

54. 225 ILCS 65/20 - 50 (1998).

55. *Id.*

56. *Alabama Board of Nursing v. Herrick,* 454 So. 2d 1041 (Ala. Civ. App. 1984).

57. *Aron D. Hempell v. Louisiana State Board of Nursing,* 713 So. 2d 1265 (1998).

58. 593 P.2d 711 (Idaho 1979).

59. ANA, *supra* note 17.

60. *Id.* at 12.

61. ANA, *supra* note 17; National Council of State Boards of Nursing, *supra* note 23.

62. *Id.*

63. *Id.*

64. See, generally, National Council of State Boards of Nursing, *supra* note 23, at 18.

65. See Chapter 8.

66. See, as examples, Sharon A. Brown and Deanna Grimes. *Nurse Practitioners and Certified Nurse-Midwives: A Meta-Analysis of Studies on Nurses in Primary Care Roles.* Washington, D.C.: American Nurses Association, 1993; Charles A. Sargent, *Nurse Practitioners and Physician Assistants in the North Central Region: Their Status and Role in Rural Primary Health Care.* Lafayette, Ind.: Purdue University, January 1987; *Nurse Practitioners, Physician Assistants and Certified Nurse-Midwives: A Policy Analysis.* Washington, D.C.: Office of Technology Assessment, December 1986; A. Catlin and M. McAuliffe, "Proliferation of Non-Physician

Providers as Reported in the Journal of the American Medical Association (JAMA) 1998," 31 *Image: Journal of Nursing Scholarship* (1999), 175–177; Mary Mundinger, Robert Kane, Elizabeth Lenz, Annette Totten, and others, "Primary Care Outcomes in Patients Treated by Nurse Practitioners or Physicians," 283(1) *JAMA* (2000), accessed January 28, 2000, at http://www.jama.ama-assn.org/issues/283nl/full/joc99696.html.

67. ANA, *supra* note 17, at 11–12.

68. *Id.*

69. For the current status of each state's treatment of advanced practice nursing, see "Annual Update of How Each State Stands on Legislative Issues Affecting Advanced Nursing Practice" which appears yearly in the January issue of *The Nurse Practitioner.*

70. See generally, "Boards of Nursing Adopt Revolutionary Change for Nursing Regulation," 18(3) *Issues* (1997), 1, 3 (National Council of State Boards of Nursing Newsletter).

71. National Council of State Boards of Nursing. "Nurse Licensure Compact," November 6, 1998, 1. The entire compact is available on the council's home page on the World Wide Web at http://www.ncsbn.org. Accessed April 2, 2000.

72. Terri Gaffney, "The Regulatory Dilemma Surrounding Interstate Practice," *Online Journal of Issues in Nursing* (May 31, 1999), at http://www. nursingworld.org. Accessed April 14, 2000.

73. Nurse Licensure Compact, *supra* note 71, at 1.

74. Pew Health Professions Commission Taskforce on Health Care Workforce Regulation. *Strengthening Consumer Protection: Priorities for Health Care Workforce Regulation.* San Francisco, Cal.: Pew Health Professions Commission, 1998, vi; 19–20 (Recommendation 6).

75. *AAOHN Supports Mutual Recognition for Nursing Regulation,* located at the National Council of State Boards of Nursing home page at: http://www.ncsbn. Accessed April 4, 2000.

76. *Air & Surface Transport Nurses Association Position Statement: Mutual Recognition Model for MultiState Licensure.* January 10, 2000. The statement can be accessed on the National Council of State Boards of Nursing home page at http://www.ncsbn.org. Accessed April 4, 2000.

77. *Position Statement of the ANA Board of Directors on the Nurse Licensure Compact.* Adopted February 17, 1999. The statement can be accessed on the American Nurses Association's home page at www.nursingworld.org. Accessed April 7, 2000.

78. *MultiState Licensure Compact.* The information about the organization's concerns about the compact can be accessed at the association's home page at http://www.napnap.org. Accessed April 17, 2000.

79. *State Compact Bill Status* (last updated on March 16, 2000). The status page can be accessed on the National Council of State Boards of Nursing home page at http://www. ncsbn.org. Accessed April 2, 2000.

80. American Nurses Association. *The American Nurses Association Proposed Licensure Models to Facilitate Practice Across State Lines,* available on the association's home page at http://www.nursingworld.org. Accessed April 9, 2000.

81. One of the major concerns about the compact is that it, as currently written, requires "absolute reciprocity among and between party states." This is an unconstitutional delegation of legislative authority in a state because it allows

another state legislature to determine the licensee's qualifications for licensure in the state in which the nurse does not reside. For an in-depth discussion of this and other issues involved in multistate licensure, see Nancy J. Brent, "Emerging Legal Issues for Nurse Managers," in *Professional Development: Issues & Opportunities for 2000 & Beyond.* Ann Scott Blouin and Mary Jo Snyder, Editors, Philadelphia, Penn.: W. B. Saunders Company (in press); Chapter 8.

82. American Nurses Association. *Competencies for Telehealth Technologies in Nursing.* Washington, D.C.: Author, 1999, 1 (citation omitted).

83. See, for example, Linda Globis, "Telenursing: Nursing by Telephone Across State Lines," 3(3) *Journal of Nursing Law* (1996), 7–17; Chapter 19.

84. *Competencies for Telehealth Technologies in Nursing, supra* note 82, at 1–2.

85. See also Laurie Stycrula, "Troubles with Telehealth: Electronic Nursing Without a License?" 12(2) *Nursing Spectrum* (1999), 8–9.

86. Gaffney, *supra* note 72, at 2–3.

87. *Id.* at 3.

88. *Id.*

89. William Roach and the Aspen Health Law and Compliance Center. *Medical Records and the Law.* 3rd Edition. Gaithersburg, Md.: Aspen Publishers, 1998, 290–327.

90. Hilary Lewis, Katheryn Ehler-Lejcher, and Barbara Youngberg, "Managing the Risks Associated with Telemedicine," in *The Risk Manager's Desk Reference.* 2nd Edition. Barbara J. Youngberg, Editor. Gaithersburg, Md.: Aspen Publishers, 1998, 363–379; Robert Roth, Joanne Jarquin, and Alice Palmer, "Confidentiality Issues Affecting Practitioners in Telemedicine: What Someone Else Does Not Know Could Hurt You," in *1999 Health Law Handbook.* Alice Gosfield, Editor. St. Paul, Minn.: West Group, 1999, 655–676; James Rosenblum, "Telemedicine Liability," in *2000 Wiley Medical Malpractice Update.* Barbara Robb, Editor. Gaithersburg, Md.: Aspen Law & Business, 2000, 1–17.

91. American Nurses Association. *Competencies for Telehealth Technologies in Nursing.* Washington, D.C.: Author, 1999.

92. *Id.* at vii.

93. American Nurses Association. *Core Principles on Telehealth: Report of the Interdisciplinary Telehealth Standards Working Group.* Washington, D.C.: Author, 1998, ix–x, 3.

94. Lewis, Ehler-Lejcher, and Youngberg, *supra* note 90, at 374–375.

95. American Nurses Association, *supra* note 93, at 19.

96. Rosenblum, *supra* note 90, at 14; Lewis, Ehler-Lejcher, and Youngberg, *supra* note 90, at 374–375.

97. Rosenblum, *supra* note 90, at 17.

98. Henry Campbell Black. *Black's Law Dictionary.* 7th Edition. St. Paul, Minn.: West Group, 1999, 1322–1333.

99. U.S.C.A. Constitution, Amendments 5 and 14 respectively.

The Nurse As Employee

16

KEY PRINCIPLES

- At-Will Employment
- Wrongful/Retaliatory Discharge
- Equal Employment Opportunity Laws
- Occupational Health and Safety
- Labor Relations
- Termination of Employment
- Employee Compensation and Benefits
- Employee Privacy and Confidentiality
- Human Resource/Personnel Records

According to recent figures, there are approximately 2,558,874 registered nurses in the United States; 83% of that number are employed.[1] The work settings of the nurses are varied: the majority work in hospitals, 8.1% in extended care facilities, and the remainder in community health, ambulatory care, and other health care delivery settings.[2]

Most nurses are employees; that is, one who (1) works for another under a contract of hire, whether express, implied, written, or oral; (2) is paid a salary or wages; and (3) is under the power or control of the employer insofar as the details and means of how the work to be done is accomplished.[3]

Being employed implies that the work performed occurs within an employer-employee relationship. That relationship is affected and influenced by many factors, not the least of which is the law. Countless federal and state statutes, rules and regulations, case law, and common law shape the employment relationship in such areas as "terms and conditions of employment," employee privacy, wages and salaries, and safety in the workplace.

This chapter will explore the employment relationship and its legal components, including employment status, fair employment practices, employee benefits, and labor relations. In addition, special considerations such as the right to refuse an assignment and employee access to personnel records will be reviewed.

EMPLOYMENT STATUS

A health care delivery system delivers patient care through its employees. Nurses compose a large segment of employees in any health care system. Generally speaking, those nurses are one of two types of employees—at-will or contractual.

Not many nurse employees have a contract of employment with an employing entity. This is due to the fact that customarily only nurse executives (e.g., the chief nurse officer), advanced nurse practitioners (a nurse anesthetist or nurse-midwife), and nurse faculty, as examples, may have contracts of employment. The rationale for having nurse executives, advanced nurse practitioners, and nurse faculty enter into an employment contract is, in part, predicated on the different roles and responsibilities of these groups.

Nurse executives, for example, may find an employment contract helpful in fulfilling responsibilities in a changing work environment without fear of losing their job.[4] Factors such as health care competition, physician discomfort, and risk taking may stifle health care executives without some assurance that their position is more secure than without the employment contract.[5] Likewise, advanced nurse practitioners, who function in a more independent role than their staff nurse colleagues, also need to be able to make decisions

without unnecessary fear of losing their job. Similarly, nurse faculty (particularly those without tenure) are often hired on a year-to-year basis (or for some other limited time frame). This type of arrangement is beneficial to the academic institution, which is able to rely on the nurse faculty's services for a particular academic time period.

In contrast, staff nurses, nurse managers, and nurses in other health care organizations rarely, if ever, are given the opportunity to negotiate a contract of employment. That is not to say that their responsibilities are less important than those who do have employment contracts. Rather, the common law has generally treated employees as at-will workers, and most nurses are no exception to this general rule.

At-Will Employment Doctrine

The at-will employment doctrine originated in England and was adopted by the American legal system as early as 1908.[6] Briefly stated, it protects both the employer's and the employee's right to terminate their relationship at any time for any reason.[7] Because the relationship is one of indefinite duration (assuming, of course, no agreement to the contrary), it can be ended "at the will" of either party for a good reason, a bad reason, or for no reason.[8] When the termination occurs pursuant to this doctrine, no legal liability will occur.[9]

Under this doctrine, then, a nurse could be terminated by the employer, and the nurse would not be able to successfully challenge the loss of the job. This would be true regardless of the (1) length of time the nurse had been an employee in the institution; (2) quality of work performed; and (3) lack of notice. The doctrine also allows a nurse to leave a position without being *legally* required to provide a requested period of notice to the employer. Although the nurse employee may want to give notice because it is professional and responsible to do so, he or she is not under a legal obligation.

The at-will employment doctrine . . . protects both the employer's and the employee's right to terminate their relationship at any time for any reason.

The at-will employment doctrine is not abso-lute, however. Several exceptions exist. They are important because under them the nurse or the employer can challenge the discontinuation of the employment relationship. The challenge to the ter-mination of employment is brought under various names, including wrongful discharge and retalia-tory discharge.

The exceptions to the at-will employment doc-trine include federal or state statutes that invalidate the doctrine; the "public policy" exception; the existence of an implied contract of employment; and a lack of "good faith and fair dealing" by the employer.[10]

Exceptions to the at-will employment doctrine include a discharge in violation of a public policy or a discriminatory termination (e.g., based on gender or religion).

Federal or State Statutes That Invalidate the Doctrine

This category of exceptions includes many fed-eral and state laws that will be discussed in detail in the following sections of this chapter. Therefore they are listed only briefly in Table 16–1.

Public Policy Exception

This exception states that an employer does not have a right to terminate an employee who refuses to participate in illegal activity at the re-quest of the employer or who exercises a protected right (e.g., filing a workers' compensation claim). This limitation on the employer's ability to termi-nate an employee "at will" is narrowly drawn by most courts, however. For a nurse employee to successfully use this challenge, the nurse must show that (1) the protected conduct is rooted in law and not the result of the nurse's definition of the "public good"; (2) a "clear mandate" of public policy exists; and (3) the concern motivating the nurse's particular conduct must be within the "public interest," not just a "private" concern.[12]

Examples of court cases illustrating these three requisites are numerous and depict varying out-comes:

- A New Jersey court upheld the firing of a nurse who worked in the dialysis unit when she refused to dialyze a patient she believed might die if the procedure was done. The nurse argued that the American Nurses Asso-ciation's *Code of Ethics* supported her refusal to perform the treatment because of its re-quirement to provide care with respect for human dignity and the nature of the health problem (Principle 1). The court held the *Code,* although possibly rising to a "public policy" protection, generally serves to protect

---

TABLE 16-1

Federal and State Statutes Nullifying At-Will Employment Doctrine

LAW	STATE OR FEDERAL	PROTECTION AFFORDED
Labor Relations Management Act (includes National Labor Relations Act of 1935 and Taft-Hartley Amendments of 1947)[11]	Federal	Union employees cannot be discharged in violation of union contract; no employee can be terminated if exercising rights of mutual aid and protection of working conditions
Whistleblowing acts	Federal & state	Public and private employees cannot be terminated for reporting certain employer conduct (e.g., illegal activity) to identified agencies
Equal employment opportunity laws	Federal & state	Employee cannot be terminated if a member of protected class and termination based on that characteristic; examples include age, gender, religion, disability
Laws requiring termination only for "just cause"	State	Employee can be terminated only for reasons listed in law (e.g., failure to do job or theft of employer's property)

Data from: Kenneth Sovereign. *Personnel Law.* 4th Edition. Upper Saddle River, N.J.: Prentice-Hall, 1999, 156–170; Robert Miller. *Problems in Health Care Law.* 7th Edition. Gaithersburg, Md.: Aspen Publishers, 1996, 240–255.

the interests of the *profession,* not the public. As such, the *Code* could not be relied on to protect the public. This was especially true in this case, the court held, in which neither the patient nor his family objected to the dialysis (*Warthen v. Toms River Community Memorial Hospital*).[13]

- A North Carolina court ruled that the firing of a nurse anesthetist was a wrongful termination because she refused to provide false testimony at a deposition when instructed to do so by her employer. The nurse anesthetist had witnessed the cardiopulmonary arrest and death of a young boy in the OR. The parents alleged negligence on the part of the anesthesiologist. When the nurse testified truthfully at the deposition, she was fired. The court opined that a firing for refusing to do something unlawful was against public policy (*Sides v. Duke University Medical Center*).[14]

- A psychiatric nurse in Illinois, concerned about the care received by patients at a psychiatric hospital, reported her concerns to a state agency responsible for monitoring the care of the mentally ill and those with guardians. She was terminated from her position. She filed a wrongful discharge suit alleging that her firing was due to the report and cited the public policy section of the Illinois statute that protected reporters from retaliation when they communicated concerns to the state agency. The employer argued that her termination was due to mistreatment of patients, insubordination, and other misconduct. The court held the nurse was wrongfully discharged as a result of sharing information with the state agency and sent the case back to the trial court. Despite this favorable ruling, the trial court did not reinstate the nurse to her former position. Because the nurse's services were of a *personal* nature (and not for *goods* or *products*), the court refused to require an employer-employee relationship to be reinstated.

Furthermore, the court held, reinstatement to a position was not a specific remedy in the reporting sections in the Illinois law relied on by the nurse. In addition, the court held that since the trial court entered a finding of fact that the employer's allegations about the nurse's conduct were true, requir-

ing reinstatement of the nurse to her position and awarding damages to her was not supportable (*Witt v. Forest Hospital*).[15]

Additional examples of wrongful discharge include terminating the nurse's employment when the nurse serves as a juror, files a workers' compensation claim, or reports information to law enforcement authorities.

Implied Contract of Employment

This exception has been used with increasing frequency in recent years to destroy the presumption of an employment relationship for an indefinite period. An employer's conduct, communications, and documents can be used by an employee to support his or her understanding that the employee was hired for a *definite* period of time. If the nurse employee is able to show sufficient evidence of a definite period of employment, the court can hold that an implied contract of employment exists. If an implied contract is found to exist, then dismissal can occur only pursuant to the terms of that implied contract.

An implied contract can be formed orally, through written documents, or through established employment practices. For example, during the job interview, a nurse may be told that if the job is done correctly, the nurse will have the position for life.[16] Or, a nurse may be assured that the position accepted would last until the nurse reaches retirement.[17] Likewise, oral assurances of promotions, bonuses, employee benefits, and a course of employer conduct over a long period of time have also been found to support terms of an implied employment contract.[18]

Written communications to employees can also be helpful in deciding if an implied contract of employment exists. In several reported cases, an internal memorandum, a letter to the employee concerning a bonus, and policies depicting standard operating procedures within the organization have been successfully used by employees to establish implied contract terms in the employment relationship.[19]

Perhaps the most widely known written document used to establish an implied contract of employment is the employee handbook or manual. Since the 1970s, courts have consistently evaluated employee handbooks for clear language of enforceable promises within the employment relationship.[20]

Although employee handbooks do not guarantee a successful challenge to an at-will termination, nurse employees have filed suits alleging violation of promises contained in them:

- The Illinois Supreme Court held that a nurse was terminated in violation of the protections afforded in the employee handbook. The nurse was fired without "prior written notice" (including three warnings) or an investigation that was required for all nonprobationary employees. The court stated that the handbook created a contract because it contained clear language offering something to the nurse employee, that she was aware of the offer, and that she accepted the offer by continuing to work as a nurse employee under those conditions (*Duldulao v. St. Mary of Nazareth Hospital*).[21]

  In a related case dealing with a change in the employee handbook concerning layoffs and "job security," the Illinois Supreme Court held that when an employer unilaterally changes terms that are *disadvantageous* to the employee without reserving the right to do so in the handbook, the changes cannot be upheld (*Doyle v. Holy Cross Hospital*).[22]

- An Arizona appellate court ordered that a case involving a director of nursing go back to the trial court for a trial on the issue of, among other things, whether the employee handbook created an employment contract. The director of nursing alleged that her termination was wrongful because the employer discharged her after she requested to be placed in her former supervisory position. The trial court had entered a summary judgment (no material issue of fact) in favor of the employer and the nurse appealed (*Liekvold v. Valley View Community Hospital*).[23]

- An LPN in Nebraska sued her employer, alleging a violation of the employee handbook's provisions concerning discharge and asking for reinstatement. Those provisions mandated certain policies and procedures to be followed in the event of termination and in the event the employee grieved that decision. According to the evidence presented, the LPN had been terminated for dishonesty because she did not renew her LPN license but falsely told the employer she had done so. The Nebraska Supreme Court held that the terms of the handbook did not guarantee the LPN continued employment. The court did hold, however, that the terms rose to the status of an implied contract governing grievances and discharge procedures (*Jeffers v. Bishop Clarkson Memorial Hospital*).[24]

It is important to note that this exception to the at-will employment doctrine has been limited in recent years. When an employee handbook or manual contains a disclaimer, prominently displayed, stating that (1) the handbook is not intended to, nor should it be interpreted to, create an express or implied contract of employment; (2) the information contained therein is "advisory only"; (3) the employer reserves the right to change or alter the terms in the handbook without notice and for any reason; and (4) the employer reserves the right to fire employees for any or no reason, courts usually rule that there is no violation of the at-will employment doctrine.[25]

Of course, when a disclaimer exists, the particular facts and circumstances of each situation are taken into account by the court. For example, in an Illinois case, the disclaimer contained in the employee handbook effectively eliminated any contract of employment between a nurse and her employer. The employer was free to discharge the nurse "automatically" when she left work without proper authorization to do so.[26]

In contrast, another court held that the one-sentence disclaimer contained in the handbook at issue in the case was not sufficient to support the ability of the hospital to discharge a nurse at will. In *Jones v. Central Peninsula General Hospital*,[27] the employer revised the handbook to include the fact that no employment contract was established. The earlier manual did not include this disclaimer. Furthermore, the revised manual contained 85 detailed pages of policies and procedures. The court held that because the manual contained many provisions relating to employee rights, the disclaimer was inadequate.[28]

Other Exceptions

A few additional exceptions to the at-will employment doctrine exist although they are not as common as the ones already discussed. One is the "constructive discharge" exception. When this occurs, the employee seemingly has voluntarily resigned from his or her position when, in actuality, a firing took place. For this exception to apply, however, the employer must make working conditions so "intolerable" that the employee really has no choice but to resign.[29]

For example, a nurse employee exposed to constant ridicule, unreasonable assignments, or harassment may resign from the position rather than continue to be subjected to that treatment. If the nurse is able to prove that the employer intentionally made working conditions such that there was no choice but to resign, the nurse may successfully win a suit alleging constructive discharge. The nurse would be entitled to damages and other remedies available to an employee who was, in fact, discharged.[30]

A similar exception is the intentional infliction of emotional distress allegation, based on tort theory. The essence of this allegation is that the employer's conduct exceeds all limitations of acceptable behavior and would offend any reasonable person.[31] Most often, these cases arise because of the conduct of a supervisor, manager, or another who has immediate control over the employee and who makes decisions concerning employment conditions.

Insults, disagreements, uncooperativeness, or termination of employment itself has been found *not* to constitute the conduct this exception seeks to prohibit.[32] In contrast, examples of conduct that would most likely result in a verdict in favor of a nurse employee against an employer include racial and sexual harassment[33] and describing an employee's spouse's behavior as "adulterous."[34]

IMPLICATIONS OF THE AT-WILL EMPLOYMENT DOCTRINE FOR NURSE EMPLOYEES

At-will employment can result in loss of employment when the employee least expects it. Because the doctrine allows for loss of a job without notice in many, if not most, instances, the nurse employee's preparation for that possibility is vital. This requires knowledge of the at-will employment law in the state where the nurse practices. In addition, it is vital that the nurse employee carefully read the employee handbook and possess a clear understanding of the conditions of the employer-employee relationship. If something is unclear, or if the nurse does not agree with a particular stipulation of employment, the nurse must inform the employer. It is best to do so in writing.

If the nurse believes termination of employment took place in violation of the at-will employment doctrine, the nurse can try to grieve the termination through the employer's internal grievance procedures. If the nurse is not successful or believes a grievance is not the course of action he or she should take, seeking legal advice concerning the termination is wise. The nurse will need to bring any documents available for the attorney to review (e.g., the employee handbook) and present the facts of the termination clearly and completely.

It is also important for the nurse to be clear about the fact that any concerns about patient care or employment practices should be resolved within the employer-employee relationship if possible. Although "whistle-blowing" and patient advocacy are valuable processes, indeed necessary in some instances, the possible outcome—the loss of a job—is not always what the former employee anticipated.

EMPLOYEE COMPENSATION AND BENEFIT PROGRAMS

Employee benefit packages and the wages or salary paid to the nurse employee can vary widely from employer to employer. There is little variation, however, in the overall management of both benefits and compensation because these areas are covered by federal and state laws. The employer must comply with the mandates established by federal and state statutes and their rules and regulations. If the employer does not comply, the employee can use various legal proceedings to obtain his or her rightful benefits under these laws.

Fair Labor Standards Act[35]

The Fair Labor Standards Act (FLSA), passed in 1938, established minimum wages, overtime pay (one and one-half the regular pay rate), and maximum hours of employment. The normal work week was defined as 40 hours in 7 days, based on an 8-hour work day. Nonprofit and for-profit employers, including state and local governments, are required to conform to the Act's mandates.[36] Employees who are considered professional, administrative, or "bona fide executives," are paid no less than $250/week, and meet statutory job responsibilities, are exempted from the minimum wage, overtime, and maximum hours of employment requirements.

In addition, the requirement of paying overtime rates to those employees who work in excess of 40 hours a week was altered for health care facility employees providing care to the ill, aged, infirm, or mentally retarded when those patients are staying on the facility's premises. The Act provides for the ability of institutions to enter into agreements with employees whereby a 14-day work week is the basis for calculating overtime wages. If agreed to, the employer must pay overtime rates to those employees who work in excess of 80 hours in the 14-day period.[37] However, the employer is required to pay overtime rates to the employee for hours worked in excess of 8 hours in any *one* day. This agreement has been called the "8-80" rule or plan.

On-call duty, in which the employee (other than those exempted above) is required to be available, either at the work site or nearby, so that reporting to work is swift when the employee is needed, is also governed by the Fair Labor Standards Act and its rules and regulations. For example, if a perioperative nurse is on call under these circumstances, he or she is usually deemed to be working while on call and is therefore paid for that time.[38] In contrast, if perioperative nurses simply leave word at work where they can be reached and can use the "on-call time" for their own purposes, payment for work on call is not required.[39]

Section 6 of the Fair Labor Standards Act was amended in 1963. The amendment, called the Equal Pay Act (EPA),[40] added the requirement that no employer could discriminate in the payment of wages on the basis of gender/sex when equal work of equal skill, equal effort, and equal responsibility was done under similar working conditions. The only exceptions to the requirement of equal pay for equal work listed in the act are seniority, a bona fide merit system, an incentive pay system, or a difference in wage based on a factor other than gender/sex.

The Equal Pay Act has been interpreted through many court decisions. For example, the equal-pay-for-equal-work standard has been interpreted to mean that the jobs being evaluated do not have to be equal, just substantially so.[41] If men are paid a different wage because they perform "extra duties," that difference is discriminatory unless women are offered the chance to perform the same jobs.[42] Also, paying men a different rate than women employees because the men work the night shift and the women work days—all doing the same work—is a violation of the Act.[43]

It is important for the reader to remember also that (1) the Fair Labor Standards Act may be supplemented or exceeded by state law mandates; (2) if employees are unionized, the union contract may provide additional protections; (3) no employee is excluded from coverage under the Equal Pay Act whereas some—"bona fide executives," for example—are not covered under the Fair Labor Standards Act.[44]

Enforcement of the Fair Labor Standards Act is done by the Wage and Hour Division of the Division of Labor Standards. The agency can investigate complaints, conduct employer audits, and interview employees.[45] The division can also bring suit on behalf of the employee, or the employee can do so. Remedies include obtaining unpaid compensation due the employee and reasonable attorney's fees and costs for the suit. If an employer "willfully" violates the federal law, fines and a prison sentence can occur.[46]

A nurse employee may elect to pursue a complaint under the state's labor department, especially if the state law provides more protection than the federal statute.

Comparable Pay for Comparable Worth

This theory attempts to provide further protection to those employees who may not be able to meet the requisites necessary under the Fair Labor Standards Act and the Equal Pay Act, but whose work is of "equal value" to the employer. The comparable worth theory rejects the notion of "equal work" and instead supports equal wages for jobs that are equally important or worthy to the employer. Under this theory, a nurse would receive as much pay as the environmental services department head, for example, because both jobs are of equal importance to the successful functioning of the institution.

The comparable worth theory became important when the number of women in the workforce doubled from 1960 to 1983 without concomitant increases in salaries and wages under the current wage and hour laws. The lack of increases in compensation for female workers, supporters argued, was due to the fact that women could not climb up the wage or salary ladder quickly because they had not been in the workforce long enough to work in jobs equal to male workers, who had been in the workforce for years. Thus, proponents argued, male workers would always be paid more than females because females could not obtain an equal or substantially equal position.[47]

Despite the potential attractiveness of this theory, it has not been supported by the courts, including the U.S. Supreme Court. Generally the claim of a female worker not receiving the same pay as a male worker has not been successful unless additional proof of the employer's intent to discriminate between male and female workers can also be shown.[48] This position is based on another federal law, Title VII and its Bennett Amendment, which will be discussed later in this chapter.

Deductions from Paycheck

Any deductions taken from an employee's paycheck must be authorized by the employee, usually through written consent. Deductions for health care insurance, a retirement plan, or a savings plan are common examples.

One deduction that can occur without the employee's consent is a wage garnishment; that is, when a court enters an order to an employer to pay a portion of the employee's (debtor's) paycheck to a creditor until the debt is paid.[49] Many federal and state laws, including the Federal Wage Garnishment Law,[50] control how those deductions take place, their amount, and notice to the employee, and they prohibit the employee from retaliating against the employer for its required compliance with the court order.

Examples of the kinds of wage garnishment that may affect a nurse employee include the nonpayment of child support and the satisfaction of a monetary award to an injured plaintiff (patient) after a professional negligence trial in which the nurse was found to be negligent.

Several other deductions occur without the employee's consent because they are part of a compulsory program of social insurance for the benefit of older workers, retired workers, disabled workers, and their dependents and survivors under the Social Security Act of 1935, as amended, and the Federal Insurance Contributions Act (FICA).[51] Covered employers and employees each pay a certain portion of the required amount from payroll taxes. The amount is regulated by Congress, and the employee's contribution is reflected as deductions on the employee's paycheck stub.

Eligibility for particular benefits under Social Security is based on meeting specific prerequisites.

Whether or not the prerequisites are met for a particular employee is "tracked" by using the employee's Social Security number. Therefore, the nurse employee needs to ensure the correct Social Security number is used for each covered employment position.

Health Insurance

Many employers offer the benefit of group health/medical insurance to employees in some form. Some employers will pay the entire cost of the employee's coverage, while others require a co-payment from the employee. The benefit may include both a basic medical plan and a major medical option. Coverage for dependents or spouses is not always provided, or if it is, there may be an additional cost to the employee. Even so, health insurance is a very important employee benefit.

Regardless of the plan provided by the employer, a federal law, the Consolidated Omnibus Budget Reconciliation Act (COBRA), requires employers with 20 or more employees and who have health care plans to continue health care benefits to employees who are terminated, laid off, or reduced in their work hours, or who divorce, separate, retire, or trigger other qualifying events. If an employee is discharged for gross misconduct (e.g., diverting controlled substances from the employer for the nurse employee's own use), or the employer terminates health insurance benefits for all employees, COBRA's continued coverage is not required.[52]

A federal law, the Consolidated Omnibus Budget Reconciliation Act (COBRA), requires employers with 20 or more employees . . . to continue health care benefits to [certain] employees [after termination of their employment status].

The employer must provide notice to the terminated or otherwise qualified employee or beneficiaries concerning their ability to continue to carry health insurance coverage. The employee must pay for the coverage, and benefits can continue for the employee for 18 months. Spouses and other dependents can obtain coverage for up to 36 months.[53]

An employee may have more protections under parallel state laws concerning the continuation of health insurance. If state laws provide less protection, however, then COBRA controls the continuation of health insurance plans.[54]

Violations of COBRA can result in fines against plan administrators. Various federal agencies, including the Department of Labor and the Internal Revenue Service, are authorized to issue interpretive regulations concerning the administration of the Act.[55]

In 1996, the federal Health Insurance Portability and Accountability Act (HIPAA)[56] was passed by Congress. Effective August 6, 1996, it allows for the "portability" of health care benefits. As a result, an employee with a "preexisting medical condition" can obtain health insurance coverage with a new employer when a change in a job occurs. The Act applies to any employer that provides medical plans for employees or their dependents directly or through insurance or reimbursement.[57]

When a "triggering event" takes place—the employee ceases to be covered under the health insurance plan or initiates coverage under COBRA, COBRA coverage has expired, or when the employee requests a notice of coverage—a written "certificate of credible coverage" must be given to the individual and his or her spouse and dependents.[58] As a result, the Act allows the determination of insurability to be portable from one group health insurance plan to another.[59]

Exclusions of preexisting conditions by the new health insurance plan are restricted under the act. For example, pregnancies cannot be excluded.[60]

Retirement Plans

Although the Social Security program is a retirement program, it is not intended to replace a retired employee's entire salary.[61] Thus, supplemental programs, both private and employer sponsored, exist. When a program is employer sponsored, it must comply with the Employee Retirement Income Security Act of 1974 (ERISA).[62]

ERISA mandates that most employers, with the exception of governmental employers and some church-sponsored plans, comply with its requirements, including nondiscrimination, the provision of a summary plan description (SPD) to employees, the vesting of benefits, and plan terminations.[63]

ERISA sets minimum protections in the area of pension plans.[64] An employer's program may provide more protections, as may some state laws governing insurance and employment benefits. It also controls other employee benefit plans, including disability, health and medical, and death benefit programs.[65]

ERISA is an important protection for employees, including nurse employees. It would prohibit, for example, the firing of a nurse immediately before the nurse would vest in an established pension program, if the firing were solely for that purpose. It also requires that the employer transfer vested benefits for the nurse employee from the current plan to the new employer plan.

ERISA does not, however, necessarily mandate certain coverage, either in terms of amounts or kinds of coverage, at least in relation to health insurance. In a 1992 case, *McGann v. H & H Music Company*,[66] the U.S. Supreme Court refused to review the Fifth Circuit Court of Appeals ruling that, with proper notice, the employer could change coverage in its self-funded health plan for AIDS from $1 million to $5,000 per benefit year.

The appeals court carefully evaluated ERISA's legislative intent and language. The Act never guaranteed particular benefits or coverage, the court opined. In this particular case, the court continued, no discrimination against the employee or employees with AIDS or a violation of other requirements occurred.[67] Therefore, the employer is free to alter benefits as it sees fit.

ERISA is enforced by the U.S. Department of Labor, the Internal Revenue Service, and the Pension Benefit Guaranty Corporation.

Workers' Compensation

Workers' compensation laws have been in existence in the United States since the late 19th and early 20th centuries.[68] At that time, the rapid growth of businesses and industry during the Industrial Revolution gave rise to safety concerns in the workplace. Many believed that caring for employees injured at work was a duty of the respective states.[69]

Workers' compensation [and unemployment compensation] laws have been in existence in the United States since the late 19th and early 20th centuries.

Employers, however, did not agree with this viewpoint, because they would have to contribute monies into a fund to cover workers' injuries. Several states attempted to pass workers' compensation laws in the early 1900s, but they were struck down as being a violation of the employer's due process rights. Wisconsin's law, passed in 1911, withstood constitutional challenge[70] and set the stage for other states to pass similar protections for workers.[71]

Currently, all states have some form of workers' compensation laws, covering all *employees* (those who are independent contractors and domestic workers are usually excluded). Federal civilian employees are covered by the Federal Employees Compensation Act,[72] and another federal law applies to maritime workers.

In either case, their purpose is to provide a means for employees who are injured during their job to obtain compensation for those injuries. Costs for coverage, whether by self-insurance or private insurance, are borne entirely by the employer. Compensation can include claims for the cost of medical care, rehabilitation, monies for the "partial" or "total disability" the worker suffers (thus rendering the employee unable to work for a particular time or unable to return to work at all), and death benefits.

Workers' compensation laws are relatively untouched by federal law. As such, they vary widely. Even so, some generalities can be identified, including the purpose of such laws, presented in Table 16–2.

Second, the types of injuries or illnesses covered by state workers' compensation laws are fairly uniform. Customarily, accidental injuries "arising out of and during the course of employment" are compensable under workers' compensation laws.[73]

TABLE 16–2

Purposes of Workers' Compensation Laws

1. Provide payment and other benefits without regard to the respective fault of the employer or employee
2. Provide payment and other benefits without regard to the financial circumstances of the employer
3. Reduce lengthy litigation, litigation costs, and attorney's fees by avoiding blame for the injury or illness
4. Reduce the economic drain on governments by having the employer pay for work-related injuries and illnesses
5. Encourage employers to continually improve working conditions to avoid paying for work-related injuries or illnesses
6. Promote honest evaluation(s) of work-related illnesses and injuries so continual improvement of working conditions occurs
7. Limit the employer's liability under the laws to injuries or illnesses that arise out of and during the course of employment
8. Require employees to give up right to sue employer for any covered work-related injury (but allows judicial review of decisions)
9. Mandate employee claims be handled through a state agency (industrial commission or workers' compensation board) rather than through the courts
10. Allow the employee to file suit against defendants other than the employer who might be responsible for the injury or illness (e.g., the manufacturer of patient equipment alleged to be the cause of the injury)

Data from: Kenneth Sovereign. *Personnel Law.* 4th Edition. Upper Saddle River, N.J.: Prentice-Hall, 1999, 238–255; Mark Rothstein, Charles Craver, Elinor Schroeder, and Elaine Shoben. *Employment Law.* 2nd Edition. Volume 2. St. Paul, Minn.: West Group, 1999, 1–193.

These requirements have understandably been the subject of much controversy in the state workers' compensation systems. Examples of injuries and illnesses seen as meeting that standard include:

- Injuries sustained by a nurse who was attacked by a patient at Florida State Hospital prior to the beginning of her shift while waiting to pick up a key for her ward[74]
- Death after suffering a heart attack at work that was the result of a nurse's stressful job[75]
- Stab wounds sustained by a nurse in a Louisiana hospital elevator on her way to work the night shift[76]
- Injuries suffered by a nursing assistant in an automobile accident on her way to an assigned patient's home for care[77]

Illnesses sustained under the same conditions would also be covered under workers' compensation laws. Such illnesses would include psychiatric or mental diseases. They would also include contagious diseases such as AIDS, hepatitis, or tuberculosis contracted as a result of caring for patients.

Preexisting medical injuries are also usually covered when those conditions are "aggravated" or "exacerbated." The distinction is important for the employee. An aggravation of a preexisting injury most often results in an acknowledgment of the entire medical problem. In contrast, an exacerbation of a preexisting injury is seen as compensable to the worker during its flare-up.[78]

Exclusions of injuries or illnesses under the state workers' compensation laws can include (1) those not arising out of and during the course of employment (for example, a nurse leaves the facility at lunch to go to the bank to cash a personal check and is injured); (2) self-inflicted injuries or illnesses (a nurse attempts suicide at his or her place of employment); (3) an injury or illness sustained under the influence of drugs or alcohol; and (4) willful misconduct or violation of a safety rule (a psychiatric nurse intentionally goes into a seclusion patient's room alone—in violation of an established unit policy—and is attacked by the patient).[79]

Unemployment Compensation

Unemployment compensation had its origins in trade union benefit plans; the earliest plan was founded in 1831 by a New York local trade union.[80] However, by the early 1900s attempts were made to require state governments to provide benefits for a limited amount of time to those employees who were out of work through no fault of their own.

In 1932, Wisconsin passed the first compulsory unemployment compensation plan. Shortly thereafter, when the federal government included unemployment compensation in the Social Security Act and stated it would set minimum standards for the programs unless states did so, all states passed laws governing their state's program.[81]

Federal involvement still exists in state unemployment compensation programs, however, mainly in the form of contributions to the state programs. Generally, the Internal Revenue Service (IRS) assesses a special payroll tax on wages paid by employers to employees, as does the state. In this framework, which exists in all but three states, money paid into the unemployment compensation system is entirely funded with *no* contributions

from employees. In two states, Alaska and New Jersey, employees *also* contribute to the fund.[82]

It is important to note that the system, although clearly established to benefit employees who are temporarily out of work, has a built-in adversarial component between employer and employee. The employer's payroll tax rate is increased by the regulatory agency or agencies as more unemployment benefits are paid out to former employees. In contrast, if an employer has few, if any, benefits paid out to former employees, the payroll tax rate remains the same. Thus, a common approach by employers is to contest unemployment compensation claims.

Like workers' compensation laws, unemployment compensation laws vary widely from state to state. Some similarities do exist, however, and they are listed in Table 16–3.

Each state unemployment compensation law also delineates those employees who are not eligible for unemployment compensation benefits. They include:

- Employees who leave work voluntarily without good reason
- Employees who are terminated for misconduct at work

TABLE 16–3

Components of Many Unemployment Compensation Laws

- Employees covered include: part-time and full-time; private, federal, state, and local government; executives, officers, and "rank-and-file"
- Workers not covered: independent contractors; children who work for their parents; individuals who work for their children or spouse; self-employed
- Employee must be out of work through no fault of own; be able to work; be willing to work; and satisfy "base period" specified in state law
- Employee cannot receive unemployment compensation until other received benefits (e.g., vacation and severance pay) no longer paid
- Benefits exist for specified period only (e.g., 36 weeks) and include a certain percentage of employee's pay
- Waiting period for benefits, if employee is eligible, must also be satisfied (e.g., 1 week after application)
- Employee must apply for benefits at local agency office; employer *does not* do so for employee
- Judicial review of final decision by agency

Data from: James W. Hunt and Patricia Strongin. *The Law of the Workplace: Rights of Employers and Employees.* 3rd Edition. Washington, D.C.: Bureau of National Affairs, 1994, 98–105; Kenneth Sovereign. *Personnel Law.* 4th Edition. Upper Saddle River, N.J.: Prentice-Hall, 1999, 256–268.

- Employees who refuse to accept suitable work without good cause
- Employees who are on strike

The ineligibility categories are understandably the focus of employer-employee contests when a former employee files for unemployment compensation. After the employee applies for benefits at the state agency (e.g., bureau of employment security or department of labor and employment), the employer receives notice of the filing and the initial determination of the agency. If the employer wishes to contest a grant of benefits, or the employee decides to contest a denial of benefits, a hearing is held with both parties present. After that determination is made, most states usually provide for additional appeals within the agency or department.

Nurse employees have been involved in unemployment compensation cases. In one case, refusing to accept suitable work without good cause was successfully argued by the former employer of a nurse who quit her job because she refused to take a position on the night shift.[83]

In *Taylor v. Burley Care Center*,[84] the charge nurse, Helen Taylor, was denied unemployment benefits because of misconduct while at work. Her employer submitted proof that Ms. Taylor refused to meet with her superiors to discuss her "poor work performance and attitude" without her sister's presence. The sister was a nurse at another facility and the director of nursing's position was that confidentiality would be breached if discussions about patients took place in front of the sister.

The director of nursing attempted to alleviate Ms. Taylor's fears of discussing her work performance with her alone by scheduling a meeting with the administrator also present. Ms. Taylor refused to meet with anyone other than her sister and the director of nursing. She was terminated and applied for benefits; they were denied.

When Ms. Taylor asked the Supreme Court of Idaho to review the denial of benefits by the state agency, the court upheld the decision. The test for misconduct in Idaho, the court held, was whether the employee's conduct fell below the standard expected by the employer and if the employer's standard was a reasonable one. In this case, both tests were met.

And, in *Clarke v. North Detroit General Hospital*,[85] two nurses who were terminated from their positions because they failed to pass the nursing board examinations were granted unemployment compensation benefits. The employer argued that they left work voluntarily without good reason attributable to the employer. The nurses argued that they did not leave voluntarily.

The Michigan Supreme Court agreed with the nurses, holding that they did not fail the examinations purposefully. In addition, it rebuffed the hospital's claims that it could not allow the nurses to continue working because only *licensed* nurses could be hired pursuant to various Michigan laws, including the Michigan nurse practice act. Although the latter was true, the court continued, that fact was not the test for denying unemployment benefits.

IMPLICATIONS OF EMPLOYEE BENEFITS FOR THE NURSE EMPLOYEE

Most employees do not have ready access to their respective rights and responsibilities in relation to employee benefits. Information about those concerns, however, can be obtained by contacting the human resource department at the workplace. The nurse can also contact the state or federal agency responsible for enforcing the particular employee benefit. The agency is listed in the telephone book, usually in the state (or federal) government section.

In addition to obtaining information when needed, the nurse employee should also review any documents given to employees by the employer concerning benefits. Any questions about coverage or exclusions can be directed to the human resource or employee benefits department of the institution.

If questions arise concerning wage and hour issues, or overtime pay, for example, those queries should be directed to the nurse's supervisor. If they are unresolved, additional information can be sought by contacting the employer's payroll department.

When the nurse is injured while working, he or she should be certain to seek treatment for the injury and to comply with any employer-required procedures (e.g., filling out specific forms, seeking additional opinions or treatments). If partially or totally disabled, the nurse should file a compensation claim. Legal counsel can be retained by the nurse if the nurse decides advice or representation is necessary (e.g., the claim is not processed in a timely manner or the nurse is pressured to accept a settlement).

If unemployment occurs, the nurse can file for unemployment compensation and obtain an agency determination concerning his or her eligibility for those benefits. It is important that the nurse supply the state agency with whatever accurate and factual information is available concerning the termination. If the case goes to a hearing, the nurse should be present and be prepared to present any additional information that supports his or her position. This would include witnesses and additional documents (e.g., a copy of the particular employee policy at issue).

EMPLOYEE PERFORMANCE AND DISCIPLINE

The employer has a right to expect that employees will conduct themselves according to certain guidelines when at work and performing their duties. Likewise, employees have a right to know the parameters of their conduct and any consequences of not meeting established guidelines. When expectations are not met, discipline of the employee can occur.

Usually the expectations and rights of the employer and employee are spelled out in writing in the employee discipline policy. In addition, the written employee grievance policy instructs the employee as to how to contest a disciplinary action and the roles of both in that process.

In some instances the written parameters of an employer-employee disciplinary policy can alter the at-will employment doctrine. That is, the methods for discipline may make it possible for the employer to terminate an employee only for "just cause" rather than for "any" or "no cause." In just-cause terminations, then, the employee's conduct must violate the rules of conduct established by the employer in order to be terminated from his or her position. The employee's argument is based on the express or implied contract of employment theory discussed earlier in the chapter.

One consistent way to evaluate employee performance and compliance with expected behaviors, and avoid successful challenges to a termination decision by the employer, is through the use of performance appraisals or employee evaluations.

> *In some instances the written parameters of an employer-employee disciplinary policy can alter the at-will employment doctrine.*

Performance Appraisals

In the clinical setting, performance evaluations are a way to ensure quality patient care.[86] They also provide valuable data in making decisions concerning nurse employee retention, promotion, and salary.[87] For both uses, however, employee evaluation must be fair and objective.

The forms of performance appraisals are varied. They include rating scales, checklists, narrative evaluations, or some combination of these formats. Regardless of their form, the instruments must (1) establish clear, measurable clinical standards; (2) be in writing; (3) provide documentation of representative performance of the staff member; (4) evaluate criteria related to the particular job the nurse is performing in the facility; and (5) provide notification of areas of needed improvement and the consequences if improvement is not seen.[88]

When the nurse employee does not measure up to established standards for clinical performance, or if improvement is not noted, corrective action may be taken against the nurse. Any action taken would be pursuant to the employer disciplinary policy and procedure and could include termination.

Disciplinary Policy and Procedure

Despite the fact that an employer is generally free to terminate an employee at will, many employers have elected to provide a means whereby an employee is given an opportunity to improve his or her conduct. The philosophy behind this approach is to aid in correcting the behavior rather than punish the employee for conduct not consistent with established requirements.[89] The policies are called various names, including corrective action or disciplinary policies. Regardless of the term used, the framework consists of a series of steps that lead to termination if improvement is not seen.

A progressive or incremental employee discipline policy provides an employee with one or more warnings concerning unacceptable conduct.[90] The system "progresses" through a series of warnings, each more serious than the former, and informs the employee that unless compliance occurs, the risk of termination is pending.[91]

Although progressive disciplinary policies vary greatly, they are usually composed of (1) notice of the unacceptable conduct subject to the corrective policy (e.g., sleeping on the job, repeated absenteeism); (2) the various steps in the policy (e.g., verbal warning, written warnings I and II); (3) the ability to suspend an employee, with or without pay, pending an investigation into any alleged conduct violative of the policy; (4) any required meetings or conferences with the employee; and (5) how prior, resolved discipline will be used in future actions against the employee (e.g., no use if a period of 1 year is completed without additional violations).

In addition, the policy often specifies when an immediate termination (also called summary termination) can take place for egregious conduct. Examples of behavior that could form the basis for immediate termination include falsification of any record used in patient care, insubordination, theft of facility property (including drugs), and a breach of patient confidentiality.

If a nurse employee believes any disciplinary action taken against him or her is unfair, unfounded, or not consistent with the employer's policies, the nurse can grieve the decision through the grievance procedure.

Grievance Policy and Procedure

A grievance procedure is any process by which an employee may question or appeal a superior's decision affecting job security.[92] The process can be informal or formal and is referred to by many names, including resolution procedures and information exchanges.

Informal systems usually consist of a policy statement in an employee handbook supporting the resolution of differences by encouraging those who are in disagreement to try to resolve their points of view. Sometimes individuals in administration are listed in ascending order for the employee to discuss his or her concerns with. In reality, these types of complaint procedures offer the employees little, if any, potential for resolution of their concerns. As a result, they may not be used by employees.

A formal employee grievance system is more common in the workplace and is composed of a series of steps the employee and employer must progress through in an attempt to resolve their respective differences. Highlights of a formal grievance system include (1) a definition of what is grievable (e.g., *any* employment decision or any decision other than termination); (2) which employees can utilize the system (e.g., probationary employees vs. nonprobationary employees); (3) the steps that must be followed by both parties and any time constraints on the initiation of those steps; (4) whether the grievance must be submitted in writing and, if so, in what manner (human resource form, other requirements); (5) employee rights (e.g., accompaniment of other employee or attorney, presentation of witnesses); and (6) whether the decision in the final step in the procedure (e.g., by outside arbitration, panel of peers randomly selected, board of directors, CEO) is binding.[93]

If the employer-established grievance procedure is fair, provides whatever due process protections should be afforded to the employee in the situation, and does not violate other employee rights (including fair employment protections), the decision will not be reversed by a court. *Khalifa v. Henry Ford Hospital*[94] illustrates this general approach by the courts.

In *Khalifa,* an employee challenged the hospital's grievance procedure by alleging that the procedure was unfair. Specifically, he took the position that the decision of the grievance council (composed of nonsupervisory employees), which was the last step in the procedure, should not be "final and binding."

The court upheld the procedure and the council's determination, holding that the procedure was fair, that the employee was given many "due process" protections (adequate notice, a right to present witnesses, and adequate time to prepare) and he was therefore bound by the council's decision.

IMPLICATIONS OF PERFORMANCE APPRAISALS AND GRIEVANCES FOR NURSE EMPLOYEES

Performance appraisals that establish unacceptable performance and adverse disciplinary actions are not enjoyable experiences for any nurse employee. Therefore, the best approach for the nurse employee is to avoid being involved in either situation. This can be attempted by knowing the employer's expectations by reviewing the employee handbook, performance requirements, and performance appraisal forms. When a work problem arises, the nurse employee should attempt to resolve the difficulty through established channels as soon as possible. Allowing a problem to escalate, whether it be a concern about nursing competency or a breakdown in the communication channels among the nursing staff, may prove fatal to the nurse employee's employment status.

If a poor performance appraisal occurs, or the nurse employee believes he or she has been disciplined unfairly, an immediate review of the employer policies and procedures governing the situation is vital. Adherence to the policies, especially in relation to required time frames and to whom a grievance should be addressed, is important. If a particular form is required for a grievance, the nurse employee should utilize that form. Most often, it can be obtained from the human resource department.

Many times a nurse employee may think that a grievance is a waste of time because the decision will not be overturned. Even if the result of the grievance does not change the original decision, making a record of why the nurse believed the original employment decision was unfair is important. Because a disciplinary action, and any grievance filed as a result, including the final disposition, is often kept in the employee's personnel file, the grievance is a way for the nurse employee to provide his or her side of the event for the record.

When formulating his or her position, the nurse employee should utilize facts to support why the corrective action is not warranted. Facts include actual happenings or events, the policy and procedure applicable to the situation and whether or not they were followed, and details left out by the employer. This approach can be utilized for *any* employment decision covered in the grievance policy, including termination or an "unfair" performance appraisal.

If a grievance procedure allows the nurse to be accompanied at any time during the process, the nurse should take advantage of that option. The person attending the procedure with the nurse employee can have various roles, depending on the employer policy. They range from acting as an advocate to functioning in a supportive capacity.

If this option is not available to the nurse, he or she may want to consider consulting with an attorney to strategize the best way in which to proceed with the grievance. This is important, not only in the grievance procedure itself, but also if the nurse employee decides to file a case against the employer for possible violations of state or federal laws that can be resolved only in the courts or other proceedings. Not raising the arguments in the grievance procedure may create problems for the nurse when seeking redress in those other forums.

The nurse who is a member of a union should consult the collective bargaining contract and contact the union representative so that whatever protections are afforded under the union contracted are utilized.

The nurse employee grieving an employment decision should obtain credible evidence, if available, concerning other employees who were not disciplined in the same manner for the same reason. Although no two situations are exactly alike, and there must be room for employer judgment and individualized discipline, the nurse employee may be able to successfully use deviations that arguably affect fairness.[95]

> [The Occupational Safety and Health Act of 1970] *was passed by Congress to ensure a healthy and safe workplace for workers.*

The nurse employee can also challenge a performance appraisal or other employment decision if principles of fairness or due process were not adhered to. For example, if the nurse was not placed on probation (as policy required) for poor clinical performance prior to a written warning or termination, grievance of those corrective actions might be successful.

LAWS GOVERNING THE EMPLOYER-EMPLOYEE RELATIONSHIP

Occupational Safety and Health Act of 1970[96]

This federal law was passed by Congress to ensure a healthy and safe workplace for workers.[97] The Act applies to employment performed in every state, the District of Columbia, Puerto Rico, the

Virgin Islands, American Samoa, Guam, Trust Territories of the Pacific Islands, the Canal Zone, Wake Island, and the outer Continental Shelf Lands.[98] Although state and federal employees are not directly covered by the Act, those employees are covered by state or other federal statutes affecting healthy and safe workplaces.

The federal law imposes two duties on covered employers: (1) to provide a workplace free from recognized hazards that are causing or likely to cause death or serious physical harm to employees (also called the employer's "general duty"); and (2) to comply with regulations promulgated by the Occupational Safety and Health Administration (OSHA) of the Department of Labor.[99]

Enforcement of the Act is the responsibility of OSHA and the secretary of labor. OSHA has the power to receive complaints, inspect work sites (with or without prior notice), interview employees during an inspection tour, and issue citations for violations of the act. If the employer does not rectify the harmful workplace violations, fines can be imposed. Those fines range from $1 to $7,000 for serious violations and from $5,000 to $70,000 for willful violations.[100] Criminal penalties for willful violations that result in death of one or more employees are also possible. Employers are granted certain due process rights in relation to alleged violations, including the right to (1) be present during an inspection tour; (2) receive written notice of any violations; (3) contest any alleged violations; and (4) appeal an adverse decision of the agency.

The Act also complements other federal employment laws protecting employees. For example, if employees call a "good faith" strike or refusal to work because of safety or health concerns, the U.S. Supreme Court has ruled that the employees cannot be disciplined by the employer.[101] Also, in *International Union UAW v. Johnson Controls, Inc.*,[102] the U.S. Supreme Court held that under Title VII, an employer could not use one of the statutory exemptions—bona fide occupational qualification (BFOQ)—to discriminate against female employees.

In *Johnson,* the employer had excluded only women who were of childbearing age from lead-exposed positions in the workplace under its fetal protection policy. Males who were also exposed to lead were not excluded. This exclusion was found to be direct, dissimilar treatment of female workers that could not be supported by the bona

fide occupational qualification defense raised by the employer.

Gender or pregnancy *may* support dissimilar treatment of females, the Court opined, but only when pregnancy or gender "actually interferes with the employee's ability to perform the job."[103] Although reproductive hazards in the workplace must be protected against, protection can occur only when it does not discriminate on the basis of gender or is necessitated by one of the employer defenses allowed by Title VII.

Clearly, the Act's protections for a healthful and safe workplace are applied to health care employees. The Act and its standards have been utilized to communicate dangers to employees handling hazardous chemicals (e.g., chemotherapeutic agents)[104] and to provide closed systems for the retrieval of patient anesthesia gases in the OR, for example.[105] Perhaps the Act's most far-reaching effect on health care employees, however, has been in the area of universal protections against bloodborne pathogens, including hepatitis and HIV.

Bloodborne Pathogen Standard

The 1991 rules were promulgated in response to recommendations from the Centers for Disease Control and Prevention (CDC) for health care workers to follow to avoid undue exposure to bloodborne contagious diseases.[106] Called "universal precautions," the guidelines included (1) treating all human blood and certain bodily fluids as if positive for HIV, HBV, and other bloodborne pathogens; (2) using gloves, masks, gowns, and eyewear whenever there was a possibility of exposure to blood or bodily fluids; and (3) following good handwashing techniques in addition to using the other suggestions.

Although many health care employers voluntarily adopted the recommendations, it was not until they became *requirements* under the Act that *all* employers covered began to utilize the standard. The requirements of the standard, along with employer and employee requisites, are listed in Table 16–4.

The standard has been met with controversy, and many employers were not happy with its mandates, especially because of the costs of providing the vaccine, gloves, and other personal protective equipment (PPE).[107] In addition, the American Dental Association (ADA) and Home Health Services and Staffing Association, Inc., filed a suit against the secretary of labor, OSHA, and the De-

TABLE 16–4

Summary of Bloodborne Pathogen Standard

EMPLOYER REQUIREMENTS	EMPLOYEE RESPONSIBILITIES
Offer hepatitis vaccine to new employees within 10 days at employer's cost; keep records or written consent/refusal	Accept or refuse vaccine in writing; employee can change mind after initial refusel
Require, in written policy, use of universal precautions	Follow universal precautions per policy
Keep written list of which employees, which jobs classes, and which tasks have occupational exposure to bloodborne pathogens	
Ensure handwashing, proper separation of food storage, smoking, and the like from areas of potential exposure; prohibit recapping, shearing, breaking, or removal of contaminated sharps unless a mechanical or one-handed technique is used by instituting work practice controls and work environment changes (e.g., sinks for handwashing, areas for eating)	Follow established policies
Require disposal of sharps, blood, and other infectious matter in leakproof and properly labeled containers with sharps in puncture-resistant, "easily accessible . . . maintained upright and routinely replaced" containers	Follow established policies
Require and supply PPE, including gloves, masks, and gowns	Use PPE per policy
Establish requirements for housekeeping re: decontamination of surfaces, protective coverage of "overtly contaminated" areas	Follow established policies
Establish requirements for proper handling of laundry (e.g., "minimum of agitation," proper labeling of contaminated laundry, use of leakproof bags/containers)	Follow established policies
Provide employee with confidential post-exposure medical care, blood test, counseling, and follow-up	Seek immediate medical treatment if exposed to blood or bodily fluid; employee can refuse, however
Use BIOHAZARD label	Be alert for label and follow required handling requirements
Provide annual in-service training on regulations with content specified in regulations; keep written records of attendance and content	Attend in-service programs and keep abreast of latest developments

PPE = Personal protective equipment.

Data from: Bloodborne Pathogen Standard, 29 C.F.R. 1910.1030; 56 Fed. Reg. 64,004; 57 Fed. Reg. 29,206 (1991); *OSHA Fact Sheet: 01/01/1992: Bloodborne Pathogens Final Standard.* January 1, 1992. Available at http://www.osha-slc.gov/OshDoc/Fact_data/FSN092-46.html. Accessed May 3, 2000.

partment of Labor challenging the standard's application to dentists and home health care agencies.[108]

The Court of Appeals for the 7th Circuit upheld the standard's application in the dental profession despite arguments by the ADA that its provisions were too costly and too cumbersome (e.g., keeping employee records for 30 years, laundering gowns at a separate facility).

The court vacated the regulation's standard for home health care and temporary medical personnel employers who do not control the work site, however. The rationale was based on a long history of decisions wherein OSHA allowed employers to use the "multi-employer work site" defense. This defense states that employers are not cited for hazards that cannot be controlled (e.g., placement of a sink for handwashing) so long as reasonable precautionary steps were taken to protect the worker.[109]

Obviously a patient's home cannot be controlled by the employer in the same way a hospital or clinic can be. The court held when work sites cannot be controlled by the employer, hospital, nursing home, or other entity specifically subject to the rule, it is not applicable to those work sites. The court did, however, uphold the "main rule."[110]

How this decision will ultimately affect home care and temporary agency employers and employees will remain to be seen. That *some type* of mandated guidelines for employee protection is needed is clear.

One of the more recent concerns surrounding the Bloodborne Pathogen Standard has been its "lack" of emphasis on needlestick risks, especially in view of this mode of transmission of bloodborne infections.[111] As a result, the Occupational Safety and Health Administration made it a priority to reduce needlestick injuries among health care workers.[112] In late 1999, the administration issued the Compliance Directive to the Pathogen Standard.[113] It details guidance for OSHA compliance officers in enforcing the Bloodborne Pathogen Standard and a 1992 update.[114] The directive also emphasizes the need for annual employer reviews of the bloodborne pathogen program, the use of safer medical devices, and postexposure treatments, not only for HIV and Hepatitis B, but for Hepatitis C as well.[115] The directive also clarifies its role when inspecting "multi-employer worksites." Although it cannot enforce such things as housekeeping requirements or ensuring the use of PPE, it will enforce "all non-site specific" requirements of the standard, including vaccination requirements, supplying PPE to employees, and a postexposure evaluation and follow-up.[116]

Workplace Exposure Statistics

One of the first three reported transmissions involving health care workers in the United States was a nurse from the University of Iowa Hospital, Barbara Fassbinder.[117] Her exposure occurred in the ED where a cut on her hand from gardening became contaminated after she applied pressure to a removed IV catheter site to stop bleeding. The patient died, and it was determined he had AIDS. Universal precautions were not "generally observed" at the time of her exposure.[118]

Work-related exposure to HIV, HBV, HCV, and TB results in increasing infection rates in health care workers annually. According to the Centers for Disease Control and Prevention (CDC), between 1985 and June of 1999, there were cumulative totals of 55 "documented" cases and 136 "possible" cases of occupational HIV transmission to U.S. health care workers.[119] Of the 55 documented cases, 49 or 89% were due to needlestick (percutaneous) injury.[120] Nurses and lab technicians were the health care workers most involved in these cases.[121]

In 1995, the CDC estimates that 800 health care workers became infected with HBV, a 95% decline from the estimated 17,000 new infections in 1983.[122] The decline is most probably due to the immunization program and universal precautions instituted by OSHA.[123]

The number of health care workers infected with Hepatitis C (HCV) is not known, although 2% to 4% of the total acute HCV infections that occur annually (26,000 in 1996) have been in health care workers exposed to blood in the workplace.[124] Interestingly, in sharp or needlestick injuries that result in contamination, one in six result from HBV, one in 20 from HCV, and one in 300 from AIDS.[125]

Tuberculosis (TB) is another contagion concern for nurses. Multi-drug-resistant strains of TB have been reported in 40 states.[126] The strains of TB have caused outbreaks in at least 21 hospitals, resulting in 18% to 35% of the exposed health care workers experiencing documented conversion tuberculin testing.[127] In one case, a registered nurse contracted multi-drug-resistant TB while caring for neurology, renal, and "overflow" TB patients from another unit in the major medical center where the registered nurse worked.[128] The nurse's treatment took 3 years, 2 of which she could not work. In addition, she required surgery to remove half of one of her lungs.[129]

Work-related exposure to HIV, HBV, HCV, and TB results in increasing infection rates in health care workers annually.

IMPLICATIONS OF THE OCCUPATIONAL SAFETY AND HEALTH ACT FOR NURSE EMPLOYEES

The American Nurses Association has supported the use of CDC guidelines, the importance of postexposure policies and practices in the event of workplace exposure to bloodborne pathogens, and the need for personnel policies concerning HIV in the workplace.[130] The nurse employee must be familiar with these statements and the responsibilities incorporated in them, including attending training programs, adherence to postexposure plans when the potential for transmission occurs, and, of course, following CDC guidelines. Because needlestick injury is the most common cause of occupationally related HIV infection,[131] the nurse must religiously follow employer policy concerning the handling of used needles.

In addition, all other employer-developed policies protecting the nurse employee must be adhered to. These policies may include such protections as regular monitoring of equipment for proper functioning, wearing certain types of shoes in particular areas of the facility (e.g., rubber soles rather than leather or plastic), and not wearing certain kinds of jewelry around patient care equipment.

A healthful and safe workplace also requires the nurse employee to participate on facility committees that develop policies for employee protection in the workplace. Reviewing any citations from OSHA (the employer is required to post them for employees to see) and keeping abreast of NIOSH Alerts can be helpful in utilizing that information to update and change policies.

If the nurse is concerned about an unhealthy or unsafe situation in the workplace, discussing the condition immediately with the nurse manager is important. If no change in the condition occurs, the nurse should seek out the nurse executive in the facility. If continued discussions do not remedy the problem, the nurse may need to factually and truthfully report concerns to the nearest OSHA office. The nurse has the option to ask that the report remain confidential when speaking with an OSHA official.

If an OSHA site inspection occurs, the nurse may be the only person in charge if it occurs on a weekend or holiday. It is best for the nurse to let the inspector know that he or she must contact the nurse executive, CEO, or other designated administration official and ask the inspector to wait on the premises until that person provides further instructions. Once the inspection begins, truthfully answering any questions the inspector may pose to the nurse concerning the work site hazard is important.

It is also important that the nurse not become complacent about workplace health and safety. Although many workplace hazards are identified and provisions for employee protection are in place, new workplace health and safety issues are continually being identified. For example, latex allergy is a relatively "new" workplace concern for health care providers. Between 1988 and 1992, the Food and Drug Administration (FDA) received more than 1,100 reports of adverse reactions to latex, including 15 deaths in both occupational and non-occupational settings.[132] It is estimated that for nurses, repeated exposure to protein allergens found in powdered latex gloves results in latex allergy for 1 in 10 nurses.[133] Symptoms include dermatitis, asthma, and anaphylaxis.[134]

The American Nurses Association, NIOSH, the FDA, and OSHA have joined efforts to ensure that this workplace threat is contained. For example, in 1998 the FDA mandated that all medical products, including latex gloves, be labeled, and that words like "hypoallergenic" and "powder-free" not be used to avoid confusion among health care workers.[135] Other efforts include attempts to introduce state legislation banning use of latex gloves and powdered gloves, ongoing continuing education on the topic, and updated information bulletins and alerts by the federal agencies involved.

If the nurse has input into which patient care products are purchased by the agency or facility, she or he should be certain to ascertain whether those products contain latex. If so, they should not be recommended for purchase. A union member should work for including the prohibition of products containing latex in the bargaining agreement. Last, education of the public and colleagues is essential in order to continue to raise their respective consciousness levels about this particular hazard in the workplace.

Equal Employment Opportunity Laws

Equal employment opportunity laws (also called antidiscrimination laws) prohibit employment policies and practices that result in different treatment of, or a disparate impact on, any protected class of applicants or employees.[136] Both state and federal laws have been passed that affect all phases of the employment process.[137]

Equal employment opportunity laws prohibit discriminatory policies and practices in the workplace.

The agency empowered to enforce most of the federal antidiscrimination laws is the Equal Employment Opportunity Commission (EEOC). Its roles also include promulgating regulations and monitoring the statutes it enforces.

If illegal discrimination is found to exist, remedies for the aggrieved individual can include reinstatement, back pay, equitable relief (an injunction to prohibit further conduct, for example), attorney's fees, and compensatory damages.

Because of the wide variances in state law, federal law will be the focus. The more familiar federal antidiscrimination laws are presented in Table 16–5.

Affirmative Action Plans

An affirmative action plan is a program established to overcome the effects of past discrimination against groups protected by antidiscrimination laws.[144] If a health care delivery system does business with, or receives funds from, the government, affirmative action is required.[145] Two executive orders, No. 11246 and No. 11375, were issued to ensure that the requirement was met. If it is violated, the Office of Federal Contract Compliance Program (OFCCP) of the Department of Labor can enforce the executive orders. The OFCCP can also share information with the Equal Employment Opportunity Commission (EEOC) when Title VII action is possible.

An affirmative action program may also be required as part of a settlement or judgment in a discrimination suit filed with the EEOC or in federal court. In addition, a policy supporting affirmative action may be voluntarily adopted by an employer.

EEOC regulations spell out the requirements of an affirmative action plan: (1) a policy specifying equal employment opportunity; (2) strategies for internal and external distribution of the policy; (3) identification of whose responsibility it is to implement the policy; (4) analysis of all job titles and descriptions; (5) a plan of action; and (6) an internal audit and reporting system of compliance with the program.[146]

Although affirmative action is agreed to, at least in theory, by most employers and society in general, its implementation is sometimes difficult. In addition, the issue of reverse discrimination— when members of groups not initially protected by antidiscrimination laws feel discriminated against because of an affirmative action plan—is also controversial. Throughout the years, the courts have not been clear about a particular approach to the reverse discrimination issue. Rather, it appears that the courts decide each situation on a case-by-case basis.[147]

Selected Cases Dealing with Equal Employment Opportunity

Many cases involving antidiscrimination laws have been decided throughout the years. Some have involved nurses as plaintiffs.

- In *Wallace v. Veterans Administration*,[148] Dorothy Wallace, an RN, won her suit against the VA Medical Center in Wichita, Kansas, after it unlawfully refused to hire her because of a restriction on her ability to administer narcotics after her successful but continuing recovery from chemical addiction. Ms. Wallace successfully argued that her addiction was a handicap covered by the Rehabilitation Act of 1973 and that she was a handicapped individual otherwise qualified for the position she applied for. The refusal of the VA to hire her because she could not pass narcotics was a violation of its duty to reasonably accommodate her.

- In *Waters v. Churchill*,[149] an RN was fired from her position at an Illinois public hospital for speaking out against the reduced quality of nursing care in the obstetrics department because of a "cross-training program" (nurses transferring to other departments than those they were trained in and usually assigned). This was held to be a possible violation of the nurse's First Amendment right of free speech and Section 1983 of the Civil Rights Act of 1866. The district court's summary judgment decision and its dismissal of the case was vacated by the U.S. Supreme Court, and the case was remanded to the trial court for further proceedings consistent with its decision.

- In *Meritor Savings Bank v. Vinson*,[150] the U.S. Supreme Court held that a female bank employee was sexually harassed in violation of Title VII when her supervisor created a "hostile (work) environment." The Court's decision is important for many reasons, but especially because it held the hostile work environment (e.g., offensive remarks, offensive pictures) violated Title VII as much as the "other type" of sexual harassment (*quid pro quo* harassment; that is, unwanted sexual advances and employment decisions based on the employee's "cooperation" with, or refusal of, those advances).[151]

- In *Buckley v. Hospital Corporation of America*,[152] the federal court reversed the trial court's summary judgment against a 62-year-old nurse supervisor who had been terminated from her position and remanded the case to the federal trial court for trial. The appeals court held that sufficient evidence

TABLE 16–5

Summary of Common Federal Equal Employment Opportunity Laws

LAW	CONDUCT PROHIBITED	COMMENTS
Civil Rights Act of 1866 and Amendments[138]	Actions occurring under "color of state law" (includes any local, state, or federal government unit)	Makes employer or employee who acts on employer's behalf personally liable; commonly referred to as Section 1981 and Section 1983 cases
Title VII of the Civil Rights Act of 1964[139]	Refusal to hire, discharge, or other discrimination against any person on basis of sex, race, color, religion, national origin; any other employment decision, including pay, benefits, promotions, job assignments based on those classes	Amendments include protections for abortion, pregnancy, sexual harassment. Exceptions/defenses to prohibitions are (1) bona fide occupational qualification (BFOQ); (2) business necessity; (3) nondiscriminatory reason for decisions. Applies to employers, labor organizations, state and local governments with 15 or more employees
Rehabilitation Act of 1973[140]	Discrimination against qualified handicapped person who can, with reasonable accommodation, perform essential job functions	Section 503 governs government contractors; Section 504 applies to any entity receiving federal financial assistance. Exceptions/defenses to prohibited conduct are (1) person not qualified; (2) accommodation required not reasonable and is undue hardship for employer or substantially increases cost for employer; (3) person not handicapped; (4) safety is a concern despite person being able to perform job essentials (BFOQ)
Age Discrimination in Employment Act[141]	Discrimination against individuals 40 years of age and older for all employment-related decisions	Applies to employers with 20 or more employees, including public employers, labor organizations, and employment agencies. Mandatory retirement also prohibited unless certain exceptions apply (e.g., not doing job or an executive in policy-making role). Exceptions/defenses include (1) age is a BFOQ; (2) decisions made on reasonable factor other than age; (3) decisions based on bona fide seniority system; (4) decisions for just cause (e.g., not performing job). Voluntary early retirement OK under act so long as requirements under amendment to act (Older Workers Benefit Protection Act) met
Civil Rights Act of 1991[142]	Conduct prohibited by antidiscrimination laws already in existence	Provides additional support with (1) availability of jury trial; (2) damages for intentional discrimination on basis of sex, disability, and religion (before only for race, national origin, and ethnicity); and other procedural protections for employees
Americans with Disabilities Act[143]	Discrimination on the basis of a disability if person qualified to perform "essential" job functions, with or without reasonable accommodation (Title I)	Applies to all employers with 15 or more employees. Exceptions/defenses include (1) individual not qualified under the Act; (2) individual a "direct threat" to health and safety of others; (3) no reasonable accommodation possible; (4) "undue" hardship on employer's part to accommodate; (5) person cannot perform essential job functions. Act also prohibits preemployment physicals, but allows them after offer of employment and if required of all applicants. Drug testing of applicants OK, but no discrimination against recovering alcoholics or drug addicts allowed. No questions about disability possible during preemployment interview, but prospective employer can ask if essential job functions can be performed

Data from: Kenneth Sovereign. *Personnel Law*. 4th Edition. Upper Saddle River, N.J.: Prentice-Hall, 1999; Henry Perritt. *Americans with Disabilities Act Handbook*, Volumes 1–3. 3rd Edition. New York: John Wiley & Sons, 1997 (with 2000–2002 cumulative supplement). Henry Perritt. *Civil Rights in the Workplace*, Volumes 1 and 2. 2nd Edition. New York: John Wiley & Sons, 1995 (with 1999 cumulative supplement).

existed for a trial on whether or not Ms. Buckley had been discharged because of her age in violation of the Age Discrimination in Employment Act (ADEA). Comments from the administrator that "new blood" was needed, younger doctors and nurses were going to be hired, and Ms. Buckley's "advanced age" was causing her anxiety and stress at work required a trial on the merits.

- In *School Board of Nassua County, Florida v. Arline*,[153] a lawsuit was filed by a teacher who was discharged from her position because she had recurring tuberculosis. She alleged she was a handicapped person under the Rehabilitation Act of 1973. The U.S. Supreme Court agreed, holding that a contagious disease is a handicap under the Act. Furthermore, the Court opined that any contagious disease must be evaluated by factual and medical evidence before a nondiscriminatory decision concerning employment can be made. The evaluation includes careful analysis of the severity of the risk to others due to the disease and the method of transmission.

- An HIV-infected pharmacist was successful in challenging a hospital's refusal to hire him because of his HIV+ status in *In re Westchester County Medical Center*.[154] Finding a violation of the Rehabilitation Act of 1973, the administrative law judge ruled that the pharmacist was not a direct threat to the health and safety of others. In addition, his HIV+ status did not prevent him from performing the duties of his position.

IMPLICATIONS OF ANTIDISCRIMINATION LAWS FOR NURSE EMPLOYEES

Equal employment laws benefit both employers and employees, and, in most instances, compliance by employers is the norm. The nurse employee should be knowledgeable about state and federal antidiscrimination laws, however, in the event there is a question about a potentially discriminatory employment decision. Furthermore, seeking a legal opinion about his or her concerns as soon as possible will help the nurse employee determine what, if any, action is best to pursue under the circumstances.

Knowing and utilizing the employer's policies and procedures for handling any potential discriminatory employment practice is also important. If a nurse believes he or she is a victim of sexual harassment, for example, following the policy adopted by the employer as to whom to notify can hopefully stop the offender's conduct. Also, requesting the appropriate administrator or employee representative for reasonable accommodation of a disability (e.g., job restructuring, scheduling days off to accommodate tests or doctor visits or changes in the physical structure of the workplace) can result in a nonadversarial resolution to the situation.

If the nurse employee experiences disinterest or nonintervention by the employer with complaints brought to its attention, the nurse employee can always seek input from the local Equal Employment Opportunity Commission office. If the commission believes there is sufficient data to support a charge of employment discrimination, it will accept the employee's charge and investigate the claim on behalf of the employee.

A nurse who applies for a position in a health care delivery system will need to be alert for any practice that is potentially discriminatory, especially when the job is not offered to the nurse. Asking questions about the nurse's marital status, age, number of children, plans for childbearing, disabilities, and religious affiliation, as examples, are prohibited by the fair employment practice laws unless they are protected by the laws' exceptions. Similarly, indirect comments about younger nurses, older nurses, and a gender preference for a particular position are not acceptable applicant inquiries.

A nurse employee 40 years of age or older who is part of a lay-off or early retirement plan, or is asked to leave his or her position, should obtain information about the protections under the Age Discrimination in Employment Act (ADEA). One specific concern is the content of the written agreement governing the plan or termination and any waivers (giving up the right to pursue legal remedies as a condition of accepting the plan or any benefits of termination) that may be included.

The Americans with Disabilities Act (ADA) may additionally protect employees, including nurse employees, against discrimination on the basis of a disability. Court decisions may also limit the Act's protection. For example, in *Downs v. Hawkeye Health Services, Inc.*,[155] the Eighth Circuit Court of Appeals ruled that a registered nurse with Hepatitis C was not "qualified" under the ADA despite his illness causing him to experience "disabling" fatigue, nausea, and chronic anxiety which resulted in his loss of his job.[156] And, in several recent U.S. Supreme Court decisions,[157] the Court has seemingly narrowed the definition of disability in the act by evaluating "mitigating" or "controlling" factors (e.g., medication, eyeglasses) and their effect on whether a person's "impairment" results in a "substantial" limitation on one or more of the individual's major life activities, including work.

National Labor Relations Act

Employees have always been concerned about job security, wages, and other aspects of working conditions, and nurse employees are no exception. Employers have been troubled by increasing costs in running their businesses, and health care entities have been no exception either. One way in which these respective concerns can be aired and resolutions obtained is through unionization and collective bargaining.

The National Labor Relations Act (NLRA),[158] also known as the *Wagner Act*, was passed by Congress to regulate private employers and employees in relation to unionization, establish the rights of employees to self-organization, provide a process for holding elections to determine union preference, and form the National Labor Relations Board (NLRB).[159] The NLRB was empowered to administer and enforce the National Labor Relations Act in terms of the election process for unionization and the unfair labor practice sections of the Act.[160]

Later amendments to the Act, the *Taft-Hartley Act of 1947* and the *Landrum-Griffin Act of 1959*, altered the original Act from a heavily pro-labor document to a more "equitably balanced" control of employers and unions.[161] In addition, the Taft-Hartley amendments also (1) brought private, nonprofit health care delivery systems and their employees under the act's protection (for-profit health care systems had been covered since 1935); (2) required unions to give a 10-day notice to the health care system before a strike, picketing, or other concerted activity takes place; (3) required unions to notify a health care facility 90 days in advance of their intention to modify or terminate an existing collective bargaining agreement; and (4) required mandatory mediation by the Federal Mediation and Conciliation Service (FMCS) on issues in dispute during bargaining contract negotiations.[162]

Another law, the (federal) *Civil Service Reform Act of 1978*,[163] and respective state laws governing public employment regulate rights and responsibilities concerning collective bargaining and unionization for those two groups of employers and employees (e.g., Veterans Administration hospitals and state and local governmental facilities).

This discussion will focus on the National Labor Relations Act, which covers any employer (and its employees) whose business affects interstate commerce. However, it is important to note that many of the same or similar protections and duties in the NLRA are also afforded by the Civil Service Reform Act and various state laws.

Sections 7 and 8 of the National Labor Relations Act (NLRA) *specify employee, employer, and union rights, responsibilities, and expected conduct when collective bargaining is contemplated or undertaken in the workplace.*

Basic Provisions of the National Labor Relations Act

The Act identifies the respective rights and responsibilities of employers, employees, and unions. Those rights and responsibilities are summarized in Table 16-6.

After a union has been elected, a bargaining agreement or contract is negotiated between the employer and the union. The contract governs the employer-employee relationship. Provisions of such contract agreements include both mandatory subjects (those required under the National Labor Relations Act) and voluntary areas (whatever the employer and union agree is important to include). Common examples of subjects included in a bargaining agreement consist of (1) the union as the exclusive bargaining unit for those employees in the unit; (2) member benefits; (3) grievance and disciplinary procedures; (4) hours of work and pay raises; (5) "union security" provisions (e.g., the work site is a "union shop" where all new employees must join the union within a specified time, or an "agency shop" where joining the union

TABLE 16–6

TABLE 16–6

Employer, Employee, and Union Rights and Responsibilities Under the NLRA

SECTION	RIGHTS/RESPONSIBILITIES	COMMENTS
7	Employees can (1) self-organize; (2) join, form, or assist labor organizations; (3) bargain collectively through representative of own choice; (4) engage in other concerted activities for purpose of collective bargaining or other mutual aid; and (5) refrain from any and all such activities	Protects all employees, not just union employees; "concerted activity" defined as employees acting together for their mutual assistance and protection concerning areas covered by Act
8	Employers cannot (1) interfere with, restrain, or coerce employees in exercise of their rights; (2) dominate or interfere with formation or administration of labor organization or contribute money or other support to it; (3) discriminate against employees in any term or condition of employment to encourage or discourage union membership or because of filing of charges or testifying under the Act; (4) refuse to bargain in good faith with employee representatives on matters subject to Act	This is the Unfair Labor Practice (ULP) section. Examples of conduct prohibited include banning wearing union insignia in facility at all times; asking employees their thoughts about union; asking applicants if they are union members; telling an employee a pay raise will take place if he or she opposes union
	Unions cannot (1) restrain or coerce employees in the exercise of rights or restrain or coerce employer in selection of representatives for purpose of collective bargaining or adjustment of grievance; (2) require employer to discriminate against an employee; (3) discriminate against any employee when membership is denied or terminated on a ground other than failure to pay dues and initiation fees required by all employees; (4) refuse to bargain in good faith with employer; (5) engage in, induce, or encourage employees to participate in a strike for the purpose of union recognition	Examples of prohibited conduct include asking employer to fire employee for not joining union; using physical or verbal threats or actual violence; charging excessive or discriminatory fees
9	Sets up union recognition rules: *voluntary recognition* by employer; *NLRB election;* and *Gissel Bargaining Order* from NLRB	Employer and union bound by rules; voluntary recognition not usual way union recognized; NLRB election is usual: petition filed; determination that union is one employees want (through union authorization cards); election held; union wins or loses
2(11)	Employer supervisors cannot be members of union if individual has authority to grant wage increases, hire, fire, settle grievances, assign work, or make recommendations concerning any of these issues	This section's application to nursing supervisors problematic; decisions made by NLRB on basis of responsibilities of nurse supervisor, not on title; nurse executive cannot be union member

Data from: Maynard Sautter, "Union Organizing, Collective Bargaining, and Strikes," in *Employment in Illinois: A Guide to Employment Laws, Regulations and Practices.* 3rd Edition. Issue 5. Carlsbad, Cal.: Lexis Law Publishing, 1999 (with regular updates); James Hunt and Patricia Strongin. *The Law of the Workplace: Rights of Employers and Employees.* 3rd Edition. Washington, D.C.: Bureau of National Affairs, 1994.

is not mandated, but all employees must pay union dues or a portion of the dues to the union); and (6) a strike or no-strike clause.

Which employees are included in a particular bargaining unit is also governed by the bargaining contract. The NLRB uses a "community of interest" test in determining the composition of any collective bargaining unit; that is, the members must have similar job functions, common supervision, and similar wages, benefits, skills, and training.[164] Professional employees, such as nurses, and non-professional employees (those whose jobs do not

require independent judgment and do not require study in an institution of higher learning) cannot be in the same bargaining unit unless a majority of the professional employees vote for inclusion in that unit.

At one time there was a question whether registered nurses should be in their own bargaining unit when they decided to unionize. The controversy surrounding this issue stemmed from the long-standing concern (voiced by employers, their professional organizations, and Congress) that the "proliferation" of bargaining units in health care would create undue difficulty for health care delivery systems trying to satisfy so many different "communities of interests."

Even so, in 1987 an NLRB rule identified eight units as acceptable for acute care hospitals: (1) RNs; (2) doctors; (3) other professionals (not doctors or RNs); (4) technical employees; (5) skilled maintenance employees; (6) security personnel; (7) business and clerical employees; and (8) all other nonprofessional employees.[165] The eight-unit rule was challenged, but in 1991 the U.S. Supreme Court unanimously upheld the rule.[166]

One of the most powerful provisions of the NLRA's concerted activity protections and any union bargaining contract is the power to exercise "economic action" against the employer. Economic pressure, of course, includes a strike; that is, a work stoppage or slow-down by employees to compel the employer to meet employees' demands.[167] Strikes by workers in health care have been controversial, and work interruptions by registered nurses are no exception. In fact, it was not until 1968 that the American Nurses Association rescinded its previous 18-year-old no-strike policy.[168] Since then, many nurses have participated in strikes throughout the country to obtain better working conditions.

IMPLICATIONS OF THE NATIONAL LABOR RELATIONS ACT FOR THE NURSE EMPLOYEE

The National Labor Relations Act and the National Labor Relations Board exist to set parameters and guidelines for employers and employees to resolve differences concerning terms and conditions of the workplace. Neither, however, are guarantees that agreement will always be reached. Therefore, one of the first things the nurse employee should be familiar with is the NLRA and any state laws that might alter his or her collective bargaining rights. For example, the nurse may practice in a "right-to-work" state (e.g., Alabama, Georgia, North Dakota, Utah, and Virginia) that prohibits union bargaining contracts from containing union or agency shop contract provisions.

Second, all employees, whether nurse managers or nurse employees, should be familiar with acceptable and unacceptable behaviors before, during, and after a union election process. Inadvertent participation in an alleged unfair labor practice can result in an undesired decision or one that is not in the best interest of all involved.

If the nurse who is a member of a union decides to vote for, and participate in, a strike, it is important that he or she understand what the ramifications of that decision might be on job status. For example, generally speaking, an employer can hire temporary employees to replace striking workers. The employer may hire those temporary employees as permanent employees if the strike is an "economic" one (over anything other than an unfair labor practice [ULP] on the employer's part) or if the strike is "unprotected" (e.g., in violation of a no-strike clause in the union contract). In contrast, if the strike is a result of an employer ULP (e.g., simply refusing to reinstate striking workers), it cannot hire the temporary employees in the striking employees' place.[169]

If a nurse is a member of a union, he or she should be very familiar with the union contract, for it governs the nurse's relationship with the employer in a different way than those who are nonunionized. For example, if the nurse faces a disciplinary action, the union representative and the contract should be consulted. The nurse's rights will be carefully spelled out in these situations, including the right to have a union representative present if requested when an investigatory interview takes place.

This rule of representative, called the *Weingarten* rule,[170] is also available to nonunion employees due to the NLRB's application of the protection to nonunion employees in recent cases.

Nurse employees who are nonunionized should keep in mind that the National Labor Relations Act does apply to them in terms of its basic provisions. Therefore, nurses who are unable to effect change in their working conditions may want to consider joining together to have protection under the National Labor Relations Act. For example, bringing employee concerns about wages to the employer by a representative selected by the employees is a good way to obtain protection under the Act.

It is interesting to note that another way nonunion employees join together to obtain better working conditions is through participation on employee committees. The character and composition of these committees have to be carefully evaluated, however, because if they fit the definition of a labor organization and are employer dominated or controlled, the employer may be found to have committed an unfair labor practice.

In *Electromation, Inc. and International Brotherhood of Teamsters, Local No. 1049, AFL-CIO and "Action Committees"*[171] the NLRB held that the action committees at issue in that case were employer established, administered, and dominated, thus resulting in "unilateral" bargaining by the employer with nonunionized employees in violation of the Act.

The *Electromation* decision was appealed to the Seventh Circuit Court of Appeals.[172] The appellate court affirmed the NLRB's decision, holding that the board had limited its decision only to committees that were employer dominated *and* had as their purpose the improvement of working conditions. The court clearly opined that "legitimate employee participation" committees that do not represent employees but rather focus on increasing company productivity, efficiency, and quality control are not prohibited by the Act.

Nurse employees should keep in mind that any employee committee that has as its purpose the improvement of working conditions, wages, and/or hours of work when the employer is involved may result in a violation of the National Labor Relations Act. Committees that are initiated by employees (or *jointly* by employees and management), have *voluntary* membership, possess a clear purpose of obtaining employee suggestions and ideas and, at the same time, improve communication between employees and management, should be able to function without a violation of the Act.[173]

Nurse employees (excluding nurse executives and other nursing administration members) who function as "supervisors" and were covered by the Act prior to 1994 may no longer be included in its protections. In *NLRB v. Health Care & Retirement Corp. of America*,[174] the U.S. Supreme Court rejected the board's test for determining whether a nurse was a supervisor. Prior to the Supreme Court decision, the board used a "patient care analysis" in making its decision.

Briefly, that analysis allowed the board to evaluate a nurse's direction of other employees on the basis of whether the direction was "incidental to the treatment" of patients. If so, then the judgment and authority exercised by that nurse would not exclude the nurse from the protection of the National Labor Relations Act because it was authority not exercised in the interest of the employer.[175] If, however, the nurse's direction and decision making were "independent" in an area other than how to care for a patient, then the nurse would be considered a supervisor and excluded from the Act's protection (see Table 16–6).

In *NLRB*, however, the U.S. Supreme Court held that since patient care is the health care employer's business, making decisions about patient care is making decisions in the interest of the employer. Thus, any nurse who makes such decisions is a supervisor and cannot enjoy the protections of the Act.

The *NLRB* decision remains controversial and confusing. The National Labor Relations Board has tried to clarify some of this confusion in its 1999 *Memorandum on Charge Nurse Supervisory Issues*.[176] It summarizes the legal issues relating to the nurse supervisor's unique role and offers guidelines for board hearing officers and agents for investigating cases, conducting representation hearings, and preparing regional director decisions.[177] It appears, however, that decisions concerning a nurse's supervisory status will continue to be made on a case-by-case basis.

Although nurse employees who are truly supervisors, however that term is ultimately defined, do not have protections under the National Labor Relations Act, there are certain circumstances in which they do have protection under Section 7 of the Act. If the employer discharges the nurse manager for any of the following reasons, the discharge is an unfair labor practice: (1) refusal to commit a ULP; (2) refusal to testify for the employer in an NLRB hearing involving union activity; (3) giving adverse testimony about the employer in an NLRB hearing; or (4) failure to prevent a union from organizing employees.[178]

SPECIAL NURSE EMPLOYEE CONSIDERATIONS

Review of Personnel Records

At least 15 states, including Illinois, New Hampshire, Pennsylvania, Utah, and Vermont, have passed laws delineating the rights of the employee and obligations of the employer in reviewing personnel records. The right of review is not absolute, however. Certain materials, such as reference letters and personal information about another employee, may not be reviewable under the state laws. Other provisions, including the right of the employee to protest certain information in the file and the number of times the employee can review the file, are also included in the state statutes.

ETHICS CONNECTION 16–1

Legislation concerning labor relations and practices is another example of coextensive relationships between ethics and law (see Chapter 3). The legislation that is identified in this chapter helps to balance the power relationships between employers and employees. Labor unions are structural units that are grounded primarily in the moral principles of distributive justice or fairness and beneficence. Labor unions' representatives negotiate with employers' management representatives to determine wages, benefits, and other conditions of employment for a period of time specified in a collective bargaining agreement or contract. Relationships between nurses and employers become more complex when nurses are represented by unions and are especially tense during contract negotiations.

Recent negotiations have focused on working conditions, particularly staffing patterns.[1,2,3] Situations such as patient safety are morally compelling issues that address nursing's primary obligation to society. Interpretive Statement 11.2 of the *Code for Nurses with Interpretive Statements*[4] morally obligates nurses to adequately represent clients and the public at large by "active participation in decisionmaking in institutional and political arenas to assure a just distribution of health care and nursing resources." Neither the code nor any of its interpretive statements may be negotiated as part of a collective bargaining agreement. The focus on staffing patterns is connected with nonmaleficence, beneficence for clients, autonomy for nursing staff, and distributive justice with respect to resource allocation and distribution.

Because safe staffing is a concern not only for the nurses but also and primarily for the welfare of the public, nurses are able to generate public interest in and support for their bargaining efforts on behalf of safe staffing. The negotiations between nurses and St. Vincent Hospital in Worcester, Massachusetts, and Tenet Health Care is an example of restructuring changes that resulted in unionization.[5] St. Vincent was a not-for-profit community hospital that became part of the Tenet for-profit chain. During the not-for-profit phase of St. Vincent's history, nurses had not been unionized. Following the corporate restructuring, nurses became concerned about staff reductions and patient safety. They unionized specifically because of staffing and safety issues. Negotiating their first contract, the nurses at St. Vincent Hospital took their issues about nurse staffing and patient safety to the community. They gathered signatures of community residents, endorsements from legislators, and support of other labor unions and nurses at other hospitals throughout Massachusetts.

When labor-management contract negotiations are contentious and stalemated, nurses have taken various job actions, including striking. Now that nurses legally are able to strike, they need to evaluate carefully the moral issues involved in strikes and other forms of job action. This is particularly the case in the health care environment, in which corporate responsibilities to shareholders may be at odds with nursing's priorities and clients' well-being. At Nyack Hospital, New York, 450 nurses went on strike for more than 4 months in 1999–2000.[6] Again, staffing and patient safety were major issues that engendered community support for the striking nurses. When employees strike, employers sometimes threaten to "lock out" or replace them. This happened during the Nyack negotiations. Management wrote letters to striking nurses informing them that they must return to work or they would risk losing their jobs. The nurses collectively burned the threatening letters during a demonstration and continued to negotiate a contract.

Although nurses and their employers historically have had complex patterns of relationships, the current climate of health care as a product designed to generate profits for corporate shareholders has created greater nurse-employer tensions. In efforts to balance economic values with the ovararching concerns for human health and welfare, nurses are taking strong positions in their collective policy, educational, and community activist initiatives.

---

[1]Anonymous. "Collectively Speaking," 6(5) *Hawaii Nurse* (September-October 1999), 8–9.

[2]Anonymous. "Community Turns Out in Support of St. Vincent Hospital Nurses," 69(5) *Massachusetts Nurse* (May 1999), 4.

[3]Anonymous. "MNA Nurses Take to the Streets for Safe Patient Care," 69(7) *Massachusetts Nurse* (August 1999), 12.

[4]American Nurses Association. *Code for Nurses with Interpretive Statements.* Kansas City, Mo.: Author, 1985.

[5]*Supra* note 2.

[6]"Tentative Agreement Reached in New York Strike," *News & Analysis @ Nurses.Com.* April 28, 2000. http://www.nurses.com/Conten...cket+News+of+the+Profession.

In addition to these protections, the nurse who is a member of a union may have additional rights to review an employment file if those rights are included in the union contract.

If a nurse works in a state in which no law or union mandates review of personnel records, the nurse must rely on any employer policy concerning examination of employment records or must utilize legal avenues (e.g., subpoena) to gain access to his or her records.

Refusing an Assignment, Including Floating Assignments

Understaffing, unsafe assignments (due to either inadequate numbers of RNs or inadequately skilled RNs) and lack of adequate training to care for a particular patient have been long-standing professional concerns for nurse employees. The concerns have been accompanied by confusion as to how to object to and rectify the particular issue impacting safe patient care.

One way in which these concerns have been translated into concrete direction for nurses is through unionization. Patient care assignments, numbers of staff per shift, other terms and conditions of work, and approaches to rectifying these problems are often carefully spelled out in the union contract. In addition, in 1987 the American Nurses Association's Cabinet on Economic and General Welfare recommended that state nurses associations develop a position statement identifying mechanisms to support a nurse's ability to exercise his or her right to accept or reject an assignment.[179] Many state nurses associations, including Massachusetts, North Carolina, and New York, did so.[180]

Nonunion employees have less clear solutions, however. As far back as 1983 only three options were identified: (1) accept the "objectionable" assignment; (2) accept the "objectionable" assignment and file a grievance or appeal; and (3) reject the "objectionable" assignment.[181]

Each of these options had consequences, including (1) being sued for professional negligence and/or facing a disciplinary action by the state licensing agency if the patient was injured, and/or (2) being disciplined for "insubordination," "abandonment of the patient," or other violations of the employer's disciplinary code.

Nurses' other alternatives to object to professionally unacceptable assignments are grounded in state or federal laws. For example, some states have "right of conscience" acts that protect a nurse's objection to a particular assignment when based on a religious or moral belief of an established, recognized religion.[182] In addition, other state statutes provide for refusal in certain care situations, such as abortion or the withholding or withdrawing of food and/or fluid.

Federal laws have been cited by nurse employees who find an assignment objectionable because of safety issues in the workplace. They include the Occupational Safety and Health Act and the Toxic and Hazardous Substances Hazard Communication Standard.[183]

Federal and state accrediting and licensing standards, such as those promulgated by the Social Security Administration (Medicare and Medicaid) and a state's public health department are also cited by the nurse employee to support an objection to a particular care assignment, especially when the protest concerns staffing and expertise of staff. Joint Commission on the Accreditation of Health Care Organizations (JCAHO) standards are relied on as well. Furthermore, in a 1993 Wisconsin case, *Winkelman v. Beliot Memorial Hospital,*[184] the Wisconsin Supreme Court affirmed the trial court's decision in favor of a nurse who utilized the Wisconsin Board of Nursing's rules and regulations when contesting her firing due to her refusal to float to a patient care area in which she was untrained and unskilled.

Although nurses have utilized these various supports for their objections for some time, all have some limitations and drawbacks. For example, in *Francis v. Memorial General Hospital,*[185] a nurse's termination due to his refusal to float from the ICU to the orthopedic floor was upheld by the New Mexico Supreme Court. The court opined that since Francis refused the offer by the hospital to orient him to any and all units he would be requested to float to, he could not claim that the employer refused to acknowledge that concern. In addition, his claims of breach of contract (there was a policy on floating, of which he was aware) and wrongful discharge were also rejected.

Employee Testing
Alcohol and Drug Screens

Nurses who practice while under the influence of drugs or alcohol are a concern in the profession.[186] To protect patients who may be harmed if

ETHICS CONNECTION 16–2

When goals and services of health care institutions are compatible with their clients' health care goals and needs, the relationships among clients, institutions, and nurses progress relatively smoothly. Such conflict-free relationships are not always the case, however. Institutional expectations frequently are contrary to nurses' assessments of the "best interests" of their clients. In today's health care climate, with its theme, "no margin, no mission," institutional conflict is becoming the norm, perhaps more than ever before.

Nurses who are employees often experience conflicts between employers' demands and professional obligations. In the 1983 edition of *Ethical Dilemmas and Nursing Practice*,[1] Davis and Aroskar traced professional-institutional conflicts both to the legacy of the Nightingale practices of indoctrinating nurses in British middle-class values of the Victorian era and to the "systematic oppression of the nursing profession."[2] They were writing at the beginning of the prospective payment era, in the waning years of fee-for-service medical practice, and before the widespread development of managed care. Then, as now, most health care institutions were bureaucratic, hierarchical corporations that expected that an employee's primary loyalty was to the employer. Nurses, however, considered that their primary moral obligation was to clients.[3] One major difference between past institutional constraints and contemporary corporate constraints is that nurses then usually knew who their employers were. Today, with fluid corporate ownership of hospitals, medical centers, long-term care facilities, and other health care institutions, nurses who were hired by one employer may find that they actually work for another. Sometimes these changes in corporate ownership and/or administrative structure are accompanied by changes in institutional missions and values. Nurses then may find themselves holding moral personal and professional values that are in conflict with the new values. These values conflicts occur more often when the merging organizations have widely divergent values, such as when a religious institution merges with a secular one.

Nurses who experience this conflict between their moral values and those of their employers have several choices. Sometimes nurses remain with the employer despite the conflicts; this choice usually is accompanied by a high degree of job-related stress. Other options include resigning, acting collectively with their colleagues and coworkers, and acting politically to secure policies that protect their clients and their practice from the injustices of market-driven health care. Nurses' options are more limited, however, if they have good reason for fearing reprisal from their employers, if they do not have the support of their families and/or colleagues, if they live in an area where there are few choices for employment, and if they cannot afford to resign. It is unreasonable to expect that individual nurses and their families will bear the burden of changing the health care systems to become more safe, effective, honorable, and just.

However, when nurses join together to work toward social change, they can influence health policy effectively and powerfully.[4, 5] Nurses have a vision of the social good. Their moral commitment is recognized by society. In a publication that is distributed to society members, Sigma Theta Tau International Honor Society of Nursing included a news brief about how respondents evaluated nurses' ethical comportment: "A 1999 annual Gallup poll on Honesty and Ethics found nearly three-quarters of Americans deem nurses' honesty and ethics as either high or very high. This ranking puts nurses at the top of the list of 45 jobs and occupations. The top five professions rated for honesty include nurses (75 percent), pharmacists (69 percent), veterinarians (63 percent), medical doctors (58 percent) and K-12 teachers (57 percent)."[6] Through their professional organizations, community action, and alliances with other professional groups and citizens who share their concerns for the health of their community, the nation, and the world, it is imperative that nurses work toward safeguarding and improving health care delivery policies and practices. Such changes are beginning to happen.

---

[1]Ann J. Davis and Mila A. Aroskar. *Ethical Dilemmas and Nursing Practice*. 2nd Edition. Norwalk, Conn.: Appleton-Century-Crofts, 1983.

[2]Davis and Aroskar's source for this second factor is JoAnn Ashley's classic study, *Hospitals, Paternalism, and the Role of the Nurse*. New York: Columbia University Press, 1976.

[3]The proposed revision for the *Code for Nurses with Interpretive Statements* is now in draft form. Its adoption in 2001 is anticipated, and it is expected to clarify and affirm that nurses' central moral commitment is to their clients, not to their employing institutions.

[4]For specific examples of political action to improve safety and effectiveness, see Ethics Connections in Chapter 4 regarding safe staffing legislation and redefining "abandonment," and in Chapter 6 regarding interdisciplinary work to reduce error in health care and medicine, particularly medication errors.

[5]See also Anonymous, "Advisory Statement on Floating Revised," 12(1) *BRN Report* [*California Board of Registered Nursing*] (Winter 1999), 4; Anonymous, "Speak Up for Safe Staffing," 71(9) *Minnesota Nursing Accent* (October 1999), 2; Anonymous, "Will Care Be There?" 71(9) *Minnesota Nursing Accent* (October 1999), 1, 3; and Anonymous, "Safe Care Campaign Continues: Legislative Agenda for Quality Care: A Vision for Nursing in the Next Century," 67(2) *Massachusetts Nurse* (February 1997), 4, 7.

[6]Sigma Theta Tau International Honor Society of Nursing. "News Briefs: Nurses Top the Charts for Honesty and Ethics," 1(2) *Excellence in Clinical Practice* (Second quarter 2000), 1.

a nurse is working while impaired and to limit their own liability, many health care employers have established drug- and alcohol-testing policies and procedures.

Employer rules for testing employees in the workplace must conform to state and federal laws. For example, the federal Drug Free Workplace Act of 1988[187] requires federal contractors, federal grant recipients, and all entities receiving grants or contracts from the federal government in excess of $25,000 to, among other things, establish a drug-free awareness program and require participation in a drug rehabilitation program for any employee convicted under a criminal drug statute.[188] Many states, including Utah, Mississippi, and Arizona, have laws concerning drug testing of employees.[189]

Employer rules for testing employees [for drug or alcohol impairment] in the workplace must conform to state and federal laws.

Also, the federal and respective state constitutions, and case law interpreting those charters, provide guidelines under the Fourth Amendment's prohibition against unreasonable searches and seizures for governmental employees and private employees whose testing is required or allowed by governmental regulations.[190]

The nurse employee should be familiar with employer-adopted policies and procedures concerning substance abuse in the workplace and testing for chemicals. Good employer policies will include the following information for employees: (1) definitions of terms such as *abuse, use,* and *impaired;* (2) conduct that is prohibited (e.g., conversion or diversion of controlled substances, falsification of patient care records); (3) the employer's response to a positive test or the employee's refusal of a test; (4) confidentiality of test results; and (5) under what circumstances testing will occur (e.g., "reasonable suspicion").[191]

If the nurse is asked to submit to a drug or alcohol test and refuses, most often the refusal will result in termination. If, on the other hand, the test is agreed to and is positive, unless the nurse can document the positive drug as legally and ther-apeutically prescribed, termination may also occur. In addition, depending on the state nurse practice act, he or she may also be reported to the state board of nursing or other regulatory agency.

The nurse employee who has a positive test may want to challenge the results of the test on several grounds through the employer's grievance procedure, if possible. An important point to raise is whether or not the testing procedure was flawed in any way. For example, regardless of whether the sample was blood, urine, or other body chemicals, the testing should be a two-stage process; that is, the first test should be used only as a "screening" test. If positive, a second, or "confirmatory" test should be done by Gas Chromatography/Mass Spectrometry (GC/MS) or a similarly reliable method.[192]

A second concern surrounding the testing procedure is whether the "chain of custody" was strictly adhered to. Without question, the sample must be accounted for *at all times* from its collection to the reporting of its result. Any break in the chain can cast doubt on the integrity of the entire process and testing results.

It is important for the nurse employee to remember that under the Americans with Disabilities Act of 1990, the testing of employees for "illegal" chemical use is not prohibited. Rather, the Act has been characterized as "neutral" on the issue of drug testing.[193] It does allow an employer to establish drug and alcohol policies that prohibit chemical use in the workplace, take disciplinary actions against employees who violate the policies, and test recovering employees to ensure they are not engaged in illegal drug or alcohol use or abuse.[194]

If the nurse employee is addicted to alcohol or illegal drugs (whether they be controlled substances, marijuana, or cocaine), it is important that the nurse seek treatment and continue in recovery after the initial regimen is concluded. This is important for two reasons. The nurse applicant or employee who is in a treatment program or has successfully completed one is protected under the Americans with Disabilities Act as an individual with a disability.

Therefore, if the nurse is "otherwise qualified" and able to perform the "essential functions of the job," with or without reasonable accommodation, the employer cannot discriminate in relation to employment. For example, if the recovering nurse would need to have time off to attend AA or NA meetings, or not administer narcotic medications to patients for a period of time after treatment, the employer would have to adjust the nurse's work schedule and assignments.

The most important consideration for undergoing treatment, however, is the fact that chemical use and abuse is self-destructive and can lead to death if intervention does not occur.[195] Many employers and nurse administrators possess positive and supportive attitudes toward chemical addiction and recovery.[196] The nurse employee can, and must, utilize those attitudes to break his or her cycle of self-devastation and reestablish himself or herself as a contributing and healthy member of society and of the nursing profession.

Polygraph/Lie Detector Tests

Employer use of the polygraph machine to detect dishonesty has been available for some time.[197] Few, if any, laws regulated its use, however, until 1988 when the *Employee Polygraph Protection Act* was passed by Congress.[198] The Act broadly prohibits the use of a "lie detector" (any mechanical or electrical device) to determine an opinion about an individual's honesty or dishonesty.[199]

The Act prohibits private employers from certain conduct, including (1) suggesting or requiring that job applicants or employees take a polygraph test; (2) asking about or using a past polygraph result; (3) refusing to hire a prospective employee who refuses to take a polygraph test; and (4) discharging or disciplining any employee who refuses to take a lie detector test, or otherwise taking action against an employee solely on the basis of the polygraph test.

The Act does contain certain exceptions to the general prohibitions against polygraph tests in the workplace. Two important ones are drug testing and public employers. Others include employer investigations in which there is economic loss or injury and when the employer is authorized to manufacture, distribute, or dispense controlled substances.[200] For hospitals and other health care delivery systems, then, the employer can administer a test to a prospective employee "having direct access" to controlled substances. It can also conduct a test on a current employee who has direct access to controlled substances as part of an ongoing investigation of "criminal or other misconduct" involving controlled substances.[201]

Even with the exceptions listed in the Act, the employer has additional restrictions. The test must be administered in accordance with the mandates in the Act, including specific information to be given the employee *before* the test is administered and his or her rights under the Act. In addition, private employers can use only polygraph machines, whereas governmental employers can use other honesty-detecting devices.[202]

The Act is enforced by the secretary of the Department of Labor. An aggrieved employee or applicant can file a suit against the employer for violations and seek reinstatement, a promotion, and back payment of lost wages and benefits. The Act also provides for civil penalties of up to $10,000. Generally, the employee's rights under the Act cannot be waived unless a written agreement is signed by all parties involved.[203]

If a nurse employee is asked to take a polygraph test, he or she should consult with an attorney as soon as possible before responding to the request. If the federal law is not followed, and an adverse employment decision occurs, the nurse and the attorney can evaluate whether or not a suit will be undertaken. Furthermore, any state law violations or union contract protecting the nurse employee will also need to be considered.

HIV Testing or Disclosure of HIV Status

HIV+ status and AIDS in the workplace have become a controversial and complex issue for both employers and employees. Much of the controversy stems from ignorance concerning the disease itself and its possible transmission to others; in this case, health care consumers.[204] Although the risk of transmission from an HIV-infected health care provider is "small," especially when the provider is not doing invasive procedures and is using appropriate infection-control procedures, the apparent transmissions of HIV to six patients by a Florida dentist—the *only* possible documented HIV provider-to-patient transmissions in the United States to date—have continued to create public concern and anxiety, especially in view of the inability to identify *how* the transmissions occurred.[205]

As a result, some employers have instituted what they see as safeguards to protect health care consumers and those who work with HIV+ coworkers or those with AIDS. These precautions include HIV screening and/or asking a health care professional to voluntarily disclose his or her HIV status or the diagnosis of AIDS to the employer.

These precautions, however well intended, are questionable under various legal challenges. To

ETHICS CONNECTION 16–3

Addiction is a common health problem in the United States. Partially because they have ready access to medications and a tendency to self-medicate, nurses and other health care professionals are at greater risk for addiction than is society at large.[1] Preventing addictive disorders is in the best interest of nurses and their families, their employers, and their clients. Unfortunately, early signs of potential addiction often go unnoticed by nurses' families and colleagues until the nurses' practice becomes impaired. Often, it is the impaired nurse's coworkers who first notice signs of drug diversion or other patterns of impaired practice. When nurses suspect that their own practice or that of a colleague is impaired, they have a moral obligation to reveal the problem while maintaining confidentiality and respecting the privacy rights of the nurse whose practice is suspected to be impaired. Disclosing the suspected impairment safeguards the well-being of clients and opens opportunities for treatment to the nurse whose practice may be or is becoming impaired. This obligation is grounded in the moral principle of beneficence and in the obligations of covenantal relationships. Ethical issues of impaired practice are communitarian ethical concerns. These issues involve not only the nurses whose practice is impaired but their families, their colleagues, their employers, state licensing regulatory bodies, and most of all, their clients. Covenantal relationships offer a way of identifying the moral obligations of all who are concerned as well as the conflicts involved.

Despite the widespread presence of addiction in nursing and health care, many nurses either do not recognize or do not report instances of impaired practice. "Many of our colleagues are at risk for this fatal illness due to the profession's denial of this problem, judgmental attitudes and lack of knowledge regarding the disease process and available treatment options."[2] Well-meaning colleagues frequently are uncomfortable about approaching and/or reporting a nurse whose practice is chemically impaired. Although they provide backup by attending to the impaired nurse's clients and making sure that they are safe and receiving appropriate care, colleagues often are reluctant to approach the impaired nurse. This occurs, in part, because of respect for the nurse's right to privacy. This practice of covering up prevents the impaired nurse from getting the kind of treatment he or she needs and may lead to tragedies that could have been prevented had coworkers intervened.

Federal and state laws and institutional policies influence how each situation is handled.[3] In general, legislation and policies recognize that addictive disorders are illnesses and that those afflicted require treatment, not punishment. Concern for safety of the public is the uppermost concern of nurse practice acts and of professional ethics. Most states and many institutions, however, have learned how to protect the public and clients while also acting with beneficence and fairness toward impaired nurses. Many states and/or professional organizations have developed peer assistance programs for impaired nurses.

Acknowledging the professional internal problem of chemically impaired practice and working toward preventing and managing it is a concern of all nurses. The Alabama State Nurses Association[4] "believes that the nursing profession has threefold responsibility" regarding practice impairment. The first responsibility is to clients; the second to maintaining professional standards through self-regulation; and the third to the nurse who requires assistance. Educational programs are being developed that help nurses become more aware of how to prevent impaired practice and how to identify and respond to manifestations of impairment in themselves and their colleagues in legally and morally responsible ways. In the United States and Canada, national, state, and provincial nurses associations have developed continuing education activities that focus on impaired practice.[5, 6]

---

[1]C. Kowalski and I. R. MacDougall. "Is Nursing a Profession in Denial?" 67(10) *Massachusetts Nurse* (November-December 1997), 8.

[2]*Id.*

[3]Margaret R. Douglas and Nancy J. Brent, "Substance Abuse and the Nurse Manager: Legal and Ethical Issues," 2(1) *Seminars for Nurse Managers,* (1994), 16–26.

[4]Anonymous, "Nurses Whose Practice Is Impaired," 25(1) *ASNA Reporter* (January 1998), 11.

[5]A. C. Bostrom, P. S. Brenner, J. L. Griffiths, M. M. Johnson, T. Volkman, and C. R. West, "Impaired Practice and the Law in Michigan," 72(7) *Michigan Nurse* (August 1999), 12–20.

[6]T. J. Butler, "Nurses: Web of Denial Project Report Summary," 26(1) *Concern* (February 1997), 17.

begin with, because a contagious disease is considered a handicap under the Rehabilitation Act of 1973 and a disability under the Americans with Disabilities Act, testing for HIV status or AIDS, or asking about this information, would have to be done *carefully*, if permitted at all. Likewise, under state and local laws prohibiting discrimination, the same procedures would be questionable.

As a result of the questionable status of such employer practices, many professional associations, including the American Nurses Association, support *voluntary* anonymous or confidential testing for HIV and the voluntary disclosure of HIV+ status, when necessary, by infected health care providers.[206] In addition, a voluntary avoidance of participation in any invasive procedures that might place a patient at risk for transmission is also recommended.[207]

Many professional associations, including the American Nurses Association, support voluntary anonymous or confidential testing for HIV and the voluntary disclosure of HIV+ status, when necessary, by infected health care providers.

The courts are dealing with the issues raised by HIV testing, HIV+ status, and AIDS in the health care industry. In 1990, an LPN whose roommate had AIDS was required to reveal the results of his HIV test. When he refused, he was fired. The federal district court upheld the firing, holding that the hospital had a "substantial interest" in maintaining the integrity of its infection control procedures. The termination was based on the LPN's refusal to reveal a possible infectious condition, which was a violation of its infection control policy, not on whether the test was negative or positive, according to the court.[208]

Because of the refusal, the court continued, the employer did not discriminate against the LPN on the basis of a "handicap" or a "disability." Furthermore, the hospital could not determine if the LPN "was otherwise qualified" and therefore was precluded from evaluating whether or not it could make the necessary accommodations to protect him and his patients.

In contrast, in another case settled prior to court action, a hospital in Kansas City, Missouri, agreed to reinstate an RN to his clinical care position after he was removed from it and placed in a position with no direct patient contact when he tested positive for HIV. The Department of Health

and Human Services also worked out an agreement with the hospital whereby its policies would be revised to conform to HHS recommendations on exposure-prone procedures and HIV+ employees.[209]

Also, in a 1993 case, *Faya v. Almaraz,*[210] the Maryland Court of Appeals held that physicians who are HIV+ have a legal duty (under an informed consent theory) to inform patients of their HIV status before operating on them.

The nurse employee who is asked to take an HIV test and reveal its results or is asked about a diagnosis of AIDS should seek the advice of an attorney as soon as possible. Hopefully, the guidance the attorney can give the nurse employee can result in a resolution that protects all the parties' respective legal rights and legal and ethical responsibilities.

Genetic Testing

Genetic testing in employment first became an issue in the early 1980s.[211] Because many were concerned that the testing would result in discrimination against certain ethnic groups due to its focus on screening for people who were genetically predisposed to certain occupational illnesses, its use was not widespread.[212] However, in recent years, despite its cost to the employer, continued concerns about the use of the results, confidentiality concerns, and the ever-present question of discriminatory motivation, genetic testing is making a comeback.

To combat the concerns surrounding genetic testing in employment, some states have passed laws prohibiting the practice. Those states include North Carolina, New York, Wisconsin, and New Jersey.[213] Likewise, it is argued that such testing would be a violation of already-existing federal laws including the Rehabilitation Act and the Americans with Disabilities Act.[214]

Despite the protective laws, some employers continue to conduct genetic testing. Employees are challenging the testing with varying results. In a 1977 case, *Smith v. Olin Chemical Corporation,*[215] an African-American employee sued his employer after being terminated from his job when his sickle-cell anemia resulted in a severe back disability. As a result of the progression of the anemia, the employee was unable to perform his job responsibilities, which required heavy manual labor.[216] The employer was able to successfully argue that the screening was necessary because lifting

---

ETHICS CONNECTION 16–4

Nurses simultaneously have personal responsibility for their own welfare and professional accountability to safeguard the health of others. These professional moral obligations are codified in the *Code for Nurses with Interpretive Statements*.[1] Thus, balancing nurses' autonomy and privacy rights with nonmaleficent and beneficent moral comportment toward clients, colleagues, and employers is an important component of decisions to self-disclose sensitive information of any kind, especially health status information. Although ethicists agree that nurses' primary obligations as professionals are to their clients,[2] they also concur that nurses do not have a duty to self-disclose information about their HIV seropositive status to their employers. Nurses do, however, have an obligation to practice in such a way that clients are protected.

Nurses are subject to all the diseases that accompany being human. When they become ill or suspect that they have a communicable disease, they sometimes experience conflict about whether or not to disclose that information to their employers. This is especially the case when nurses have sexually transmitted diseases such as HIV/AIDS. The question of whether seropositive nurses should disclose their HIV status to their employers is an issue that has complex implications for nurses, their clients, and employers.

Law and ethics generally are consistent in supporting confidentiality and privacy rights of seropositive individuals. For the most part, disclosure of an individual's HIV status requires consent. Furthermore, people who are HIV infected are protected under the Americans with Disabilities Act. However, it is harmful and, in some states, unlawful to knowingly expose other people to HIV/AIDS. Thus, there is tension between the right to privacy and the need to know. HIV-infected nurses are not immune from this tension and carefully weigh benefits and burdens of disclosing their status versus keeping silent.

Although there is considerable evidence that health care workers face risks to livelihood and/or social isolation if they disclose their HIV status to employers, there is little evidence that clients are at risk from health care workers who test positive for HIV. Professional accountability requires that individual nurses use moral and clinical judgment in assessing risks and responsibilities regarding self-disclosure. Both the Centers for Disease Control and Prevention[3] and the American Nurses Association[4] also agree that there should not be mandatory practice restrictions for HIV-infected nurses. Good moral and clinical judgment would require that nurses practice universal precautions and voluntarily refrain from participating in invasive procedures that place patients at risk.

---

[1]American Nurses Association. *Code for Nurses with Interpretive Statements.* Kansas City, Mo.: Author, 1985.
[2]Margaret A. Burkhardt and Alvita K. Nathaniel. *Ethics & Issues in Contemporary Nursing.* Detroit: Delmar Publishers, 1998.
[3]Centers for Disease Control and Prevention, 10(1) *HIV/AIDS Surveillance Report* (1998), 14.
[4]American Nurses Association. *Position Statement: HIV Infected Nurse, Ethical Obligations and Disclosure.* Washington, D.C.: Author, 1992.

---

and doing manual labor was "job related" and the ability to do so a "business necessity." As a result, the court found no violation of Title VII.

In *Norman-Bloodsaw v. Lawrence Berkeley Laboratory*,[217] several employees applying for a position underwent a preemployment medical examination during which blood and urine samples were taken. Without their knowledge or consent, the samples were tested for pregnancy, syphilis, and sickle cell trait.[218] Seven current and former employees sued under the federal and state constitutions, Title VII, and the Americans with Disabilities Act. The federal district court dismissed the suit, holding that the employees had answered "highly personal" questions on the medical questionnaire and knew that blood and urine tests were part of the examination. As a result, the court held, the

additional "intrusion" of performing the genetic tests was minimal.[219]

The Ninth Circuit Court of Appeals reversed the federal district court's decision and remanded the case to the court for a trial on the Title VII claims and the constitutional violations. The dismissal of the ADA claim was upheld because under the ADA, preplacement medical examinations can "be of unlimited scope and need not be job-related."[220]

If the nurse, whether as an employee or as a job applicant, is asked to take a genetic test, it will be important for him or her to obtain legal advice immediately. The law in the nurse's state may explicitly prohibit such testing, or may allow it but not allow any employment decisions to be made on the basis of the results. Even if the testing is allowed, it may be that the procedure is done only on specific groups of employees or applicants (e.g., women, African-Americans), which may be a clear violation of state and federal antidiscrimination laws. Third, the nurse should carefully review, and share with the attorney, the consent form used to authorize the test. Is the form clear? Is the consent being asked for too broad or unspecific? How will releases of the results be handled? Where are the results of the laboratory tests kept? Who has access to the test results?

Many answers to these, or other, questions surrounding genetic testing in employment remain unclear. Employees will certainly continue to challenge the procedure.

Family and Medical Leave Act of 1993

The Family and Medical Leave Act (FMLA),[221] effective August 5, 1993, requires employers with 50 or more employees to grant up to 12 weeks of unpaid leave annually for the birth or adoption of a child, to care for a spouse or immediate family member with a serious health condition, or when unable to work because of a serious health condition."[222] The employer is required to maintain any preexisting health coverage during the leave, and when the worker is ready to return to work, reinstate the employee to the same or an equivalent job.[223]

The Act also requires the employee to provide the employer with 30 days' notice concerning the leave, if possible. In addition, to be eligible for the leave, the employee must have worked at least 12 months for the employer and have worked at least 1,250 hours in the year *prior* to the leave.

The nurse employee should review the employer's policy and procedures concerning the Family and Medical Leave Act and raise any questions with its human resource department. If a leave is necessary, as much notice as possible should be given to the employer. Because intermittent leaves are possible in certain situations under the FMLA, a clear understanding of the requirements of this option is necessary if it is being considered.

It is important for the nurse to know that the employer may request "certification" of the need for the leave from the employee's health care provider. Generally, employees taking a leave under the Act must be restored to their position or equivalent position when they return to work. If the nurse em-

---

ETHICS CONNECTION 16–5

Under the current system of disclosure of medical information, nurses must be very cautious about revealing their own health status to their employers. Currently, personal health care information is not well protected from those who want to access it and have the technical skills to do so. This situation will continue to get worse before it improves. As Etzioni notes, "personal medical information is now bought and sold on the open market. Companies use it to make hiring and firing decisions. . . ."[1] In a communitarian ethical approach to resolution of the widespread abuse of medical records, Etzioni describes three layers or circles of information access and use. The center or inner circle includes direct providers of treatment to clients. Generally, the people who provide such direct, intimate care need to have access to information and "share a culture that respects confidentiality and is sensitive to privacy issues." Health insurance and managed care corporations are at the intermediate level or circle. The danger is that although people in this level currently require access to information about specific clients, profit is their primary motivation, and they have not been grounded in the health care culture that respects confidentiality. Finally, the outer circle includes those who have legal access to medical records and do not intend to use them for the good of the clients, but to limit access to goods and services or to publicly expose health care information. This outer circle includes employers, life insurance companies, and the media. Etzioni proposes ways of modifying access to information so that the parties within each circle have the information they require, and no more.

[1]Amitai Etzioni, "Medical Records," 29(2) *Hastings Center Report* (March/April 1999), 14–23.

---

ployee does not return to work after the leave time is utilized, however, the employer can recoup from the employee the money paid for health benefits during the leave unless (1) the leave was taken due to a serious health problem; or (2) the inability to return to work on time was due to circumstances beyond the control of the employee.[224]

Refusal of Nurse to Care for a Particular Patient Because of Diagnosis, Race, or Other Discriminatory Reason

Health care delivery systems cannot discriminate against any individual on the basis of such protected classes as race, color, religion, national origin, or disability. Nor can nurse employees engage in such conduct. This prohibition is grounded in ethics as well as in the law.

A nurse employee's conduct can result in the health care employer also being sued if discriminatory conduct by the nurse is alleged. For example, under the Americans with Disabilities Act's public accommodation requirements (Title III), a refusal to care for a patient because of the presence of a disability (e.g., AIDS) could result in an alleged violation by both the nurse and the institution. Title III of the Act requires, among other things, that those with a disability not be denied the "full and equal enjoyment" of goods, services, facilities, privileges, advantages, or accommodations of any place of public accommodation.[225] In short, those with disabilities must be given an equal opportunity to obtain the same results as nondisabled people.[226]

In a 1998 case, the U.S. Supreme Court underscored the protections of Title III of the ADA. In *Bragdon v. Abbott*,[227] the Court held that Ms. Abbott, who had AIDS but was asymptomatic, was protected under the Act. Her dentist, Dr. Randon Bragdon, was told of her diagnosis by Ms. Abbott when she went to see him for a dental examination. The dentist found a cavity but he refused to fill it in his office as was his custom. He informed Ms. Abbott that he would do so only in a hospital, and that any additional costs and his fees would be her responsibility.[228]

In its decision, the Court, among other determinations, ruled that one of the Act's exceptions—that of the person with a disability posing a significant risk of a "direct threat" to the health and safety of others—did not apply in this case. The individual raising this defense for not treating a person with a disability bears the burden of proof that the risk exists, and it must be based on scientific evidence, not irrational fears, stereotypes, or generalizations.[229] According to the Court, the dentist's refusal to provide care to Ms. Abbott in his office was discriminatory.[230] Clearly, the lesson of this case is that a health care provider, including a nurse, "can not make subjective assessments of risk (when deciding whether to treat a disabled patient) but must rely on objective scientific data."[231]

Other courts have decided cases relating to a nurse's or other health care worker's refusal to provide services in the employment setting under other theories.

For example, in *Armstrong v. Flowers Hospital, Inc.*,[232] the Eleventh Circuit Court of Appeals ruled against a pregnant nurse who refused to care for an AIDS patient and sought relief under Title VII of the Civil Rights Act when she was fired from her position.

Ms. Armstrong, a home health care nurse in the hospital's home care department, based her refusal on the fact that she was in the first trimester of her pregnancy, suffered from gestational diabetes, and was worried about the opportunistic infections common in AIDS patients.[233] The employer's policy was to fire any employee who refused to care for patients with AIDS. When Ms. Armstrong refused to change her mind, she was fired according to the policy. Armstrong then filed a complaint with the Equal Employment Opportunity Commission alleging discrimination on the basis of gender (pregnancy).

The appeals court upheld the federal trial court's opinion that the employer had no duty to provide special or preferential treatment to every pregnant nurse under Title VII. Furthermore, the court continued, the employer's policy applied equally to pregnant and nonpregnant employees.[234]

In another case involving a laboratory staff technician,[235] Dorothy Stepp refused to work on laboratory specimens that had biohazard warning labels on them, despite the employer's clear compliance with the Centers for Disease Control and Prevention guidelines. Her refusal was based on her belief that AIDS was a plague from God.[236] Ms. Stepp was suspended for 3 days because the refusal was seen as insubordination.

Upon return from the suspension, Ms. Stepp continued to refuse to work with contaminated specimens and was discharged. She sought unemployment compensation and was denied payments because she was fired for "just cause." The decision of the unemployment compensation board was affirmed by all levels of its review procedures.

Ms. Stepp then filed suit for a review of those decisions by the Indiana judicial system. Her allegations were based on OSHA regulations that allowed a refusal if based on a "reasonable apprehension" of death or serious injury due to an unsafe workplace.

The Indiana court upheld the decision of the unemployment compensation department. It rejected Ms. Stepp's argument concerning the justification of the refusal and the unsafe workplace. Rather, it held, the refusal was based on her religious beliefs. Furthermore, the court continued, she had been adequately and properly warned about the consequences of her refusal. Therefore, the employer was justified in firing her based on her refusal to do a "required task."

It is important to note that despite these decisions, the employer cannot ignore an employee's concerns about infectious diseases. In *Doe v. State of New York*,[237] a nurse employed by the state correctional facility successfully sued her employer when she attempted to restrain an HIV+ inmate who suffered a seizure. Correctional officers did not respond to the nurse's requests for help, and during the struggle, she accidently stuck herself with an IV needle she was trying to reattach when it became dislodged during the struggle. Ms. Doe tested positive for HIV 1 year after the needlestick.

The court ruled that the guards were negligent in not intervening to help the nurse and awarded her nearly $5 million.

The nurse employee who is concerned about an individual's contagious disease status or any other characteristic that is protected against discrimination should seriously evaluate his or her position if a refusal to provide care is contemplated. Generally such a refusal will not be protected. As a result, the nurse employee will probably not be successful in challenging a host of repercussions that will take place after the refusal, including termination, refusal of unemployment compensation, and possible disciplinary action by the state licensing authority.

If the refusal of care is seen as necessary by the nurse, he or she will need to base that denial on solid legal ground (e.g., unsafe workplace or lack of personal protective equipment). Regardless of the legal foundation upon which such a refusal may rest, however, there are ethical ramifications to the decision as well.

The American Nurses Association supports an ethical model for refusal by asking the nurse to differentiate when the benefit to the patient is a moral duty and when it becomes a moral option.[238] The equation for decision making includes the step of evaluating the risk to the nurse, if any, in providing care to a particular patient.[239] Other ethical theories, including the ethics of care, require careful inquiry into any contemplated or actual refusal to administer treatment to another.[240]

SUMMARY OF PRINCIPLES AND APPLICATIONS

The employer-employee relationship is constantly evolving, despite its long-standing existence. As new laws are passed and new social issues emerge, the relationship will continue to be shaped by those events. The nurse employee cannot ignore the many changes that will continue to occur in his or her relationship with employers. Therefore, it is important for the nurse employee to:

- Keep abreast of changes in the laws of the workplace
- Understand the at-will employment doctrine and its exceptions
- Be familiar with employee benefits and the nurse's obligations under them
- Regularly examine his or her personnel file
- Regularly review the employee handbook
- Utilize employee protection laws, whether state or federal in origin, to ensure a safe workplace
- Adhere to universal precautions when providing care to patients
- Adhere to all Centers for Disease Control and Prevention standards/guidelines, other state and federal agency alerts and directives, and employer policies concerning a safe and healthful workplace
- Understand antidiscrimination laws as they apply to both the nurse and the consumer of health care
- Compare and contrast the benefits and drawbacks of union vs. nonunion membership
- Consult with an attorney when a questionable workplace issue arises (e.g., HIV testing)
- Understand that refusing to care for any patient places the nurse at legal risk (unless the refusal is justified) and compromises the ethical duty to care for patients

TOPICS FOR FURTHER INQUIRY

1. Design a study to evaluate nurses' attitudes toward unionization.
2. Interview nurses in particular specialty areas of nursing (e.g., coronary care units, mental health units) con-

cerning their respective attitudes toward caring for patients with contagious diseases.

3. Design a study to evaluate the effectiveness of employee handbooks in informing nurse employees about their rights and responsibilities in the workplace.

4. Compare and contrast several health care providers' experiences (including nurses') in applying for workers' compensation claims for patient care–related injuries.

REFERENCES

1. Jo Ann Klein, "Facts About Nurses in the United States: Part I and I," citing the March 1996 Nursing Sample Survey of the Division of Nursing, Department of Health and Human Services, located at http://www.nursingnetwork.com/facts.htm. Accessed April 28, 2000.
2. *Id.*
3. Henry Campbell Black. *Black's Law Dictionary.* 7th Edition. St. Paul, Minn.: West Group, 1999, 543.
4. See, generally, "Employment Contract Formation and Implementation," in Kurt Decker and Thomas Felix. *Drafting and Revising Employment Contracts.* New York: John Wiley & Sons, 1991, 21–50 (with regular updates).
5. *Id.*
6. *Adair v. United States,* 208 U.S. 161 (1908).
7. Henry Campbell Black, *supra* note 3, at 545.
8. Kenneth Sovereign. *Personnel Law.* 4th Edition. Upper Saddle River, N.J.: Prentice-Hall, 1999, 156–157.
9. *Id.*
10. *Id.* at 159–170. See also Alfred G. Feliu. *Primer on Individual Employee Rights.* 2nd Edition. Washington, D.C.: Bureau of National Affairs, 1996, 183–225.
11. 29 U.S.C.A. Sections 141–187 (1973, 1992 Supp.); Act of July 5, 1935, ch. 372, 49 Stat. 449; Act of June 23, 1947, ch. 120, 61 Stat. 136.
12. Feliu, *supra* note 10, at 183–201.
13. 488 A.2d 229 (N.J. App. Div.), *cert. denied,* 501 A.2d 926 (1985).
14. 328 S.E.2d 818 (N.C. App.), *rev. denied,* 333 S.E.2d 490, and *rev. denied,* 335 S.E.2d 13 (1985). In *Marello v. Carter,* 640 N.Y.S.2d 679 (1996), two *student nurses'* reporting of a registered nurse's abuse of a patient was protected. The registered nurse was terminated from her position and the court upheld the termination based on the student nurses' honest and clear testimony.
15. 450 N.E.2d 811 (Ill. Ct. App. 1st Dist. 1983). Likewise, a case involving the reporting of Medicare fraud, *Spierling v. First American,* 737 A.2d 1250 (Pa. 1999), the Superior Court of Pennsylvania ruled against a registered nurse who reported past incidents of Medicare fraud to the federal government. Shortly thereafter, she was terminated from her position as a nursing supervisor. Ms. Spierling filed a retaliatory discharge suit against her employer, but the termination was upheld. The court opined that the nurse was under no duty to report instances of past fraud. Interestingly, the employer, First American Home Health Services, was indicted for improperly claiming Medicare reimbursement for personal expenses, lobbying, and other costs not covered under Medicare. The employer was later convicted of Medicare fraud. David

Tammelleo, "Whistleblower Fired for Reporting Medicare Fraud," 40(9) *Nursing Law's Regan Report* (2000), 1.
16. For a case where this kind of communication was held to support an implied contract of employment, see *Varis v. Arnot-Ogden Memorial Hospital,* 891 F.2d 51 (2d Cir. 1989).
17. See, for example, *Eales v. Tanana Valley Medical-Surgical Group,* 663 P.2d 985 (Alaska 1983).
18. Feliu, *supra* note 10, at 48–55.
19. *Id.* at 48–53.
20. *Id.* at 43–47.
21. 505 N.E.2d 314 (Ill. 1987).
22. 708 N.E.2d 1140 (1999), *rehearing denied* March 29, 1999.
23. 688 P.2d 201 (Ariz. App. 1983), *vacated,* 688 P.2d 170 (1985).
24. 387 N.W.2d 692 (Neb. 1986).
25. Feliu, *supra* note 10, at 22–26.
26. *Daymon v. Hardin County General Hospital,* 569 N.E.2d 316 (Ct. App.), *appeal denied,* 580 N.E.2d 111 (1991).
27. 779 P.2d 783 (Alaska 1989).
28. *Id.*
29. Sovereign, *supra* note 8, at 167–170.
30. *Id.* at 167.
31. Feliu, *supra* note 10, at 214–217.
32. *Id.*
33. *Id.,* citing *Agarwal v. Johnson,* 25 Cal. 3d 932 (1979) and *Shrout v. Black Clawson Co.,* 689 F. Supp. 774 (S.D.C. Ohio 1988).
34. *Id.,* citing *Keehr v. Consolidated Freightways of Delaware, Inc.,* 825 F.2d 133 (7th Cir. 1987).
35. 29 U.S.C. Sections 201–219.
36. Robert D. Miller. *Problems in Health Care Law.* 7th Edition. Rockville, Md.: Aspen Publishers, 1996, 251.
37. *Id.* at 157.
38. Maynard G. Sautter. *Employment in Illinois: A Guide to Employment Laws, Regulations and Practices.* 3rd Edition. Issue 4. Carlsbad, Cal.: Lexis Law Publishing, 1999, 4-26 (with regular updates).
39. *Id.* at 4-27, *citing* C.F.R. Section 778.115.
40. 29 U.S.C. Section 206 *et seq.*
41. *Schultz v. Wheaton Glass Co.,* 421 F.2d 259 (3rd Cir.), *cert. denied,* 398 U.S. 905, *on remand to,* 319 F. Supp. 229 (D.N.J. 1970), *aff'd in part, vacated in part, remanded by,* 446 F.2d 527 (3rd Cir. 1971).
42. *Id.*
43. *Corning Glass Works v. Brennan,* 417 U.S. 188 (1974).
44. Sautter, *supra* note 38, at 8-31.
45. 29 U.S.C. Section 211.
46. 29 U.S.C. Section 216(a).
47. Sautter, *supra* note 38, at 8-30.
48. Black, *supra* note 3, at 689.
49. 15 U.S.C.A. Sections 201–219.
50. 42 U.S.C. Sections 301–1397(e).
51. *Id.*
52. Pub. L. No. 99-272, 100 Stat. 82, *as amended;* 29 U.S.C. Section 601–608.
53. *Id.*
54. *Id.*
55. *Id.*
56. 29 U.S.C.A. Section 1181 *et seq.*

57. Christopher Kerns, Carol J. Gerner, and Ciara Ryan. *Health Care Liability Deskbook*. 4th Edition. St. Paul, Minn.: West Group, 1998, 12–26 (with regular updates).

58. *Id.* at 12–29.

59. Sautter, *supra* note 38, at 5-35.

60. Kerns, Gerner, and Ryan, *supra* note 57, at 12–28.

61. James W. Hunt and Patricia Strongin. *The Law of the Workplace: Rights of Employers and Employees*. 3rd Edition. Washington, D.C.: Bureau of National Affairs, 1994, 202.

62. 29 U.S.C. 1001 *et seq.*; 29 C.F.R. Section 2509–2677 (1974).

63. Miller, *supra* note 36, at 157. See also Mark Rothstein, Charles Craver, Elinor Schroeder, and Elaine Shoben. *Employment Law*. 2nd Edition. Volume I. St. Paul, Minn.: West Group, 1999, 459–517.

64. Hunt and Strongin, *supra* note 61, at 211.

65. *Id.* at 53.

66. 946 F.2d 401 (5th Cir. 1991), *cert. denied sub nom. Greenberg v. H & H Music Company*, 506 U.S. 981 (1992).

67. 946 F.2d 401, 407–408 (1992).

68. Rothstein, Craver, Schroeder, and Shoben, *supra* note 63, Volume II, at 2–8.

69. Sovereign, *supra* note 8, at 239.

70. *Id.*

71. *Id.*

72. 5 U.S.C. Section 8101 *et seq.*

73. Sovereign, *supra* note 8, at 242–245.

74. *Johns v. State Dept. of Health & Rehab.*, 485 So. 2d 857 (Fla. Dist. Ct. App.), *rev. denied*, 492 So. 2d 1333 (1986).

75. *Herman v. Miners' Hospital*, 807 P.2d 734 (1991). In a more recent case, *Kovalchick v. South Baldevin Hospital*, 695 So. 2d 1199 (Ala. 1997), a registered nurse's heart attack was initially held not compensable under Alabama's Workers' Compensation law by a trial court. The Alabama Court of Civil Appeals, however, reversed the dismissal of the case by the trial court and remanded the case to the trial court for a hearing on the issue of causation. If the nurse could show that there was a causal connection between her heart attack and her job in the ED, coverage would exist.

76. *Mundy v. Dept. of Health & Human Resources*, 580 So. 2d 493 (La. Ct. App.), *writ granted*, 586 So. 2d 519 (1991), *rev'd*, 593 So. 2d 346, *remanded to*, 609 So. 2d 909 (La. Ct. App. 1992), *writ granted*, 613 So. 2d 960, *aff'd.* 620 So. 2d 811 (1993).

77. *Alsten Kimberly Quality Care v. Petty*, 934 S.W.2d 956 (1996).

78. See, generally, Sautter, *supra* note 38, at 11-5.

79. *Id.* at 11-3–11-4.

80. Sovereign, *supra* note 8, at 256–257.

81. *Id.* at 257.

82. Hunt and Strongin, *supra* note 61, at 98.

83. *Baptist Medical Center v. Stolte*, 475 So. 2d 959 (Fla. Dist. Ct. App. 1985), *rev. denied sub nom. Unemployment Appeals Comm'n v. Baptist Medical Center*, 486 So. 2d 598 (1986).

84. 828 P.2d 821 (1991).

85. 470 N.W.2d 393 (1991).

86. See generally, Howard Rowland and Beatrice Rowland. *Nursing Administration Handbook*. 4th Edition. Gaithersburg, Md.: Aspen Publishers, 1997, 579–610.

87. *Id.*

88. *Id.*

89. Kurt Decker and Thomas Felix II. *Drafting and Revising Employment Handbooks*. New York: John Wiley & Sons, 1991, 249 (with regular updates).

90. Rowland and Rowland, *supra* note 86, at 553, 555–556.

91. *Id.*

92. Black, *supra* note 3, at 709.

93. See generally, Decker and Felix, *supra* note 89, at 258–266.

94. 401 N.W.2d 884 (Mich. App. 1987).

95. Feliu, *supra* note 10, at 61–65.

96. Pub. L. No. 91-596, 84 Stat. 1590, 29 U.S.C. Sections 651–678, *as amended.*

97. Sovereign, *supra* note 8, at 228.

98. Mark Rothstein. *Occupational Health and Safety Law*. 4th Edition. St. Paul, Minn.: West Group, 1999, 11 (with 2000 Supplement).

99. *Id.* at 8, *citing* the Act at 29 U.S.C. Section 654.

100. Omnibus Budget Reconciliation Act of 1990, Pub. L. No. 101-508, 104 Stat. 1388 (November 5, 1990).

101. *NLRB v. Washington Aluminum Company*, 370 U.S. 9 (1962).

102. 499 U.S. 187 (1991).

103. *Id.* at 203.

104. 42 U.S.C. Sections 11001–11050; 29 C.F.R. Section 1910.1200 (1987). See also a compilation of hazardous medications information developed by OSHA at http://www.osha.scl.gov/SLTC/hazardousmedications/index.html. Accessed November 18, 1998; Denise DelGaudio and Menonna Quinn, "Chemotherapy: Potential Occupational Hazards," 98(11) *AJN* (1998), 59–65.

105. Another governmental agency, the National Institute for Occupational Safety and Health (NIOSH), has also been active in ensuring a safe workplace. For example, it publishes *Hazard Controls* to alert workers about workplace dangers and offers solutions based on research studies that "show reduced worker exposure to hazardous agents or activities." See, for example, *Control of Smoke from Laser/Electric Surgical Procedures* (1998), 1–2. Available at http://www.cdc.gov.niosh. Accessed April 30, 2000. NIOSH is a part of the Centers for Disease Control and Prevention (CDC) and is empowered by OSHA to conduct research, recommend new standards, conduct inspections, and question employers and employees for research purposes. Rothstein, Craver, Schroeder, and Shoben, *supra* note 63, Volume II, at 634–635.

106. 29 C.F.R. Section 1910.1030; 56 Fed. Reg. 64,004, 57 Fed. Reg. 29,206 (1991).

107. "OSHA Stiffens Bloodborne Rules, Decrees Free Hepatitis B Vaccine," *AJN* (January 1992) 82–84.

108. *American Dental Association v. Martin, et al,* 984 F.2d 823 (7th Cir.), *cert. denied*, 114 S. Ct. 172 (1993).

109. "OSHA Rule Upheld for Dentists, Partly Vacated for Home Health Industry," 2(5) *BNA's Health Law Reporter* (February 4, 1993), 132.

110. *ADA v. Martin, supra* note 108.

111. "OSHA to Request Information on Needlestick Prevention, Jeffress Says," 7(33) *BNA's Health Law Reporter* (1998), 1297.

112. *Id.*

113. OSHA Compliance Directive (CPL 2-2.44D). *Enforcement Procedures for the Occupational Exposure to Bloodborne Pathogens.* November 5, 1999. The directive is available on the Internet at http://www.osha-slc.gov/OshDoc/Directive-data/CPL_2–2_44D.html. Accessed May 3, 2000.

114. *Id.* at 3.

115. "OSHA Revises Bloodborne Pathogens Compliance Directive," *OSHA National News Release,* November 5, 1999, at http://www.osha.gov/media/oshanews/nov/99/national-19991105.html, 1-3. Accessed May 3, 2000.

116. OSHA Compliance Directive, *supra* note 113, at 5–7. In November 1999, NIOSH also published its ALERT on needlestick injuries in the health care setting. *NIOSH ALERT: Preventing Needlestick Injuries in Health Care Settings.* November 1999. The publication—DHHS(NIOSH) Publication No. 2000-108—can be ordered through NIOSH at its Publications Dissemination Office, 4676 Columbia Parkway, Cincinnati, OH 45226-1998 or on its home page at http://www.cdc/gov/niosh.

117. "Nurse Infected with HIV Virus Urges Others to Take Care," 90(7) *AJN* (1990), 86.

118. *Id.*

119. *NIOSH ALERT, supra* note 115, at 4.

120. *Id.*

121. *Id.*

122. *Id.*

123. *Id.*

124. *Id.* at 5. The CDC has published guidelines for the prevention of transmission of tuberculosis at 29 C.F.R. 1910.139. It recently published additional guidelines when respirators are used to minimize TB exposure. *TB Respiratory Protection Program in Health Care Facilities: Administrator's Guide.* September 1999.

125. Susan Wilburn, "Preventing Needlestick Injuries," 99(1) *AJN* (1999), 71.

126. National Institute for Safety and Health. "Case Studies." Located at http://www.cdc.gov/niosh/tb-case/html. Accessed May 4, 2000.

127. *Id.*

128. *Id.*

129. *Id.*

130. See, for example, Position Statement on Personnel Policies and HIV in the Workplace (1991); Position Statement on Post-Exposure Programs in the Event of Occupational Exposure to HIV/HBV (1991); Position Statement on Availability of Equipment and Safety Procedures to Prevent Transmission of Bloodborne Diseases (1991), in American Nurses Association, *Compendium of HIV/AIDS Positions, Policies, and Documents.* Washington, D.C.: Author, 1992.

131. American Nurses Association. *HIV, Hepatitis-B, Hepatitis-C, Blood-Borne Diseases: Nurses' Risks, Rights, and Responsibilities.* Washington, D.C.: Author (1992) (Workplace Information Series Brochure WP-2); *NIOSH ALERT, supra* note 116.

132. Cheryl Peterson, "FDA Requires Warning Statement," 97(12) *AJN* (1997), 16 (Washington Watch section).

133. Michelle Slattery, "The Epidemic Hazards of Nursing," 98(11) *AJN* (1998), 50 (Issues Update section).

134. *Id.*

135. *Id.*

136. Sovereign, *supra* note 8, at 33–34.

137. *Id.* at 33.

138. 42 U.S.C. Sections 1981, 1983.

139. 42 U.S.C. Sections 2000e-4 through e9.

140. 29 U.S.C.A. Sections 701–794.

141. 29 U.S.C.A. Sections 621–634, 663(a).

142. Pub. L. No. 102-166, 105 Stat. 1071 (1991).

143. 42 U.S.C. Sections 12101–12213 (1991).

144. Sautter, *supra* note 38, at 8-50.

145. Affirmative Action Guidelines, EEOC, *Federal Register,* Volume 44 (January 19, 1979).

146. 41 C.F.R. Sections 60-2.13(a) and 60-2.20; 60-2.13(b) and 60-2.21; 60-2.13(c) and 60-2.22; Sections 60-2.11(a); 60-2.13(f) and 60-2.24; Sections 60-2.13(g) and 60-2.25.

147. Sovereign, *supra* note 8, at 126–130.

148. 683 F. Supp. 758 (D. Kan. 1988).

149. 511 U.S. 661 (1994).

150. 477 U.S. 57 (1986).

151. See generally, Alba Conte. *Sexual Harrassment in the Workplace: Law and Practice.* Volumes 1 and 2. 3rd Edition. New York: Panel Publication, 1994 (with 2000 cumulative supplement).

152. 758 F.2d 1525 (11th Cir. 1985).

153. 480 U.S. 273 (1987), *rehearing denied,* 481 U.S. 1024 (1987), *on remand to,* 692 F. Supp. 1286 (M.D. Fla. 1988).

154. No. 91-504-2, Decision No. CR 191 (Department of Health and Human Services, Departmental Appeals Board, Civil Remedies Division, April 20, 1992); decision upheld, No. 91-504-2, DAB Decision No. 1357 (Department of Health and Human Services Civil Rights Reviewing Authority, September 25, 1992).

155. 148 F.3d 948 (8th Cir. 1998).

156. Henry J. Perritt. *Americans with Disabilities Act Handbook.* Volumes 1–3. 3rd Edition. New York: John Wiley & Sons, 1997, 59 (with 2000–2002 cumulative supplement).

157. *Albertsons, Inc. v. Kirkingburg,* 119 S. Ct. 2162 (1999); *Murphy v. United Parcel Service, Inc.,* 119 S. Ct. 2133 (1999).

158. 29 U.S.C. Section 151–169.

159. Sautter, *supra* note 38 at 10-3.

160. 29 U.S.C. Sections 153, 158, 159, 160, 161.

161. Sautter, *supra* note 38, at 10-3.

162. 29 U.S.C. Sections 158(g), 158(d) and 183.

163. 5 U.S.C. Sections 7101–7135.

164. Black, *supra* note 3, at 273–274.

165. 29 C.F.R. Section 130.30, *as added by* 54 Fed. Reg. 16,347–16,348 (April 21, 1989).

166. *American Hospital Association v. NLRB,* 499 U.S. 606 (1991).

167. Black, *supra* note 3, at 1435.

168. *ANA's Economic & General Welfare Program: A Historical Perspective.* Kansas City, Mo.: ANA, 1981, 5.

169. See, for example, *Waterbury Hospital v. NLRB,* 950 F.2d 849 (Ct. 1991).

170. *NLRB v. J. Weingarten, Inc.,* 420 U.S. 251 (1975), *on remand to,* 511 F.2d 1163 (5th Cir. 1975).

171. 309 N.L.R.B. 163, Case No. 25-CA-19818 (December 16, 1992).

172. *Electromation, Inc. v. National Labor Relations Board,* 35 F.3d 1148 (1996).

173. Sovereign, *supra* note 8, at 274–277.

174. 511 U.S. 571 (1994).
175. *Newton-Wellesley Hospital,* 94 N.L.R.B. 699, 700 (1975).
176. *NLRB Guideline Memorandum on Charge Nurse Supervisory Issues* (OM 99-44), August 24, 1999, reprinted in 8(35) *BNA's Health Law Reporter* (1999), 1459–1471.
177. *Id.* at 1459.
178. *NLRB v. Talladega Cotton Factory, Inc.,* 213 F.2d 209 (5th Cir. 1954); *NLRB v. Miami Coca-Cola Bottling Co.,* 702 F.2d 1 (1st Cir. 1983).
179. American Nurses Association. Report to the Board of Directors from the Cabinet on Economic and General Welfare. *Right to Accept or Reject an Assignment.* ANA (1987).
180. Massachusetts Nurses Association. Mechanisms to Support Nurses' Abilities to Exercise Their Right to Accept or Reject an Assignment: Position Statement (November 9, 1982); North Carolina Nurses Association. Guidelines for the Registered Nurse in Giving, Accepting, or Rejecting a Work Assignment (1986); New York State Nurses Association. Protesting of Assignment—Documentation of Practice Situation (May 1985).
181. Alan MacDonald, "Commentary on Nurses' Right to Accept or Reject Assignment," *Massachusetts Nurse* (February 1983).
182. See, for example, 745 Illinois Complied Statutes Annotated (ILCS) 70/1 *et seq.* (1977), *as amended.*
183. OSHA Hazard Communication Standard, 29 C.F.R. Section 1910.1200 (1993).
184. 483 N.W.2d 211 (1992).
185. 726 P.2d 852 (N.M. 1986).
186. Madeline Naegle and Ann Solari-Twadell, "Impaired Practice: Still an Issue," 10(2) *Journal of Addictions Nursing* (1998), 61–62 (editorial).
187. 41 U.S.C. Sections 707–707.
188. Rothstein and others, *supra* note 63, at 97.
189. *Id.* at 105–107.
190. See generally, Kevin Zeese. *Drug Testing Legal Manual and Practice Aids.* 2nd Edition. Deerfield, Ill.: Clark Boardman Callaghan, 1996 (with regular updates).
191. See, as examples, Sovereign, *supra* note 8, 79–84; Sautter, *supra* note 38, 7-11–7-12.
192. Zeese, *supra* note 190, Volume 1, at 2-2, 2-3.
193. 42 U.S.C. Section 12114(d)(2).
194. 42 U.S.C. Section 12114(c)(5); 12114 (a) & (b).
195. See, for example, Sally Hutchinson, "Chemically Dependent Nurses: The Trajectory toward Self-Annihilation," 35(4) *Nursing Research* (July/August 1986), 196–201.
196. George B. Smith, "Attitudes of Nurse Managers and Assistant Nurse Managers towards Chemically Impaired Colleagues," 24(4) *Image: Journal of Nursing Scholarship* (1992), 295–300; J. Lloyd Lachicotte and Judith Alexander, "Management Attitudes and Nurse Impairment," 21(9) *Nursing Management* (September 1990), 102–110; Carol Kowalski and Margaret Rancourt, "Profile of the Nurse Participating in a Substance Abuse Program of a Board of Registration in Nursing in a New England State," 9(1) *Journal of Addictions Nursing* (1997), 22–29; Margaret Douglas and Nancy J. Brent, "Substance Abuse and the Nurse Manager: Ethical and Legal Issues," 2(1) *Seminars for Nurse Managers* (1994), 16–26.
197. Sovereign, *supra* note 8, at 193.
198. 29 U.S.C. Section 2001 *et seq.*
199. *Id.*
200. 29 U.S.C. Section 2006(d).
201. *Id.* at 2006(f).
202. Sautter, *supra* note 38, at 7–14.
203. 29 U.S.C. Section 2005.
204. Sovereign, *supra* note 8, at 86–87.
205. C. Ciesielski, D. Marianos, C. Y. Ou, and others, "Transmission of Human Immunodeficiency Virus in a Dental Practice," 116 *Ann. Intern. Med.* (1992), 798–805. See also, Schaffner and others, "A Surgeon with AIDS: Lack of Evidence of Transmission to Patients," 264 *JAMA* 467 (1990) (753 patients treated by surgeon with no transmission); Parker and others, "Management of Patients Treated by a Surgeon with HIV Infection," 113 *Lancet* (January 13, 1990) (76 out of 339 patients who asked for HIV testing were HIV negative); David Webber. *AIDS and the Law.* 2nd Edition. New York: John Wiley & Sons, 1992 (with 1996 Cumulative Supplement No. 1), 95; Rothstein and others, *supra* note 63, at 86.
206. American Nurses Association. *HIV Infected Nurse, Ethical Obligations and Disclosure.* Washington, D.C.: Author, 1992, available on the World Wide Web at http://www.nursingworld.org (American Nurses Association home page), accessed May 4, 2000; American Medical Association. *HIV Testing.* Chicago, Ill.: Author, 1994, available on the American Medical Association's home page at http://www.ama-assn.org, accessed May 4, 2000; American Medical Association. *Physicians and Infectious Disease.* Chicago, Ill.: Author, 1996, available on the association's home page listed above.
207. See references cited in note 206.
208. *Leckelt v. Board of Commissioners,* 909 F.2d 820 (5th Cir. 1990), *affirmed,* 909 F.2d 820 (5th Cir. 1990), *aff'g.* 714 F. Supp. 1377 (E.D. La. 1989).
209. "Hospital to Reinstate HIV-Positive Nurse to a Clinical Care Position," 1(1) *BNA's Health Law Reporter* (December 21, 1992), 411 (News and Developments department).
210. 620 A.2d 327 (Md. 1993).
211. Rothstein and others, *supra* note 63, Volume 1, at 91.
212. *Id.* at 92
213. *Id.* at 92–93.
214. Feliu, *supra* note 10, at 180–182.
215. 555 F.2d 1283 (5th Cir. 1977).
216. Feliu, *supra* note 10, at 181.
217. 135 F.3d 1260 (9th Cir. 1998).
218. Rothstein and others, *supra* note 63, Volume 1, at 94.
219. *Id.*
220. *Id., citing* 135 F.3d 1260, 1273.
221. 29 U.S.C. Section 2601 *et seq.*
222. Kerns, Gerner, and Ryan, *supra* note 57, at 12-21–12-22.
223. 29 U.S.C. Section 2601.
224. Kerns, Gerner, and Ryan, *supra* note 57, at 12-22.
225. 42 U.S.C. Section 12102(a); 28 C.F.R. Section 36.201(a).
226. Lawrence Gostin, Chai Feldblum, and David Webber, "Disability Discrimination in America," 281(8) *JAMA* (1999), 745–752. See also, Susan Laughlin, "Compliance with Title III of the ADA," 5(3) *Journal of Nursing Law* (1998), 51–62.
227. 118 S. Ct. 1196 (1998).
228. Gostin, Feldblum, and Webber, *supra* note 226, at 745.

229. *Id.* at 746 (citations omitted).

230. *Id.*

231. *Id.* at 747.

232. 812 F. Supp. 1183 (M.D. Ala. 1993), Call No. 93-6502 (October 3, 1994).

233. "Court Dismisses Complaint of Pregnant Nurse Who Refused to Treat AIDS Patient," 2(20) *BNA's Health Law Reporter* (May 20, 1993), 641.

234. "Home Care Nurse Who Refused to Treat HIV Patient Fails in Pregnancy Bias Claim," 3(40) *BNA's Health Law Reporter* (October 13, 1994), 1445.

235. *Stepp v. Review Board of the Indiana Employment Security Division,* 521 N.E.2d 350 (Ind. App. Ct. 1988).

236. Winifred Carson, "AIDS and the Nurse—A Legal Update," *American Nurse* (March 1993), 18.

237. 588 N.Y.S.2d 698 (Ct. Cl. 1992), 595 N.Y.S.2d 592 (N.Y. App. Div. 1993), *rev'g in part,* 588 N.Y.S.2d 698 (Ct. Cl. 1992).

238. ANA. *Position Statement Regarding Risk v. Responsibility in Providing Nursing Care.* Kansas City, Mo.: Author, 1994.

239. *Id.*

240. See Chapter 3.

The Nurse in the Acute Care Setting

In one study analyzing adverse events in hospitals in two states. . . . the emergency department had the highest proportion . . . of negligent adverse events.

At one time, hospitals were the most familiar type of health care delivery system in the United States. In fact, until the 1980s, the growth of hospitals and hospital services thrived.[1] Since then, however, hospitals have seen a decline in their occupancy rates, discharge rates, and length of stays.[2] In addition, downsizing, mergers, and closures continue to occur.[3] Costs in acute care continue to rise, and, as a result, increased competition from less expensive delivery entities such as health maintenance organizations (HMOs) and preferred provider organizations (PPOs) has occurred.[4] Even so, hospitals still provide a wide array of services to those who need them, including emergency care, surgery, specialty care (ICU/CCU), and labor and delivery services. Moreover, hospitals are the major employers of nursing personnel.[5]

Recent statistics indicate that hospitals employ 1.3 million registered nurses and 175,000 licensed practical nurses.[6] This chapter will explore only a few of the many legal issues of interest to the staff nurse working in acute care in the following practice areas: emergency nursing, perioperative nursing, and adult psychiatric/mental health nursing.

NURSING IN THE EMERGENCY DEPARTMENT

Emergency department (ED) nursing is a highly challenging, complex, and rapid-paced nursing practice. It is also an area of high liability.[7] In one study analyzing adverse events in hospitals in two states, 30% were due to negligence. Of the 30%, the emergency department had the highest proportion—52.6%—of negligent adverse events.[8]

Many reasons account for the potential for malpractice claims in the ED. To begin with, large numbers of individuals utilize the emergency department as a primary health clinic or in lieu of a physician's office. Because there is little, if any, continuity of care, follow-up is often nonexistent. The lack of follow-up care can result in further injury or death to the patient.[9]

Second, EDs often treat individuals with severe trauma, including gunshot wounds and multiple injuries due to vehicular accidents. Trauma injuries are not always easily identified, at least initially. An expected or unexpected change in the patient's condition requires prompt intervention by the ED team. When the intervention does not work, and a patient allegedly suffers further injury or death as a result, a malpractice or wrongful death suit often follows.

These more traditional areas of liability for the ED, as well as recent case and statutory law, have resulted in ED nurses' involvement in lawsuits.

Duty to Provide Care

The duty of a hospital to provide emergency care is a long-standing one established by case law and federal and state statutory law and respective rules and regulations. The earliest federal law passed by Congress establishing the duty was the Hill-Burton Act of 1946.[10] Among other obligations, it mandated that hospitals receiving money for construction and modernization of their facilities could not refuse to provide emergency care to those who could not pay for those services or whenever the hospital had an "uncompensated care obligation."[11]

Many states also passed statutes requiring hospitals to provide emergency care, including Illinois, Florida, Tennessee, and Wyoming. Illinois' act was passed in 1927 and has been used as a model for subsequent state laws. Even so, the particulars of the acts vary considerably.

One of the early cases ensconcing the duty to provide emergency care was *Wilmington General Hospital v. Manlove*,[12] decided in 1961. When Mr. and Mrs. Manlove brought their child to the ED with diarrhea and an elevated temperature, the nurse on duty in the ED informed the Manloves that, pursuant to hospital policy, no care could be provided by physicians at the hospital until the attending doctor was consulted. The ED nurse attempted to contact the pediatrician but could not reach him. As a result, no care was given to the infant and the Manloves were sent home with instructions to return to the pediatric clinic in the morning. The Manloves did make an appointment for their son to see the pediatrician that evening, but that afternoon, Darien Manlove died of bronchial pneumonia.

The parents brought suit against the hospital. The trial court denied the request by the hospital for a summary judgment. That decision was appealed, and the Delaware Supreme Court affirmed the trial court decision and sent the case back to the trial court for further proceedings to determine if the hospital had been negligent in not responding to the emergency condition of the infant. The court's theory in underscoring its decision was that if a hospital has an ED, there is a duty to provide care and treatment to all those who need services *when an emergency exists.*

One of the problems in the *Manlove* case was the lack of an assessment of the infant's condition. According to the nurse involved in the case, despite the parents' voiced concerns, the child was not in any apparent distress. Even so, the child died.

Thus, one of the other rules of law in relation to the duty to treat that has emerged from the *Manlove* case is the duty to evaluate the patient to determine if a true emergency exists. That evaluation involves a decision whether the nontreatment of the patient may result in a threat to the patient's well-being or life. If the answer is affirmative, treatment must occur. If a delay will not result in harm to the patient, then an "emergency" does not exist, and there is no obligation to provide care. In short, the rule clearly focuses on the individual's *condition* at the time he or she arrives in the ED.

In 1986, Congress passed another law further expanding and defining the duty to provide emergency care. The Emergency Medical Treatment and Active Labor Act (EMTALA)[13] prohibited facilities receiving Medicare and Medicaid funds from "dumping" patients out of their emergency rooms when they could not pay. The Act requires hospitals to (1) medically screen a patient for the existence of an emergency medical condition and (2) stabilize the patient's condition. If transfer of the patient is required, the transfer can occur only after the condition is stabilized, the patient or the patient's legal representative gives informed consent for the transfer, there is a facility to accept the transfer, and the physician documents and certifies certain factors (e.g., the benefits of transfer outweigh the risks of transfer).[14]

The Emergency Medical Treatment and Active Labor Act also defines an emergency medical condition and active labor. An emergency medical condition is one with acute symptoms of such severity that the absence of medical care "could reasonably be expected" to result in (1) serious jeopardy to the health of the patient (including the woman and unborn child); (2) serious impairment of bodily functions; (3) serious dysfunction of any bodily part or organ; or (4) with a woman in active labor, sufficient time to effect a safe transfer before delivery is not possible, or the transfer may pose a threat to the health and safety of both the woman and fetus.[15]

Violations of the Emergency Medical Treatment and Active Labor Act can result in termination of the facility's participation in the Medicare and Medicaid programs. In addition, the Act provides for civil penalties against the offender facility. Also, the injured party may sue for any "personal injury" under the laws of the state in which the hospital exists and may seek "equitable relief" (e.g., an injunction) as well.[16]

In fact, several cases have been filed alleging violations of the Emergency Medical Treatment and Active Labor Act. In one case, *Stevison by Collins v. Enid Health Systems, Inc.*,[17] Mrs. Stevison brought her 13-year-old daughter to the ED at Enid Hospital for abdominal pain. According to Mrs. Stevison, the ED nurse told her that her daughter could not be seen unless a $50.00 payment was made. Because Mrs. Stevison was on welfare, she could not pay the required fee. The nurse testified that she told Mrs. Stevison that welfare did not cover ED visits, and she would be billed for any care and treatment for her daughter.

Despite conflicting stories, it was undisputed that Mrs. Stevison and the daughter left without receiving treatment. The next day, the daughter suffered a ruptured appendix, had the appendix removed at another hospital owned by the defendant hospital, and her postoperative recovery was prolonged and more painful than normal. In addition, due to the rupture, the daughter's ability to have children was probably compromised.

Mrs. Stevison filed suit in federal court alleging that no screening of her daughter's condition took place as required by the EMTALA. The jury returned a verdict in favor of the hospital, and Mrs. Stevison appealed. The Court of Appeals for the Tenth Circuit reversed the lower court decision. The court held that the hospital had the burden of proof of supporting its contention that Mrs. Stevison "withdrew" her request for treatment after being told of the $50.00 payment. Although the EMTALA does provide that no violation of the Act occurs if a patient refuses screening and treatment after it is offered, the ED must establish this fact by a preponderance of the evidence. The court based its rationale on the intent of the Act; that is, to deter "patient-dumping" of indigent patients who do not have health insurance or cannot pay for ED services.

In today's climate of managed care and reduced costs, cases like the *Stevison by Collins* case take on new meaning. One concern is the use of "gatekeepers" for managed health care plans that authorize or deny payment by insurance plans for emergency care. When a denial or a delay in the authorization of payment for an ED visit occurs and the patient decides to refuse care and leaves the ED, careful documentation of the denial must be made in the medical record.[18] Also, in order to avoid liability under the EMTALA, the patient must be informed that emergency care *is* available from the ED and staff. The only issue is who will be responsible for the care—the insurance company or the patient.[19]

Also, in *Johnson v. University of Chicago Hospitals*,[20] the Seventh Circuit Court of Appeals held that the EMTALA does not apply to situations in which the patient does not physically enter the ED for treatment and telemetry services alone are used to divert the patient to another facility. According to the three-judge panel, a hospital-operated telemetry system is distinct from the same hospital's ED.[21]

In the *Johnson* case, a 1-month-old infant stopped breathing and was transported by ambulance to the University of Chicago Hospital. The ambulance personnel were in touch with the hospital's telemetry nurse. When the ambulance was within five blocks of the ED, the nurse informed the ambulance that the pediatric unit was full, they were on "by-pass" status, and the child would have to be taken to another hospital. The child was taken to St. Bernard Hospital's ED but had to be transported again to Cook County Hospital because St. Bernard had no pediatric ICU. The child died after being transferred to Cook County Hospital.

Although the appeals court held that several causes of action could be brought against the University of Chicago Hospital under Illinois laws, none could be brought under the Emergency Medical Treatment and Active Labor Act.

As a result of *Johnson* and another case[22] with similar facts, the Health Care Financing Administration (HCFA) defined in its regulations when an individual "comes to" the ED. Essentially, whenever a person presents himself or herself anywhere on hospital property (whether it be a sidewalk, a parking lot, or in a hospital-owned ambulance), the person has "come to" the ED for EMTALA purposes.[23] If an individual is in a non-hospital-owned ambulance, the person has not "come to" the ED unless the ambulance is on hospital property.[24] Phone contact alone with the ED from the non-hospital ambulance does not constitute "presence" in the ED.

If the non-hospital-owned ambulance staff disregard any instructions by the hospital staff to take the patient to another facility and bring the patient to the hospital, however, then the person is regarded as having "come to" that ED. As a result, he must be treated in accordance with the EMTALA.[25]

Triage

Triage in the ED is sorting patients and setting treatment priorities according to medical need.[26] Many times this process is done by ED nurses with the help of physician-based standing orders and written protocols. Triage is important for many reasons, including providing an immediate response to a patient's needs and in controlling patient flow throughout the ED.

Triage in the ED is sorting patients and setting treatment priorities according to medical need.

The manner in which triage occurs is varied. It can occur on the telephone, in the ED waiting room, or when several patients arrive at the ED via ambulance. Regardless of form, triage decisions can result in potential liability for the nurse making treatment priority choices.

In some instances, the ED nurse's liability results from a failure to carry out triage on the patient at all, as in the *Manlove* case discussed earlier. In other situations, the nurse performs triage but does so negligently. In *Ramsey v. Physician's Memorial Hospital*,[27] for example, the ED nurse evaluated two young boys who were brought to the ED by their mother. Both had symptoms of high fever and a rash. The mother told the ED nurse that she had removed two ticks from one of her sons. The ED nurse failed to inform the physician of this fact and told him only of her physical findings. As a result, the physician diagnosed measles. Unfortunately, one of the children had Rocky Mountain spotted fever and died.

Other cases involving negligent triage by ED nurses include *Lunsford v. Board of Nurse Examiners for State of Texas*[28] (nurse failed to properly assess patient's heart condition; told patient to drive himself to another hospital and he died en route) and *Thomas v. Corso*[29] (nurse failed to report vital signs of automobile accident victim to physician and underestimated injuries and patient's voiced complaints, resulting in his death).

Duty to Report Certain Patient Conditions

To protect the public health and safety, states have passed laws that require the reporting of certain events to an identified state agency. EDs and ED personnel, including nurses, are almost always included as mandated reporters in these laws. Although the respective state laws can vary widely as to what situations must be reported, some of the more common events include:

- Child abuse and neglect
- Communicable diseases (e.g., tuberculosis, AIDS, sexually transmitted diseases)
- Person dead on arrival in the ED
- Gunshot wounds, stab wounds, or other injuries due to violence
- Sexual assaults
- Food poisoning
- Industrial accidents[30]

Staffing/Administration of Emergency Department

Adequate staffing of the ED is essential because of the fast-paced, unpredictable nature of ED nursing. Moreover, because of the complex cases and patient conditions treated in the ED, it is important that staff be qualified, competent, and adequately trained as well. As in many health care delivery settings, one single, universal staffing system does not exist.[31] Rather, a number of factors must be evaluated on a regular basis in order to ensure safe care and, at the same time, maintain an ED that is operationally efficient.[32] The Emergency Nurses Association has developed guidelines to help nurse administrators in the ED to help plan staffing patterns.[33] Factors that must be evaluated include staff mix (e.g., RN, LPN), physician staff, patient volume, patient mix (e.g., obstetrical, psychiatric, cultural diversity), patient acuity, and type of triage system.[34] Needless to say, the registered professional nurse is an "essential element in the delivery of quality, cost efficient care."[35]

In addition, risk management principles support ED staff qualifications consistent with a level I ED; that is, providing comprehensive services with at least one physician experienced in emergency medicine on duty 24 hours a day.[36] The physician should be board certified in emergency medicine. If that is not possible, at a minimum all ED physicians should be certified in Advanced Cardiac Life Support (ACLS) and have some training in a specialty relevant to emergency medicine.[37] Nursing staff should be ACLS certified as well and seek certification in emergency nursing.[38]

The non-RN caregivers who are used [in the ED] include emergency medical technicians, . . . paramedics, emergency department technicians, and orderlies.

Some health care delivery organizations have redesigned the ED to include alternate staffing options.[39] EDs are using non-RN caregivers to provide direct patient care.[40] The non-RN caregivers who are used include emergency medical technicians (EMTs), paramedics, emergency department technicians, and orderlies.[41] Although the non-RN staff members may, at least superficially, increase staff numbers in the ED, they cannot perform professional nursing activities as defined in a state nurse practice act.[42] Rather, their respective jobs must be well defined through written job descriptions, they must be supervised by the registered nurse in the ED, they must be evaluated in terms of patient care outcomes, and they must comply with established standards of care.[43] Under no circumstances should the non-RN caregiver in the ED *replace* the emergency department registered nurse.[44] Moreover, the ratio of non-RN staff to registered nurses in the ED must be carefully established in order to maintain quality care to patients in the ED.[45]

IMPLICATIONS FOR EMERGENCY DEPARTMENT NURSES

The ED nurse must help the ED establish and maintain clear and complete policies and procedures concerning the nurse's role in the assessment and treatment of patients who come to the ED for care. The policies must reflect the ED's duty to provide care when a true emergency exists. Furthermore, it should be established hospital policy that no patient is refused care based on his or her inability to pay. If the ED nurse believes a patient is refused care on the basis of this factor, the ED nurse should discuss this with the ED physician and contact the ED nursing supervisor immediately, and an incident report should be filed with the hospital risk manager.

Likewise, a patient should not be refused care or transferred to another facility in violation of the EMTALA. The ED nurse will need to ensure this does not happen by discussing the Act with the ED physician when refusal or transfer is being contemplated[46] and notify the nursing supervisor immediately.

When a decision is made to transfer a patient consistent with the Emergency Medical Treatment and Active Labor Act, the ED record should also reflect any treatment given to stabilize the patient and the patient's condition upon transfer.

Any decision concerning noncare of a patient in the ED must be carefully documented. If the patient refuses care, or leaves against medical advice (AMA), a complete and factual entry should be made by the ED nurse in the ED record. Some EDs have developed AMA forms for the patient to sign that state that the patient has refused

care and releases the ED, ED staff, and hospital from any liability due to his or her decision to leave.

The teaching of the patient/family in the ED must be carefully done and documented fully in the ED record. When teaching is not documented, whether they were given instructions can be the basis of a suit, particularly when an injury or death occurs. For example, in one reported case, *Crawford v. Earl Long Hospital*,[47] a deceased man's mother filed a suit against the hospital alleging that no patient care instructions were given to her after her adult son was treated in the ED when hit on the head with a baseball bat and stabbed in a fight. The patient was not admitted to the hospital, and therefore, according to hospital policy, a responsible adult—the mother of the patient, with whom he was living—was called to come to the ED to get oral discharge instructions. At the time the case arose, it was not the accepted standard of care to provide either the patient or the family written discharge instructions.

Although the nurse testified at trial that she had specifically called the mother to come into the ED and had given her instructions about the care to give to her son after discharge (e.g., check pupil size and orientation of son), the nurse did not document the instructions in the ED record. The jury returned a verdict in favor of the hospital because it believed the nurse's testimony. The appellate court upheld the verdict for the hospital. If the nurse had only documented the instructions given, the mother could not have alleged that the teaching was not done.

To help ED nurses with discharge instructions, many EDs have developed teaching forms that provide a ready way in which to include and document needed instructions given to the patient and/or family. Whether the ED nurse documents teaching with a form or narratively, the nurse will also want to be certain to discuss with the patient and/or family the ramifications on the health and well-being of the patient if the instructions are not followed. In *LeBlanc v. Northern Colfax County Hospital*,[48] the death of a patient after being seen in the ED was alleged to have been caused by the ED nurse's inadequate instructions concerning the pain the patient was experiencing after being kicked in the stomach. Because the patient did not have any medical knowledge, the ED nurse's instructions to the patient to "come back to the ED if the pain persists" may not have been clear

ETHICS CONNECTION 17–1

Nursing, unlike medicine, consistently has sought to be inclusive, providing career opportunities for individuals from diverse socioeconomic, cultural, and ethnic backgrounds. Periodically, this inclusiveness has been misinterpreted as vagueness of boundaries and has resulted in intrusions by other disciplines, especially medicine, into nursing practice. As nursing practice has become more autonomous and free of institutional and physician control, efforts to replace nurses as primary caregivers have been made. In the late 1980s, for example, the American Medical Association (AMA) proposed the creation of registered care technologists (RCTs) who would provide direct patient care and report to physicians.

Efforts at cost control also have led to the creation of other categories of personnel who would not be licensed but would be used to assist in the provision of patient care. The American Nurses Association defines this category of unlicensed assistive personnel (UAPs) as unlicensed individuals who are "trained to function in an assistive role to the licensed nurse in the provision of patient/client activities as delegated by the nurse. The activities can be generally categorized as either direct or indirect care."[1] This direct care category of personnel includes "nurse aides, orderlies, assistants, attendants, or technicians."

The increased use of UAPs has concerned nurses for several reasons, including patient safety and nurses' accountability for the actions of UAPs without control of their education or scope of responsibilities. Medication administration by UAPs is of special concern to nurses. In addition, nurses generally have not been well educated in supervisory or delegation skills. In 1997, Shoffner reviewed the confusion and complexities surrounding employment of UAPs. She wrote, "Evidence seems to be growing that the UAP is being used for the delivery of care in settings and with patients where only RNs or LPNs would have been considered the appropriate provider in the past."[2] Nurses' moral concerns about patient safety, their own welfare, and professional erosion through intrusions by UAP advocates into the scope of nursing practice led to political action. Through their professional organizations, nurses across the nation became politically active in efforts to support or hinder passage of state legislation regarding UAPs.[3, 4, 5, 6]

The ANA has developed position statements on UAPs[7] and on the education of Registered Nurses regarding working with UAPs.[8] Delegation is defined as "the transfer of responsibility for the performance of an activity from one person to another while retaining accountability for the outcome."[1] Any nursing intervention that requires independent, specialized, nursing knowledge, skill or judgement can not be delegated."[9]

Interpretive Statement 6.4 of the *Code for Nurses with Interpretive Statements*[10] addresses "delegation of nursing activities" and clearly indicates that nurses have accountability for delegating nursing care activities, "regardless of employer policy or directives." This statement is another illustration of how important it is becoming to further develop communitarian ethics. The statement has the potential to place acute care nurses in opposition to their employers, depending upon the organizational culture of the institution in which the nurse works. Basic nursing education and workplace education programs have a moral obligation of fairness and beneficence to better prepare nurses to develop the knowledge and skills that are necessary for safely and effectively delegating activities to UAPs.

[1]American Nurses Association. *Registered Nurse Utilization of Unlicensed Assistive Personnel*. Washington, D.C.: Author, 1992.

[2]D. Shoffner. "Unlicensed Assistive Personnel: Helpful or Harmful?" 60(2) *Tennessee Nurse* (April 1997), 13–15.

[3]Anonymous. "Bill Introduced to Regulate Unlicensed Assistive Personnel," 51(5) *Pennsylvania Nurse* (May 1996), 16.

[4]Anonymous. "Governor Signs Nursing Practice Act," 42(2) *New Mexico Nurse* (Summer, 1997), 1–4.

[5]Anonymous. "Practice Alert: WVNA Warns Nurses," 1(2) *West Virginia Nurse* (Summer 1997), 3.

[6]Anonymous. "6000 Unlicensed Persons Certified to Administer Medications," 65(8) *Massachusetts Nurse* (September 1995), 1, 3.

[7]ANA, *supra* note 1.

[8]American Nurses Association. *Position Statements: Registered Nurse Education Relating to the Utilization of Unlicensed Assistive Personnel*. Washington, D.C.: Author, 1992.

[9]ANA, *supra* note 1.

[10]American Nurses Association. *Code for Nurses with Interpretive Statements*. Kansas City, Mo.: Author, 1985.

enough for the patient to act upon. The patient delayed going back to the ED for 6 days despite his continued pain. The pain resulted from a lacerated liver and gastrointestinal bleeding due to a ruptured ulcer, which, combined with no food, the ingestion of unprescribed Darvon, and only small amounts of liquid, caused his death.

To help ED nurses with discharge instructions, many EDs have developed teaching forms . . .

The appellate court reversed the trial court's summary judgment for the hospital (based on its finding that the patient's death was due to his delay in seeking treatment and not on the nurse's instructions) and sent the case back to the trial court for a trial. Although the case settled out of court, it may well be an indication that discussing and documenting implications if treatment recommendations are not followed is a good risk management approach for the ED nurse.

Many times the ED will receive a telephone call from an individual requesting medical advice over the phone. The call may be from an individual never seen in the ED before, or it may be from a patient who was treated in the ED but sent home because admission was not necessary. The ED nurse must be very careful about giving telephone advice in this manner. It is more prudent to encourage the individual to come into the ED or see his or her physician as soon as possible.[49] Similarly, if a person asks whether or not a visit to the ED is necessary, the ED nurse should err on the side of encouraging the individual to be seen in the ED.

Policies and procedures for proper reporting of required events in the ED are also important. The development of forms to help the ED nurse with his or her responsibilities in this regard can also be very helpful.

If the ED nurse works in a setting where EMTs, paramedics, or other non-RN care providers work, the nurse will need to be very clear about the state nurse practice act requirements concerning working with non-RN staff. The ED nurse should carefully review any delegation, supervision, and other requirements in order to be in compliance with the practice act and with standards of care.

PERIOPERATIVE NURSING

The American Association of Operating Room Nurses (AORN) represents 43,000 registered nurses who practice perioperative nursing, teach perioperative nursing, manage this specialty area, do research, or are enrolled in an educational program in perioperative nursing.[50] The perioperative nurse fulfills various roles in the perioperative department, including that of circulating nurse, monitor and caregiver for the patient in the postanesthesia area, and RN first assistant (RNFA). Perioperative nursing is, by its very nature, complex and demanding. Because a patient's condition can change rapidly during or after surgery, adverse patient outcomes are always a possibility. Often the adverse outcomes result from a breakdown in the patient's continuity of care during the surgical process.[51]

Adverse Patient Outcomes in Perioperative Nursing

Many of the allegations of professional negligence in the perioperative area involve the administration of anesthesia or the negligent monitoring of patients who are under anesthesia[52] or who are recovering from anesthesia in the postanesthesia care unit (PACU). Several malpractice cases involving the certified registered nurse anesthetist are discussed in Chapter 21. Examples of other cases against perioperative nurses are presented in Table 17–1.

The RN First Assistant

The RN first assistant (RNFA) in the perioperative setting possesses an expanded role. Although the RN first assistant's role may be prescribed by the state nurse practice act, it is also often molded by the health care facility's policies and procedures. The American Association of Operating Room Nurses (AORN) revised official statement on the RN first assistant[53] provides a consistent definition of what the first assistant does and defines the association's qualifications for the nurse in this role.

The RN first assistant at surgery collaborates with the surgeon and the health care team in performing a safe operation with optimal outcomes for the patient.

TABLE 17-1

Malpractice Cases Involving Perioperative Nurses

CASE NAME	ALLEGATION	DECISION
Goldsby v. Evangelical Deaconess Hospital (1978)[1]	Failure to follow nursing monitoring procedures postop caused patient death	Judgment against hospital due to postanesthesia nurse's negligence
Laidlow v. Lion Gate Hospital (1969)[2]	Failure of postanesthesia nurses and supervisor to provide adequate supervision and nurses caused patient arrest, resulting in permanent brain damage to patient	Judgment against hospital due to nurses' and supervisor's conduct
Evoma v. Falco (1991)[3]	Failure of postanesthesia nurse to ask what drug patient was given during surgery, to ensure patient would be monitored when leaving PACU, and to recognize patient was not breathing, resulting in initial comatose state and then death of patient over a year later	PACU nurse's conduct 100% responsible for patient injury; court verdict for patient's estate
Robinson v. N.E. Alabama Regional Medical Center (1989)[4]	Nurse in OR counted sponges incorrectly after vaginal hysterectomy, resulting in patient's pain, nausea, vomiting, inability to sleep, and dizziness for 5 months postop	Verdict for patient and against hospital in amount of $250,000
Dickerson v. Fatehi (1997)[5]	Failure of scrub and/or circulating nurse to do needle count after surgery; undiscovered 18 gauge needle and "metal detector," causing patient severe pain and additional surgery to remove needle and marker	Summary judgment for nurses and surgeon reversed and remanded for trial. *Res ipsa loquitur* doctrine applicable to all defendants
Chin v. St. Barnabas Medical Center (1999)[6]	One or both circulating nurses incorrectly connected Hystero-Flo Pump to Hysteroscope, resulting in embolism and death of patient from air introduced into uterus	Case remanded to trial court only to review percentage of liability determinations; jury determined nurses, physician, and hospital negligent and awarded $2 million to be "apportioned" among defendants

[1] 74-004-754 (N.M. 1978)
[2] 70 W.W.R. 727 (1969)
[3] 589 A.2d 653 (N.J. 1991)
[4] 548 So. 2d 439 (Ala. 1989)
[5] 484 S.E.2d (Va. 1997)
[6] 734 A.2d 778 (N.J. 1999)

The RN first assistant at surgery collaborates with the surgeon and the health care team in performing a safe operation with optimal outcomes for the patient.[54] He or she practices in collaboration with and at the direction of the surgeon during the patient's "intraoperative phase" of the perioperative experience.[55] The RN first assistant's scope of practice is firmly grounded in perioperative nursing practice but is a "refinement" of that nursing specialty.[56] Responsibilities of the RN first assistant include handling tissue, suturing, and providing hemostasis.[57]

The American Association of Operating Room Nurses recommends that the RN first assistant be certified in operating room nursing (CNOR) and possess diversified scrub and circulating proficiency. In addition, the first assistant should complete a formal education program that includes didactic and supervised clinical experience and learning.[58] The formal programs must include all content from the *Core Curriculum for the RN First Assistant*[59] and take place in academic institutions accredited by the Association of Colleges and Schools.[60] Obviously the ultimate goal is certification (certified RN first assistant; CRNFA) or a degree as an RN first assistant.

Staffing/Administration of Perioperative Department

Surgery scheduling is an essential component of efficient and effective provision of services in perioperative care. So, too, is the scheduling of qualified staff. In the operating room (OR) itself, for example, the basic requirement should be that at least one RN will function as circulating nurse in each OR. Moreover, the RN is an essential staff member in the OR.[61]

Other factors that must be taken into consideration when scheduling staff include the number of patients who will be moving through the perioperative area on a given day, the number of OR suites, the types of procedures that will be performed, whether registry/outside contract personnel will be necessary, and the method of staffing used (e.g., fixed or variable).[62]

The use of ancillary, unlicensed assistive personnel can help staffing concerns by their respective provision of assistive and support services to the perioperative nursing staff. They cannot, however, substitute for the perioperative nurse or perform perioperative nursing functions.

IMPLICATIONS FOR PERIOPERATIVE NURSES

All perioperative nurses must be certain to provide nonnegligent care consistent with established standards of care for this specialty practice.[63] Although assessment, observation, and evaluation are important responsibilities for all perioperative nurses, they are very important in the PACU. As the court stated in the *Laidlow* case presented in Table 17–1:

> The patient in this room requires the greatest attention because it is fraught with the greatest potential dangers to the patient. This hazard carries with it . . . a high degree of duty owed by the hospital to the patient. . . . There should be no relaxing of vigilance if one is to comply with the standard of care required in this room. . . .[64]

ETHICS CONNECTION 17–2

Both administrators and acute care nurses deplore the shortage of experienced nurses who are competent and flexible and have well developed critical thinking skills. Nationwide, patients and the public share nurses' concerns about staffing patterns and skill mix.[1] The use of unlicensed assistive personnel (UAPs) is increasing, as is the use of agency nurses and mandatory overtime. Nurses are beginning to gather data to explore their contention that current staffing shortages place patients in danger.[2]

Evidence-based staffing information tends to support their concerns regarding adverse patient outcomes, including falls, medication errors, and nosocomial infections.[3] Results of several studies have found significant inverse relationships between adverse patient outcomes and nurse staffing. The more adequate the staffing pattern, the less often did adverse outcomes occur. For example, in a stratified probability sample of 589 acute-care hospitals in 10 states, Kovner and Gergen[4] examined the relationship of nurse staffing and adverse events. Hospital-level data were matched to American Hospital Association data on community hospital characteristics. They found a large, significant relationship between nurse staffing and postoperative urinary tract infection ($p < .0001$) and between nurse staffing and postoperative pneumonia ($p < .001$). Statistically significant relationships also were found between nurse staffing and postoperative thrombosis ($p < .01$) and nurse staffing and postoperative pulmonary compromise ($p < .05$).

Thus, failure to provide adequate nurse staffing does harm patients in measurable ways. Inadequate nurse staffing patterns and practices are immoral, a breach of the moral principle of nonmaleficence. Adequate nursing staff patterns and practices, on the other hand, are related to uncomplicated postoperative recovery. Adequate nurse staffing is a beneficent and fair practice.

It is not easy, however, to specify precisely what are the appropriate staffing patterns and skill mix. Research funds need to be allocated for studies that will inform staffing patterns and practices. The Kovner and Gergen study is an example of outcomes research that has the potential to contribute to the development or refinement of practice guidelines. Although the relationships between outcomes research and clinical judgment are being explored, this approach of outcomes research or evidence-based practice has critics, particularly in medicine,[5] who are concerned that it may interfere with their autonomy and clinical judgment.

---

[1]S. Tabone, "Staff Models for the Next Millennium," 73(5) *Texas Nursing* (May 1999), 6–7.
[2]N. McGuckin, "Nurses Report 1999 Workplace Trends," 6(4) *Hawaii Nurse* (July-August 1999), 1–3.
[3]*Id.*
[4]C. Kovner and P. J. Gergen, "Nurse Staffing Levels and Adverse Events Following Surgery in U.S. Hospitals," 30(4) *Image: The Journal of Nursing Scholarship* (1998), 315–321.
[5]Fred Gifford, "Outcomes Research and Practice Guidelines: Upstream Issues for Downstream Users," 26(2) *Hastings Center Report* (March-April 1996), 38–46.

That standard of care includes not leaving the post-anesthesia patient alone with no monitoring as well as monitoring the patient effectively.

Monitoring the patient well, in addition to performing all of the other responsibilities in perioperative nursing, requires adequate numbers of personnel in the perioperative areas as well as adequately trained staff. The Association of Operating Room Nurses recommends a 1:1 perioperative RN to patient ratio during operative and other invasive procedures.[65] The perioperative nurse will need to voice any concerns about inadequate staffing to the nurse manager in the perioperative suite. Using Association of Operating Room Nurses' guidelines, as well as licensing requirements and accreditation suggestions, may help rectify any staffing issues.

The documentation of the care given to the perioperative patient must be complete, factual, and timely. Utilizing well-developed documentation forms can enhance the effectiveness of required documentation. Likewise, well-formulated and accessible policies and procedures are invaluable.[66] The perioperative nurse needs to focus on specific areas that include when and how the patient was monitored, the identification of persons who provided perioperative care to the patient, the continual assessment of the patient's condition preoperatively, intraoperatively, and postoperatively, any significant or unusual occurrences, the interventions taken during the patient's stay in the perioperative area, notification of the patient's surgeon or others if a change in the patient's condition occurred, and, of course, the patient's condition and status upon leaving the perioperative suite.[67]

It is important that when the perioperative nurse is functioning as an RN first assistant, he or she should assume only that role. For example, the RN first assistant should not also function as the scrub nurse while first assisting.[68] Current certification in both OR nursing and as a first assistant is essential. It is also important that the RN first assistant comply with any policies and procedures required of the institution concerning the role of the first assistant.

RN first assistants will also need to work to change nursing practice acts in states in which the RN first assistant is not recognized. Moreover, if the hospital in which the RN first assistant works provides a mechanism for the RN first assistant to obtain clinical privileges, that procedure should

be used so that the RN first assistant can function effectively in the role and consistent with his or her education and clinical background.

Assistive workers in the perioperative area can be utilized to aid the nurse consistent with the assistive worker's job description, the state nurse practice act, and other regulatory requirements. The perioperative nurse will need to be clear about what the nursing profession, the professional associations, and the law allow the nurse to delegate to the assistive worker. The nurse can then use that information to delegate certain patient care tasks to the competent assistive worker without violating those guidelines. For example, the Association of Operating Room Nurses clearly states that assessment, diagnosis, outcome, identification, planning, and evaluation of the patient—all "core activities" of perioperative nursing—cannot be delegated to assistive workers.[69] In deciding what perioperative patient care might be delegated to the unlicensed assistive worker, the amount of supervision the RN will be able to provide, the competency of the worker, the complexity of the patient's condition, and the ratio of RNs to assistive workers based on patient need are some of the factors that must be evaluated.[70]

All perioperative nurses will need to be ever vigilant in guarding against any intrusion into their practice. Reorganizing or restructuring the hospital or perioperative area, using surgical technicians to replace RN first assistants, laying off qualified perioperative nurses and replacing them with assistive workers, and requiring more professional responsibilities of the nurse without hiring adequate numbers of qualified staff are all examples of ways in which perioperative nursing practice can be, and is being, threatened.

The perioperative nurse will also need to be involved in research concerning the role of the nurse in providing quality care to patients. Documented research findings are helpful, not only in stemming the tide against intrusion by others into perioperative nursing practice, but also for convincing legislators to provide, or continue to provide, the legal basis for perioperative nursing practice.

PSYCHIATRIC/MENTAL HEALTH NURSING

The nurse who works in psychiatric/mental health nursing must not only be knowledgeable about general legal issues in the provision of care to patients (e.g., informed consent/refusal of treatment, documentation) but must also be mindful of the application of those general legal issues to this specialty area of practice. Many of the applications faced by the nurse when caring for the client who has psychiatric difficulties are relatively newer than general legal rights and issues. It was not until the 1960s that legal rights of the mentally ill were finally recognized by the courts and state and federal governments.[71] With those established rights came concomitant responsibilities for health care providers, including psychiatric/mental health nurses.

It was not until the 1960s that legal rights of the mentally ill were finally recognized by the courts and state and federal governments.

The legal responsibilities of psychiatric nurses are further compounded by the fact that the law has in many instances provided more legal protections for those with psychiatric problems because of the very nature of the illness and the treatment required. For example, the very fact that someone requires admission to a psychiatric unit for care can stigmatize that person. Moreover, if the individual does not consent to admission and an involuntary admission is necessary, many constitutional issues must be carefully handled, not the least of which are numerous constitutional due process protections.[72]

Table 17–2 lists the types of admissions possible and the constitutional issues raised by those admissions.

Duty to Protect the Patient from Harm

Once admitted to a hospital psychiatric unit, the recipient of mental health care requires a thorough assessment, careful monitoring, and a sound plan of care throughout his or her stay in the unit. This is especially so for the psychiatric patient who may be suicidal. The psychiatric nurse must ensure the patient's safety in accordance with established standards of care.[73] When the assessment, monitoring, or plan of care does not meet established

standards of care and a patient is injured or dies, the nurse may be liable.

For example, in *Johnson v. Grant Hospital*,[74] a woman patient in the psychiatric unit told several staff members about her suicidal thoughts one evening. The nurse supervisor informed the patient's psychiatrist of the patient's conversations with staff. The psychiatrist ordered the patient secluded for the remainder of the evening. The next day, the day nurse, unaware of the patient's suicidal thoughts, assigned the patient to a newly hired staff member. After leaving the seclusion room with the new staff member, the patient was left alone for a few moments. She was able to jump to her death through a nearby window of the unit. The court returned a verdict against the hospital, holding that it was the staff's duty to protect the patient from potential harm.

The duty to protect also extends to the use of seclusion and restraints. The purpose of seclusion and restraints is to manage aggressive or self-destructive behavior when other measures (e.g., the therapeutic relationship or medication) do not work.[75] Notwithstanding the necessity of both methods in certain situations, utilizing them negligently, or failing to utilize them when needed, can result in injury or death to a patient.

In *Pisel v. Stamford Hospital*,[76] a patient in a seclusion room on a steel-frame bed suffered brain damage after being left in the seclusion room without proper monitoring. The patient was able to wedge her neck between one raised side rail and the mattress, which decreased blood flow to her head. In entering a judgment against the hospital, the court held that, among other things, the staff and hospital had been negligent in (1) secluding the patient with the bed frame in the seclusion room; (2) failing to monitor the patient properly; and (3) improperly designing and locating the seclusion room, which could not be clearly seen from the nursing station.[77]

Duty to Maintain Patient Confidentiality

All nurses have a legal and ethical responsibility to protect patient confidentiality and privacy. The responsibility for psychiatric patients is even more encompassing. Specific state and federal statutes[78] govern the release of patient information to others when that takes place other than with the patient's consent. The state statute may be called a "confidentiality act," or the protections may be

TABLE 17–2

Types of Psychiatric Admissions

NAME	REQUIREMENTS FOR USE	WHEN DISCHARGE POSSIBLE	CONSTITUTIONAL ISSUES
Informal	Patient identifies need and signs informal admission form	Whenever patient chooses to leave, unless involuntary admission procedures initiated by hospital or mental health care provider	None if patient is admitted and discharged without difficulties
Voluntary	Patient, or legal representative, consents to admission	Whenever patient chooses to leave *after* time specified in mental health code (e.g., 5 days), unless involuntary admission procedures initiated by hospital or mental health care provider	14th Amendment (due process, liberty, privacy [right to refuse treatment])
Involuntary A. Emergency certificate B. Judicial commitment C. Other	Most states require that individual be a danger to self or others and be mentally ill; other criteria might include inability to care for own basic needs	Whenever patient no longer mentally ill or danger to self or others or can care for own basic needs. Determined by hospital, physician, or other mental health care provider or court, depending on how patient was involuntarily committed	14th Amendment (due process, liberty, privacy [right to refuse treatment]); 8th Amendment (cruel and unusual punishment, especially if certain treatment required); 14th Amendment (equal protection). Courts have characterized treatment issues, especially involuntary confinement against one's consent, as the right to a least restrictive alternative placement (LRA). LRA also has been extended to type of treatment; that is, treatment that is effective but that does not overly inhibit personal liberties

Data from Joseph Smith. *Medical Malpractice: Psychiatric Care.* New York: McGraw-Hill Book Company, 1986 (with 1998 cumulative supplement); Ralph Chandler, Richard Enslen, and Peter Renstrom. *Constitutional Law Deskbook: Individual Rights.* 2nd Edition. Rochester, N.Y.: Lawyers Cooperative Publishing, 1993 (with May 1999 supplement).

included in a general statute dealing with mental health care. Although the contents of the state statutes vary, most include:

- Written consent from patient or legal representative required for release of records or information
- Provisions when written consent from patient or legal representative not possible (e.g., upon death of patient)
- Information necessary for written consent to be honored
- Guidelines for patient access to and review of own records
- Situations in which information or records can be released without patient's written consent (e.g., when the patient must be involun-

tarily committed for psychiatric care, when child abuse or neglect is suspected)[79]

When the guidelines for protecting patient confidentiality are not followed, liability can result for breaching the patient's confidentiality. The reverse is also true; that is, when there is a requirement to release information and it does not happen, a breach of the psychiatric/mental health nurse's duty can also occur.

In *Tarasoff v. Regents of the University of California*,[80] a graduate student who was being seen in the school mental health clinic told his psychologist-therapist that he intended to kill a woman student. The psychologist, concerned about what his patient had told him, especially in light of his duty to maintain confidentiality, shared his concerns with others on the clinic staff. It was decided that because of the nature of the communication, the psychologist needed to inform the police about the threat. The police brought the graduate student to the police station and questioned him but did not detain him because they did not think he was irrational.

No one attempted to notify the woman student or her family. Nor did anyone initiate commitment proceedings against the male patient. The patient did stab Tanya Tarasoff to death several days later.

The parents of Ms. Tarasoff brought a suit against the mental health professionals and the university, alleging negligence in their handling of the situation. The California Supreme Court returned a decision against the university and its clinic staff and opined:

> Once a therapist does in fact determine, or under applicable professional standards should have determined, that a patient poses a serious danger of violence to others, he bears a duty to exercise reasonable care to protect the foreseeable victim of that danger. While the discharge of this duty of due care will necessarily vary with the facts of each case, in each instance the adequacy of the therapist's conduct must be measured against the traditional standard of reasonable care under the circumstances.[81]

The court's requirement that a mental health professional protect a foreseeable victim based on the circumstances of the situation has been characterized as the "duty to warn third parties" of potential injury or death. This characterization is probably inaccurate, because the duty established in the opinion is much broader. In some instances, for example, the duty of the health care provider may indeed be to warn the intended victim. In other instances, it may be more appropriate to initiate involuntary admission proceedings against the person threatening another. Or, a combination of these two actions may be necessary. Therefore the duty is more accurately characterized as the "duty to inform third parties."

The *Tarasoff* decision was adopted by many other jurisdictions through case decisions and through amendments to state mental health codes/laws. Its adoption provides a legal basis for the mental health professional, including the psychiatric/mental health nurse, to share patient information when confronted with this type of situation without incurring liability for a breach of confidentiality.

Privilege

In addition to confidentiality of mental health information and treatment, psychiatric patients are also protected within the context of judicial proceedings against the release without the patient's consent of any information obtained during the relationship between the patient and the mental health professional. Unlike the duty to maintain confidentiality, which is clearly borne by the mental health professional, the protection of privilege is owned by the patient.[82] Therefore, it is the patient who determines when the privilege can be waived.

The . . . requirement that a mental health professional protect a foreseeable victim based on the circumstances of the situation has been characterized as the "duty to warn third parties" . . .

Privilege is established in respective state statutes. It can be found, for example, in specific mental health "confidentiality statutes" or in other provisions of state law. In Illinois, for example, the Mental Health and Developmental Disabilities Confidentiality Act contains specific provisions concerning when mental health providers, including nurses, can refuse to testify in judicial and administrative proceedings by asserting this privilege on their own, or on behalf of the recipient of mental health services.[83] Other states protect the patient's privilege in civil practice rules concerning testimony or in licensing acts.

The protection of privilege, like the protection of confidentiality, is not absolute. Exceptions to the right of the patient to refuse to allow the nurse to testify in judicial or administrative proceedings include many of the same exceptions concerning the confidentiality of mental health records. They include (1) when child abuse or neglect is reasonably suspected; (2) when a person needs to be involuntarily admitted to a psychiatric facility; (3) when a patient introduces his or her own mental condition into any court or administrative proceeding; and (4) during investigations and trials for homicide or murder.[84]

Presumption of Competency of the Psychiatric Patient

When an individual is admitted to a psychiatric facility, the patient retains all abilities to make decisions on his or her own behalf, including treatment decisions. In other words, there is a presumption of competency of the psychiatric patient. This presumption extends to both voluntary and involuntary patients. The presumption of competency is usually codified in the state mental health code or it may be established as a result of case law. In either situation, the psychiatric client retains the right to make decisions and carry out other responsibilities that nonpsychiatric patients possess (e.g., enter into a contract, obtain a divorce, sell stock).

In some instances, a patient receiving mental health services may not be able to enjoy the protections of this presumption. The diagnosed illness may impair his or her ability to make appropriate decisions. If the patient's competency is a concern for mental health professionals working with the patient, then a guardianship proceeding may need to be initiated to judicially appoint another to make decisions for the patient. This is especially so when no other legal mechanism exists to appoint a surrogate decision maker (e.g., durable power of attorney).

State guardianship statutes define the requirements necessary for a guardian to be appointed for the person alleged to be legally incompetent (the ward). For example, many require the presence of a physical or emotional illness that seriously affects the person's ability to make decisions.[85] A judge hears evidence concerning the person's inability to make decisions. Such evidence includes testimony from family members as well as treating mental health professionals.

If a guardian is appointed, the role of the guardian and his or her powers will be carefully spelled out by the court. For example, the guardian may be a "personal" guardian or an "estate" guardian. The powers of the guardian may be "limited" or "plenary."

Insofar as treatment issues are concerned, the guardian must have powers of a personal guardian; that is, to give informed consent for treatment/nontreatment and make decisions surrounding other life choices. In contrast, "estate" guardians are responsible for making financial decisions concerning the ward (e.g., selling property, paying bills). In either case, the guardian must always act consistent with the state guardianship statute and the best interest of the ward.

A guardianship is not necessarily permanent. State statutes provide for judicial oversight of the guardianship to ensure that it meets the needs of the ward. The court can remove a guardian at any time. Likewise, a petition for restoration of competency can be filed by the ward.[86] The ward must prove he or she is able to handle his or her own affairs by competent (relevant and material) evidence.

IMPLICATIONS FOR PSYCHIATRIC/MENTAL HEALTH NURSES

The type of psychiatric unit in which the psychiatric/mental health nurse practices will affect some of the practice decisions needed to comply with the legal obligations protecting the psychiatric client. When a patient is admitted to the unit, the nurse must ensure that all necessary documentation is in the patient's record concerning the type of admission for that patient. For example, if the patient is a voluntary patient, the form for that admission should be complete and signed by the patient. Both voluntary and involuntary patients should receive a written list of rights consistent with the state's mental health code.

Immediately upon admission, but also throughout the patient's stay in the unit, careful, complete, and adequate monitoring of the patient's condition will be necessary. Because safety of the patient and others on the unit is paramount, any acting-out behavior, violent behavior, or expressions of suicidal thinking must be immediately handled. Doing so will require thorough knowledge of the state mental health laws in this area and the institution's policies concerning medication administration, seclusion, restraint, and suicide precautions. The psychiatric/mental health nurse will need to carefully document any behavior observed and notify the psychiatrist and others on the mental health team as soon as possible.

When intervening with violent behavior or suicidal ideation, the nurse will need to obtain orders from the psychiatrist or other mental health team member for the institution of seclusion, restraint, or medication. However, if there is an emergency that requires immediate intervention, the psychiatric/mental health nurse can initiate whatever care is needed so long as that initiation is consistent with his or her institution's policies and procedures and state law. For example, it may be possible for the nurse to place a patient in restraints without an order beforehand if an emergency exists in which the patient is physically harmful to himself or herself or is physically abusing others.[87] In such an event, any proper notification to other mental health team members, including the psychiatrist, will need to occur.

Because the procedure for placing a patient in restraints can be potentially injurious to both the patient and staff, the Health Care Financing Administration (HCFA) now requires that only staff trained in restraint application be permitted to place patients in restraints.[88] In-service training is also required on a continual basis for this procedure and for placing a patient in seclusion.

The psychiatric/mental health nurse will need to constantly monitor the patient who is in restraints or seclusion and document carefully the time and manner of monitoring. The use of a form or checklist that contains the required monitoring times and other information for use by the nursing staff can help the mental health team comply with this duty.

Proper and complete documentation of the need for restraint and seclusion is also important in the event the patient decides to charge the nurse and others with false imprisonment. Several successful cases alleging this intentional tort have been filed.[89]

When the psychiatric/mental health nurse is faced with releasing information about the patient as a recipient of mental health services, his or her treatment, or any other information surrounding the provision of mental health services, the nurse must consult applicable state and federal laws and institutional policies. If the nurse has a clinical concern that a threat voiced by a patient against another may indeed occur, notification of the psychiatrist or other health care provider is vital so that how to handle the situation can be determined. Whatever the decision, complete documentation in the patient's record as to the course of action taken is necessary.

If asked to testify in any judicial or administrative proceeding, the psychiatric/mental health nurse will want to obtain the advice of the institution's attorney and/or an attorney of his or her own to ascertain the best approach to take concerning the testimony. Under no circumstance should the nurse simply agree to testify, show up at the trial or hearing, or respond to a subpoena requesting treatment records without first obtaining advice from an attorney.

Consent for psychiatric/mental health treatment should be obtained from the patient unless

---

ETHICS CONNECTION 17–3

Skilled ethical comportment is becoming increasingly important to nurses who work in acute care settings. With decreases in nurse staffing, changes in corporate structure and organizational culture, and increasingly ill patients, acute care nurses experience ethical concerns on a daily basis. Individualistic ethics does not adequately address the scope of the issues that they face. In acute care nursing as in other aspects of nursing practice, communitarian ethics offers an alternative or complementary approach to nursing practice.

Blake and Guare[1] studied nurses in acute care settings to determine what those nurses thought were the central ethical concerns in their practice. Not surprisingly, most of the issues that nurses identified were related to organizational culture and institutional ethics. Nurses in acute care settings specifically were concerned about end-of-life issues, including Do Not Resuscitate Orders, futile treatment, preserving human dignity, cultural practices, and respect for autonomy. Pain management of patients whose physicians under- or inappropriately medicated them was an institutional problem, as was truth-telling. Truth-telling with respect to reporting medication errors and other incidents was a problem in organizations that adopted a punitive rather than an educative approach to error. Nurses in such organizations also were less forthcoming about reporting suspected impaired practice.

Blake and Guare suggest ways of improving organizational culture so that nurses will be supported in their ethical comportment. "Given the present climate of scarce resources and ongoing restructuring, health care organizations cannot afford errors in judgment or internal conflicts associated with ethical decision making. An effort to determine the best way to support ethical decision making among nurses must be developed and implemented. Nurse managers can become key players in reengineering current processes in ethical decisionmaking."[2]

---

[1]C. Blake and R. E. Guare. "Nurses' Reflections on Ethical Decision Making: Implications for Leaders, 28(4) *Journal of the New York Nurses Association* (December 1997), 13–16.
[2]*Id.*

a guardian has been appointed to perform this role or some other legally recognized surrogate decision maker exists for that purpose. If there is a question of a patient's competency (or decision-making ability) to provide consent or refusal of treatment, the psychiatric/mental health nurse should notify the psychiatrist, nurse manager, and others on the team to decide how to proceed. If a guardianship petition is filed, the nurse may well be asked to testify at the guardianship hearing concerning the patient's conduct and behavior while in the psychiatric unit. Again, it is essential for the nurse to obtain legal advice before testifying concerning the patient and his or her conduct while in treatment.

SUMMARY OF PRINCIPLES AND APPLICATIONS

Practicing in the acute care setting is varied, challenging, and exciting. Regardless of the changes in health care delivery, hospitals are here to stay. There is no doubt that as hospitals continue to exist, nurses in hospitals will continue to exist because nursing and nursing services are central to the provision of hospital care.[90] Even so, the character of nursing in acute care settings will probably continue to change. With that change will come increasing concerns for the provision of quality care, nursing staff satisfaction, and liability concerns. The nurse in the acute care setting may be able to resolve some of these concerns in the three nursing practice areas presented by:

- Keeping up to date about the many laws and regulations that affect the nurse's specific area of practice

- Providing care in accordance with standards of care established by the profession, professional associations, and the law

- Advocating for safe nursing staffing patterns, in terms of both numbers of staff and competency of staff

- Resisting encroachment of nursing practice

- Delegating to and supervising unlicensed assistive workers in accordance with state laws, regulatory guidelines, and professional nursing association mandates

- Guarding the patient's right to confidentiality and the patient's right of testimonial privilege

- Continuing to attend in-service training, continuing education programs, and formal nursing educational

programs to achieve additional knowledge in his or her area of practice

- Utilizing appropriate resources, including legal resources, for guidance when a difficult practice issue arises

TOPICS FOR FURTHER INQUIRY

1. Conduct a survey of emergency or perioperative departments in at least two hospitals in your community. Evaluate the use of assistive workers in those units. The survey can include interviews of staff (including nursing management), job descriptions, or other indicia concerning use of non-RN caregivers. Suggest how improvements in the use of RNs in the units could occur. Suggest how the assistive worker could be used in a better manner to assist the RN.

2. Compare and contrast at least five nurse practice acts for their respective support of RN first assistants. Determine how the acts define the role; what rules, if any, have been promulgated to further define the role; and other provisions unique to this role.

3. Identify case decisions in your state concerning the duty of mental health care providers to warn third parties of potential injury by a psychiatric patient. Determine if any psychiatric/mental health nurses were involved in any of the cases, and if so, under what circumstances. Identify any themes the cases might show (e.g., types of violence involved, how a communication was handled), and from them, draft a "model" statute concerning the duty to warn third parties. Contrast the mental health provider duty to warn with his or her ethical duties in this situation.

4. Interview a nurse in a hospital ED for his or her opinion concerning triage in the facility. Areas for consideration might include what factors the nurse uses when doing triage, how the triage system was developed, and what limitations exist when the nurse carries out triage (e.g., scope of practice concerns). Then develop a policy and procedure for triage based on the information obtained from the interview.

REFERENCES

1. Anthony Kovner and Steven Jonas, Editors. "Hospitals," in *Health Care Delivery in the United States.* 6th Edition. New York: Springer Publishing Company, 1999, 157–160.
2. *Id.*
3. American Nurses Association. *The Acute Care Nurse in Transition.* Washington, D.C.: 1996, vii.

4. *Id.*

5. U.S. Department of Labor, Bureau of Labor Statistics. "Registered Nurses," *Occupational Outlook Handbook* 3, 5. Available on the World Wide Web at http://stats.bls.gov/oco/ocos083.htm. Accessed May 9, 2000.

6. Kovner and Jonas, *supra* note 1, at 81.

7. Paul A. Craig, "Risk Management Issues in the Emergency Department," in *The Risk Manager's Desk Reference.* 2nd Edition. Barbara J. Youngberg, Editor. Gaithersburg, Md.: Aspen Publishers, 1998, 295.

8. Institute of Medicine. Committee on Quality of Health Care in America. *To Err Is Human: Building a Safer Health System.* Linda Kohn, Janet Corrigan, and Molla Donaldson, Editors. Washington, D.C.: National Academy Press, 2000, 37.

9. Craig, *supra* note 7.

10. Hospital Survey and Construction Act of 1946, 60 Stat. 1040, codified at various sections of 24 U.S.C., 33 U.S.C., 41 U.S.C., 46 U.S.C. and 49 U.S.C.

11. Robert Miller. *Problems in Health Care Law.* 7th Edition. Gaithersburg, Md.: Aspen Publishers, 1996, 360.

12. 174 A.2d 135 (1961).

13. 42 U.S.C. Section 1395dd(a) *et seq.*

14. 42 U.S.C. Sections 1395dd(3)(A), 1395dd(c)(1), and 1395dd(b)(2).

15. 42 U.S.C. Section 1395dd(e)(1).

16. 42 U.S.C. Section 1395dd(d)(2)(A).

17. 920 F.2d 710 (Okla. 1990).

18. Mikel Rothenberg, "Emergency Medical Malpractice in a Nutshell—What's New," in *1999 Wiley Medical Malpractice Update.* Melvin Shiffman, Editor. Gaithersburg, Md.: Aspen Law & Business, 2000, 159.

19. *Id.*

20. 982 F.2d 230 (7th Cir. 1992).

21. *Id.*

22. *Arrington v. Wong,* 1998 WL 661343 (Dist. Ct. Hawaii 1998).

23. Christopher Kerns, Carol Gerner, and Ciara Ryan. *Health Care Liability Deskbook.* 4th Edition. St. Paul, Minn.: West Group, 1998, 5-2 (with regular updates).

24. *Id.*

25. *Id.*

26. Craig, *supra* note 7, at 296.

27. 373 A.2d 26 (Md. App. 1977).

28. 648 S.W.2d 391 (Ct. App. Texas 1983).

29. 288 A.2d 379 (Md. 1972).

30. William Roach, Jr., and the Aspen Health Law Center, "Access to Medical Records Information," in *Medical Records and the Law.* 3rd Edition. Gaithersburg, Md.: Aspen Publishers, 1998, 88–139.

31. Emergency Nurses Association. *Position Statement: Staffing and Productivity in the Emergency Care Setting.* 1999, 1-2. Available on the association's Web page at http://www.ena.org. Accessed May 9, 2000.

32. *Id.* at 1.

33. Emergency Nurses Association. *The 1998 National Emergency Department Database Report.* Des Plaines, Ill.: Author, 1999.

34. Emergency Nurses Association, *supra* note 31, *Addendum: Key Assessment Criteria.*

35. Emergency Nurses Association, *supra* note 31, at 1.

36. Craig, *supra* note 7, at 295–296.

37. *Id.*

38. *Id.*

39. Emergency Nurses Association. *Position Statement: The Use of Non-Registered Nurse (Non-RN) Caregivers in Emergency Care.* 1999, 1. Available on the association's Web page at http://www.ena.org. Accessed May 9, 2000.

40. *Id.*

41. *Id.*

42. *Id.*

43. *Id.* at 1–2.

44. *Id.* at 2.

45. *Id.*

46. See, for example, *Burditt v. U.S. Dept. of Health and Human Services,* 934 F.2d 1362 (5th Cir. 1991), which affirmed a $20,000 penalty against the emergency department physician for, among other things, transferring a patient in active labor in violation of the Act. A nurse in the ED at the time of the incident attempted to inform Dr. Burditt that his intention to transfer the patient would be in violation of the Act, and gave him a copy of it, but he did not read it. See also *Scott v. Hutchinson,* 959 F. Supp. 1351 (1997), where the use of required hospital forms surrounding the nonemergent transfer of a patient resulted in no liability under the EMTALA.

47. 431 So. 2d 40 (La. 1983).

48. 672 P.2d 667 (1983).

49. See *Starkey v. St. Rita's Medical Center,* 690 N.E.2d 57 (Ohio 1997), where a "hotline" nurse's advice to a wife whose husband experienced a heart attack was the focus of the suit.

50. American Association of Operating Room Nurses. "About Us." Available on the association's Web site at http://www.aorn.org. Accessed May 12, 2000.

51. See generally, Janet Pitts Beckmann. *Nursing Negligence: Analyzing Malpractice in the Hospital Setting.* Thousand Oaks, Cal.: Sage Publications, 1999, 120–157.

52. Barbara J. Youngberg, "Risk Management Issues Associated with Anesthesia," in *The Risk Manager's Desk Reference.* 2nd Edition. Barbara Youngberg, Editor. Gaithersburg, Md.: Aspen Publishers, 1998, 266.

53. American Association of Operating Room Nurses. *Revised AORN Official Statement on RN First Assistants.* 1998. Available on the association's Web site at http://www.aorn.org. Accessed May 12, 2000.

54. *Id.* at 1.

55. *Id.*

56. *Id.*

57. *Id.*

58. *Id.* at 2. See also *AORN Recommended Education Standards for RN First Assistant Programs.* 1996, on the association's Web site. Accessed May 12, 2000.

59. *Id.*

60. *Id.*

61. American Association of Operating Room Nurses. *Position Statement: Statement on Mandate for the Registered Professional Nurse in the Perioperative Practice Setting.* 1997. Available on the association's Web site. Accessed May 12, 2000.

62. See generally, Victoria Steelman, "Issues in Perioperative Nursing," in *Current Issues in Nursing.* 5th Edition. Joanne McCloskey and Helen Kennedy Grace, Editors. St. Louis, Mo.: Mosley, 1997, 264–269.

63. See, for example, AORN's *Standards, Recommended Practices and Guidelines* available through the association on its Web site.

64. "Negligence in the Recovery Room," 66(26) *Canadian Nurse* (July 1970), 4.

65. American Association of Operating Room Nurses. *Position Statement: AORN Official Statement on Unlicensed Assistive Personnel.* 1995. Available on the association's Web site. Accessed May 12, 2000.

66. Youngberg, *supra* note 52, at 274–276; Linda Zinser-Eagle and Sue Meiner, "Recording Patient Care in Perioperative Nursing," in *Nursing Documentation: Legal Focus Across Practice Settings.* Sue Meiner, Editor. Thousand Oaks, Cal.: Sage Publications, 1999, 153–174.

67. Youngberg, *supra* note 52; Zinser-Eagle and Meiner, *supra* note 66.

68. American Association of Operating Room Nurses, *supra* note 50, 1.

69. American Association of Operating Room Nurses, *supra* note 65, 1.

70. *Id.*

71. See generally, Robert Levy and Leonard Rubenstein. *The Rights of People with Mental Disabilities.* Carbondale, Ill.: Southern Illinois University Press, 1996.

72. *Id.*; *O'Connor v. Donaldson,* 422 U.S. 563 (1975); *Wyatt v. Stickley,* now *Wyatt v. Alderholt,* 344 F. Supp. 373 (M.D. Ala. 1972), *enforcing* 344 F. Supp. 387 (M.D. Ala. 1971), *enforcing* 325 F. Supp. 781 (M.D. Ala. 1971), *aff'd in part, modified in part,* 503 F. 2d 1305 (5th Cir. 1974).

73. See, for example, American Nurses Association. *Statement on Psychiatric-Mental Health Clinical Nursing Practice and Standards of Care of Psychiatric-Mental Health Nursing Practice.* Washington, D.C.: Author, 1994.

74. 286 N.E.2d 308 (1972).

75. See, as examples, Ann Burgess and Helen Harner, "From the Other Side of the Door: Patient Views of Seclusion," 37(3) *Journal of Psychosocial Nursing and Mental Health Services* (1999), 13–22; Joint Commission on Accreditation of Health Care Organizations. *CAMBC Behavioral Health Care Supplement.* 2000. Available on the association's Web site at http://www.jcaho.org. Accessed April 1, 2000; U.S. General Accounting Office. *Mental Health: Improper Restraint or Seclusion Use Places People at Risk.* Washington, D.C.: U.S. Government Printing Office, 1999.

76. 430 A.2d 1 (1980).

77. *Id.*

78. The federal statute is the Mental Health Systems Act of 1980, Pub. L. No. 96-398, 94 Stat. 1564 (October 7, 1980).

79. See, for example, 740 ILCS 110/1 *et seq.* (1979), *as amended,* for Illinois' protections. The Act is called the Illinois Mental Health Confidentiality Act.

80. 529 P.2d 553 (Cal. 1974), *vacated, reheard en banc and aff'd.,* 551 P.2d 334 (1976).

81. *Id.* at 345.

82. Joseph T. Smith. *Medical Malpractice: Psychiatric Care.* New York: McGraw-Hill, 1986, 529–530 (with 1998 cumulative supplement).

83. 740 ICLS 110/10 (1979), *as amended.*

84. See, for example, Illinois Mental Health and Developmental Disabilities Confidentiality Act, 740 ILCS 110/1 *et seq.* (1979), *as amended;* Levy and Rubenstein, *supra* note 71, at 308–313.

85. See Chapter 19.

86. *Id.*

87. See, for example, Illinois' Mental Health Code, 405 ICLS 5/2-107.1 (1979), *as amended.*

88. 42 U.S.C. Section 482.13 (1999). See also Chapter 19.

89. W. Page Keeton, Editor. *Prosser and Keaton on Torts.* 5th Edition. St. Paul, Minn.: West, 1984, 47–54 (with 1988 pocket part).

90. Kovner and Jonas, *supra* note 1, at 83.

The Nurse as Administrator

18

KEY PRINCIPLES

- Liability
- Professional Negligence
- Negligent Supervision
- Board of Directors
- Employment Contract
- Severance Agreement/Benefit

An administrator is a person who manages affairs of any kind.[1] Administration and management involve many functions, some of which include directing, regulating, governing, and supervising.

In the mid 1880s, Florence Nightingale defined the major role of the nurse administrator as that of educating others in the care of the sick and ill.[2] Since that first definition, the role has been further expanded to include 10 major roles identified for any executive by Mintzberg.[3] Categorized into three major areas—interpersonal, informational, and decisional—the roles are figurehead, leader, liaison, monitor, disseminator, spokesperson, entrepreneur, disturbance handler, resource allocator, and negotiator.[4]

In the mid 1880s, Florence Nightingale defined the major role of the nurse administrator as that of educating others in the care of the sick and ill.

The nurse administrator performs these various roles in many health care delivery settings, including hospitals, home health care agencies, and psychiatric/mental health facilities. Moreover, the nurse administrator may perform the roles at various levels within the health care delivery system. For example, the nurse administrator may hold an executive position as part of senior administration. Most often, the nurse administrator's title in that role is chief nurse executive (CNE) or chief nurse officer (CNO) and the position is described as, for example, vice president of nursing services.

In contrast, the nurse administrator may hold a position as a nurse manager, either at a first- or middle-level position, whose responsibilities include patient care concerns (e.g., staff scheduling and coordinating nursing activities) and who reports to the nurse executive.[5] Titles of nurse managers may include head nurse, nursing supervisor, and clinical nurse manager.

Moreover, nurse administrators perform their various roles in nursing departments that are organized differently. A nurse administrator may be employed in a decentralized agency or one that is more bureaucratic.[6] Shared governance or a participative management framework, described by Barnum and Kerfoot as authority structures, also affect the nurse administrator's role.[7]

Regardless of which role a nurse has in administration and which organizational structure is present, the roles of both the nurse executive and the nurse manager are in a state of flux.[8] Factors that have affected nursing administration practice include increased governmental involvement in the nursing services provided to patients, work redesign, telehealth, managed care, and the use of computers in nursing administration.[9] This chapter will briefly focus on some of the many legal issues affecting nurse administrators in this time of change.

THE NURSE MANAGER

Nurse managers perform a variety of activities as part of their role: recruiting, selecting, and retaining personnel; staffing; and planning and monitoring the budget for their defined area.[10] There is no doubt that these responsibilities may result in liability for the nurse manager.

Selection of Nursing Staff

A major responsibility of nurse managers is the hiring of nursing staff. This role requires excellent interpersonal skills during the interviewing of prospective employees. It also requires awareness of employment and other laws affecting this aspect of a potential employment relationship. The nurse manager cannot ask about or attempt to obtain information from the applicant that may violate state or federal antidiscrimination and employment laws.

For example, asking a female applicant about her marital status or plans for having children is a violation of Title VII when the answers are used to make employment decisions, as discussed in Chapter 16. Similarly, asking an applicant about disability-related issues prior to giving the applicant a conditional job offer is a violation of the Americans with Disabilities Act, also discussed in Chapter 16.

Guidelines are available to the nurse manager for review and for use when interviewing prospective staff. The guidelines include rules and regulations promulgated by the Equal Employment Opportunity Commission (EEOC) and other agencies published in the Code of Federal Regulations (C.F.R.), EEOC and other agency enforcement guidance documents, textbooks dealing with antidiscrimination and personnel law, and nursing journal articles that highlight this type of information for their readers (e.g., *American Association of Occupational Health Nursing Journal, Healthcare Law, Ethics & Regulation*).

Negligent Supervision

One of the important roles—indeed duties—of the nurse manager is the provision of adequate supervision of staff nurses for whom he or she is responsible.[11] When adequate supervision does not occur and a patient is injured, the patient may allege that the nurse manager's supervision of the nurse providing the direct patient care in the situation was negligent. Liability for negligent supervision may be based upon several types of conduct of the nurse manager. For example, if the nurse manager delegates patient care to a nurse who is unable to perform the care, and/or if the nurse manager fails to personally supervise the nurse providing care when the manager knew, or should have known, that supervision was necessary, liability may be imposed on the nurse manager.[12] Liability may also be found by a court when the nurse manager does not take the necessary steps to avoid patient injury when he or she was present and able to intervene. And, if the nurse manager does not properly allocate the time of available staff and an injury occurs, the nurse manager may be responsible for his or her own negligent judgment in the nurse manager role.[13]

Liability for negligent supervision may be based upon several types of conduct of the nurse manager.

The liability of the nurse manager for negligent supervision does not arise under the *respondeat superior* theory discussed in Chapter 4. The nurse manager is not the employer of the nursing staff that he or she manages and supervises. Rather, the liability is based on the nurse manager's breach of his or her own duties as a nurse manager. As a result, when negligent supervision is alleged, the standard of care that will be used to measure the nurse manager's conduct will be that of other ordinary, reasonable, and prudent nurse managers in the same or similar circumstances.

Because the nurse manager is an employee of a particular facility, the nurse manager's alleged negligent supervision can, of course, allow the patient to also name the employer as a defendant under *respondeat superior*. Table 18–1 lists several cases against nurse managers.

Managing Employee Issues

Because the nurse manager is responsible for the supervision of the nursing staff, he or she must be well versed in the many employment, and other,

---

TABLE 18–1

Cases Involving Nurse Managers

CASE NAME	TYPE OF FACILITY	ALLEGATIONS	COMMENTS
Moon Lake Convalescent Ctr. v. Margolis (1989)[1]	Nursing home	DON breached duty to maintain policy concerning bathing of residents and policy for excessive bath temperatures	Decision for resident; DON helped with bathing of resident but did not follow policy for safe bathing; resident injured and burned; court also found DON and home liable because no policy established for safe temperatures when bathing residents
Bowers v. Olch (1953)[2]	Hospital OR	Supervising nurse in OR responsible, along with hospital and surgeon, for leaving needle in patient's abdomen during surgery	Supervising nurse not responsible for injury; she had properly assigned two competent nurses to assist surgeon during surgery; supervisor not present during surgery so could not intervene
State v. Washington Sanitarium and Hospital (1960)[3]	Psychiatric hospital	Supervising nurse and hospital negligent in not preventing patient's suicide when they allowed him to wander on unit rather than keep hydrotherapy appointment	No liability on part of nurse or hospital; patient gave no indication that he was suicidal; psychiatrist had no orders for suicide precautions

[1] 535 N.E.2d 956 (1989).
[2] 260 P.2d 997 (1953).
[3] 165 A.2d 764 (1960).

ETHICS CONNECTION 18–1

Nurse administrators are accountable for the quality of nursing care and for protecting patients from harm that may result from incompetent or impaired nursing practice. These and other workplace issues are becoming more difficult as administrators and managers face the "conflicting demands of providing quality care with limited resources."[1] Implicitly, nurse managers are asked to act in ways that they cannot morally condone.[2] Writing about institutional and organizational ethics, Badzek and her colleagues note that nurse administrators "have become dispirited" with organizations that do not have values congruent with their own. Maintaining confidentiality and privacy of nursing staff while assuring safety and effectiveness of care is one of the practical moral issues that administrators confront.

Using the case of a nurse whose practice is impaired because she is diverting drugs, Badzek and her colleagues discuss the practices of nurse managers in making ethical decisions related to confidentiality and client safety. They emphasize the factors to be considered in deciding when there are "morally compelling reasons to override confidentiality." This and other case studies[3] that illustrate day-to-day moral tensions will be useful for administrators and managers who are challenged to expand their ethical decision-making skills in rapidly changing health care systems.

[1] Laurie A. Badzek, Kathleen Mitchell, Sandra E. Marra, and Marjorie M. Bower, "Administrative Ethics and Confidentiality and Privacy Issues." *Online Journal of Issues in Nursing.* December 31, 1998. Available at http://www.nursingworld.org/ojin/topic8/topic8__2htm

[2] J. L. Badaracco and A. Webb, "Business Ethics: A View from the Trenches," *California Management Review* 37(1995), 8–21.

[3] Margaret R. Douglas and Nancy J. Brent, "Substance Abuse and the Nurse Manager: Legal and Ethical Issues," 2(1) *Seminars for Nurse Managers* (1994), 16–26.

court dismissed the allegations of slander against the head nurse.[15]

Moreover, the nurse manager will be faced with the possibility of increasing involvement in such lawsuits for additional causes of action alleged by staff, including sexual harassment under Title VII,[16] invasions of workplace privacy,[17] and "English-only" work rules.[18]

IMPLICATIONS FOR NURSE MANAGERS

The nurse manager can maintain some control over involvement in lawsuits alleging negligent supervision or a violation of staff rights by instituting a sound management style that has a proactive risk management focus.[19] When hiring new staff, for example, careful attention to the questions asked during the interviewing process is essential. Information that may be seen as discriminatory or an intrusion into the applicant's privacy cannot be requested by the nurse manager. Rather, the information obtained, and the decision to hire or not hire an applicant, must be based on a careful analysis of the applicant's skill, experience, and ability to work within the demands of the unit or agency milieu.

Adequate orientation of new staff is essential. The orientation plan may be a formalized program or a less formal preceptor-type plan.[20] In-service programs are also essential to provide ongoing improvement and enhancement of the nursing staff's capabilities.[21]

> *The nurse manager can maintain some control over involvement in lawsuits alleging negligent supervision or a violation of staff rights by instituting a sound management style that has a proactive risk management focus.*

The supervision of nursing staff by the nurse manager must be consistent and in accordance with standards of care. When a problem is identified, whether concerning the quality of the care provided by the nursing staff member or the interpersonal relationships on the unit or in the agency,

laws that affect the manager–staff nurse relationship. These laws were presented in earlier chapters. It is clear that nurse managers are often involved in suits alleging violations of these laws.

For example, in *Watson v. Idaho Falls Consolidated Hospitals,*[14] a nurse's aide alleged that the head nurse on her unit had intentionally interfered with the aide's employment relationship, had inflicted emotional distress, and had given reasons for her termination that were slanderous. The prompt intervention by the nurse manager is essential. Not only will prompt intervention hopefully rectify the problem, it may also avoid additional problems for the nurse manager. In *Ethridge v. Arizona State Board of Nursing*,[22] a nurse manager was held accountable and was disciplined by the board of nursing for her failure to respond to the nursing staff's concerns about, among other things, possible drug diversion and falsification of records at the hospital. The Arizona State Board of Nursing held that the nurse manager's failure to intervene in the staff concerns, and especially her failure to report a staff nurse's diversion of Valium to the board, was unprofessional conduct under the Arizona Nurse Practice Act. Ms. Ethridge was censured, and her professional nurse license was placed on 12 months' probation.

The nurse manager must also develop effective policies and procedures for the staff working in the facility or on his or her unit. They must reflect current practice and be reviewed and updated as needed.[23]

When a patient or family member expresses unhappiness with patient care, the nurse manager should respond to those concerns immediately and in a caring manner.[24] Research has indicated that doing so may avoid the filing of a suit, even when an injury to the patient has occurred.[25]

The nurse manager's communication with staff is also an important preventive measure.[26] Open lines of communication at all times can aid in resolution of potential difficulties before they become a legal risk within the health care delivery system or influence the quality of care provided by nursing staff.[27] In addition, communication patterns that stress feedback, participation, tolerance for new ways of providing patient care, and solving problems when they arise contribute to a "satisfied" nursing staff.[28]

Open lines of communication and nurse manager support and leadership during any restructuring, merger, or redesign of the facility will also help avoid patient care problems and enhance staff morale. By allowing staff to help in the planning of any necessary changes, providing a safe environment in which to express anxieties and concerns, providing time for any new training or changes that must be "learned," displaying "manager-empowering" behavior, and mentoring those who are implementing the restructuring, the nurse manager can provide a framework for a less problematic change in the workplace.[29]

ETHICS CONNECTION 18–2

"At a time when fiscal constraints within the health care industry are increasing, nurses and other health care professionals are troubled by the ethical dilemmas in practice that are associated, in part, with downsizing and displacement."[1] One of the most difficult tasks that fall to administrators and to managers is the action of terminating nurses' employment. This is difficult enough when the nurses are dismissed for cause. In recent years, however, corporate downsizing has led to the termination of large numbers of nurses from institutions across the country. It often falls to nurse administrators to decide which nurses will remain on staff and which will lose their positions. Not only can this be devastating to the nurses being terminated, it also can be morally agonizing to the nurse administrators. Although it may not be possible for the administrators to alter the fact that nursing positions will be lost and nurses will be terminated, they have a moral obligation to influence how the termination is done. They can help to assure that the termination process is fair and just and that, whenever possible, support is provided to both the nurses who have been terminated and those who remain. It is demoralizing for nurses or anyone else to be treated as objects rather than persons, as means rather than ends. Moral principles of justice and beneficence are relevant to how the terminations are managed. It is critically important that the employee's humanity and service to the institution be acknowledged.

---

[1]C. Blake and R. E. Guare. "Nurses' Reflections on Ethical Decision Making: Implications for Leaders," 28(4) *Journal of the New York Nurses Association* (December 1997), 13–16.

THE CHIEF NURSE EXECUTIVE

The chief nurse executive has always possessed a very important role within the health care delivery system. Whether planning strategy, evaluating the overall quality of nursing care within an entity, or allocating human and fiscal resources, the chief nurse executive's role in the organization, the community, and the profession cannot be underestimated.[30] Even so, the role of the chief nurse executive is evolving from a focus on nursing services in traditional settings to an even broader accountability for patient care services in integrated community-based practice.[31] Termed a "continuum" of care, it will require the chief nurse executive to expand his or her expertise in this area.[32]

The chief nurse executive has always possessed a very important role within the health care delivery system.

As the chief nurse executive develops skills and expertise in the continuum of care, the traditional skills and expertise of the chief nurse executive will continue to be needed. Moreover, both the traditional and new responsibilities and roles will create legal concerns for the nurse executive.

Board of Directors Membership

Most often a health care facility's organizational structure is that of a corporation. Incorporated pursuant to state law, the corporation may be a for-profit or not-for-profit entity. A corporation must be managed by a governing body, referred to as a board of directors or a board of trustees.[33] The board has major functions, including oversight, policy formation, and assuring the financial viability of the organization.[34] Through these and other functions the board manages and fulfills the obligations of the organization and is legally accountable for its decisions.

Board membership may vary from organization to organization. Even so, it is recommended that the membership be composed of representatives from the entity itself and the community it serves.[35] Often the chief nurse executive is a member of the board.

With board membership comes the potential for liability if the board breaches any of its duties. Boards of health care facilities have many duties. One is, of course, to ensure that the health care delivered by the corporation's employees is non-negligent. If this duty is breached, the board and its members may be sued under the doctrine of *respondeat superior* and/or *corporate negligence*. This duty includes (1) selecting a capable and competent administrator; (2) complying with any applicable statutes, rules, and regulations pertaining to the delivery of health care; (3) providing adequate and capable health care delivery staff; and (4) providing adequate facilities.[36] Additional board member management responsibilities include the establishment of institutional goals, policies, and procedures; the appointment of the chief operating officer (COO); and the preservation of assets of the corporation.[37]

When an alleged breach of any of these duties and responsibilities occurs, the chief nurse executive member may be named in the suit, particularly if the nurse executive had voting privileges on the board. Suits have been filed against boards of directors. The landmark case establishing the doctrine of corporate negligence was *Darling v. Charleston Community Hospital*[38] discussed in Chapter 4. Other selected cases appear in Table 18–2.

IMPLICATIONS FOR THE CHIEF NURSE EXECUTIVE

Sitting on the board of one's health care facility is an important role for the nurse executive. However, it is also a responsibility, and the nurse executive will need to be knowledgeable about liability issues inherent in the role. In addition, familiarity with the organization's by-laws and articles of incorporation is essential.[39] Being an active participant on the board is also required.

Sitting on the board of one's health care facility is an important role for the nurse executive.

If the chief nurse executive has voting privileges as a board member, he or she will need to carefully review each decision that is to be made before casting the vote. This will be especially important with any patient care issues. Because the nurse executive has a unique perspective in relation to patient care concerns, he or she will be seen by other board members as an expert in this area.[40] As a result, the nurse executive's contribution to the decision-making process can have a long-lasting effect on the character of the corporation.[41]

The chief nurse executive will also want to determine if liability insurance coverage for board members (called directors and officers or D & O

TABLE 18-2

Selected Cases of Corporate Negligence

CASE NAME	ALLEGATIONS	DECISION	COMMENTS
Montgomery Health Care Facility v. Ballard (1990)[1]	Understaffing caused death of resident due to infected bedsores	Court decided for estate of deceased resident; upheld $2 million punitive award against parent corporation that owned nursing home	Three nurses were witnesses and testified about short-staffing; one nurse testified that she told supervisor more staff was needed, but none was provided
Johnson v. Misericordia Hospital (1981)[2]	Permanent paralysis of right thigh due to surgeon severing right femoral artery	Decision for injured 18-year-old and against hospital based on failure of hospital to carefully screen surgeon prior to admission to medical staff	Plaintiff had settled case against surgeon, so hospital was only defendant
Czubinsky v. Doctors Hospital (1983)[3]	Postanesthesia patient's cardiac arrest resulted in permanent brain injury due to postanesthesia nurse leaving area when monitoring should have been ongoing	Judgment for patient based on failure of hospital to provide adequate staff to monitor postoperative patients	Court reversed verdict of jury in favor of hospital, ruling that injuries were directly related to lack of adequate staff

[1]565 So.2d 221 (1990).
[2]301 N.W.2d 156 (1981).
[3]188 Cal. Rptr. 685 (1983).

liability insurance) is provided by the health care facility. D & O liability insurance coverage is an important protection for board members. The D & O liability insurance provided should include indemnification of the board member for all liabilities and expenses, including attorney fees, fines and penalties, and any funds paid to satisfy judgments.[42] Most often, coverage will occur only if the board member acted in good faith and reasonably believed his or her action was lawful and in the best interests of the corporation.[43]

If the nurse executive is not provided with liability insurance by the health care facility, it can be purchased personally. However, it is expensive, and a careful and thorough comparison of rates will be necessary.

The nurse executive will also want to talk with other nurse colleagues who sit on governing boards to gain as much insight into that experience as possible. Even though it is a vicarious way in which to begin to examine the role, it provides an excellent opportunity to begin to understand and develop the role of the chief nurse executive as a board member.

Employment Concerns of the Chief Nurse Executive

One of the many responsibilities the chief nurse executive has is the management of organized nursing services within the health care facility or agency. This includes defining the qualifications of staff and developing policies and programs to attract and retain competent nursing staff.[44] This process requires a thorough knowledge of employment and labor law, including the many nuances of the at-will employment doctrine.

The nurse executive has, however, unfortunately failed in many instances to use this knowledge to develop a realistic plan to maintain his or her own employment in the health care delivery system in which he or she works. Despite holding a senior administrative position, few chief nurse executives may have employment contracts.[45] They, too, are employees at will and can face termination at any time during their employment in the health care delivery system.

As a result of the turbulent nature of health care today—mergers, work redesign, and managed care, to name a few—the trend of unwanted terminations will probably continue to be experienced by chief nurse executives.

Despite holding a senior administrative position, few chief nurse executives may have employment contracts.

If the nurse executive is terminated as an at-will employee, there may be little legal recourse for the nurse. Several cases involving an attempt by nurse administrators and executives to challenge the terminations have been reported in recent years. In *Frank v. South Suburban Hospital Foundation*,[46] the nursing supervisor of the oncology unit filed a suit against her employer after being terminated for not carrying out a physician's order she believed to be harmful to a patient and for performing carotid massage on the unmonitored patient. Ms. Frank alleged the hospital wrongfully terminated her. The appellate court, however, upheld the summary judgment for the hospital and held that Ms. Frank was an at-will employee with no guarantee of continued employment. Moreover, the court opined, the employee handbook created no contract of employment for Ms. Frank.

It is important to note that whether or not Ms. Frank's actions helped or hindered the patient had no bearing on the decision of the court.[47] Because at-will employees can be terminated for "a good reason, a bad reason or no reason at all,"[48] the issue was not relevant to the termination.

Likewise, in *Bourgeous v. Horizon Healthcare Corporation*,[49] the director of nursing at one of Horizon Healthcare's nursing centers was terminated from her employment during the 90-day probationary period required of all at-will employees. During her initial tenure at the center, Ms. Bourgeous maintained that she was orally told that she would be groomed for a medical consultant role and the director of nursing position was a prerequisite for that role. However, shortly after assuming the director of nursing position, Ms. Bourgeous felt she was not given adequate training for her role, complained that the facility was understaffed, and discovered that unlicensed personnel were providing physical therapy to residents. After meeting with officials from the center, she was asked to resign. Ms. Bourgeous refused and was terminated from the director of nursing position.

Ms. Bourgeous filed a suit against the center and alleged wrongful termination. The court entered a directed verdict in favor of the center and the Supreme Court of New Mexico affirmed that decision. In addition to illustrating the at-will employment doctrine, this decision also supports the important principle that, generally, relying on oral representations concerning continued employment is legally risky.[50]

If the chief nurse executive is terminated for an unlawful reason, however, he or she may be able to successfully challenge the unwanted termination. Unlawful reasons include a discriminatory motive, such as making the decision on the basis of a disability, age, or gender as presented in Chapter 16.

IMPLICATIONS FOR THE CHIEF NURSE EXECUTIVE

There is no doubt that the chief nurse executive should obtain a contract of employment for any senior administrative position. The contract should contain provisions concerning the position to be filled, the term (length) of the contract, salary (including any bonuses and how those will be determined), vacation, benefits (e.g., health insurance, computers, paid professional association dues), and sick pay.[51] The proposed contract should be reviewed by the nurse executive's attorney. It may be necessary for the nurse executive's attorney and the attorney for the health care facility to amend, change, or add provisions in the proposed contract.

In addition to the general provisions in the employment contract, the attorney for the nurse executive will want to review the contract for specific paragraphs. One will be the existence of any restrictive covenants. Restrictive covenants prohibit the employee from working for a competing employer or starting a competing business either during or after employment with the current employer.[52] To be legally enforceable, they must be reasonable (e.g., length of time, geographic area covered), protect a legitimate employer interest, be supported by valid consideration (e.g., the salary and other benefits the nurse executive is contracting for in the position), not be against public policy or harmful to the public, and be part of the employment contract.[53]

A second provision of concern for the nurse executive will be the conditions of termination of the employment contract before the term of employment is completed. The best protection for the nurse executive will be language that requires a "for-cause" or "just-cause" termination, with some requirement of notice when the employer decides to exercise its ability to end the employment contract. Examples of for-cause or just-cause terminations include negligence, failure to perform job responsibilities, addiction to drugs or alcohol, and conviction of a crime.[54]

Obviously the requirement of a documented reason for terminating the nurse executive's employment provides job security. Moreover, if the employer does not abide by the contract terms and terminates the nurse executive in violation of those terms, the nurse can sue the employer for breach of the employment contract.

Another important provision in the nurse executive's employment contract should be one governing severance benefits in the event the employment contract is not renewed at its end, or if the nurse executive's employment is terminated prior to the end of the contract. Although severance benefits are not always mandated by state law, if validly contracted for, they are legally enforceable. Even so, nearly 2,000 recent survey responses from organizations indicated that 83% of the responding organizations had a severance policy or practice.[55] Only 79% of the respondents who have a policy in place have it in writing.[56]

Although severance benefits are not always mandated by state law, if validly contracted for, they are legally enforceable.

One purpose of a severance arrangement is to provide financial support for the former employee until he or she finds another position. Therefore, the nurse executive will want to obtain the best severance benefit package possible at the time of hiring. Some elements of a good severance arrangement include a severance payment, outplacement services, and continued benefits coverage during the severance period (e.g., health care insurance, pension credit), and a positive reference from the former employer.[57]

If the nurse executive is not able to negotiate an employment contract that includes a severance arrangement, and an unwanted termination does occur, the nurse executive should attempt to negotiate a severance agreement with the employer at that time. The employer may see a negotiated exit as advantageous in terms of controlling future litigation,[58] particularly if a broad waiver of any right to sue the employer is agreed to by the nurse executive and included in the severance agreement. However, without an obligation to provide severance benefits, the employer may see a negotiated severance agreement as unnecessary, especially if it believes there was no discrimination or other unlawful conduct on its part.

If the chief nurse executive is concerned that his or her involuntary job loss may be due to some discriminatory motive, a consultation with an attorney should be obtained. Although discrimination suits are costly and are not quickly resolved, it may be the only recourse the chief nurse executive has for a violation of his or her rights. The chief nurse executive will want to consider this option even when her unwanted termination is not the only one within an organization. For example, in a case filed under Title VII involving allegations of racial discrimination as the motive for a large number of job terminations (not involving a nurse executive), the federal court evaluated such factors as how the hospital determined which positions would be eliminated, the process by which the terminations were effectuated, and the transferability of duties.[59] These factors must be carefully evaluated by the chief nurse executive who is part of a large reduction in force, especially in view of the fact that many nurse executives are women and over 40 years of age.[60]

SUMMARY OF PRINCIPLES AND APPLICATIONS

Nurse administrators are in a time of transition, not only in terms of the health care systems within which they are employed, but also in terms of their own roles and responsibilities. As if those changes were not enough to contend with, nurse administrators must also help the staff they govern prepare for the same changes.[61] Because nurse administrators balance many roles in diverse set-

tings at various levels, these as well as other requirements can be met. However, they must be met proactively and innovatively.[62] The nurse administrator can do so by:

- Performing the nurse administrator role—whether as a nurse manager or chief nurse executive—consistent with applicable professional standards
- Continuing to develop skills and expertise in the many roles required by the nurse administrator
- Remaining sensitive to the many concerns staff nurses and other nurse colleagues have concerning the many changes they face in their nursing practice
- Evaluating carefully the role of a board member before accepting the responsibilities inherent in that role
- Obtaining advanced educational preparation for the role of nurse manager or chief nurse executive
- Keeping abreast of the latest developments in the law that impact upon the nurse administrator's practice
- Negotiating a contract of employment, either in the nurse executive's current position or before a new position is accepted
- Reviewing carefully any contract of employment or severance agreement before signing
- Obtaining legal advice when necessary to make informed decisions concerning employment and any involuntary separations
- Participating in research to identify trends and continuing issues faced by nurse administrators in their various roles in health care delivery

TOPICS FOR FURTHER INQUIRY

1. Develop a research tool to measure one of the major roles of the nurse executive identified by Mintzberg. Limit the use of the tool to a select group of nurse executive functions. Compare and contrast the findings.

2. Using available public records from the state regulatory agency, identify disciplinary actions against nurse administrators. Determine the frequency of the types of actions in the sample studied. Identify ways in which the nurse administrators could have avoided the disciplinary action taken against them.

3. Develop a questionnaire for use with chief nurse executives to explore their role on a health care facility board. Design the questionnaire to evaluate a particular aspect of the role of board member. Elicit both

legal and ethical implications of the role evaluated. Analyze the results for similarities and differences.

4. Investigate how many discrimination suits have been filed by nurse administrators against former employers in a given period since 1990. Identify how many of the nurse administrators included in the study were offered severance benefits that contained a waiver of their right to sue the employer if they accepted the benefits. Determine how many of the suits filed were decided in favor of the nurse administrator.

REFERENCES

1. *The Random House College Dictionary.* Revised Edition. New York: Random House, Inc., 1998, 18.
2. Barbara Volk Tebbitt, "Nurse Executives: Who Are They, What Do They Do, and What Challenges Do They Face?" in *Current Issues in Nursing.* Joanne McCloskey and Helen Grace, Editors. 5th Edition. St. Louis: C.V. Mosby, 1997, 25–26.
3. Henry Mintzberg, "The Manager's Job: Folklore and Fact," 53(4) *Harvard Business Review* (1975), 49–61.
4. *Id.* at 92–93.
5. Eunice Turner. *Scope and Standards for Nurse Administrators.* Washington, D.C.: American Nurses Publishing, 1996.
6. "Governance Structures," in Barbara Stevens Barnum and Karlene Kerfoot. *The Nurse as Executive.* 4th Edition. Gaithersburg, Md.: Aspen Publishers, 1995, 59–63.
7. *Id.* at 61–62.
8. Tebbitt, *supra* note 2, at 30–33; American Organization of Nurse Executives. *The Evolving Nurse Executive Practice.* Chicago, Ill.: Author, 1996. Available on the organization's Web site at http://www.aone.org. Accessed May 15, 2000; Norma Geddes, Jeanne Sayler, and Barbara Mark, "Nursing in the Nineties: Managing the Uncertainties," 29(5) *JONA* (1999), 40–48.
9. Geddes, Sayler, and Mark, *supra* note 8; see also American Nurses Association. *Competencies for Telehealth Technologies in Nursing.* Washington, D.C.: Author, 1999.
10. American Nurses Association. *Scope and Standards for Nurse Administrators.* Washington, D.C.: Author, 1995, 7–8.
11. Helen Schaag, "The Role of the Nurse in Maintaining Quality and Managing Risk," in *Take Control: A Guide to Risk Management.* Linda Shinn, Editor. Chicago, Ill.: Kirke-Van Orsdel, Inc. and Chicago Insurance Company, 1998, 1–18.
12. *Id.*
13. Robert D. Miller. *Problems in Hospital Law.* 7th Edition. Gaithersburg, Md.: Aspen Publishers, 1996, 332–333.
14. 720 P.2d 632 (1986).
15. *Id.*
16. See, generally, Alba Conte. *Sexual Harrassment in the Workplace: Law and Practice.* 3rd Edition. Volumes I and II. Gaithersburg, Md.: Panel Publishers, 2000.
17. See, as examples, Kurt H. Decker, "Employee Privacy Interests and Employer Restrictions Outside the Workplace," in *1998 Wiley Employment Law Update.* Henry Perritt, Editor. New York: Aspen Law & Business, 1998, 1–40; "E-Mail Communications: Employers' Friend or Foe?" in *The 1997 Executive File: Hot Employment Issues.* Brentwood, Tenn.: M. Lee Smith Publishers, 1997, 71–72.
18. See Rafael Gely, "Workplace English-Only Rules," in *1999 Employment Law Update.* Henry Perritt, Editor. Gaithersburg, Md.: Panel Publishers, 1999, 35–63.
19. Schaag, *supra* note 11.
20. Miller, *supra* note 13, at 235.
21. Barbara Brunt, "The Importance of Lifelong Learning in Managing Risks," in *Take Control: A Guide to Risk Management,* supra note 11, 1–28.
22. 796 P.2d 899 (1990).
23. Howard Roland and Beatrice Rowland. *Nursing Administration Handbook.* 4th Edition. Gaithersburg, Md.: Aspen Publishers, 1997, 165–181.
24. See generally, Ann Scott Blouin and Nancy J. Brent, "Creating Value for Patients: A Legal Perspective," 28(6) *JONA* (1998) 7–9.
25. *Id.* (citations omitted).
26. See generally, Janet Pitts Beckmann. *Nursing Negligence: Analyzing Malpractice in the Hospital Setting.* Thousand Oaks, Cal.: Sage Publishers, 1996.
27. *Id.*
28. Rowland and Rowland, *supra* note 23, at 491–511.
29. Heather Spence Laschinger, Carol Wong, Linda McMahon, and Carl Kaufmann, "Leader Behavior Impact on Staff Nurse Empowerment, Job Tension, and Work Effectiveness," 29(5) *JONA* (1999), 28–39. For an interesting article on the effects on redesign on *nurse managers,* see Gail Ingersoll, Jo-Ann Cook, Sarah Fogel, Margaret Applegate, and Betsy Frank, "The Effect of Patient-Focused Redesign on Midlevel Nurse Managers' Role Responsibilities and Work Environment," 29(5) *JONA* (1999), 21–27.
30. American Nurses Association, *supra* note 10, at 6–8.
31. American Organization of Nurse Executives, *supra* note 8, at 1.
32. *Id.*
33. George Pozgar, *Legal Aspects of Health Care Administration.* 7th Edition. Gaithersburg, Md.: Aspen Publishers, 1999, 155–156.
34. *Id.*
35. See generally, Miller, *supra* note 13, at 17–42.
36. Pozgar, *supra* note 33, at 165–178.
37. Miller, *supra* note 13, at 17–39.
38. 211 N.E.2d 253 (1965), *cert. denied,* 383 U.S. 946 (1966).
39. Pozgar, *supra* note 33, at 165.
40. Rowland and Rowland, *supra* note 23, at 114–115.
41. *Id.*
42. Pozgar, *supra* note 33, at 435–436. See also Vickey Masta-Gornic, "A Basic Insurance Primer," in *The Risk Manager's Desk Reference.* 2nd Edition. Barbara Youngberg, Editor. Gaithersburg, Md.: Aspen Publishers, 1998, 205–207.
43. Miller, *supra* note 13, at 30.
44. Tebbitt, *supra* note 2, at 26–28.
45. For example, in one small sample of 11 chief nurse executives who left their positions involuntarily, none had an explicit contract of employment. Three did have an implied employment contract in their letter of offer or letter of hire. Ann Scott Blouin and Nancy J. Brent, "Nurse Administrators in Job Transition: Stories from the Front," 22(12) *JONA* (December 1992), 13–14, 27.
46. 628 N.E.2d 943 (1993).

47. A. David Tammelleo, "Nurse Supervisor Challenges Doctor's Orders: Termination," 34(11) *Regan Report on Nursing Law* (April 1994), 2.

48. Henry Perritt. *Employee Dismissal Law and Practice.* 4rd Edition. Volume I. New York: John Wiley & Sons, 1998, 3 (with 2000 cumulative supplement).

49. 872 P.2d 852 (1994).

50. Perritt, *supra* note 48, at 319–511.

51. See Kurt Decker and Thomas Felix. *Drafting and Revising Employment Contracts.* New York: John Wiley & Sons, 1991 (with periodic updates); Kenneth Sovereign. *Personnel Law.* 4th Edition. Upper Saddle River, N.J.: Prentice-Hall, 1999.

52. Decker and Felix, *supra* note 51, at 105.

53. *Id.* at 105. See also Steven Harvey, "Enforcing the Noncompete and Confidential Duties of High Level Executives," in *1998 Wiley Employment Law Update.* Henry Perritt, Editor. New York: Aspen Law & Business, 1998, 151–184.

54. *Id.* at 135–141.

55. Lee Hecht Harrison. *Severance and Separation Benefits—An Update to Our Severance Study.* Available on Lee Hecht Harrison's Web site at http://www.lhh.com. Accessed May 16, 2000.

56. *Id.*

57. *Id.;* "How to Write and Negotiate a Severance Agreement," in *The 1999 Executive File: Hot Employment Issues.* Brentwood, Tenn.: M. Lee Smith Publishers, 1999, 13–14.

58. *1999 Executive File, supra* note 57.

59. *Khouri v. Frank Cuneo Hospital,* 929 F.2d 703 (7th Cir. 1991).

60. See generally, American College of Healthcare Executives. "Still Don't Trust Anyone Over 30?" Available on the college's Web site at http://www.ache.org. Accessed May 15, 2000.

61. Laschinger, Wong, McMahon, and Kaufmann, *supra* note 29.

62. Tibbett, *supra* note 2.

The Nurse in the Community

19

Mary Linn Green, JD, MS, RN

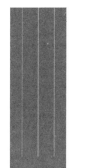
KEY PRINCIPLES

- Negligence/Professional Negligence
- Liability
- Immunity from Suit
- Abandonment (of patient)
- Elder Abuse
- Elder Neglect
- Guardianship
- Telenursing/Telephone Triage
- Workplace Health and Safety
- Restraints
- Seclusion

The role of the nurse in the community is gaining more importance with each passing year. As the demographics of our society change, nurses are increasingly being called upon to fulfill roles which were once reserved to the patient's relatives. From elderly patients with no relatives and in need of home care services, to schoolchildren from broken homes who may be victims of abuse or neglect, community-based nurses are being called upon to provide ever-increasing services and to act as advocates for their patients.

Added to these societal changes are scientific and technological advances which seem to be occurring at breakneck speed. Community-based nurses are asked to provide increasingly more complex care and perform highly technological procedures. The explosive growth of information technology has changed the future of health care and will have far-reaching implications for the nurse in the community.

As the roles of nurses in the community become increasingly independent and autonomous, there will be a commensurate increase in their responsibility, accountability, and potential liability. It has been postulated that health care settings outside of acute care will see more malpractice cases because of increased liability arising out of technology, paradigm shifts in health care delivery to home and community-based settings, and the continuing trend toward litigation.[1] Although most authorities expect to see a great deal of increase in malpractice cases involving nurses outside of the traditional hospital setting, a recent study has revealed that they compose only a small percentage of cases actually filed at the present time. In a study of 381 reported state and appellate court cases involving nursing negligence over a 7-year period, only 12.4% of the cases involved areas outside the hospital setting. These areas included nursing homes (5.8%), correctional facilities (1.5%), home health care agencies (2.1%), occupational centers (0.5%), medical clinics/physician offices (1.6%), staffing agencies (0.7%) and hospice agencies (0.2%).[2]

It is becoming ever more important for community-based nurses to understand the legal implications of their respective roles, and the legal process as it pertains not only to the nurses, but their patients as well. This chapter will explore various types of community-based nursing and pertinent legal issues within each specialty. The problem of abuse and neglect of the elderly, as

The author would like to acknowledge Judy Balcitis, RN, Director of Clinical Services at Visiting Nurses Association, Rockford, Illinois, for her invaluable help with the chapter. Her generosity in meeting with the author to discuss current issues in home health nursing and the sharing of information and policies from the VNA are greatly appreciated.

well as the legal process of guardianship, will also be addressed.

HOME HEALTH CARE NURSING

Home health care has undergone explosive growth within the last few decades. The National Association for Home Care reports that 7 million people received home care in 1995, and that home care is the fastest growing segment of the health care industry.[3] Patient care provided in the home is a good alternative, because it is generally less expensive than institutional care. A 1996 study by the General Accounting Office (GAO) evaluated both the benefits and costs of home health care. The study analyzed the number of home health visits from 1989 to 1993, and found that patients with 60 or more visits per year increased from 10% to 25%. Correspondingly, spending increased from $2.7 billion in 1989 to $12.7 billion in 1994.[4]

In the face of this burgeoning growth, certain legal issues have surfaced which are common to

---

ETHICS CONNECTION 19–1

Nurses in community health and community-based practice provide a wide range of services to clients. With the tendency for only acutely ill individuals to be treated in hospitals, many more nurses are practicing in the community than in the past. Not all nurses in the community are community health nurses. Community health nurses generally consider their clients to be populations and communities, rather than individuals and families. Community-based nurses, on the other hand, generally provide care to individuals and families who already have experienced some interruptions in their usual health patterns.

Community health nurses make a significant contribution to attaining the national health objectives identified in *Healthy People 2010*. *Healthy People 2010* is the prevention agenda for the United States. The goals of this agenda are to (1) increase quality and years of healthy life and (2) eliminate health disparities.[1] These national goals are related directly to moral principles of beneficence and distributive justice. They also are an expression of the covenant that the federal government has with its people. Community health nurses have been working toward attainment of such goals for well over a century. As nurses who have always "thought upstream," community health nurses look at patterns of health and work collaboratively with community groups and others to improve health and health care.

Individualistic ethics, thus, is limited in informing skilled moral comportment of community health nurses. Communitarian ethics offers an alternative approach. Communitarian ethics respects the inherent worth of individuals and acknowledges that humans are embedded in relationships. Campbell[2] proposes a radical revision of health care ethics. He "shifts the locus of health from the individual body to the community of persons who share common vulnerabilities and resources,"[3] and calls for "fresh symbols of health."[4] In particular, Campbell urges that health care professionals let go of the power that they have over clients and participate in a health care system of shared freedom. Frank,[5] in a review of Campbell's book, notes that Campbell's notion of communal ethic "is best expressed in his quotation of a poem by W. H. Auden. Auden describes a street urchin who could not imagine a world where 'one could weep,/Because another wept.' Here is the morality of social membership that mainstream ethics often ignores: the other's cause to weep is my cause as well. When those 'others' are given voices and their suffering is made present and real, then ethical thinking has to change, or at least ethicists have to confront themselves in a new way." Community health nurses know this compassion, or suffering with, others. They are committed to the entire community, but have special concerns for vulnerable populations and people that are underserved in the health care system. Like nurses in other practice roles, settings, and specialties, however, nurses in the community are experiencing the consequences of restructuring and reductions in staff. Thus, nurses in the community have unique ethical concerns but also experience many of the ethical problems that all nurses share.

---

[1]Office of Disease Prevention and Health Promotion. U.S. Department of Health and Human Services. *Healthy People 2010*. Washington, D.C.: Author,. See also Web site: http://www.health.gov/healthypeople/PrevAgenda/whatishp.htm

[2]Alistair V. Campbell. *Health as Liberation: Medicine, Theology, and the Quest for Justice*. Cleveland, Ohio: Pilgrim, 1995.

[3]Arthur W. Frank. "A Common Health: Redrawing the Moral Map," 113 *Christian Century* (May 1, 1996), 486–490.

[4]Campbell, *supra* note 2.

[5]Frank, *supra* note 3.

most home health care agencies and staff. These issues include safety, injuries, communication, personnel, advanced technology, reimbursement, and termination of services.

Safety

A major area of concern for home health care staff is the environment into which they are sent to care for patients. This has always been a concern in large metropolitan and high crime areas but has also become a problem in smaller communities due to the increasing prevalence of alcohol abuse, illegal drugs, and firearms.[5] Home health care staff usually work alone, often work early morning or late night hours, and work in community settings or homes which involve extensive contact with the public. Violence in patients' homes and threats to staff are becoming more common.

In response to these threats to staff safety, many home health care agencies have developed programs for orientation and annually train staff to recognize potentially dangerous or violent situations and how to respond appropriately to them. For example, if a patient or family members are verbally or physically abusive, or appear intoxicated, the staff are advised not to make the home visit.

Most home health care agencies also have specific policies and procedures which address safety in the field and give guidance for action if problems arise. In community situations, staff are encouraged to stay on high-traffic, well-lighted streets if at all possible. If night visits are necessary, staff are encouraged to ask the patient to turn on the outside light and meet them at the door of the most accessible entrance. Staff may also request a police escort if it is absolutely necessary to visit a patient in an unsafe area.

In patients' homes, such problems as unruly pets may be encountered. Staff should request that pets be properly secured prior to the visit if they hinder work or safety. Most agencies provide staff with cellular phones to keep with them at all times, in case emergency help must be summoned.

Transportation also poses multiple safety risks for the home health care employee. Agencies must verify employees' driving records and insurance coverage prior to employment and annually. Staff should have routine maintenance performed on their vehicles and carry emergency equipment with them. Home health care staff must take re-

sponsibility to maintain their own safety by practicing preventative actions.[6]

Injuries to both staff and patients are another area of legal concern in home health care.

Injuries

Injuries to both staff and patients are another area of legal concern in home health care. Staff can be exposed to such things as infectious diseases and wastes, needle stick injuries, and bloodborne pathogens. Most agencies have policies which specifically address isolation techniques, universal precautions, and preventative measures.[7]

Injuries to the back from moving patients are some of the most frequent staff injuries. These often occur because of the lack of staff training in proper body mechanics for lifting and moving patients. Problems also arise when staff have inadequate assistance in moving patients and still attempt to do so, causing not only staff injuries but patient injuries as well.[8] In *Gustin v. Physician's Home Services,*[9] the patient had a regular home health aide who was familiar with her needs. A substitute home health aide who was unfamiliar with the patient was sent by the agency. The home health aide dropped the patient and fell on top of her. The substitute employee was found to be negligent, and the case was settled in the patient's favor. Patient injuries are the cause of most litigation against home care agencies. Both patient and staff injuries are monitored and evaluated as part of the agencies' quality improvement programs, so that problems can be addressed with staff and future potential injuries avoided.

Communication

Communication among health care providers is essential to all patient care. In no other area of health care is communication as essential as in home health care. Home care workers most often give patient care alone and are geographically separated from the agency, their coworkers, and the patient's physician. Thorough documentation and communication of the patient's problems, conditions, and care are of the utmost importance.

The patient's plan of care and any changes in the patient's condition must be communicated to the patient's physician and relatives. In *Lauth v. Olsten Home Healthcare, Inc.*,[10] the patient was cared for by home health care services in a group home in which she lived. Over a period of time, she suffered deterioration, including weight loss, decubitus ulcers, urinary tract infections, and leg and foot contractures. The home health staff did not report her problems to her physician or family and failed to fully document her care. The home care agency was found negligent, and a verdict was rendered in favor of the plaintiff.

Communication among the home care staff and reporting and documentation of the patient's condition among coworkers is imperative. In *Milazzo v. Olsten Home Healthcare, Inc.*,[11] a home care agency CNA was hired as a sitter by the patient's family to care for her while in the hospital recovering from brain surgery. The CNA noticed that the patient suddenly began leaning to the left and was unable to stand, but did not report this change in condition to the hospital RN, physician, or patient's family. The patient suffered brain injury, with resultant paralysis and impaired memory. The home care agency was found negligent for the actions of the CNA, and a verdict was rendered in favor of the plaintiff.

Communication among the staff and patient and family is necessary to assess the patient's physical and mental condition and identify any actual or potential problems. This information must be clearly documented in the medical record and reported to agency coworkers. In *Wesser v. Homer Care Homemaking Services*,[12] a home health aide was hired to care for a patient who needed close observation. Her family related that the patient was likely to hurt herself, but this was not documented, nor was the patient's mental status. The patient jumped out of the window in the presence of the aide. The family brought suit, and a verdict was returned in their favor.

Communication with the patient's physician should be ongoing, and any questions concerning care must be clarified. Because most communication occurs via telephone, all orders should be double-checked and verified with the physician when they are received. The physician must be kept apprised of the patient's condition, and any changes must be communicated to the physician in a timely manner. If the home care staff has difficulty in contacting the patient's physician concerning a patient problem requiring attention, the staff should go up the agency "chain of command" to obtain assistance in resolving the problem.

Personnel

Home health care agencies face personnel issues which are somewhat different from those of hospitals and clinics, due to the type of patient care provided. Home care agency staff work independently and are geographically separated from one another. Employees are usually not directly supervised during patient care and must be knowledgeable about the procedures they perform before being sent out to the patient. Three areas of particular importance as they relate to home care agencies are hiring, training, and supervision of personnel.

Prior to the hiring of employees, the home care agency must carefully screen each individual to determine any history of problems. Background checks, fingerprinting, and thorough reference checks are necessary to determine any prior dishonesty or problem behaviors. This is particularly important for unlicensed employees who will be sent into patients' homes under unsupervised conditions.[13] In *Morrett v. Kimberly Services, Inc.*,[14] the agency hired two home health workers without conducting adequate background screening. Although the workers had prior convictions, the agency did not require any testing or references before employing them. While employed by the agency, these workers accessed patient files and information. After leaving the agency's employment, they broke into an elderly patient's home, tied her up, and assaulted and robbed her. The agency was found to be guilty of negligent hiring, and a verdict was rendered for the plaintiff.

Another area of concern [in home health care] is the delegation of duties to staff and the supervision of their performance.

Once the agency has screened and hired new employees, they must be adequately oriented and trained for their positions. There should be a formalized orientation program for all employees, with emphasis on job descriptions and patient care policies. Each new employee should be assigned a preceptor and receive a handbook which outlines expected conduct and disciplinary procedures. New staff members must be familiarized with policies and procedures which set guidelines for patient care and act as a resource for them if they are unfamiliar with a particular procedure.[15] In-service education regarding new policies and procedures should be provided routinely to all employees. In *Fink v. Kimberly Services, Inc.*,[16] a quadriplegic patient was injured when he was dropped by a home health aide while being transferred from his bed to wheelchair. The agency was found negligent for failure to properly train, educate, and supervise the aide concerning proper body mechanics and transfer techniques.

Another area of concern is the delegation of duties to staff and the supervision of their performance. Home care agencies employ staff at various levels of training and capabilities. Careful attention must be given to what tasks and procedures must be performed by RNs, and what may be delegated to staff with less training. This must comply with each state's laws concerning the scope of nursing practice. The agency should develop guidelines for supervision of staff which include observation and supervisory visits to monitor staff performance and competence.[17] In *Roach v. Kelly Health Care, Inc.*,[18] the daughter of an elderly patient who had a stroke arranged for the home care agency to provide 24-hour live-in care. CNAs were sent to provide the care with little RN supervision. The CNAs were not qualified to provide the care they did, which should have been provided by home health aides. The patient fell, was injured, and eventually died, and the daughter sued the agency. The court found that there was evidence of negligence by the agency for the use of unqualified personnel and failure to supervise the CNAs.

Home care agencies which have thorough personnel policies and procedures for screening, evaluation, education, and supervision of all levels of staff will be in a better position to avoid liability based upon personnel issues than those agencies which do not.

Advanced Technology

Due to advances in technology, home care agency staff are called upon to perform procedures and utilize equipment which were once only available in the hospital setting. Increasingly, home care nurses are giving transfusions of blood products, chemotherapy, and intravenous medications such as Heparin and Dobutamine to patients in their homes. Highly technological types of equipment such as ventilators, infusion pumps, and fetal heart monitors are being utilized in patients' homes. Nursing staff must be thoroughly trained and proficient in the performance of these highly technological procedures and use of this complex equipment. In addition to receiving in-depth training, a 24-hour resource helpline should be available to the staff for any questions or problems.

Besides learning about this new technology and equipment themselves, staff must also train the patient and caregiver how to use it and recognize any problems. The ability of the patient and caregiver to perform a procedure or use a piece of equipment must be carefully assessed and any problems addressed. This should always be thoroughly documented by the staff in the patient's medical record.

Many home care agencies actually select and supply the equipment and products which are utilized by the patient. The agency staff are responsible for maintaining the equipment and detecting any problems with it. The agency must have up-to-date product information and warranties. Products and equipment should never be used past expiration or replacement dates. If equipment or a product causes injury to the patient, the home health agency may be liable. Any equipment malfunction should be reported to the manufacturer. The staff should take it out of service and maintain its condition until it can be inspected. It should never be thrown away or destroyed, as it may become important evidence at a later date.[19]

Due to the continuous advancements in health care technology, home care nurses can look forward to utilizing even more complex and highly specialized procedures and equipment for their patients in the future.

Reimbursement

The Balanced Budget Act of 1997 made dramatic changes in the reimbursement system for Medicare home services. The law reduced projected federal government spending on the Medicare program by making numerous changes to the way in which the program operates. Prior to this legislation, home health services were paid on a cost-based reimbursement system. The agencies would actually incur the costs for home health services and be reimbursed after Medicare determined the costs reported were reasonable and necessary.[20] One of the cost-saving measures is the introduction of an interim payment system, which will ultimately lead to a prospective payment system for home health care. The interim payment system will remain in effect until the new prospective payment system is implemented.[21]

The Health Care Financing Administration has developed an outcome and assessment information set (OASIS system), which is a comprehensive system of functional assessments to be utilized for all Medicare patients. This comprehensive assessment is to be completed for all patients no later than 5 days after the start of care. Assessments are then to be done every 60 days thereafter, or within 48 hours of the patient's return to the home from a hospital admission of 24 hours or more, and at discharge.[22] The Health Care Financing Administration will utilize the information collected by the OASIS system as a basis for the development of a finalized prospective payment system for home health care. Home care agencies must comply with these federal government mandates and understand the impact they will have on reimbursement for care.

When an agency terminates services to a patient, it must be based on the lack of continued need for the services,

---

Termination of Services

In light of the changes and limitations in Medicare reimbursement to home care agencies, termination of services to patients is expected to increase. When an agency terminates services to a patient, it must be based on the lack of continued need for the services, not solely on the patient's ability to pay or insurance coverage.[23] If the agency terminates the patient's care, it could be found guilty of abandonment under certain circumstances.

The basis of an abandonment claim is that the home health agency has assumed a duty to care for the patient, breached the duty, and caused an injury to the patient.[24] In order for a patient to successfully bring a claim for abandonment against an agency, he or she must prove (1) the agency unilaterally terminated the provider-patient relationship (2) without reasonable notice and (3) when further attention was needed by the patient. Whether notice is reasonable depends upon the facts and circumstances of each case. Notice must be given in writing to the patient, and a copy placed in the patient's record. The patient's physician must also be notified of the agency's decision.[25] Some states have applicable state licensure requirements which relate to patient admission and discharge. In some states there are specific standards in terms of the timing of notice, the parties with a right to notice, and the basis for terminating care of home care patients.[26]

Admission denials and discharge determinations should never be based upon the mistaken belief that a patient has exceeded his or her Medicare or insurance company payment limit. Rather, these decisions should be based upon whether the agency has sufficient clinical resources to meet the needs of the individual patient, as well as the rest of its patients.[27] In *Ready v. Personal Health Care Services Corp.*,[28] a home care agency decided to terminate services to a 3-year-old child because they mistakenly believed that she had run out of benefits. The child died, and the parents sued the home care agency. A verdict was rendered for the parents, who received $13 million in emotional and punitive damages.

Home care agencies should have policies and procedures in place which address the issues of termination of services without abandonment of the patient. If services are terminated, agencies should make reasonable efforts to transfer the patient to an alternative caregiver to meet continuing care needs. All of the agencies' actions should be thoroughly documented.[29]

The issue of termination of services to patients is expected to become a more critical one in the future, as Medicare and insurance benefits become increasingly restricted and limited. Home care agencies must have policies and procedures in place to effectively deal with this problem and decrease their liability as much as it is feasible to do so.

As home health care continues its rapid growth in future years, it can be expected to face even more legal issues with greater complexity. Comprehensive risk management and quality improvement programs are needed to address these issues.

PUBLIC HEALTH NURSING

Public health agencies are separate and distinct entities from home health care agencies. Because they are public rather than private agencies, their roles carry different expectations. Public health agencies are government based and most commonly exist on city and county levels. These agencies are charged with the responsibility of protecting the public's health through the enforcement of primarily state and some federal laws, and thus public health nurses must be familiar with state and federal health codes. Another responsibility is to report and treat communicable diseases, such as tuberculosis or sexually transmitted diseases, for the protection of the public's health, as defined by state health codes.

Because these agencies are public ones, their employees are given qualified legal immunities under the legal principle of sovereign immunity. Where a nurse employed by a private home care agency can be held liable for simple negligence, a nurse employed by a public health agency cannot, based upon governmental tort immunity. However, if a public health nurse is found to have been grossly negligent, such that the nurse's actions were "willful and wanton," or the nurse intentionally caused the patient harm, the nurse will not be granted this immunity. Each state possesses a statute which governs tort immunity for public or governmental entities and their employees, such as public health departments and the nurses who work in them.

Because . . . [public health] agencies are public ones, their employees are given qualified legal immunities under the legal principle of sovereign immunity.

In state after state, courts have dismissed claims against public health departments and their employees, based upon governmental tort immunity. In *Hudson v. Rausa*,[30] a factory worker had been prescribed INH by the county health department to prevent the spread of tuberculosis in the factory where he worked. He developed hepatic and renal failure from the medication and died. His widow brought suit against the supervisor of nurses and the physician director of the county health department for negligence. The trial court granted summary judgment for both of the defendants. The Mississippi Supreme Court affirmed this ruling and found that the nurse's and doctor's actions were covered by qualified immunity as public officials.

In *Matteo v. City of Philadelphia Department of Public Health Family Medical Services*,[31] a child suffered brain damage as a result of a D.P.T. immunization given by department of public health employees. The parents brought suit against the city department of public health and a department doctor. The trial court entered judgment in favor of the city department of public health and held that it was entitled to immunity provided by the Pennsylvania Political Subdivision Tort Claims Act. The Pennsylvania appellate court affirmed the trial court's ruling that governmental immunity applied.

In *Jamieson v. Luce–Mackinac–Alger School-craft District Health Department*,[32] a patient went to the district health department about a positive tuberculosis skin test and saw the nurse. She was put on the department protocol for exposed tuberculosis patients, which included preventive chemotherapy, INH and vitamin B_6, and a chest X ray. The doctor read her chest X ray as negative. Two years later, a chest X ray revealed a lung mass which was malignant, and the patient eventually died of cancer. Her family brought suit against the district health department, nurse, and doctor for failure to diagnose and treat her lung cancer. The trial court granted summary judgment for the defendants and held that the district health department, nurse, and doctor were entitled to governmental tort immunity pursuant to state law. The nurse and doctor were given immunity, unless it could be proven that their conduct was "willful and wanton." The court defined "willful and wanton" as conduct which shows an intent to harm, or such indifference to whether harm will result as to be equivalent to a willingness that it does. The Michigan Appellate Court affirmed the trial court's finding that the nurse's and doctor's conduct was not willful and wanton.

In *Headley v. Berman*,[33] a patient went to a public clinic for the treatment of inactive tuberculosis. The Boston City Hospital Pulmonary/TB Clinic was established by the City of Boston with public health department approval. The patient was given INH and monthly check-ups at the clinic. She developed hepatitis from the medication and died. Her family brought suit against the clinic doctors and nurse who were involved in her treatment. The trial court granted the defendants' motion for summary judgment. The Massachusetts Supreme Court affirmed and held that because the antituberculosis treatment program was established under the auspices of the Massachusetts Department of Public Health, its doctor and nurse employees were entitled to governmental immunity under the state statute.

The case law overwhelmingly reveals that public health departments and their employees have been granted governmental tort immunity in cases where it has been raised as a defense under state laws. However, if a state does not have such an immunity statute, or the issue is not raised and immunity is not claimed, the public health agency employees will be treated by the courts in the same manner as private home health agency employees. In *Bass v. Barksdale*,[34] a patient brought suit against a public health department nurse, and doctor employees of the department and her private doctor for blindness. Her blindness was caused by the medications which she received for the treatment of tuberculosis. No governmental immunity defense was raised by the public health department and its employees. A verdict of $300,000 was rendered against the defendant nurse and doctors, and the court ordered judgment against the public health department. The case was reversed by the Tennessee appellate court and remanded for a new trial due to an error in jury instructions by the court. The issue of qualified immunity was not raised in this case, and a much different outcome was reached than in the other cases previously discussed.

It is important for the nurse who works in public health to know whether a state statute grants governmental tort immunity, and whether the agency for which the nurse works is considered to be a governmental entity to which this immunity would apply. In addition, an understanding of how the courts have decided cases governing the immunity granted in the statute is also important.

TELENURSING

In the past few decades, there has been an explosive growth in the telecommunications industry. Increasingly, nurses are using telecommunications technology to provide patient care. Telenursing is the process by which nurses provide care to patients via telecommunication devices such as the telephone, the Internet, two-way conferencing, and even two-way video.

The telephone is by far the most commonly used device which nurses have been using to communicate with patients for many years. More recently, nursing call centers and hotlines have been developed to provide telenursing services. These are based in hospitals, or sponsored by health care systems, managed care organizations, and even insurance companies. Their purpose is to provide patients with access to registered nurses who can help the callers make more informed and cost-effective health care decisions. Some of the services which are provided by nursing call centers are making physician referrals, providing general health information, scheduling hospital and physician appointments, and managing medical emergencies.[35]

This interaction between the nurse and patient via telephone is commonly referred to as telephone triage. Health care organizations utilize nursing telephone triage to increase referrals to the system and to help contain costs. Patients are referred to physicians and services within the organization for care, thus increasing revenues to the system. Patients also receive health care information via telephone triage at much less cost than unnecessary visits to the emergency room or doctor's office.[36] The practice of telenursing, and telephone triage nursing in particular, raises some very definite legal issues. These include licensure, standards of care, and the use of guidelines and protocols.

Licensure

The practice of telenursing has raised several licensure issues for nurses who engage in it. No specific statutory laws mandate who should perform telephone triage. Most state nurse practice acts define the scope of and limitations imposed on various levels of nursing practice: registered nurses, licensed practical nurses, and allied health care professionals are some examples. These state nurse practice acts provide the best guidance in determining who should answer telephone triage calls. The scope of nursing practice varies from state to state, and each specific state nurse practice act should be consulted to determine how it would apply to telephone triage nursing. Many state nurse practice acts seem to suggest that only registered nurses should be utilized to answer telephone triage calls.[37]

Another licensure issue is whether the nurse is appropriately licensed to practice telenursing where it occurs geographically. When telecommunications devices are used to provide nursing services (e.g., nursing assessment, evaluation, or judgment), those services constitute the practice of nursing—whether they are provided by telephone or by videoconferencing.[38] The National Council of State Boards of Nursing's position is that a nurse who interacts with a patient at a remote site to electronically receive the patient's health status data, initiate and transmit therapeutic interventions and regimens, and monitor and record the patient's response and outcome, is engaging in the practice of nursing. The nurse may be located in one state and the patient in another state where the nurse is not licensed. Most of the literature on telenursing suggests that the practice of nursing takes place where the patient is located.[39] State licensure boards and various professional organizations have considered the issue, and the weight of authority indicates that the nurse should be licensed in his or her home state and the state where the patient is located.[40]

Licensure issues in telenursing are also discussed in depth in Chapter 15.

Standard of Care

Standards of care for telenursing have only recently been developed by such organizations as the American Academy of Ambulatory Care Nursing. However, there may be conflicts as to which standard of care should apply to a certain situation: the state where the nurse is located or the state where the patient is located. In the absence of any clearly designated standards of care, the telephone triage nurse would be expected to exercise that degree of care ordinarily used by other reasonably well qualified telephone triage nurses.

If telephone triage nurses were to form a designated specialty group, a higher standard of care could potentially be imposed. Health care organizations and nurses should use a conservative approach in drafting policies, procedures, and guidelines, and in staffing and training their telephone triage nurses.[41]

Guidelines and Protocols

Appropriate guidelines and protocols must be developed by providers of telephone triage nursing. These guidelines and protocols identify appropriate advice to be given for a particular problem and can establish a standard of care for a particular practice setting. The American Accreditation HealthCare Commission/URAC, an accrediting body which sets standards for health care organizations, including those health care entities which provide 24-hour telephone triage and health information services, requires that clinical decision support tools be used for managing calls. These clinical decision support tools must be developed with the assistance of physicians and other health care providers in that particular clinical specialty and must be reviewed and updated on at least an annual basis. These clinical decision support tools will guide the nurse through the assessment and decision-making process with the patient.[42]

Even when guidelines, protocols, and clinical decision support tools are utilized by a health care organization, they should not be blindly followed by the telephone triage nurse without the exercise of independent nursing judgment. The nurse may use his or her independent nursing judgment to override guidelines which are inappropriate in a particular patient situation. A highly skilled and trained nurse is needed to assess patient situations, even with the assistance of the guidelines and protocols.[43]

Telenursing and nursing call centers have recently begun to be the targets of professional negligence lawsuits brought by patients. The case of *Shannon v. McNulty*[44] involved a failure to diagnose and treat Sheena Shannon's preterm labor, which allegedly resulted in the death of her severely premature infant. She was instructed by her HMO to call the physician she had selected as her obstetrician, Dr. McNulty, or to call the HMO Nursing Call Line if she had any medical questions or if she was experiencing a medical emergency. She saw the doctor on a monthly basis and utilized the HMO Nursing Call Line for medical advice on several occasions during her early pregnancy.

On October 2, 1992, she began experiencing abdominal pain and contacted the doctor. The doctor examined her on October 5th, told her that her pain was from a fibroid tumor, and instructed her to rest. She called the doctor four times between October 7th and October 9th, with continued complaints of abdominal pain and other complaints. On October 10th, she called the HMO Nursing Call Line complaining of severe irregular abdominal pain and the doctor's lack of response to her complaint. The triage nurse told her to again contact the doctor, which she did not do. She again contacted the HMO Nursing Call Line on October 11th, reporting that her symptoms were worse. The triage nurse again instructed her to call the doctor. She did call the doctor, who told her she was not in preterm labor. On October 12th, she again phoned the HMO Nursing Call Line with increasing complaints of abdominal pain and her doctor's continued lack of response to her complaints. This time, her call was directed to an in-house orthopedic surgeon, who advised her to go to the emergency department. After arriving at the hospital, she delivered a severely premature infant who died two days later.

There were two claims against the HMO: (1) vicarious liability for the negligence of its employee nurses for their failure to refer her for a cervical examination and fetal stress test; and (2) direct corporate liability based upon the absence of protocols or policies related to providing medical advice over the telephone to HMO subscribers. The Shannons were required to present expert testimony to show that the HMO nurses deviated from the standard of care for telephone triage, and this deviation resulted in harm to the Shannons. The Shannons' expert witness (a doctor with experience in a health care organization that provided telephone triage) testified that the triage nurses did not meet the standard of care. The nurses should have responded to her calls on October 10th, 11th, and 12th with immediate referrals to a physician or hospital for a cervical examination and a fetal stress test. The nurses also had a duty to follow up with Mrs. Shannon's obstetrician to determine if she received appropriate care in response to her complaints.

The Shannon decision is important to claims of negligence against a health care organization for the actions of its telephone triage nurses. Although the trial court granted a nonsuit to the defendant HMO, the Pennsylvania Superior Court disagreed. The Superior Court held that the HMO was responsible to oversee that the dispensing of advice by the nurses would be performed in a medically reasonable manner and was subject to corporate liability for breach of that duty. The case was sent back to the trial court for a new trial.

The Shannon case is a good example of the liabilities in telenursing. Nurses who work in this area should become familiar with their potential liability and also check their professional liability insurance regarding coverage for telenursing activities. As new telecommunications technology is developed, so too will innovative nurses come up with methods to utilize and apply this technology to patient care situations.

VOLUNTEER NURSING

Many nurses serve as volunteers in a number of different capacities. From performing health screenings at fairs, to working in first-aid booths at festivals, to serving as nurses at their childrens' camps, nurses can be found giving of their professional time as a community service. Because they are working as volunteers, and not paid, many nurses believe that there is no potential professional liability in these activities. However, this may not be true, as one recent case illustrates.

In *Boccasile v. Cajun Music, Ltd.*,[45] a widow brought a wrongful death action against a nurse and a physician who volunteered to staff a first aid booth at a festival and unsuccessfully treated her husband for an allergic reaction. The decedent husband attended a music festival and had a severe allergic reaction to the seafood which was in the gumbo he sampled, causing anaphylactic shock. A physician's assistant who was also attending the festival was the first person to come to his aid. The volunteer doctor and other members of the first aid crew left the first aid tent to go and render emergency assistance. The volunteer nurse stayed at the first aid tent, so as not to leave it unstaffed.

When the doctor first approached the decedent, he was still standing. She told him she was a doctor and asked if he needed any help. He told her he had eaten some seafood, was having an allergic reaction, and needed a shot. The doctor asked him to come with her to the first aid tent, but he replied that he was unable to do so. He sat down on the ground and repeated that he needed a shot. While the doctor stayed with him, other members of the crew returned to the first aid tent to get an adrenaline injector and call an ambulance.

While waiting for the injector, the doctor continued to speak with him, and he again refused to go to the first aid tent. He was talking in full sentences without difficulty and was not retracting or using any accessory muscles to breathe. He was not wheezing, gasping, or coughing, and showed no signs of respiratory distress. In a few minutes, someone returned with an Epipen. The doctor administered the epinephrine into his exposed thigh. Although the doctor requested a second injector, none was available.

The nurse was relieved by another volunteer and left the first aid tent to see if she could be of assistance at the scene. She knew nothing about his condition, but he was lying on the ground when she arrived. The doctor had already administered the Epipen, and she was told that an ambulance had been called. The nurse remained with him until the ambulance arrived.

After the doctor had injected him with the Epipen, he said he did not feel it, complained that he felt worse, and continued to request a shot. Because she had no more injectors, she administered the Epipen in his thigh a second time. Although it felt to her as though it fired a second time, he said he was unable to feel the second shot. He could not catch his breath and said, "I am going." Then his eyes rolled upward and he lost consciousness. He went into arrest. CPR was initiated by the doctor and physician's assistant. Although they were able to get a weak pulse briefly, there were no respirations. The ambulance arrived, and the doctor, believing that the physician's assistant was really also a doctor, let him accompany the decedent to the hospital. Despite further resuscitation efforts in the ambulance and at the hospital, he never regained consciousness and died the next day.

His widow sued the nurse and doctor, alleging negligence, including gross willful and wanton negligence in rendering medical assistance to the decedent. The nurse allegedly responded inadequately to the medical emergency by arriving at the scene without any medical equipment, thus delaying the epinephrine administration. The doctor allegedly responded inadequately to the decedent's condition by failing to initially bring any medical equipment with her, failing to administer sufficient epinephrine, failing to establish an adequate airway, failing to check on the medical equipment available in the first aid tent, and failing to accompany the decedent in the ambulance.

Both the nurse and doctor filed motions for summary judgment based upon Rhode Island's Good Samaritan statute, which were granted by the trial court. The court found that they were medical volunteers rendering gratuitous services and therefore entitled to the protection of the Rhode Island Good Samaritan statute. The court further found that the facts did not support an action for negligence, much less gross negligence. The plaintiff appealed, and the Rhode Island Supreme Court ruled in favor of the defendants. The plaintiff failed to provide any expert evidence to support the professional negligence claims against the health care providers. The Rhode Island Supreme Court noted that there must be expert testimony to establish the prevailing standard of care and proof of failure to meet the standard and that the negligence was the proximate cause of the patient's injury. The judgment of the trial court was affirmed.

The defense of the nurse and doctor was based upon the state's Good Samaritan statute. In 1995, the Rhode Island statute was amended to include the term "anaphylactic shock":

> No person who voluntarily and gratuitously renders emergency assistance to a person in need thereof including the administration of life-saving treatment to those persons suffering from anaphylactic shock shall be liable for civil damages which result from acts or omissions by such persons rendering the emergency care, which may constitute ordinary negligence. (R.I. Gen. Laws, 1956)[46]

The addition of the term "anaphylactic shock" to this law was a direct result of the *Boccasile* case.[47] Each state has its own Good Samaritan statute, which tend to vary somewhat from state to state. Most of these statutes require that, for the law to be invoked, an emergency situation must exist and the provider of care must act in "good faith."[48]

The current state of the law suggests that if nurses render professional nursing services to a person, even though on a free-of-charge and volunteer basis, they could be held professionally liable for [professional] negligence.

As the *Boccasile* case illustrates, it is important for nurses to become familiar with the Good Samaritan statute in the state in which they practice. However, even with the protection afforded by this statute, it will most likely apply only to emergency situations. If a care situation arose which was not considered "emergent," nurses would not receive this protection. Not all of the volunteer activities in which nurses engage will involve emergency situations.

Nurses frequently volunteer to conduct health screenings, such as blood pressure or blood sugar checks, at community events. These activities usually also include health education by the nurses concerning various diseases. If they participate in these screenings, nurses should have set parameters for which referrals to physicians or even emergency rooms are necessary. Nurses could potentially be held liable if they detect an abnormality at a health screening and do not provide appropriate follow-up and referral for the patient.

The current state of the law suggests that if nurses render professional nursing services to a person, even though on a free-of-charge and volunteer basis, they could be held professionally liable for negligence. The professional liability insurance provided by nurses' employers does not cover volunteer activities outside of the scope of the nurses' job responsibilities. It would be prudent for nurses who engage in volunteer nursing activities to carefully evaluate purchasing a personal professional liability insurance policy, which might cover them in these situations. Nurses must be aware that, even with a charitable intent, volunteer nursing activities can involve professional liability.

SCHOOL NURSING

School nursing is a well-established and significant specialty of community-based nursing practice. School nursing began in the United States in 1902, when a nurse named Lina Rogers was placed in four New York City schools. She and 25 additional nurses who were hired one month later reduced the number of children who were excluded from school for communicable diseases from over 10,000 in September 1902 to a little over 1,000 in September 1903.[49] School nursing has steadily evolved since its inception, so that today school nurses function as public health nurses for the school population. It is not uncommon for school nurses to provide such highly technical services as blood glucose level monitoring, catheterizations, and even tracheostomy and ventilator care for their students. School nurses are independent practitioners and are commonly the only health care providers whom the student sees on a regular basis.[50]

School nurses are granted certain immunities similar to those of public health nurses, which were discussed previously. State tort immunity statutes apply to school districts and their employees as local governmental units. These statutes grant immunity from prosecution to school district employees, including nurses, for ordinary negligence. These statutes do not provide immunity for "willful and wanton" negligence, which is commonly defined as a reckless disregard for the student's safety. School nurses should become familiar with the governmental tort immunity statute in the state in which they practice, to determine the immunities which specifically apply to their own state and situation. In addition, a review of the state's school code, which may also grant immunities, is important.

Screenings

School nurses currently provide a multitude of health services to a diverse population of students. They monitor mandated immunizations and exclude students from school if they do not meet the local and state immunization requirements. They provide health counseling and education on a variety of different issues. They are responsible for assisting in ensuring a safe school environment. They communicate with and make referrals to community-based resources, such as the local and state health departments and boards.[51]

School nurses perform yearly state-mandated screenings of vision, hearing, height, weight, and scoliosis. If abnormalities are detected, and the student's parents are not notified, the nurses may encounter possible liability. In *Koltes v. Visting Nurses Association,*[52] a student brought a personal injury action against his grade school and high school, claiming that the schools negligently failed to notify his parents that he had scoliosis. The spinal condition was revealed during periodic screenings conducted by licensed nurses at the schools. These nurses were employed by the V.N.A., which had contracted with the county to provide health services to the schools. The trial court granted the schools' motion for summary judgment and held as a matter of law that the schools did not have a duty to supervise the V.N.A. nurses who were not their employees, nor did the schools need to take any affirmative steps to ensure that the nurses were carrying out their professional responsibilities to inform the student's parents of the scoliosis which was discovered during the periodic screenings. The Nebraska Supreme Court affirmed the trial court's decision and found that there was no agency relationship between the schools and the V.N.A. The nurses were licensed professionals who were performing services pursuant to a contractual agreement between the V.N.A. and the county, and the schools had a right to rely upon V.N.A. and its nurses to perform their duties in a competent manner. The V.N.A. was held vicariously liable for the actions of its nurses in not notifying the student's parents about his scoliosis. If these nurses had been employed by the schools, the case against the schools would not have been dismissed in this manner. School nurses must keep in mind that students' parents must be notified of abnormal findings discovered in health screenings.

Medication Administration

Another service which school nurses provide is medication administration and monitoring. Increasingly, students receive long-term medication treatment for disorders such as seizures, attention deficit disorders, and diabetes. State law governs the administration of medications in schools, but some states do not have explicit regulations on the subject. Schools should develop policies and procedures for the administration of medications during school hours with the input of school nurses. Nurses should take certain precautions with medications in schools: they should not give medication with which they are unfamiliar; medications should be carefully labeled to avoid giving them to

the wrong student; and administered medication should be noted daily in the student's health record.[53]

Skilled Nursing Care

School nurses provide skilled nursing care and case management for students with special health care needs, including individualized health care plans. Various trends have contributed to making the public school system more accessible to students with long-term health care needs. Technological advances have not only prolonged the lives of children with disabilities and chronic illnesses but have also facilitated their ability to function in the community. Insurance policies, federal mandates, and federal and state case law require that children with long-term care needs are to be given services in the least restrictive environment possible. Some of the most frequently occurring health care needs are medication administration, diapering, and respiratory treatments. The most common medical conditions requiring services are asthma, attention deficits, and seizures. The most frequently occurring chronic conditions encountered by school nurses with students are asthma, hearing loss, learning disabilities, migraines, seizures, attention deficit disorders, and diabetes.[54]

A student's chronic illness can also be exacerbated by injury, which may be difficult for the school nurse to detect. In *Hopkins v. Spring Independent School District,*[55] an elementary school student with cerebral palsy was left unsupervised in a classroom. She was pushed into a stack of chairs by another student and received a severe blow to the head. When the teacher returned to the classroom, she was told of the incident. The student claimed she had mild convulsions, cold sweats, and became dazed and incoherent. She remained in the classroom until the occupational therapist took her to therapy. The student told the occupational therapist that she had a headache, and the therapist took her to the school nurse. The school nurse told the student that she should remain in school and did not notify her parents. At the end of the day, the student got on the school bus and had severe convulsions on the bus. The bus driver radioed his supervisor to have a school nurse at the next bus stop, but one was not provided. The driver was told to take the student to her day care center as usual, and after she arrived there, she received treatment. Her mother filed suit against the school district, nurse, teacher, driver, and principal for personal injuries and decreased life expectancy for her daughter due to their alleged negligence. The trial court granted motions for summary judgment for all of the defendants, including the nurse. The Texas Appellate Court affirmed and based its decision on the Texas Tort Claims Act, which provided that local governmental units and their employees acting in governmental capacities were immune from prosecution for their alleged negligence resulting in bodily injuries or death.

Assistive Personnel

In order to provide services to students with complex health care needs and contain costs, school districts are hiring caregivers who are less expensive than registered nurses. These caregivers are referred to as unlicensed assistive personnel (UAPs), nursing assistants or aides, or health technicians.[56] In 1995, the National Association of School Nurses drafted a position paper which states that the school nurse has the sole responsibility and authority within the school setting to delegate nursing services which promote the health and safety of children. State law, national standards, local policies, and the judgment of the nurse govern the structure and process of this delegation. The National Council of State Boards of Nursing has also taken the position that UAPs should assist registered nurses but not replace them. According to council guidelines, it is inappropriate for an employer to require registered nurses to delegate duties when, in the nurses' professional judgment, it is unsafe to do so.[57] It remains the responsibility of the school nurse to delegate tasks appropriately to these assistive personnel.

While UAPs can supply clerical help and perform tasks as delegated by the school nurse, it is the [school] nurse who remains responsible for the care delivered to the student.

If the actions or inactions of the assistive personnel result in harm to a student, the school nurse could incur professional liability. In *Nance v. Matthews*,[58] the child was a disabled student in an elementary school. The child had recent bladder surgery and needed to be catheterized at school on a particular day. Although the aide was informed of the need to catheterize the student, she failed to do so. The mother of the student filed an action against the aide, the school nurse, the school principal, and the supervisor of special education for damages from injuries arising from the aide's refusal to catheterize the student. The mother alleged that the aide was guilty of negligence and willful and wanton conduct toward the student. She further alleged that the school nurse, principal, and supervisor of special education negligently supervised the aide in her care of the student. The trial court dismissed the claims against all of the defendants except the aide, based upon their qualified immunity as public employees under the Alabama state constitution. The appellate court affirmed, but the case did proceed against the aide. Without the immunity afforded to the school nurse by this particular state law, the nurse could very well have been found liable for negligent supervision of the aide. School nurses are well advised to use care in supervising and delegating tasks to assistive personnel. While UAPs can supply clerical help and perform tasks as delegated by the school nurse, it is the nurse who remains responsible for the care delivered to the student.[59]

Emergency Care

The area of school nursing which holds the most potential for professional liability is that of acute and emergency care. School accidents and injuries are one of the most common reasons for which students visit the school nurse. The school nurse must be capable of providing good emergency care and also be able to determine which injuries are minor and which require referral for medical treatment.[60] There are numerous cases in which the school nurse's care of the student's injuries form the basis of liability. In *Peck v. Board of Education of City of Mount Vernon*,[61] a student's parents brought a wrongful death action against the Mount Vernon Board of Education, a teacher, and the school nurse. Their son was accidentally kicked in the head in gym class. He complained of pain and dizziness but had no loss of consciousness. He was admitted to the hospital within two hours after the accident, where he eventually died from a skull fracture and cranial bleed. The jury rendered a verdict in favor of the parents, and the defendants appealed. The appellate court found that there was insufficient evidence to support a finding that the defendants unreasonably delayed the student's medical treatment, or that the delay was causally related to his death, and dismissed the case.

In *Kersey v. Harbin*,[62] a 13-year-old student became involved in a fight with his classmate on the way to gym class. He either fell or was dropped on the floor, and asked to see the school nurse. The nurse found no apparent sign of extreme injury and allowed the student to return to gym class. The student became worse; he returned to the nurse's office, and the nurse called his parents. His parents took him to his doctor, and he died shortly thereafter of a skull fracture with massive cerebral hemorrhage. The parents brought a wrongful death action against the school nurse, two gym teachers, the principal, and the superintendent of public schools. The school nurse filed a motion for summary judgment, which was granted due to insufficient evidence by which to prove a case of negligence against her.

In *Duross v. Freeman*,[63] a middle school student was in a science class which was supervised by the science teacher. She participated in an experiment with potassium hydroxide, a caustic chemical compound. The chemical was crystalline and did not burn until it interacted with the moisture of her skin. Because it was an alkaline substance, the effects of the burn were not felt until the injury had progressed. Later in the day, the student went to the school nurse but allegedly there was not time to treat her. By the time she reached home, the injury was severe, and her parents immediately took her for medical treatment. The parents brought suit on behalf of the student against the school nurse and the science teacher for delay in treating the injury and negligent supervision of the science class. They claimed that the student received severe, permanent, disabling, and disfiguring injuries, requiring future reconstructive surgery. The trial court granted the defendants' motion for summary judgment and dismissed the case. The appellate court affirmed and held that the student was precluded from pursuing negligence claims against the nurse and teacher based upon the immunities provided under the Texas Education Code.

In *Cook v. Hubbard Exempted Village Board of Education*,[64] a high school student's ankle was hurt in a fight. He was assessed by the school nurse, who did not suspect a fracture and did not call an ambulance. The student was picked up by a family member and later taken to a hospital where he was diagnosed with a fractured ankle. The student and his parents brought suit against the school nurse, the principal, and the board of education. The trial court granted the defendants' motions for summary judgment and dismissed the case against them. The appellate court affirmed and noted that the Ohio State Governmental Tort Immunity Statute provided that school district employees were not liable unless their conduct was reckless or wanton, or their actions were made in bad faith or led to additional injury to the student. The court held that the school nurse's actions fell within the scope of the statutory immunity provided by the state and precluded the student's case against her.

In *Grandalski v. Lyons Township High School District 204*,[65] a 15-year-old high school student was injured when she fell on her head while performing a gymnastics maneuver in physical education class. The student had taken gymnastics training since she was 3 years old. She was performing the maneuver in which she was injured on her own and not at her teacher's request. After her fall, she complained of pain. The school nurse came to the gym, examined her, and found that she had no numbness or tingling and could move all her extremities. The nurse took the student to her office in a wheelchair and called her mother. Her mother took her to the emergency room, where she was diagnosed with a cervical fracture and eventually underwent a spinal fusion. The parents brought suit against the school district on the student's behalf, alleging, among other things, that the nurse and teacher were negligent in their medical treatment of their daughter. The specific allegations of negligence concerning the nurse were that she failed to immobilize the student's neck, failed to properly assess the neck injury, and failed to request an ambulance to transport her to the hospital. The trial court granted the school district's motion to dismiss based upon the immunity provided under the Illinois Local Governmental and Governmental Employee's Tort Immunity Act. The appellate court affirmed the dismissal of the case.

These cases illustrate various situations in which school nurses are called upon to exercise considerable professional judgment in a nonmedical setting. When confronted with student accidents and injuries, school nurses must assess the situation to determine if the student requires treatment and/or transfer for medical attention. In assessing and rendering care for traumatic injuries, school nurses will be held to an emergency nursing standard of care. The majority of school nurses' potential liability in the lawsuits which are filed seems to be based upon underassessing the severity of the student's injuries and not transferring the student for medical attention. Even though nurses who are employees of public school districts are granted certain immunities from lawsuits based upon ordinary professional negligence, school nurses must be certain to provide nursing care to students consistent with established standards of school nursing practice.

ETHICS CONNECTION 19–2

School nurses are in a unique position to influence the health of children, their families, and communities. School nurses frequently confront issues including substance abuse, child abuse and neglect, tobacco smoking, teenage pregnancy, sexually transmitted diseases, and violence committed by children. Apart from working to prevent and manage such health issues, school nurses are challenged to practice ethically by balancing benefits and burdens of some commonly encountered issues. One of the most difficult of these issues is determining the limits and boundaries of confidentiality. Respecting the children's and families' privacy while deciding what confidential information should be disclosed and to whom is an ethical concern for school nurses.

In the United States, the age of majority for health care decision making is 18, although in some states, exceptions are made for mature and/or emancipated minors. This chronological determination of decisional capacity is an area where ethics and law differ somewhat. "No reliable or validated test presently exists to determine whether any individual of any age has the capacity to make decisions in any particular situation."[1] Consequently, there is a continuum of positions on moral involvement of parents and children about the children's health care decisions. At one extreme, parents are considered to be the exclusive moral agents for their own children.[2] At the other extreme, proponents of children's moral rights argue that even young children have a right to participate in decisions that affect them.[3,4] School nurses recognize that decisional capacity is a developmental process that includes many factors, including cognitive, psychological, economic, and moral factors. Some young children are able to make responsible decisions regarding self-disclosure of disorders such as epilepsy, for example, while some 18-year-olds do not exercise responsible moral judgment regarding protected sexual activity, use of recreational drugs, or bringing weapons to school.

Such a broad span of individual children's decisional capacity coupled with federal and state legislation and school board and institutional policies and practices require very skilled ethical comportment on the part of school nurses. They must prudently and reflectively balance the benefits and burdens of disclosure, especially when the public health and well-being are concerned. Teen pregnancy and substance abuse are examples of public health concerns in which balancing benefits and burdens of disclosure is necessary. Morally, health care providers—including school nurses—counsel the children or adolescents to self-report but may warn that if the child does not self-disclose, the nurse will need to report the situation to the appropriate individuals or agencies.

School nurses are becoming more involved in prevention of the common mental, physical, and social health problems of school-age children. They work collaboratively with classroom teachers, Parent Teacher Associations, school boards, health departments, and other community groups to develop educational and screening programs. Although most school nurses tend to have very heavy workloads and little time for communicating with one another, the National Association of School Nurses (NASN) maintains an active Internet Web site.[5] Standards of practice, educational forums, and position statements on school nursing and school health are available through the NASN site, as well as the table of contents of recent issues of the *Journal of School Nursing*. This journal recently added a column on legal and ethical issues for school nurses.

---

[1] Jeremy Sugarman. *20 Common Problems: Ethics in Primary Care.* St. Louis: McGraw-Hill, 2000.

[2] L. F. Ross. *Children, Families, and Health Care Decision-Making.* Oxford, UK: Oxford University Press, 1998.

[3] J. Holt. *Escape from Childhood.* New York: Dutton, 1974.

[4] H. Cohen. *Equal Rights for Children.* Totowa, N.J.: Rowman and Littlefield, 1980.

[5] See the National Association of School Nurses Web site: http://www.nasn.org/ Two federal sites also are important for school nurses and children: http://www.cdc.gov/nccdphp/dash/guide.htm includes School Health Program Guidelines and http://www.hhs.gov/kids has topics of interest for "kids" and adults.

Child Abuse and Neglect

Another area in which school nurses have legal responsibilities is in assessing for and reporting child abuse and neglect. All states have child abuse and neglect statutes, which include nurses among those groups of professionals who must report known abuse, even if the child or parent requests confidentiality. Failure to report child abuse can subject the nurse to civil and/or criminal penalties. In many cases, school nurses will be in a unique position to first identify abuse and/or neglect in the students with whom they work. They provide the first line of defense in recognizing and reporting child abuse and neglect, due to the daily nature of their contacts with students. School nurses should become familiar with the child abuse and neglect statutes in the state in which they practice, to ensure a working knowledge of their required reporting procedures.

School nursing will continue to provide an ever-increasing multitude and diversity of health-related services to students of all ages and backgrounds. It is the most significant of the community-based nursing specialties in contributing to the health and well-being of children and adolescents.

OCCUPATIONAL HEALTH NURSING

Occupational health nursing is another significant specialty of community-based nursing practice. Nurses serve in various roles in diverse types of work environments, from small companies to large industries. Some common legal issues which confront nurses in this specialty are workers' compensation, workplace safety, the Occupational Safety and Health Act (OSHA), and confidentiality.

Workers' Compensation

Workers' compensation acts are state laws. These statutes provide compensation to workers for job-related injuries sustained as a result of their employment, without having to prove fault on the part of the employer. When an employee sustains an on-the-job injury, that employee may be eligible for compensation whether or not the employer was at fault. Workers' compensation acts are based upon the relationship between the employee and the employer, rather than negligence. An employee

who is entitled to a workers' compensation award is barred from bringing a negligence action against the employer, which serves as a shield against liability for the employer. In return for compensation that is certain, the employee gives up the right to sue the employer for damages. The compensation, or award, which the employee receives is typically lower than that which he or she might have received from a jury, but the award is more certain.[66] The requirements for an employee to collect compensation are straightforward: (1) there must be an employer-employee relationship; (2) the injury or illness must be one covered by the compensation act; and (3) there must be a connection between the injury and the employment.[67]

Occupational health nurses may be open to liability for injuries which are compensated under workers' compensation acts. This would depend upon the nurse's status as either an employee or an independent contractor, and if the workers' compensation statute in the state protects fellow employees from separate liability. Nurses who are considered independent contractors can be sued for negligence in treating employees, even if the employee's injuries are covered by workers' compensation.[68]

In *McDaniel v. Sage,*[69] the Indiana appellate court held that a nurse employed by the company acted as an independent contractor when the nurse administered an injection to a company employee. The employee's medical malpractice action against the nurse was not precluded by the "fellow employee" rule of Indiana's Worker Compensation Act. The court found that the nurse's liability arose from the nurse-patient relationship with the employee and not the employer-employee relationship which the Worker Compensation Act was designed to regulate.

Other jurisdictions have held that nurses are fellow employees and acting within the scope of their job description in rendering care to employees. In this capacity, the workers' compensation act would bar an independent medical negligence action against the nurse. In *Jenkins v. Sabourin,*[70] an employee was injured by a fellow employee on the job and received care from nurses at the employer's clinic. The Wisconsin Supreme Court held that the employees were prohibited from bringing a third-party action against the employer for contribution in the negligence suit. The exclusivity of the remedy of the worker compensation act barred an action for negligence against the employer for the medical attention which was provided to the injured employee. The court found that the function of providing medical care to employees was undertaken by the employer because of the employment relationship. Therefore, the employee was prohibited from maintaining a separate negligence suit against the employer for the actions of the nurses.

Occupational health nurses may become involved in rendering care to employees who have been injured on the job. Thorough and complete documentation of the extent of the injury and the care rendered is absolutely essential. Nurses should become familiar with the workers' compensation act in the state in which they practice. They should also determine whether their role as a nurse is considered to be that of an independent contractor or a fellow employee for purposes of professional liability, separate from the state workers' compensation act.

Workplace Safety

Occupational health nurses are frequently charged with the responsibility of monitoring the safety of the workplace. This includes not only the assessment of physical conditions in the workplace but also providing education to the employees concerning safety practices. In *Rounds v. Standex International*,[71] the New Hampshire Supreme Court held that the duty to maintain a safe workplace rests exclusively with the employer, and the employer's duty is nondelegable.

The employer cannot mandate that an employee work in a place or conditions which pose objectively substantial risks of death, disease, or serious bodily injury to the employee. In *Parsons v. United Technologies Corporation*,[72] an employee was allowed to bring a wrongful discharge claim against his former employer for terminating him because he refused to work under unsafe conditions. The employer was a corporation which manufactured, distributed, and serviced helicopters, and the employee was an instructor of aircraft maintenance. The employer assigned the employee to a work project located at a military installation in an independent sheikhdom in the Persian Gulf. The military installation had been serving as a staging ground for allied warplanes during the Persian Gulf War. The employee refused the work assignment due to safety concerns and a travel advisory which had been issued by the U.S. State Department, and he was immediately terminated by the employer. The Supreme Court of Connecticut held that the employee could state a claim that he had been wrongfully discharged in violation of public policy requiring employers to provide a safe workplace.

In some jurisdictions, the responsibility for workplace safety rests jointly with both the employer and the employee. In *Whittaker v. McClure*,[73] a worker's injury was found to have been substantially caused by her willful violation of a safety rule. The Supreme Court of Kentucky imposed a penalty reduction in the award paid to the employee by the employer. The court found that according to the Kentucky Occupational Health and Safety Act (KOSHA), the responsibility for workplace safety is shared by employers and employees. The employer's obligation is to provide a place of employment that is free from recognized hazards to employees' health and safety. The employees' obligation is to comply with health and safety provisions.

Occupational health nurses serve a dual role in workplace safety. They assess the workplace for unsafe or hazardous conditions and serve as a catalyst in rectifying these dangers. Additionally, they monitor the employees in their work situations to determine whether they comply with the employer's rules and regulations related to health and safety.

The Occupational Safety and Health Act (OSHA)

The Occupational Safety and Health Act of 1970 (OSHA)[74] was enacted by Congress to assure safe and healthful working conditions for all workers in the United States. This federal law covers nearly all workers and requires the employer to protect employee safety, to maintain records concerning employee health and safety, and to report employee injury, illness, or death due to work-related causes. The states may regulate workplace safety issues which are not already addressed by an existing federal standard. However, for any workplace safety issues for which an OSHA standard is in effect, the state law is preempted by OSHA.[75]

The identity of a person who files a complaint under OSHA is confidential, and the name is protected from release. In addition, the Act prohibits an employer from retaliating against an employee for making a report to the Occupational Safety and Health Administration, which enforces the Act.

Occupational health nurses must have a working familiarity with OSHA rules and regulations, and how they apply to their particular workplace. They should also become familiar with any additional state statutes which regulate workplace safety in the state in which they practice.

Confidentiality

Many employers require that medical examinations and drug testing be completed on individuals prior to employing them. Depending upon the job and the employer, employees will also periodically be given medical examinations and drug testing during the course of their employment. Occupational health nurses are usually involved in the employee examination, testing, and screening process. Confidentiality of patient information is a key concern, and the employee-patient must be able to trust the occupational health nurse to maintain confidentiality. A nurse could be held liable by a patient for invasion of privacy by the public disclosure of private information. However, this does not include sharing information with other health care providers who are directly involved in the patient's care.[76]

The American Association of Occupational Health Nurses (AAOHN) Code of Ethics states: "The occupational health nurse strives to safeguard the employee's right to privacy by protecting confidential information and releasing information only upon written consent of the employee or as required by law."[77] Problems can arise as to how much information should be released to the employer. Many times, the occupational health nurse is expected to provide the employer with all of the medical information which is related to the employee's job duties.[78] The nurse must carefully determine what information, if any, is necessary to provide. It would be prudent for the nurse to obtain a signed release of information from the employee prior to providing information to the employer.

Confidentiality of patient information is a key concern, and the employee-patient must be able to trust the occupational health nurse to maintain confidentiality.

However, there are circumstances in which private and confidential patient information must be released. State public health codes require reporting the occurrence of communicable and sexually transmitted diseases to state departments of public health. State statutes also mandate reporting child and elder abuse to the state agency responsible for protecting minors. The Occupational Safety and Health Act, and the regulations to enforce the Act, may require the release of information about individual patients, and both contain standards for access to patients' medical records.[79]

Occupational health nurses should become familiar with what employee-patient information may be disclosed to the employer in their own particular workplace situation. Nurses should also become familiar with the state and federal statutes which mandate reporting of confidential information in the state in which they practice. In addition, the occupational health nurse must also be familiar with his or her responsibilities in maintaining the confidentiality of employee health data. Prior to releasing any confidential employee-patient information, nurses should obtain a written, signed consent for release of information from the patient. The release should designate what information may be released and to whom, and the form should be retained by the nurse.[80]

In the future, occupational health nurses will continue to serve in many important roles related to employee safety and wellness. As the workplace in the United States continues to change demographically, so too will the role of occupational health nursing in response to these workers' needs.

ELDER CARE NURSING

Nurses in the community will frequently encounter and help to care for the elderly. One of the dominant demographic trends in the United States in the 20th century has been the aging of the population. The elderly are the fastest growing segment in the U.S. population, and the percentage of elderly is projected to reach 21.8% by the year 2030. The proportion of those over 85 years old is growing faster than the number of elderly in general, and the elderly population is predominantly female.[81] As a group, the elderly are more likely than younger patients to have some form of interaction with the legal system. The legal issues which most affect older adults are elder abuse and neglect, the process of guardianship, and the use of physical restraints by caregivers. It is extremely important for nurses who work with the elderly to have some familiarity with these legal issues and processes.

Elder Abuse and Neglect

The elderly are often among the poorest, frailest, and most isolated members of the community. Many have limited financial resources, physical health, or competency—all of which provide ripe opportunities for physical, emotional, and financial abuse.[82] Despite congressional and scholarly estimates that 1 to 2 million cases of elder mistreatment occur every year, few cases are reported to state authorities, and only a minute number result in criminal prosecution or civil litigation.[83] The exact extent cannot be determined with precision, but elder abuse is at least as prevalent as child abuse and far less likely to be reported. Elder abuse occurs in all segments of the population, irrespective of race, sex, ethnicity, or socioeconomic background. It most often occurs in private residences against persons with limited contact with outsiders and thus remains a largely hidden problem.[84]

Mistreatment of the elderly is most commonly equated with physical abuse. However, it also includes less dramatic actions such as psychological or emotional abuse, financial exploitation, and neglect of caretaking obligations. Mistreatment is generally characterized as abuse or neglect. Whether behavior is labeled as abusive or neglectful may depend on the frequency, duration, and severity of the mistreatment. Abuse may encompass several types of behavior: physical abuse (nonaccidental physical pain or injury), psychological abuse (the willful infliction of severe mental anguish), and financial abuse (the unauthorized or exploitative use of funds, property, or resources). Neglect is generally defined as the willful or passive failure of caregivers to fulfill their caretaking duties. Self-neglect is conduct by an older person which threatens his or her own safety or health.[85]

The legal system protects the elderly in two ways. The first is through criminal laws which outlaw abuse and neglect and prescribe punish-

ments for it. The second is through legal mandates which require professionals to report reasonably suspected instances of abuse and neglect. Compliance with these mandatory reporting laws by nurses and other health professionals is critical in stemming the incidence of elder abuse.[86] In 1974, protective services for adults became a state-mandated program under Title XX of the Social Security Act. This created an Adult Protective Services system on the state level, which provides services for the elderly living in the community to maintain independence and avoid abuse and exploitation. These state-funded Adult Protective Services agencies are a primary referral source for reports of elder abuse and neglect. Presently, all 50 states have statutes specifically aimed at protecting the elderly. These statutes are very diverse, but typically have two components: (1) a coordinated provision of services for the elderly who are at risk, and (2) the actual or potential power of the state or local agencies to intervene to protect endangered individuals.[87]

Victims of elder abuse and neglect may be difficult to assist for a number of reasons.

Most states mandate that a wide variety of professionals, including nurses, report known or suspected cases of elder abuse, although a few states still make reporting voluntary. Mandatory reporting laws generally provide three things. First, certain professionals or any persons with a reasonable belief or suspicion of elder abuse are required to report that information to designated public authorities. Nurses are one of the designated groups of professionals who are required to report. Second, immunity from liability is provided for those who report in good faith. Third, reports of abuse initiate investigative and treatment services by Adult Protective Services or other agencies.[88] Almost all states guarantee anonymity or confidentiality to reporters of abuse. A failure to report elder abuse to public authorities can subject nurses and other designated professionals to criminal and civil liabilities. Disciplinary actions against nurses by the state licensing agency and malpractice suits can be brought for failure to report.

The perpetrators of elder abuse and neglect can be held both criminally and civilly liable. Some states now allow a civil case against a health care provider to be brought under the state's elder abuse laws. In *Delaney v. Baker*,[89] the daughter of a nursing home resident brought suit against the nursing home for both professional negligence and neglect under the state elder abuse statute. The plaintiff put her 88-year-old mother in a nursing home after she had fallen and fractured her ankle. Less than 4 months later, the mother died while still a resident at the nursing home. At the time of her death, she had Stage III and Stage IV decubitus ulcers on her ankles, feet, and buttocks. There were accusations that the patient had been frequently left lying in her own feces for an extended period of time. The alleged neglect was apparently partly the result of staffing shortages, rapid turnover of staff, and inadequate training of employees. There was evidence of numerous violations of medical monitoring and record-keeping regulations, which prevented necessary information from being transmitted to the patient's physician in a timely manner. The patient's daughter persistently complained to the nursing staff, administration, and a nursing home ombudsman about the neglect of her mother. The nursing home had been cited for patient neglect by the California Department of Health Services before the patient's admission. After this patient's death, the nursing home was given a Class A Citation and fined. (This citation is given only when the inadequate care would create a substantial probability that death or serious physical harm would result to the nursing home residents.)

The patient's daughter filed suit against the nursing home and two administrators on theories of negligence, willful misconduct, and neglect of an elder under California state law. The jury awarded damages to the plaintiff, and the defendants appealed. The California Supreme Court held that a health care provider who engages in reckless neglect of an elder adult is subject to the Elder Abuse Act. The health care provider can be held liable for elder abuse, and not simply professional negligence. To be held liable under the Elder Abuse Act, the plaintiff must prove by clear and convincing evidence that the defendant is guilty of recklessness, which is more than simple negligence. Recklessness is a conscious choice of a course of action with the knowledge of the serious danger to others involved in it. In order to be found guilty of neglect under the California Elder Abuse Act, the plaintiff must prove that the nursing home acted recklessly and not simply negligently.[90] The *Delaney* case reflects the fact that courts are beginning to hold health care providers liable for elder abuse and neglect under state abuse statutes, in addition to the providers' liability for professional negligence.

Victims of elder abuse and neglect may be difficult to assist for a number of reasons. They may be isolated in nursing homes or other institutions or at home from those who could assist them. They often are dependent upon their abusers for emotional and physical assistance. They may be unable to seek help due to dementia or other physical limitations.[91] Nurses and other health care professionals are in strategic positions in offices, clinics, hospitals, and community agencies where the elders and their caregivers may appear. They are in a unique position to identify the signs and symptoms of elder abuse and neglect. The professional nature of their relationship with the elderly patient increases the probability that the patient will confide in them if appropriate interviewing and screening techniques are utilized.[92] Nurses and other health professionals should take advantage of these opportunities to make a significant contribution to the treatment and prevention of elder abuse and neglect.

Nurses should become familiar with elder abuse and neglect statutes in the state in which they practice. They should have a working knowledge of how the statutes define abuse and neglect, and to whom suspected cases should be reported. They should also determine if it is mandatory to report elder abuse and/or neglect, and the civil or criminal penalties for not reporting. Finally, nurses should contribute their professional knowledge to help develop solutions for the prevention of elder abuse and neglect.

Guardianship

As the elderly continue to have longer lifespans, the incidence of their inability to function independently is also on the increase. It is estimated that currently, over 50% of cognitively impaired elders are cared for at home. If the elder has not made plans while competent and communicated his or her wishes to the appropriate persons, then a guardianship may be the only option available to handle the legal and financial decisions which must be made.[93] Guardianship arises under the power of each state to care for its citizens who cannot care for themselves. In cases where the elderly are unable to care for themselves, the state can appoint a guardian, most often a relative. If no suitable guardian is available, the state itself becomes the guardian of the elderly person, known as the ward. Guardianship is accomplished when a petitioner (usually a relative) asks the court to determine whether the elderly person is competent to handle his or her own affairs. If the court decides that the elder is not competent to do so, the judge will appoint a guardian who will have the duty and power to make decisions for the elder.[94]

A recent study conducted by Weisensee and others explored the problems and events which gave rise to filing for guardianships for the elderly. The ages of the petitioners ranged from 35 to 85, with 59 being the average. The majority of the petitioners were female and married. Their most common relationship to the elderly ward was daughter (23%), son (16.4%), and niece (11.5%). The ages of the elderly wards ranged from 65 to 99, with 84 being the average. The majority of the elderly wards were female and widowed.[95] The most frequent problems with the elderly ward which made the petitioners seek guardianship were memory problems (93%), difficulty holding a sensible conversation (78%), problems with financial matters (77%), needing help with bathing and dressing (77%), and needing help with cooking and household activities (60%).[96]

Guardianship arises under the power of each state to care for its citizens who cannot care for themselves.

Yet another recent study by Kjervik and others examined the "trigger" events which most frequently lead to the establishment of guardianships for the elderly. The most frequent classification was cognitive/emotional and included such things as problems with management of finances, confusion, refusal of assistance, inability to recognize their own lawyer, falling, burning themselves, bizarre behavior, and unsanitary living conditions and poor hygiene. The second most frequent classification of "trigger" events was situational and

included such things as loss of a caregiver, hospital-mandated guardianship because of surgery, being a victim of unscrupulous persons, and preservation of the person's estate. The least frequent classification was physical, which were all medically related.[97] This study concluded that if the elderly person's mind was intact, there was usually no need to seek guardianship.[98]

Guardianship becomes necessary when events and behaviors such as those listed above threaten the well-being of the elderly person. However, as a legal mechanism, it severely limits the person's autonomy. When a person is declared incompetent and a guardian is appointed, the ward loses many rudimentary rights. These include the right to marry or divorce; to vote; to make or revoke a will; to manage his or her own money; to drive; to buy, sell, or lease property; to decide where to live; and to consent to or refuse medical treatment.[99]

The specific process of guardianship is controlled by the law of each individual state. Even so, there are many similarities in the processes. The process is initiated when a petition for guardianship is filed with the court. The majority of states allow "any interested person" to file the petition for guardianship. Illinois, for example, allows any "reputable" person to file a petition, and the statute does not indicate a preference for a family member, state social agency, or medical practitioner.[100] Even elderly people themselves can file petitions on their own behalf.

The person who files the petition requesting guardianship need not be the person who would serve as guardian if the elderly person is found to be incapacitated. The standards for who may serve as petitioner and who may serve as guardian are not the same.[101] In Illinois, a guardian is required to be 18 or older, a U.S. resident, "not of unsound mind," not adjudged disabled (that is, not a ward), free of felony convictions, and one whom the court finds is capable of providing an active and suitable program of guardianship.[102]

The alleged disabled person has the constitutional right to be given notice that guardianship proceedings have been initiated. Most state statutes include this right to notice. Illinois, for example, requires that the person about whom the guardianship proceedings have been initiated be personally served with the summons and copy of the petition at least two weeks prior to the hearing.

Many states require notice also be given to the person's close family as well.[103]

Many states, such as Illinois, require that a report be filed with the petition for guardianship. This report must include certain information which will help the judge determine whether the elderly person is incapacitated. This information includes a description of the disability; a recent physical and mental evaluation; an opinion about the scope of the proposed guardianship; and the signatures of all the persons who evaluated the disabled person, one of whom must be a licensed physician. There is no requirement that the elderly person who is the subject of the report receive a copy of it.[104]

The elderly person who is alleged incompetent has a right to be represented by an attorney in the guardianship proceedings. In most states, the judge will appoint an attorney to represent the elderly person, either at that person's request or upon the judge's decision that the person would be best served by having one. The attorney's role is to represent the elderly person and pursue his or her wishes.[105] In addition to appointing an attorney to represent the elderly person, the judge may also appoint a *guardian ad litem*. This is a second attorney who independently evaluates the elderly person and the situation and advises the judge as to the person's ability to manage his or her affairs or estate. If the guardian *ad litem* determines that the elderly person is not competent to handle his or her own affairs, the *guardian ad litem* will recommend to the judge how the person's affairs should be handled.[106]

When an individual requires the appointment of a guardian, the person is said to be "incompetent" or "incapacitated."

A court hearing is set before the judge, and evidence is presented by the petitioner and the elderly person. Various witnesses may testify as to the elderly person's condition and situation. The burden of proof required to prove incapacity or incompetence varies by state. In some cases, a jury may make the determination instead of a judge. The issue to be decided is whether the elderly person has the ability to care for his or her own person and estate. In Illinois, the statute directs the judge to inquire about the level of the person's general intellectual and physical functioning, the impairment of adaptive behavior in a person with a developmental disability, the nature and severity of any mental illness, the capacity of the person to make responsible decisions concerning his or her person, and the capacity of the person to manage his or her estate and financial affairs.[107]

When an individual requires the appointment of a guardian, the person is said to be "incompetent" or "incapacitated." This varies from state to state, but the current trend is to use "incapacitated." This term seems to carry less stigma and focuses more on the inability to manage one's affairs, unlike "incompetency," which suggests a mental deficiency.[108] If the elderly person is judged to be incapacitated or incompetent, the judge will appoint either a guardian or a conservator for him or her. A conservator is basically a limited guardian who only controls the elderly person's property, not the person. A guardian, if a plenary guardian, has the property power of the conservator as well as power over the elderly person himself or herself.[109] Most states require some type of reporting back to the court by the guardian as to the status of the ward. However, the frequency and depth of this reporting varies greatly from state to state, with no uniform standard.

Nurses who provide services to elderly patients may become involved in guardianship proceedings. An assessment that the elderly person is unable to care for his or her person may serve as the impetus to evaluate the situation in more depth. Nurses may be called upon to assist in identifying a potential guardian for the elderly person and possibly even to testify at the guardianship hearing. Nurses should become familiar with the guardianship process in the state in which they practice and local attorneys who have expertise in this area of the law.

Of particular concern is the inappropriate use of restrictive devices as a means of coercion, discipline, convenience, or punishment by caregivers.

Physical Restraints

The use of physical restraints by caregivers is becoming a more frequent issue with the elderly. Of particular concern is the inappropriate use of restrictive devices as a means of coercion, discipline, convenience, or punishment by caregivers. The Food and Drug Administration (FDA) estimates that at least 100 deaths from the improper use of restraints occur annually. There is also evidence that the use of restraints is associated with adverse effects such as longer hospitalizations, higher mortality and morbidity rates, and threats to a person's psycho-social well-being.[110]

For a number of years, there have been statutes governing the use of physical restraints. These statutes vary from state to state and may be included in various types of regulations. In Illinois, for example, the use of restraints for patients with mental health and developmental disabilities is governed by the Mental Health and Developmental Disabilities Code.[111] In addition, the Nursing Home Care Act contains requirements which govern when restraints are used in nursing homes.[112] The Joint Commission on Accreditation of Healthcare Organizations (JCAHO) also has restraint standards.[113]

In 1999, the Health Care Financing Administration (HCFA) promulgated an interim final rule concerning patients' rights.[114] The rule applies to all Medicare- and Medicaid-participating health care facilities, including short-term, long-term, rehabilitation, children's psychiatric, and alcohol-drug facilities. This interim final rule contains standards regarding restraints and seclusion, which are patterned after the JCAHO standards but go beyond the commission's requirements.[115]

According to the interim final rule, a physical restraint is defined as "any manual method or physical or mechanical device, material, or equipment attached or adjacent to the patient's body that they cannot easily remove that restricts freedom of movement or normal access to one's body."[116] A drug used as a restraint is defined as "a medication used to control behavior or to restrict the patient's freedom of movement and is not a standard treatment for the patient's medical or psychiatric condition."[117] Seclusion is defined as "the involuntary confinement of a person in a room or an area where the person is physically prevented from leaving."[118]

The two standards which specifically apply to restraints and seclusion are Standard #5—

Restraints in Acute Medical and Surgical Care, and Standard #6—Seclusion and Restraint for Behavior Management.[119] The drafters of these standards discovered a pattern of differences between an intervention used in the provision of acute medical and surgical care, and one used to manage behavioral symptoms. Therefore, these two situations are dealt with separately.

Standard #5—Restraints in Acute Medical and Surgical Care—provides that a restraint can be used only if needed to improve the patient's well-being, and less restrictive interventions were ineffective to protect the patient or others from harm. The restraint must be ordered by a physician or other licensed independent practitioner permitted by the state and hospital to order a restraint. The order cannot be either a standing one or a PRN one. If the restraint is not ordered by a patient's treating physician, a consultation about the restraint with that physician must occur as soon as possible, and there must be a written modification to the patient's plan of care. The restraint is to be implemented in the least restrictive manner possible, be in accordance with safe and appropriate restraining techniques, and end at the earliest possible time. The condition of the restrained patient must be continually assessed, monitored, and reevaluated. All staff having direct patient contact must have ongoing education in the proper and safe use of restraints.[120]

Standard #6—Seclusion and Restraint for Behavior Management—contains many of the same provisions as Standard #5. In addition, it discusses the use of seclusion and provides specific recommendations for the monitoring and evaluation of a patient who is secluded or restrained for behavior management. Seclusion or a restraint can be used only in emergency situations if needed to ensure the patient's physical safety, to protect the patient or others from harm, and when less restrictive interventions have been ineffective. The use of a restraint or seclusion must be pursuant to the order of a physician or other licensed independent practitioner permitted by the state and hospital to order seclusion or restraint. The standard sets forth requirements for the type and timing of orders, as well as notification of the patient's treating physician. These requirements may be superseded by existing state laws that are more restrictive. A restraint and seclusion may not be used simultaneously unless the patient is continually monitored by staff, either face to face or via video and audio

ETHICS CONNECTION 19–3

Nurses in the community generally work more autonomously and with less collegial support than do nurses in hospitals and medical center settings. Thus, ethical concerns in community nursing practice traditionally have tended to emphasize individual issues related to the dilemmas that nurses face in the delivery of health care. This focus, too, is changing. Ethics in community nursing practice is shifting away from individualistic ethics toward communitarian ethics. Increasing attention is being paid to the ethical stance of the community institutions, both for-profit and not-for-profit. Contrary to the strategy of expecting that individuals are responsible for the ethical character of their organizations,[1] McCurdy proposes a shared moral responsibility between individuals and their organizations that seems particularly apt in community nursing practice. Nurses in the community are embedded in complex sets of relationships. Case managers, for example, work with homemakers and other caregivers and organizations. To expect that the individual nurse is the primary moral agent in such a complex set of relationships disregards the moral nature of the institution. Community organizations can support or hinder the nurses' ethical comportment, depending upon what kind of ethical climate is created in the organization itself.[2]

Using community-based agencies that focus on health care services for elders, McCurdy presents some of the structures, processes, issues, and practices to be considered in developing "an ethical organization." To McCurdy, the term "ethical organization" means more than establishing and monitoring institutional and employee adherence to a code of conduct or a set of rules. It means continual reflection about moral responsibilities, including the issues that should be addressed, who within the institution and in the larger community should participate in the conversation about moral responsibilities, and an openness to reconsidering established practices as circumstances change. "Thus, above all, the ethical organization is one that is continually alert to and reflective about ethical questions, with an eye to establishing—where possible—standards or accepted ways of approaching issues, while also recognizing the provisional, reviewable nature of the standards and practices that it develops."[3] Such an organization provides community health nurses and others working in the community with a moral community within which to consider practice and policy issues.

Creating an ethics group, such as a committee or forum, is an important step in developing a moral community. McCurdy recommends that the ethics group, which should include nurses as members, develop a list of core "values and virtues" related to the organization's mission. In a home care agency that has a high population of elderly clients, for example, such values might include "client self-determination, client safety and protection, client dignity and self-respect, compassion, professionalism, family integrity, caring attitudes and practices, and stewardship of agency resources."[4]

The ethics group would have several functions, including the most important one of helping to create the general ethical climate in the organization, "moral ecology."[5] Part of the ethical climate would include how the organization treats its employees, especially those who are least well paid. In addition, the ethics group then could serve as ethical counselors to nurses and others in the community who have specific issues to address. Concerns of an agency that provides care to elders include boundary issues in which family members might be concerned that a homemaker is displacing the family or financially exploiting the client; issues of client safety and confidentiality, particularly when reporting elder abuse or neglect; and how to respect clients' self-determination when their living conditions are widely divergent from and unacceptable to the nurses.

Nurses in the community generally have a strong commitment to social justice, and an ethical community-based organization has a strong commitment to political advocacy. When nurses participate in creating an ethical organization, they are in a more powerful position to advocate for those in the community who are most vulnerable and underserved. This advocacy role is consistent with Interpretive Statement 11.2 of the *Code for Nurses with Interpretive Statements.* "For the benefit of the individual client and the public at large, nursing's goals and commitments need adequate representation. Nurses should ensure this representation by active participation in decision making in institutional and political arenas to assure a just distribution of health care and nursing resources."[6]

---

[1]As is the case in Interpretive Statement 11.2 of the *Code for Nurses with Interpretive Statements,* which obligates nurses to be moral agents regardless of their "employer policy directives." American Nurses Association. *Code for Nurses with Interpretive Statements.* Kansas City, MO: Author, 1985.

[2]David B. McCurdy. Creating an Ethical Organization. *Generations,* 22(3), 26–31 (Fall), 1998.

[3]*Id.*

[4]*Id.*

[5]*Id.*

[6]American Nurses Association, *supra* note 1.

equipment. The condition of the patient must be continually assessed, monitored, and reevaluated. All staff having direct patient contact must have ongoing education in the proper and safe use of seclusion and restraint application and techniques, and alternative methods for handling behaviors and situations which were traditionally handled with restraints and seclusion. If a patient dies while in restraints or seclusion, or where a patient's death is a result of restraint or seclusion, the facility must report this to the Health Care Financing Administration (HCFA).[121]

These two new standards have been designated by HCFA as minimum protections. Even more stringent protections may be found in state laws. Nurses who work with restraints and seclusion must become familiar with the institutional policy related to the use of restraint and seclusion in the facility in which they work. They should also become familiar with state statutes which govern the use of restraints in the state in which they practice.

The issue of elder abuse and neglect, the process of guardianship, and the use of physical restraints by caregivers are pertinent legal issues affecting the elderly. This is by no means an exhaustive list of legal issues which confront them. As the elderly population in the United States continues to increase, so too will the amount and variety of legal issues which confront them.

SUMMARY OF PRINCIPLES AND APPLICATIONS

The role of the nurse in the community is gaining more importance with each passing year. As the demographics of our society change, nurses are increasingly being called upon to fulfill roles which were once reserved to the patient's relatives. From elderly patients to schoolchildren, community-based nurses are being called upon to provide ever-increasing services and to act as advocates for their patients. These nurses are asked to provide increasingly more complex care and perform highly technological procedures. The explosive growth of information technology has changed the future of health care and will have far-reaching implications for the nurse in the community. As the roles of nurses in the community become increasingly independent and autonomous, there will be a commensurate increase in their responsibility, accountability, and potential liability. It is becoming increasingly important

for community-based nurses to understand the legal implications of their respective roles and the legal process as it pertains not only to the nurses but their patients as well.

Therefore, the following guidelines are important for the nurse in the community.

Nurses who work in home health care should:

- Take personal responsibility to maintain their own safety by practicing preventive actions
- Monitor patient and staff injuries, and address any problems to avoid future potential injuries
- Keep open lines of communication with the patient, family, and patient's physician
- Carefully orient, train, and supervise staff in the performance of their duties
- Become thoroughly trained and proficient in the performance of highly technological procedures and use of complex equipment, as well as train the patient and caregiver in these areas
- Be aware of changes in reimbursement for home services and standards for compliance
- Become familiar with the agency's policies and procedures in relation to termination of services to patients

Nurses who work in the area of public health should:

- Determine whether a state statute grants governmental tort immunity, and whether the agency for which the nurse works is considered to be a governmental entity to which this immunity would apply
- Be familiar with state and federal regulations concerning reporting of various diseases

Nurses who work in the area of telenursing should:

- Be familiar with the nurse practice act in the state in which they practice and how it applies to telephone triage nursing
- Obtain licensure in all of the states where they provide telenursing services, both the state in which they work and the states in which potential patients reside
- Check their professional liability insurance regarding coverage for telenursing activities

Nurses who serve as volunteers should:

- Become familiar with the Good Samaritan statute in the state in which they practice
- Set parameters for referrals to physicians and hospitals which will occur if they participate in health screenings

- Consider obtaining a personal professional liability insurance policy which would cover volunteer nursing activities

Nurses who work in schools should:

- Notify the student's parents of abnormal findings discovered in health screenings
- Take precautions with medications in schools by becoming familiar with the medications they are giving, carefully labeling each student's medication, and noting administered medication(s) in the student's health record
- Use care in supervising and delegating tasks to assistive personnel, and realize that the nurse remains responsible for the care delivered to the student
- When confronted with student accidents and injuries, carefully assess the situation and refer and transfer for medical attention, as well as notification of the parents
- Become familiar with the child abuse and neglect statutes in the state in which they practice, to ensure a working knowledge of their required reporting procedures

Nurses who work in occupational health should:

- Become familiar with the workers' compensation act in the state in which they practice, and determine whether their role as a nurse is considered to be that of an independent contractor or fellow employee for purposes of professional liability, separate from the workers' compensation act
- Assess the workplace for unsafe or hazardous conditions, and serve as a catalyst in rectifying these dangers
- Monitor employees in their work situations to determine whether they comply with their employer's rules and regulations related to health and safety
- Have a working familiarity with the Occupational Safety and Health Act rules and regulations, and how they apply to their particular workplace
- Become familiar with any additional state statutes which regulate workplace safety in the state in which they practice
- Become familiar with what employee-patient information may be disclosed to the employer in their own particular workplace situation
- Obtain the written consent for release of information from the employee-patient prior to releasing any confidential information

Community nurses who work with the elderly should:

- Become familiar with elder abuse and neglect statutes in the state in which they practice
- Have a working knowledge of how the statutes define abuse and neglect, and to whom suspected cases should be reported
- Become familiar with the guardianship process in the state in which they practice and with local attorneys who have expertise in this area of the law
- Become familiar with state and federal statutes which govern the use of restraints in the state in which they practice

TOPICS FOR FURTHER INQUIRY

1. Interview nurses in at least two states who work in the local public health agencies regarding their knowledge about what communicable diseases must be reported to the state public health department.

2. Research the various telenursing services available in the region in which you live, and determine if these services are covered by the state nurse practice act. If the services are not covered, identify needed changes in the act for inclusion of the services.

3. Contact nurses who volunteer to perform health screenings at a local health fair, and determine what parameters these nurses use to refer patients to physicians or hospitals for further care. Evaluate which parameters are consistent with acceptable standards of nursing practice.

4. Interview a school nurse to determine the amount and type of nursing care provided to students. Evaluate the school nurse's use of UAPs by determining what student care activities are delegated to these assistive helpers.

5. Research your state's statutes on the process of guardianship, and interview a local attorney who specializes in this area regarding how he or she believes the law works to protect an individual's rights during the guardianship process.

REFERENCES

1. Bonnie Faherty, "Medical Malpractice and Adverse Reactions Against Nurses: Five Years of Information from the National Practitioner Data Bank," 5(1) *Journal of Nursing Law* (1998), 20.
2. Mabel H. Smith-Pittman, "Nurses and Litigation: 1990–1997," 5(2) *Journal of Nursing Law* (1998), 12.
3. Linda J. Gobis, "Licensing and Liability: Crossing Borders with Telemedicine," *Caring Magazine* (July 1997), 18.

4. Gina M. Reese and Joseph H. Hafkenschiel, "Hot Topics in Home Health Care," 20 *Whittier Law Review* (1998), 366.

5. Kathleen M. Abbott, "Home Care and Nursing Risk Management," 3(3) *Journal of Nursing Law* (1996), 44.

6. See, for example, Visiting Nurses Association of Rockford, Ill., "Field Staff Safety," Administrative Policy No. 3.8.1 (Rev. 12/98).

7. See, for example, Visiting Nurses Association of Rockford, Ill., "Safety for Employees," Administrative Policy No. 3.8 (Rev. 12/98). See, generally, Fay Rozovsky, *Liability and Risk Management in Home Health Care.* Gaithersburg, Md.: Aspen Publishers, 1998.

8. Abbott, *supra* note 5, at 34.

9. No. 900901993; LPR Pub. No. 141680; UT 1994.

10. 678 So. 2d 447 (Fla. App. 2 Dist. 1996).

11. 708 So. 2d 1108 (La. App. 5 Cir. 1998).

12. No. 18743/84; LPR Pub. No. 152626; N.Y. 1994.

13. Abbott, *supra* note 5, at 46.

14. No. 127096; Verdictum Juris No. 10 Mar 127068, CA 1996.

15. Nancy J. Brent, "Risk Management and Legal Issues in Home Care: The Utilization of Nursing Staff," 28(8) *J.O.G.N.N.* (October 1994), 663. See also Rozovsky, *supra* note 7.

16. No. 91-1179; LPR Pub. No. 122690; FLA 1993.

17. Abbott, *supra* note 5, at 47.

18. 87 Or. App. 495, 742 P.2d 1190 (Or. App. 1987).

19. Abbott, *supra* note 5, at 45–46.

20. Reese and Hafkenschiel, *supra* note 4, at 374.

21. Marilyn D. Harris, "The Impact of the Balanced Budget Act of 1997 on Home Healthcare Agencies and Nurses," 16(7) *Home Healthcare Nurse* (July 1998), 436.

22. 42 C.F.R. Part 484, Section 484.55; 64 3784, Fed. Reg. January 25, 1999, Rules and Regulations.

23. Abbott, *supra* note 5, at 49.

24. William Dombi and Mary St. Pierre, "Interim Payment System and Risk Management," 18(6) *Caring Magazine* (June 1999), 35.

25. Elizabeth E. Hogue, "Child Neglect in Home Care: Weighing Legal and Ethical Issues," 19(5) *Pediatric Nursing* (Sept.–Oct. 1993), 497.

26. Dombi and St. Pierre, *supra* note 24, at 36.

27. Dombi and St. Pierre, *supra* note 24, at 37.

28. No. 842472; LPR Pub. No. 0072991; CA 1991.

29. Dombi and St. Pierre, *supra* note 24.

30. 462 So. 2d 689 (Miss. 1984).

31. 512 A.2d 796 (Pa. Commn. 1986).

32. 497 N.W.2d 551 (Mich. App. 1993).

33. 646 N.E.2d 1051 (Mass. 1995).

34. 671 S.W.2d 476 (Tenn. App. 1984).

35. Susan D. Laughlin, "Telenursing," 6(2) *Journal of Nursing Law* (1999), 43. See also American Nurses Association. *Competencies for Telehealth Technologies in Nursing.* Washington, D.C.: Author, 1999.

36. Carol M. Stock, "Standardization of Telephone Triage: Is It Time?" 2(2) *Journal of Nursing Law* (1995), 19.

37. Stock, *supra* note 36, at 19–20.

38. Gobis, *supra* note 3, at 19.

39. Laughlin, *supra* note 35, at 46.

40. Gobis, *supra* note 3, at 19.

41. Stock, *supra* note 36, at 23. See also American Nurses Association. *Core Principles on Telehealth.* Washington, D.C.: Author, 1998.

42. Laughlin, *supra* note 35, at 45–46.

43. Stock, *supra* note 36, at 23–24.

44. 718 A.2d 828 (Pa. Super. Ct. 1998).

45. 694 A.2d 686 (R.I.) 1997.

46. R.I. Gen. Laws Section 9-1-27.1 (1995).

47. Joyce K. Laben and Elizabeth G. Rudolph, "Volunteering for First-Aid Booths: Potential Liability?" 4(4) *Journal of Nursing Law* (1997), 54.

48. *Id.*

49. Sarah D. Cohn, "Legal Issues in School Nursing Practice," *Law, Medicine, & Health Care* (October 1984), 219.

50. Joan C. Borgatti, "School Nursing Today," *Nursing Spectrum* (July 12, 1999), 20.

51. *Id.* See also National Association of School Nurses. *School Nursing Practice: Roles and Standards.* Scarborough, Maine: Author, 1993.

52. 256 Neb. 740, 591 N.W.2d 578 (Neb. 1999).

53. American Association of School Nurses. *Medication Administration in the School Setting.* Scarborough, Maine: Author, 1997. The position statement can be accessed on the association's Web page at http://www.nasn.org.

54. Vivian E. Ott and Margaret J. Stafford, "Using Unlicensed Assistive Personnel in School Settings," 6(1) *Insight* (National Council of State Boards of Nursing) (Winter/Spring 1997), 1.

55. 706 S.W.2d 325 (Tex. App. 14 Dist. 1986). See also National Council of State Boards of Nursing. *Delegation Concepts and Decision-Making Process.* Chicago, Ill.: Author, 1995. The publication can be obtained on the council's Web site at http://www.ncsbn.org.

56. Ott and Stafford, *supra* note 54, at 1.

57. Ott and Stafford, *supra* note 54, at 11.

58. 622 So. 2d 297 (Ala. 1993).

59. Ott and Stafford, *supra* note 57.

60. See, generally, American Association of School Nurses. *Preparing a Response to Emergency Problems.* Scarborough, Maine: Author, 1998.

61. 30 N.Y.2d 700, 283 N.E.2d 618 (N.Y. Ct. App. 1972).

62. 591 S.W.2d 745 (Mo. App. 1979).

63. 831 S.W.2d 354 (Tex. App. - San Antonio 1992).

64. 116 Ohio App. 3d 564, 688 N.E.2d 1058 (Ohio App. 1996).

65. 711 N.E.2d 372 (Ill. App. 1 Dist. 1999).

66. Faye D. Ivey and Mark W. Morris, "Liability Issues for Occupational Health Nurses," 41(1) *AAOHN Journal* (January 1993), 18.

67. *Id.* at 19. See also Mark Rothstein, Charles Craver, Elinor Schroeder, and Elaine Shoben. *Employment Law.* Volume 2. 2nd Edition. St. Paul, Minn.: West Group, 1999, 1–193.

68. *Id.*

69. 419 N.E.2d 1322 (Ind. App. 1981).

70. 311 N.W.2d 600 (Wis. 1981).

71. 550 A.2d 98 (N.H. 1988).

72. 700 A.2d 655 (Conn. 1997).

73. 891 S.W.2d 80 (Ky. 1995).

74. 29 U.S.C. 651 (1970).

75. *Ben Robinson Company v. Texas Workers' Compensation Commission,* 934 S.W.2d 149, 158 (Tex. App. - Austin 1996).

76. Ivey and Morris, *supra* note 66, at 20.

77. AAOHN. *Code of Ethics.* Atlanta, Ga.: Author, August 1991.

78. Ivey and Morris, *supra* note 76.

79. Ivey and Morris, *supra* note 66. See also Mark Rothstein. *Occupational Safety and Health Law.* 4th Edition. St. Paul, Minn.: West Group, 1998 (with regular updates).

80. Ivey and Morris, *supra* note 66.

81. Seymour Moskowitz, "Saving Granny from the Wolf: Elder Abuse and Neglect—The Legal Framework," 31(77) *Connecticut Law Review* (1998), 85–86.

82. Suzanne J. Levitt and Rebecca J. O'Neill, "A Call for a Functional Multidisciplinary Approach to Intervention in Cases of Elder Abuse, Neglect, and Exploitation—One Legal Clinic's Experience," *Elder Law Journal* (Spring 1997), 196; See also Marshall Kapp. *Geriatrics and the Law: Understanding Patient Rights and Professional Responsibilities.* 3rd Edition. New York: Springer Publishing Company, 1999.

83. Moskowitz, *supra* note 81, at 78.

84. Moskowitz, *supra* note 81, at 78–79.

85. Moskowitz, *supra* note 81, at 90–91.

86. Moskowitz, *supra* note 81, at 80–81.

87. Moskowitz, *supra* note 81, at 83–85.

88. Moskowitz, *supra* note 81, at 107–108. See also Sherry Greenberg, Gloria Ramsey, Ethel Mitty, and Terry Fulner, "Elder Mistreatment: Case Law and Ethical Issues in Assessment, Reporting, and Management," 6(3) *Journal of Nursing Law* (1999), 7–20.

89. 971 P.2d 986 (Cal. 1999).

90. A. David Tammelleo, Editor, "'Reckless' Neglect of Elders Violates Elder Abuse Act," 39(11) *Regan Report on Nursing Law* (April 1999), 1.

91. Leavitt and O'Neill, *supra* note 82.

92. Moskowitz, *supra* note 81, at 108.

93. Mary G. Weisensee, Joanne B. Anderson, and Diane K. Kjervik, "Family Members' Retrospective Views of Events Surrounding the Petition for a Conservatorship or Guardianship," 3(3) *Journal of Nursing Law* (1996), 19–20.

94. Mark D. Andrews, "The Elderly in Guardianship: A Crisis of Constitutional Proportions," *Elder Law Journal* (Spring 1997), 79.

95. Weisensee, Anderson, and Kjervik, *supra* note 93, at 21.

96. *Id.* at 28–29.

97. Diane K. Kjervik, Earline W. Miller, Janice M. Wheeler, and Mary G. Weisensee, "Events that Trigger the Decisions to Seek Proxy Decision-Making Arrangements for Older Persons: Caregiver and Lawyers' Views," 6(1) *Journal of Nursing Law* (1999), 22.

98. *Id.* at 23.

99. Andrews, *supra* note 94, at 76.

100. Andrews, *supra* note 94, at 87.

101. *Id.*

102. 755 ILCS 5/11a - 5(a) (1987).

103. Andrews, *supra* note 94, at 88.

104. 755 ILCS 5/11a - 8 (1998).

105. Andrews, *supra* note 94, at 90–91.

106. Andrews, *supra* note 94, at 80.

107. 755 ILCS 5/11a - 11(e) (1995).

108. Andrews, *supra* note 106.

109. Andrews, *supra* note 106.

110. 64 Fed. Reg. 36,078, July 2, 1999.

111. 405 ILCS 5/2-108 (1993).

112. 210 ILCS 45/2-106 (1993).

113. Federal Register, *supra* note 110, at 36,080.

114. 42 C.F.R. 482.13 (1999).

115. American Hospital Association, "Final Rule on 'Patients Rights': New Restraint and Seclusion Standards as Part of Medicare Conditions of Participation," *AHA Regulatory Advisory* (July 29, 1999), 2.

116. American Society for Healthcare Risk Management, "Health Care Financing Administration Imposes New Patients' Rights Conditions of Participation Requirements for Hospitals Effective August 2, 1999 (Final Interim Rule)," *ASHRM Member Alert* (July 20, 1999), 3.

117. *Id.*

118. *Id.* at 4.

119. *Id.* at 3–4.

120. *Id.*

121. *Id.* at 4–5.

The Nurse in the Academic Setting **20**

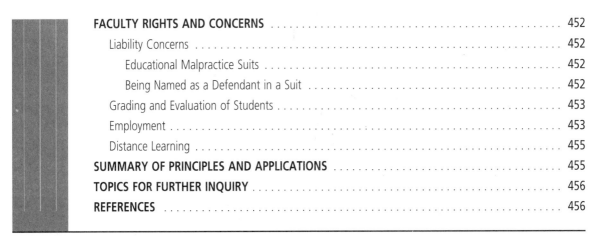

KEY PRINCIPLES

- Due Process
- Public Academic Institution
- Private Academic Institution
- Constitutional Protections
- Disciplinary Dismissal
- Academic Dismissal
- Academic Freedom of Faculty
- Tenure

Nurses in the academic setting find themselves in one of two roles—that of the student and that of the faculty member. Both students and faculty have specific rights and responsibilities supported by law. Regardless of which role the nurse holds, those rights and responsibilities are important to adhere to.

This chapter will explore selected areas of both roles and examine applicable laws. The chapter will begin with the student, whether the student be in a 2- or 4-year collegiate program, a 3-year diploma program, or a graduate degree program (M.S. or terminal degree). Likewise, the faculty member's rights and responsibilities will be analyzed from general principles of law that apply to any type of educational program the nurse may be teaching in.

HISTORICAL DEVELOPMENT OF STUDENT RIGHTS AND FACULTY RESPONSIBILITIES

At one time, students in postsecondary educational settings had few, if any, enforceable legal rights in relation to the academic institution and its administration and faculty.[1] The reasons for this lack of rights were rooted in a number of theories espoused by society and the judicial system concerning the student's relationship with the academic institution. Most often the student's inability to challenge any action by the institution focused on the institution's decisions about suspending or terminating the student from a program or from the school because of disciplinary and academic actions.

> *At one time, students in postsecondary educational settings had few, if any, enforceable legal rights in relation to the academic institution and its administration and faculty.*

One theory that was utilized in keeping the student from having any enforceable legal rights against the institution was the *beneficiary theory*. The student, a beneficiary of the knowledge and wisdom imparted by the faculty, was unable to challenge any action because the student should not question what was being given to him or her as a gift. The *privilege theory* utilized the same reasoning: The student was privileged to be in the academic setting and therefore should not be armed with the legal ability to challenge any adverse decision.

Perhaps the most successful theory utilized by the academic institution to support its decisions was the *in loco parentis doctrine,* which means "in the place of the parent."[2] In the academic setting, the institution acted as the parents in disciplining the student, an action that might result in suspending, terminating, or dismissing a student from the school or program for academic reasons. Because the student could not challenge a parent's action against him or her, the academic institution's decision could not be questioned because it stood in the place of the parent.[3]

The *in loco parentis* doctrine was very helpful in shielding any challenges to an educational institution's decisions concerning dismissals or suspensions for disciplinary reasons (e.g., a breach of rules of conduct or dormitory rules). It was not helpful, however, when the decision to terminate or dismiss a student was based on an academic reason, for parents have never had the responsibility to grade their children in an academic setting. Thus the school could not really state that it had taken over a function of the parents. This, and other developments in society, set the stage for slow but dramatic changes in a student's right to question the educational institution's actions against him or her.

The Due Process Cases

The U.S. Constitution includes the Fourteenth Amendment, which protects certain individual rights from being restricted by state government. The Fourteenth Amendment states that, among other things, no state can deprive a person of life, liberty, or property without due process of law.[4] This portion of the amendment has been at the center of a multitude of lawsuits that have attempted to define both what due process is and what life, liberty, and property include. The courts generally define due process as what is *fair* under the circumstances. In addition, rather than enumerate every situation that might arise and what would be *fair* in every instance, the courts customarily look at the right that might be limited or eliminated by the state government and then ask the question: What process is due to ensure that fairness will prevail? As a result, the individual charged with a crime that carries with it the pos-

sibility of incarceration would receive more due process protections than would a student who is threatened with expulsion from an academic institution. However, in either case, the due process protections are mandated only when the state (government) is involved in possible restriction of an individual's rights guaranteed by the Fourteenth Amendment. This application is often referred to as "state action" or an action "under the color of state law."[5]

> *The courts generally define due process as what is fair under the circumstances.*

What is and what is not state action is not always easily resolved. This is also true with whether an academic institution is a public (state) or a private school.

Generally a public academic institution is one that is affiliated with a state government; in other words, a state school. As such, the school is supported by state revenues. In contrast, a private school is one that is *not* supported by state revenues but rather receives its financial support from private funding.

If a school is a public one, the power of the state and federal government over faculty and students and their constitutional rights is limited by the Constitution. Private academic institutions do not have the same requirement of abiding by constitutional limitations on their actions but cannot act in a manner that is arbitrary, capricious, or discriminatory when making decisions about students and faculty.

It is possible, though, that an academic institution, even if private, does receive state funds in some manner. If that is the case, it may be that the school must abide by the due process requirements of the Fourteenth Amendment required of public schools in dismissing students for misconduct.

Dixon v. State of Alabama

One of the most important initial cases to delineate the due process rights of students in their relationship with the academic institution was *Dixon v. Alabama State Board of Education.*[6] In

Dixon, six students at the Alabama State College for Negroes in Montgomery, Alabama, were expelled from the college without notice and without a hearing for "misconduct." Although never clearly specified, it was believed that the misconduct engaged in by the six students was their participation in several off-campus civil rights demonstrations.[7] The students, after receiving a letter from the college president indicating the board of education's unanimous decision to expel them, filed a case asking the federal district court to grant them a preliminary and permanent injunction restraining the board of education and other college officials from prohibiting them from attending college. The district court upheld the dismissals and denied the students' requested relief. On appeal, the U.S. Court of Appeals for the Fifth Circuit reversed the district court and remanded the case to the circuit court for further proceedings consistent with its opinion.

The appeals court, in reversing the trial court's decision, held that the due process protections guaranteed in the Fourteenth Amendment of the U.S. Constitution required a state academic institution to give notice to students concerning their possible expulsion and a hearing prior to the expulsion. In so holding, the court also listed the following standards that should be followed when providing that notice and hearing: (1) the notice should be specific as to the allegations and basis for the potential expulsion; and (2) the nature of the hearing, which is adversarial, should depend on the circumstances of each situation but should allow an opportunity for both sides to present in detail their respective positions.[8]

The *Dixon* court also held that the students must be given the names of witnesses against them and what each witness would be testifying to, an opportunity to present their own defenses to the allegations, and, if the hearing was not to be held before the board of education, a written copy of its findings and decision in the case.[9]

Dixon, then, paved the way for clear due process protections for students in postsecondary public academic institutions when threatened with expulsion for misconduct or, stated in another way, when a disciplinary action was being taken against them. A disciplinary dismissal against a student is a serious matter because it results from a violation of a code of conduct or rules and regulations. Because the behavior complained of allegedly violates standards of conduct, a disciplinary

dismissal has the potential for a long-lasting effect on the student's reputation. *Dixon,* however, was clearly limited to those two prerequisites. Other case law decisions established additional protections and further defined their limitations.

Goss v. Lopez

Although the *Dixon* case was a landmark one in terms of protecting public students' rights of due process vis-à-vis the institution and its faculty, *Goss v. Lopez*[10] firmly solidified them. Decided by the U.S. Supreme Court, the *Goss* decision required *all* public academic institutions, whether they be grade schools, high schools, or colleges and universities, to provide due process protections to their students.

In *Goss,* nine public high school students filed a class action against the Columbus Board of Education and many administrators, alleging that without a hearing they were all suspended from their respective schools for "misconduct" for up to 10 days. Although their respective suspensions were possible under an Ohio statute, the students alleged that the statute was unconstitutional in that it allowed a school principal and other public school administrator to suspend a student without a hearing.[11] Alleging that this lack of a hearing before a suspension was a violation of their procedural due process rights guaranteed by the Fourteenth Amendment to the U.S. Constitution, they also sought to enjoin the public school administrators from suspending more students and asked the court to require the schools to remove any reference concerning their suspensions from their respective files.

At the federal district court trial, a three-judge court held that the students were denied due process, and the Ohio statute permitting a suspension to occur without a prior hearing, or within a reasonable time period after the suspensions, was unconstitutional. It ordered that any and all references to the students' suspensions be removed from their school files.

The court also listed what was minimally necessary for a school to do in an emergency situation that might require suspension before a hearing could be held. Those minimum requirements were notice of the suspension proceedings sent to the parents of the student within 24 hours of the decision to hold them; a hearing within 72 hours of the suspension, with the student present; and the right of the student to make a statement in his or her defense, to have statements of the charges against him or her, but not to have an attorney present.[12] In all nonemergency situations, however, the three-judge court held that notice and a hearing prior to suspension were required.

On a direct appeal by the defendants to the U.S. Supreme Court, the Court affirmed the three-judge court's holding. In doing so, the Court held that the property right created by Ohio statutes for a free public education to all residents between the ages of 5 and 21 years of age and the state's requirement of compulsory attendance in school for a certain period of time could not be taken away in violation of the Fourteenth Amendment's requirement of due process.

The Court also discussed a person's interest in liberty, as guaranteed by the Fourteenth Amendment. Because a suspension may result in damage to a student's reputation or good name throughout his or her school career and beyond, therefore affecting his or her ability to freely choose future life options, the Constitution demanded adherence to due process protections, regardless of the length of the suspension.[13]

Last, but not least, the Court, in determining what process is due under these circumstances, held that some kind of notice and hearing is necessary before a suspension takes place. These requirements are essential to protect the student's due process rights and, in the words of the Court, "provide a meaningful hedge against erroneous action."[14]

> *Both the* Dixon *and* Goss *courts limited their decisions . . . to disciplinary actions.*

Both the *Dixon* and *Goss* courts limited their decisions to public institutions and to disciplinary actions. What rights, if any, did a student have when an academic decision resulted in dismissal from a program, course of study, or academic institution? Although difficult to define clearly, an academic dismissal by faculty is based on poor academic performance by a student. In other words, the student does not meet established criteria to successfully pass a course or clinical placement, or does not meet established criteria to enable the student to successfully continue in the course or program of study. For example, a student who fails to maintain a C average in a nursing program pursuant to the program's requirements may be dismissed.

Until the U.S. Supreme Court decided *Board of Curators of the University of Missouri v. Horowitz*[15] in 1978, rights of students faced with academic dismissal, whether enrolled in a public or private postsecondary institution, were unclear.

University of Missouri v. Horowitz

In *Horowitz,* the respondent, Charlotte Horowitz, was admitted to the University of Missouri's Medical School (a public institution) with advanced standing. Her academic record was impressive: a bachelor of science degree from Barnard College, a master of science degree in psychology from Columbia University, a year of study in pharmacology at Duke University, a year's attendance at the Women's Medical College of Pennsylvania (withdrawing in good standing after 1 year because of illness), and more than 5 years of research in psychopharmacology at the National Institute of Mental Health.[16] After her first year in medical school, however, she was informed by the dean in writing that she was being placed on probation because of dissatisfaction by several faculty members with her clinical performance during her pediatrics rotation. The probationary status was based on several deficiencies, including poor relationships with others, erratic attendance during the clinical rotation, and poor personal hygiene (inadequate handwashing and poor grooming). Ms. Horowitz was informed that she needed to improve in these areas, but that, with the Council on Evaluation's recommendation, she would be allowed to advance to the next "rotational unit" in the curriculum.

Ms. Horowitz continued in the medical school program on probation during her second and third years, but the faculty was still "dissatisfied" with her performance. As a result, in January of 1973, the Council on Evaluation recommended that she not graduate in May of 1973. Ms. Horowitz was informed in writing of this decision and was also informed that, if she did not agree with it, she could take a set of oral and practical examinations with seven physicians who had no prior contact with her in order to have them evaluate her academic performance and make recommendations as to her continuing as a student in the program.

The oral and practical examinations were taken, and two of the physicians voted to have her graduate on schedule, two said she should be dismissed immediately, and the remaining physicians said she should not graduate in May but continue on probation until further evaluations concerning her clinical progress could be carried out and reviewed.[17] Based on the physicians' evaluations, the council voted not to allow her to graduate in May and informed her of this decision.

When the council met again in May of 1973, it deliberated about whether or not Ms. Horowitz should be allowed to continue in the program beyond June of 1973. Because of the lack of major improvements in her performance, the council voted to dismiss her from the school. When another negative evaluation of Ms. Horowitz's performance in the emergency rotation was received, the council unanimously recommended that she be dropped from school. The recommendation was approved by the Coordinating Committee and the dean, and the dean notified the student in writing on July 6, 1973, that she was dismissed from the school. Ms. Horowitz appealed the decision in writing to the university provost for health sciences, but the decision was upheld.

Ms. Horowitz then filed a case in the U.S. District Court for the Western District of Missouri and alleged that her civil rights were violated, citing 42 U.S.C. Section 1983.[18] The complaint also alleged that she was not afforded procedural due process rights prior to her dismissal from the school. After a full trial, the district court held that Ms. Horowitz had been given all the rights guaranteed to her by the Fourteenth Amendment and dismissed the complaint. The student appealed the decision. The Eighth Circuit Court of Appeals held that a dismissal from a medical school can have serious consequences for the student's ability to obtain a job in medicine, and therefore a hearing was required prior to dismissal. The court based this rationale on the Fourteenth Amendment's protection of "liberty"; in other words, the ability of this student to be free to obtain and change employment freely and the infringement of that right by the university (a public institution) in dismissing her from their program.[19]

The university appealed the Eighth Circuit's decision, and the U.S. Supreme Court granted certiorari. By accepting the case for review, the Supreme Court would decide for the first time what procedures must be given to a student at a state educational institution whose dismissal may constitute a deprivation of "liberty" or "property" within the meaning of the Fourteenth Amendment.[20]

The U.S. Supreme Court unanimously reversed the judgment of the appeals court. To begin with, it held that the action taken by the university was an *academic* one. As such, no hearing was required prior to the dismissal. The Court supported this holding by discussing the difference between disciplinary decisions, which require objective fact-finding and a subsequent decision based on those facts, and academic decisions, which are based more on a subjective determination of a student's abilities and on a "continuing relationship between faculty and students."[21] Furthermore, the Court held that, because the student-faculty relationship is not an adversarial one, it is based on the expert evaluation of the faculty member who decides about student progress that is cumulative in nature. Historically such decisions have not been judicially scrutinized unless they are arbitrary or capricious. Courts are generally "ill equipped" to evaluate academic performance and therefore will not, as a rule, intrude into academic decision making.

In addition to its holding that the university's action was an academic one, the Court also held that there was no need to determine if there was a violation of Ms. Horowitz's "property" or "liberty" interests under the Fourteenth Amendment, because she had not alleged a violation of any "property" right in the courts below. The "liberty" interest allegation was unfounded, the Court held, because the dismissal was communicated not publicly but to her alone, and because, assuming for the sake of argument it did exist, Ms. Horowitz had been given as much due process as the Fourteenth Amendment would require.[22]

Horowitz, then, set clear parameters for all academic institutions—whether public or private—to abide by when making decisions concerning the academic performance of students. No hearing is *required* prior to dismissal for academic reasons (although it can be afforded if the school elects to do so). Adequate notice must be given to the student concerning his or her academic performance, what must be improved upon, under what time guidelines, and the impact on continuation in the program if the suggestions are not met. The decision to dismiss the student must not be disseminated publicly, and only careful and delib-

ETHICS CONNECTION 20–1

Learning the foundations of skilled ethical comportment is important not only to nursing practice but to retention of nurses as well. Profound prolonged moral distress contributes to nurses leaving nursing. Knowing how to think about and negotiate resolution of ethical situations can make a difference in the moral distress that nurses and nursing students experience. Thus, grounding in ethics education is critically important to the development of skilled ethical comportment in clinical nursing practice.

Historically, the ethics of teaching ethics consistently has been a concern for nurses in academic settings, both faculty and students. Educators experienced conflict about teaching nursing students to be moral agents and patient advocates in institutions that sometimes made it very difficult to practice in the advocate role. This moral conflict about the teaching of ethics was highlighted in Yarling and McElmurry's[1] classic article that revealed the institutional constraints on morally responsible nursing practice. Various versions of the *Code for Nurses with Interpretive Statements*[2] reinforced this conflict by urging nurses to practice ethically regardless of external constraints. Nursing students experienced a powerlessness in being able to recognize clinical moral issues but not always being able to resolve them because of hindrances within institutional bureaucratic systems. At that time, the ethical focus was an individualistic one that did not place a burden on the organization to conduct itself ethically.

As nursing autonomy increased, nursing faculty became concerned about which of the various approaches to bioethics would be most appropriate to teach and learn. Early approaches to teaching ethics had focused on indoctrinating students with the "virtues" of professional nursing practice. The moral character of any given nurse was compared to the moral ideal of the virtuous nurse. Student nurses were expected to comport themselves in a professional manner and were taught that confidentiality, respect for authority, punctuality, professional appearance, and the like were important characteristics of nursing. Most nursing students were single young women who lived at the schools and were governed by strict rules not only during class and clinical practice but in the dormitories as well. Susan Reverby's[3] reflections on nursing history reveal how nurses were "ordered to care" in a society that does not value caring.

With the emphasis on science and technology in the latter half of the 20th century, nursing education focused on scientific foundations of practice. At about the same time, the field of bioethics was developing.[4] Bioethics focused initially and primarily on medical ethics; nursing ethics was considered to be a subset of bioethics. Beauchamp and Childress's principlist model of ethics became the dominant model of biomedical ethics.[5] This model was derived from philosophical ethics rather than theological ethics and provided a structure for analysis of clinical situations through casuistry (case analysis). This individualistic principlist model was useful for several reasons. It helped students to develop analytical skills and offered a common language for ethical discourse in clinical practice. Principlist ethics was limited, though, in its usefulness for ethical decision making. Case analysis often yielded better understanding of the facets of a case but allowed for competing decisions to be morally grounded in different moral principles. Thus, case analysis based on moral principles did not point to one preferred course of nursing action.

By the beginning of the 1990s, nursing ethics began to emerge as a separate branch of bioethics rather than as a subset of biomedical ethics (see Chapter 3). Referred to as the ethic of care, nursing ethics clearly is grounded in relationship rather than exclusively in philosophical ethical theory and moral principles. The ethic of care, when considered as covenantal relationships, is more closely aligned with theological ethics than with philosophical ethics. Bioethics, too, is shifting away from a focus on the moral claims of individuals to a communal ethics that looks at shared rather than competing moral interests. This current transition to communitarian ethics is congruent with the shift in nursing education from primarily hospital-based care that emphasizes individual patients to a community-based approach that considers clients to be in relationship with others and that pays more attention to aggregate care.

With the compatibility of communitarian ethics and the ethic of care with community-based nursing practice, it would seem that the ethics of teaching ethics is self-evident. There is another trend, however, that may pose danger for ethics education in some schools of nursing. Outcome-based curricula are teleological approaches to curriculum design and implementation that focus primarily on specific sets of outcomes such as critical thinking, therapeutic nursing interventions, and communication. These curricula are so packed with content and clinical practice experiences that there is a danger of losing an emphasis on ethics education in some schools. There is an emerging tendency for faculty to expect that students will learn ethics from the philosophy department as part of college or university core requirements. Faculty, then, are expected to integrate ethics throughout the curriculum. Sometimes this is effective. More often, it is not. "What is everyone's job is no one's job" may be relevant for ethics education in emerging curricula. Some schools have found creative, effective ways to teach ethics despite the intense curricula in most schools of nursing. The Joseph and Rose Kennedy Institute of Ethics at Georgetown University has been collecting syllabi on ethics education since the 1980s. Faculty and students may review these syllabi for relevance to ethics education in their own academic settings.[6]

[1]Rod Yarling and Beverly McElmurry, "The Moral Foundation of Nursing," 8(2) *Advances in Nursing Science* (1986), 63–73.

[2]American Nurses Association. *Code for Nurses with Interpretive Statements.* Kansas City, MO: Author, 1985.

[3]Susan Reverby. *Ordered to Care: The Dilemma of American Nursing* 1850–1945. New York: Cambridge University Press, 1987; Albert R. Jonsen. *The Birth of Bioethics.* New York: Oxford University Press, 1998.

[4]*Id.*

[5]Thomas F. Beauchamp and James L. Childress. *Principles of Biomedical Ethics.* 4th Edition. New York: Oxford University Press, 1994.

[6]Syllabi are on deposit at the National Center for Bioethics Literature, Kennedy Reference Center for Bioethics Literature, Kennedy Institute of Ethics, Georgetown University, Box 571212, Washington, DC 20057-1212; Web site is http://www.georgetown.edu/research/nrcbl/syllabus.

erate decisions by faculty concerning academic dismissals will be protected by the "hands-off" policy of the courts.

What remains unclear after Horowitz, however, is what constitutes an academic, as opposed to a disciplinary, action or decision by the faculty . . .

What remains unclear after *Horowitz,* however, is what constitutes an academic, as opposed to a disciplinary, action or decision by the faculty of the academic institution. This lack of clarity has not been corrected in subsequent cases, and, as a result, faculty and students must struggle with this issue on a regular basis. One way in which this concern is often resolved is by applying the due process principles discussed by the courts in *Dixon* and *Goss* whenever there is doubt about whether a decision is disciplinary or academic. The rationale for such an application is based on the idea that a court cannot fault an institution for providing more protections than are necessary in a certain situation.

The Contract Theory

The cases and theory presented thus far have dealt with dismissals from public academic institutions and have been based on constitutional protections afforded students. Other safeguards, however, were being concomitantly developed, especially for students in private institutions. One

very important theory was the contract theory; that is, the application of traditional contract law to the relationship between the student and the academic institution. Briefly, this theory supports an express or implied contract between the student and academic entity based on written documents (e.g., the student catalog) or oral representations or promises (an academic advisor's statement that a particular course could be substituted for another course, for example). If breach of contract occurs, then the student, for example, could be dismissed from the school for not maintaining the required grade point average, or conversely, the student could sue the school for dismissal in violation of the express or implied grade point average "provisions" of the contract.

Although the contract theory can be used by students in both private and public institutions, it is most often utilized by students in private academic settings because, as has been discussed, constitutional protections are not as readily available to those students. Furthermore, as stated by the *Dixon* court, the law has followed the "well-settled rule that the relations between a student and a private university are a matter of contract."[23] The contract theory has been applied in various situations and has proved to be flexible for both student and the academic institution,[24] not only with dismissals but in all aspects of the student-institution relationship, as will be developed more fully in this chapter.

SPECIFIC STUDENT RIGHTS AND FACULTY RESPONSIBILITIES

Admission and Readmission

Whether public or private, academic institutions must abide by guidelines unique to the character of the institution when deciding about student admissions to the school and/or a specific program of study. Public academic institutions must abide by state and federal constitutional mandates. Private schools must adhere to express or implied requirements set forth in school publications or by faculty and staff. In addition, both public and private schools receiving state or federal funding or covered by state or federal statutory law prohibiting discrimination, bias, or other conduct in their decisions concerning admission must comply with those requirements. If not, the institution may face not only a lawsuit by the student allegedly aggrieved by the decision but also loss of funding and other sanctions if the allegations are substantiated.

Nondiscrimination is one tenet that must be adhered to by academic institutions in admission and readmission decisions. This requirement stems not only from statutory (state and/or federal) laws but also from case law. Table 20–1 summarizes selected cases dealing with discrimination issues litigated by students in relation to admission and readmission.

IMPLICATIONS FOR NURSING STUDENTS AND FACULTY

The decisions included in Table 20–1 and recent decisions further refining the parameters of admission and readmission can be helpful to nursing students and faculty. For example, the *Bakke* decision stands for the prohibition of utilizing race as one of the only factors in deciding admissions to academic institutions. It also stands for the importance of admission programs being as individualized as possible, whatever their format. In subsequent years, however, the prohibition in *Bakke* has been challenged in several cases.[25] In addition, the U.S. Supreme Court did not review an appeals court decision which upheld the validity of California Proposition 209. The proposition amended the California Constitution and prohibited state and local agencies, including public institutions of higher learning, from using preferences based on race or gender in admissions or in other decisions.[26] Because of continuing legal challenges pertaining to admissions and readmissions into nursing and other educational programs, keeping abreast of the latest developments in this area is essential.

Like race discrimination, sex/gender discrimination will be carefully scrutinized by the judicial system. State academic institutions must be able to conclusively show that any admission policy that favors members of one gender over another can pass the constitutional tests enumerated in *Hogan* and subsequent decisions.

The *Davis* decision is also important for students and faculty but must be relied on cautiously. To begin with, it was based on the applicant's desire to enter a professional school that consisted of classroom *and* clinical components. The outcome may have been different if the program applied to was composed only of classroom requirements. Any requirements that are set by the academic institution must be essential ones for participation in that program. Additionally, *Davis* does not stand for the principle that a court would not require less burdensome accommodations to be made by an academic institution for a handicapped student so that he or she could participate in an academic program. Likewise, "auxiliary aids" (e.g., hearing aids or interpreters) and "support services" may be required in certain instances. Last, but by no means least, although there may be no *legal* obligation for a program to accommodate an otherwise qualified applicant, a college or university is not prohibited from doing so voluntarily. However, in deciding to do so, the academic institution would have to establish clear-cut policies and procedures to ensure even-handed decision making in regard to every qualified handicapped student who was considered.

It is important to note that the Americans with Disabilities Act (ADA)[27] may be used along with the Rehabilitation Act, or perhaps alone, in challenging decisions by academic institutions because Title III of the ADA clearly prohibits places of "public accommodation" (privately owned establishments that make goods, services, or programs available to the public)[28] from discriminating against individuals with disabilities. Likewise, Title II, which governs governmental entities, prohibits the same conduct.[29] Therefore, academic institutions would violate either of these two provisions with discriminatory admission or readmission policies and decisions.

. . . the Americans with Disabilities Act (ADA) may be used along with the Rehabilitation Act, or perhaps

alone, in challenging decisions by academic institutions . . .

Although not presented in Table 20–1, nondiscrimination on the basis of age is another important canon that the academic institution must adhere to when deciding about applicants. Generally, as with the other protected categories already discussed, age cannot be used to deny admission to a college or university program. In addition to state laws prohibiting discrimination on the basis of age, the federal Age Discrimination Act of 1975[30] forbids discrimination on the basis of age for those public and private programs or activities receiving federal funds. Exceptions include when an age requirement is vital to the "normal operation" of the program receiving the funds, or when the age requirement conforms with a statutory purpose for which the program or activity is receiving the funds. Those exceptions are carefully monitored by the courts, and it is safe to say that any decision based solely on age will be carefully questioned by the courts if challenged.

Perhaps the best way an academic institution can avoid any unnecessary liability for discriminatory decision making concerning admission is to have well-drafted policies. A statement that the postsecondary institution does not discriminate and adheres to all applicable state and federal laws concerning nondiscrimination is helpful. It is also important that any and all policies concerning the process, including admission classifications, advanced standing, tuition and fees, and withdrawal from the school or program, be nondiscriminatory.

The general position statement and the academic policies statement should appear in all school academic catalogs and in department or specific program handbooks as well. Not only does this approach make clear the school's position in relation to nondiscrimination, it also provides notice to the potential applicant of the requirements necessary for admission to the college or program. As a result, whether a public or private institution, the school has met its legal and ethical obligations to inform the potential applicant of the rules that will be adhered to during the admission decision-making phase. Likewise, the student is equipped with information necessary to make choices concerning applying for admission, making up defi-ciencies before doing so, or deciding to forgo applying to that particular school.

Clear-cut statements and policies concerning readmissions to an academic institution or program are also important to include in the various documents given to applicants or students.

In addition to the requirement of nondiscrimination, decisions concerning readmissions must unquestionably follow catalogs and other documents delineating the process. If the institution fails to follow these written guidelines, the student may allege a breach of the language in the documents and proceed to court on the contract theory, as in the *Babb* case.

Although courts will look at whether an educational institution's conduct is arbitrary or capricious when that is alleged by a litigant, in *Babb* that was not an issue. Rather, as the court said, the issue was one of contract law and whether the nursing program breached the contract provisions. Carefully drafted catalogs and other written documents governing students and their relationship with the academic institution are essential. The written material must be clear and unambiguous and state what is intended by the academic institution. Clarity aids both the student and the academic institution, as either can be easily held to those mandates by the courts.

Carefully drafted catalogs and other written documents governing students and their relationship with the academic institution are essential.

Many academic institutions, concerned about decisions based on contract theory, often place disclaimers in school catalogs and other written documents stating, in effect, that the document does not create an express or implied contract and that the institution reserves the right to make changes in curriculum, course content, fees, and other areas at any time those changes are necessary or desirable. Although there is no guarantee that such a disclaimer would result in a judgment in favor of the postsecondary school, its inclusion in catalogs and other documents is one issue a court would consider when allegations of breach of contract against the academic entity are raised.

TABLE 20–1

Selected Cases on Discrimination in Admission and Readmission in Education

CASE NAME/DATE	DISCRIMINATION ALLEGED	BASIS OF SUIT	DECISION AND COMMENT
Brown v. Board of Education (1954)[1]	Race	14th Amendment Equal Protection Clause	Supreme Court decision for plaintiff, who was black and attempted to get into an all-white public school. Public schools cannot discriminate against an individual when making admission decisions on basis of race unless state has a "compelling state interest" in doing so. Here, no interest found. First case to set precedent for all public schools even though decision based on grades 1–12. Federally supported in Title VII of the Civil Rights Act of 1964, Title IX of the Education Amendments of 1972, and 42 U.S.C. Section 1981.
Regents of the University of California v. Bakke (1978)[2]	Race	University affirmative action programs (specifically designed by the university to provide a separate admission system for minority students); 14th Amendment Equal Protection Clause; California Constitution; Civil Rights Act of 1964	Supreme Court invalidated special admission programs and decided in favor of Bakke; Court held programs were a "racial quota"; ordered that Bakke be admitted to medical program and enjoined school from considering race in its admission programs; case called the "reverse discrimination" case because Bakke was white and minorities admitted were nonwhite.
Mississippi University for Women v. Hogan (1982)[3]	Sex/Gender	14th Amendment Equal Protection Clause; Title IX of the Education Amendments of 1972; university's female-only admission policy	Supreme Court decision for Hogan, who applied to school of nursing's B.S. program but was denied admission because he was male; Court held that university's policy did not serve important "governmental objectives" required when single-sex policies challenged under 14th Amendment; Hogan decision dealt with public university; public and private universities also must not discriminate on the basis of gender/sex under Title IX of the Education Amendments of 1972 (includes marital status, family status, and pregnancy).

Case	Issue	Legal Basis	Decision
Southeast Community College v. Davis (1979)[4]	Handicap (bilateral sensorineural hearing loss)	Section 504 of Rehabilitation Act of 1973; 14th Amendment (Due Process and Equal Protection)	Supreme Court decision in favor of college; Court held that although Rehabilitation Act prohibits discrimination when school receives federal funding if student is "otherwise qualified" and can be "reasonably accommodated," student here not "otherwise qualified" and accommodation required was too extensive, especially considering clinical component of school program; to require school to admit this student would be costly and might compromise the quality of the program.
University of Texas Health Sciences Center at Houston v. Babb (1982)[5]	Change in school of nursing catalog discriminated against student; required withdrawal and reapplication to program under "new" catalog that contained adverse requirements for student in comparison to initial catalog	Contract theory	Decision for student; appeals court held school catalog a written contract between student and school; because student only requested her cumulative grade point average be determined by initial catalog, ruling based on that request.
United States v. Commonwealth of Virginia (1996)[6]	Sex/Gender	14th Amendment Equal Protection Clause; Virginia Military Institute's (VMI) male-only admission policy	Supreme Court decision against VMI; institute failed to prove that male-only policy served "important governmental objectives" discussed 14 years ago in *Hogan*; VMI's attempt to establish a "comparable educational program" for women at Virginia Military Institute for Women (VMIW) *not* equal to VMI program.

[1] 347 U.S. 483 (1954)
[2] 438 U.S. 265 (1978)
[3] 458 U.S. 718 (1982)
[4] 442 U.S. 397 (1979)
[5] 646 S.W. 2d 502 (1982)
[6] 116 U.S. 2264 (1996)

ETHICS CONNECTION 20–2

Attempts to teach nursing students to practice ethically will be futile if the academic setting itself has not attended to its institutional ethics. The mission statements of the college or university and the school of nursing should clearly convey the institutional goals to the students and faculty. Institutional policies and practices should be consistent with the mission and with standards and criteria of accrediting organizations. Although academic freedom is intended to protect both students and faculty in the search for truth, there are power imbalances in which students generally are more vulnerable than faculty. Just policies provide students with avenues of appeal or grievance when they believe that they have been unfairly treated. Such policies should be published and made available to all students. Examples of such policies include appeal processes, grievance procedures, progression, evaluation and grading policies, policies regarding drug testing, learning disabilities, and compliance with the *Americans with Disabilities Act*.

Privacy rights often are threatened when nursing students begin clinical practice courses. Increased computerization of students' academic records and personal data create possibilities for breaching privacy rights. In addition, the volume of personal data that is required by the clinical practice settings seems to increase annually. Some states require that hospitals and other health care institutions do criminal background checks of everyone who practices there, including students. Institutional policies and practices that are fair and beneficent while respecting the autonomy of students and faculty and safeguarding their privacy create a context in which ethical comportment can develop and flourish.

Advancement in the School or Program

The main goal of a student admitted to a school and/or specific program is to successfully complete all program and school requirements in a timely manner in order to graduate, sit for and pass nursing boards, and begin professional life as a nurse. However, that goal can be fraught with obstacles as students progress through their academic career, for their success is dependent upon evaluation in the form of grades, in both the classroom and the clinical setting. Generally speaking, as was discussed in the *Horowitz* case, the court will not interfere or second-guess academic decision mak-

ing by faculty, for the court is not experienced in evaluating success or failure in the academic setting. Despite that general posture, the court will scrutinize decisions by faculty or administration if they (1) are arbitrary, malicious, capricious, or not in accordance with adopted policies or procedures; (2) show bad faith; or (3) violate a student's constitutional or other rights.

Academic and Clinical Grading

In *Clements v. County of Nassau*,[31] Helen Clements, age 51, enrolled in the state-supported Nassau County Community College's licensed practical nursing program. A former laboratory technician and active member of many health-related community groups, Ms. Clements was not new to health care delivery. Her first year of the 2-year program went well academically, although there seemed to be a clash between her alleged attitude of "thinking she knew more than she actually did" and faculty allegedly "resenting (her) from the beginning" because of her knowledge and experience in aspects of health care.

During the second year of the program, Ms. Clements contaminated the newborn nursery during her pediatric rotation. Although she was told of the error and acknowledged it, Ms. Clements was allowed to continue in the rotation and program. However, several months later, she failed her clinical evaluation because she did not "maintain cleanliness." The F in her clinical evaluation resulted in an F for the entire course.[32]

Clements appealed her grade to the dean of health sciences, and despite a school policy allowing only two chances to obtain a passing grade, the dean provided Ms. Clements with another chance to rectify her grade and pass the course. This included being assigned to another instructor and successfully completing an additional clinical test in addition to the one she failed earlier. Clements passed the course with a B.

During the final clinical course, however, she again failed to maintain the sterile procedure required when changing a dressing, did not realize her mistake, and therefore did not correct it. The instructor made the judgment that Clements did not "understand sterile technique," and the student was allowed to withdraw with a W grade rather than receive an F for the course. The instructor also recommended that Clements "take time off" from school to improve her clinical skills and return to retake the course in a year. Although

Clements did not disagree with the instructor's judgment, she was very unhappy about the recommendation that she leave the program for a year. When she approached the dean again concerning this latest recommendation, the dean refused to take any corrective action and agreed that she should drop out of school for the year. Ms. Clements then went to the vice president for academic affairs, who intervened on her behalf and allowed her to enroll in the fall semester.[33]

In addition to seeing the vice president for academic affairs, Ms. Clements had seen other administrators at the college since her difficulties began, had also written the New York State Education Department, and had contacted her senator. Her complaints to these various individuals and organizations were, among other things, that she was being harassed.

Ms. Clements began the fall 1983 term in clinical. Unfortunately, while giving a soapsuds enema to a patient, she did not provide for the patient's "safety needs," and was given an F in the course. Because this was the second failure for the student, she was unable to continue in it. Ms. Clements grieved the grade on the grounds that it was "unfair" to fail her on the second day of the course and because of the faculty's "inaccurate anecdotal records" about her. The first three steps of the grievance process were concluded, but the final step did not take place until April of 1985. The hearing, conducted by an ad hoc committee of the college academic standing committee, decided in favor of Ms. Clements and recommended that she be allowed to repeat the final course. Because the college's policy concerning grades is vested in the faculty, the nursing faculty member who gave Ms. Clements the F refused to change it.

Ms. Clements then filed suit in the U.S. District Court for the Eastern District of New York and alleged that, under The Civil Rights Act of 1871 (42 U.S.C. Section 1983), the college and faculty violated her civil rights by not making judgments about her clinical performance but rather on the basis of "personal animus and ill will" and "acted in concert" to force her out of the college's licensed practical nursing program. Thus, she alleged, her Fourteenth Amendment due process and equal protection rights were breached. She also alleged other causes of action, including contract and tort violations. The district court entered a summary judgment in favor of the college, and Clements appealed.

The appeals court upheld the entry of the summary judgment for the college. Citing *Horowitz* and a subsequent case supporting that decision, the court stated that courts will not overturn academic decisions unless there is a clear departure from "accepted academic norms so as to demonstrate that the person or committee responsible did not actually exercise professional judgment."[34] Furthermore, the court said, the faculty and college were more than "sympathetic" to her situation and gave her many opportunities to rectify her behavior, which she simply did not do. In addition, no due process or equal protection violations took place, for the college's grievance process was more than adequate, and Ms. Clements was not subjected to academic standards that were additional to those similarly situated. Last, the anecdotal records kept by the faculty were not used in grading nor were they disseminated to the public. Thus, no liberty interest deprivation was present.

In a similar case, *Southwell v. University of the Incarnate Word*,[35] a nursing student's allegations that her failure to pass a required course and therefore maintain a C grade in order to stay enrolled in the program was a decision arrived at "unfairly." The allegations were not upheld by the Texas Court of Appeals for the Fourth District. The court held that Ms. Southwell's failure to pass the course was based on the faculty member's "daily assessments" of the student's performance and were therefore entitled to be relied upon when deciding that the student would not pass the course and would be dropped from the program.

The *Clements* and *Southwell* cases are important ones because they continue to support a faculty's right to make judgments concerning grades, both in the classroom and in the clinical area. However, any such judgment will be measured by current academic norms. Thus, for both the student and faculty, well-developed evaluation forms concerning student progress that constitute the basis of the student's clinical grade are vital. They must be criterion based and contain behavioral objectives that can be measured. The student must be given a copy of the evaluation tool on the first day of class so that he or she has notice about what will be the basis of the grade. The evaluation process must be an ongoing one throughout the student's clinical rotation. If the student is not meeting clinical objectives, then he or she must be warned, told how to improve his or her difficulties, given any time constraints within which that improvement must occur, and be informed about what will take place if the required improvement does not occur (for example, suspension, request for withdrawal, failing grade). Any policies requiring a written form to be sent to a specific college or program dean or department concerning the poor clinical performance should be complied with and a copy given to the student. Anecdotal records can and should be kept by faculty. However, they do not substitute for the utilization of the evaluation form and other documents and procedures set by the academic program concerning evaluation. Also, as the *Clements* court cautioned, they cannot be untrue or abused.

Academic evaluation of students also consists of the faculty member's judgment concerning the student's classroom performance. As with clinical evaluations, the decision concerning grading must be in accordance with acceptable standards utilized by faculty generally. Moreover, the decision-making process must be as fair and equitable as possible. Thus, at the initiation of the course the student should be informed of what is to be expected of him or her. This is best accomplished by utilizing a syllabus that spells out the respective responsibilities of *both* the student and faculty member. Information in the syllabus for any course includes (1) name of the course; (2) credit hours earned; (3) method of grading; (4) grading scale; and (5) topics to be covered, dates of coverage, and required preparation for each class. Objectives that form the basis of the grade, and that the student is required to fulfill, must be included in the syllabus. Likewise, if the course requires projects, papers, and/or examination, the dates those required projects are due are an essential feature to include in the syllabus.

The faculty member should go over the syllabus with the students on the first day of class to ensure that they are clear about its contents. In addition, the students should be given an opportunity to ask any questions or clarify any requirements that are unclear. The opportunity to raise questions or seek clarification should continue throughout the course, however, and the faculty member should inform students of his or her office hours during the semester or quarter, either orally or by placing that information in the syllabus.

It is important that the faculty member adhere to the syllabus. If it needs to be altered or corrected, these changes must be discussed with the students as soon as possible. Changes that might ad-versely affect the student will be ones that will require special care and consideration. Most often, changes in grading criteria, or changes in the evaluation of the student in terms of his or her grade, will be the kinds of changes most often seen as adversely affecting the student, especially from the student's perspective. The syllabus clearly becomes a "contract" between the student and the faculty member and therefore can be used to challenge any deviations from its provisions. Moreover, the student can also allege that even if the terms of the syllabus were adhered to, they were applied in an arbitrary or capricious manner.[36]

In *Lyons v. Salve Regina College,*[37] for example, a senior nursing student who had received mostly As and Bs was absent for several days from a course that included a clinical component. As a result of her absences, which occurred not because of her own illness but rather so she could be with a friend who was hospitalized, the faculty member teaching the class and clinical course assured Ms. Lyons that she would receive an "Incomplete" rather than an F for the course.[38] The student continued in the course, finished all other course requirements, and took the final examination. When she received her grades, however, she had been given an "F" for the course.

Ms. Lyons appealed the grade through the school's grievance procedure listed in various documents of the college, including its catalog. These documents clearly stated that once the grievance was submitted to the appeals committee, its recommendation would be submitted to the dean. During the time the committee was deliberating her situation, Ms. Lyons received a letter from the dean informing her she could conditionally register for other classes, but that registration would be rescinded if the committee's recommendation was not in her favor.

The three-faculty-member committee recommended two to one in favor of Ms. Lyons; that is, that she receive an Incomplete and be allowed to make up the course deficiencies due to her absences. The third member voted to let the F stand, but to allow Ms. Lyons to apply for reinstatement. The dean dismissed the student from the program, and Ms. Lyons filed suit in the federal District Court in Rhode Island and asked the court to interpret the language in the school documents concerning the dean's and the committee's role in the grievance procedure.

The trial court held that the school catalog, the appeal committee hearing procedures, and the letter from the dean did constitute a contract between Ms. Lyons and the school.[39] Furthermore, the court held that based on those documents as a contract, the committee, not the dean, was empowered to make the final decision in this matter. The school appealed the decision, and the appellate court reversed the trial court, stating that the lower court had applied contract law too strictly. Because the relationship of the student and academic institution is unique, a rigid application of contract law cannot occur. In this instance, the court continued, the dean had the final say in whether or not a student continued in the nursing program. Even so, the court cautioned that a school catalog and other documents can be viewed as evidence of a contract between the school and student.

In *McIntosh v. Borough of Manhattan Community College*,[40] the New York Court of Appeals considered a student's allegation that the faculty's refusal to round off her 69.713 failing grade to a 70.000 passing grade was arbitrary and capricious. Citing *Horowitz*, the court stated that since the faculty member had not acted as the student alleged, no judicial review of the decision concerning the grade would occur.

Disciplinary Actions

A second obstacle for a student as he or she progresses through the academic program is conduct that the academic program considers a violation of its established code of acceptable behavior. Often formalized in "codes of conduct" or expected behaviors listed in school catalogs and other school documents, the prohibited behaviors cover, as examples, cheating and/or plagiarism, the use of alcoholic beverages on campus, participation in criminal activity, and in professional programs, unethical conduct not consistent with the profession's standards.

Dismissals for disciplinary reasons are subject to different rules of judicial review than are academic dismissals. The *Dixon* and *Goss* decisions are still "good law," and their continued applicability can be seen in subsequent case decisions. *Jones v. Board of Governors of the University of North Carolina*[41] is one such case illustrating the courts' continued application of those decisions. Nancy Jones, a nursing student in the university's program, was allegedly involved in cheating on an

examination by obtaining answers to two of the questions from the faculty member teaching the course and changing a paper before turning it in. Five days after the alleged incidents took place, Jones was informed by the dean of the School of Nursing that she had been accused of cheating and could either take an F for the course or have a hearing before the University Student Court, which was composed of three students. Ms. Jones asked for, and had, a hearing before the Student Court, which found her guilty of "academic dishonesty."[42]

Consistent with university procedures, Jones appealed the decision to the university chancellor and asked for a new hearing before the Chancellor's Hearing Panel, which was composed of three university faculty members. The chancellor and the panel decided that the hearing conducted by the Student Court was not a fair one and required a new hearing to be conducted by the panel in which both sides could present evidence on the alleged conduct of Ms. Jones. After the hearing occurred, the panel made its recommendation of "not guilty" and shared its decision with the chancellor. The university's legal counsel filed an objection to this determination with the chancellor. The chancellor asked the vice chancellor of academic affairs to review the hearing transcript and the objection of the University attorney. He did so, and decided that Ms. Jones was guilty of the alleged misconduct. He then upheld the Student Court's recommendation: that Ms. Jones receive an F in the course and be placed on disciplinary probation for a semester. Because she did not receive a passing grade in the course, Ms. Jones' registration was cancelled for the next semester because every student in the nursing program was required to pass all previous courses before being allowed to register and continue with subsequent courses.[43]

Nancy Jones filed suit in the U.S. District Court for the Western District of North Carolina, alleging that, under 42 U.S.C. Section 1983, the university had violated her procedural due process rights. She also asked for an injunction to reinstate her as a student in good standing until the suit was resolved on its merits. The district court granted this latter request, and the university appealed the decision to issue an injunction, alleging that doing so was an abuse of the court's discretion.

In addition to discussing its role in issuing injunctions, the court again outlined its role in evaluating decisions by faculty and administration.

Although "great deference" must be given to educational institutions, the court, citing *Goss*, stated that it must continue to ensure that "rudimentary precautions against unfair or mistaken findings of misconduct and arbitrary exclusion from school does not occur."[44] In this instance, the court continued, Ms. Jones will suffer "irreparable injury" by having to wait out a decision by the university—her education would be interrupted, she would be deprived of the opportunity to graduate with her classmates, and her goal of becoming a nurse would be delayed. In contrast, the university would not be harmed by having the student reinstated pending resolution of the case. In fact, the court pointed out, the confused and arguably irregular proceedings that took place, which were in stark divergence from established procedures, clearly deprived Ms. Jones of her due process rights as supported in *Goss*.

Although the *Jones* case was not decided on its merits at the appeals level, the opinion is an important one in supporting the right of the student to obtain a fair hearing on the facts surrounding his or her particular case. For Ms. Jones, that meant upholding the decision to allow her to be reinstated pending a full and fair hearing concerning the alleged misconduct and whether dismissal for disciplinary reasons would be warranted.

In another interesting case, *Slaughter v. Brigham Young University*,[45] a private university's actions were evaluated by a federal district court. After a hearing, the university dismissed a doctoral student for using his professor's name as a coauthor of articles the student had written before being admitted as a student in the program. Prior to using the faculty member's name as a coauthor, the student could not get the papers published. The university cited its rules of conduct, which stated that the student should observe "high principles of honor, integrity and morality," and be honest in all behavior, as the basis for its dismissal.

The federal court held that the university's rules of conduct were reasonable, clear, and well defined. Furthermore, the court held that all of the student's due process protections were afforded to him and therefore upheld the decision of the university.[46]

Physical or Mental Incapacity

A third obstacle that may stand in the way of a student's main goal in the academic environment is a physical or mental incapacity that prevents the student from successfully completing the program of study. Earlier this chapter discussed the general prohibition against making admission and readmission decisions solely on the basis of a handicap and presented the general limitations on such decisions. Likewise, limitations also exist for subsequent decisions based on a health problem that hinders the student's academic and clinical performance. These limitations do not mean that a faculty member cannot make a decision based on the existence of a mental or physical problem. Rather, they mean that the decisions must be careful and deliberate and clearly conform to existing state and federal laws protecting any student who may fall under their respective protections.[47]

Curriculum/Catalog Changes

Another obstacle facing students as they progress through their academic experience may be a change in the curriculum. Generally speaking, changes in the curriculum must be done in a timely manner and give students adequate notice of the change and how it will affect them. This notice is especially important if the effect is an adverse one; for example, not graduating as planned or needing additional coursework that requires more cost to the student. Moreover, viable options must be provided for the student to comply with the "new requirements" without detriment.[48] When such conditions are allegedly not met by the educational entity and are challenged by students, the court must define how the institution's need for change can be balanced with fairness vis-à-vis the student body.

Another obstacle facing students as they progress through their academic experience may be a change in the curriculum.

In *Atkinson v. Traetta*,[49] six nursing students at Queensborough Community College were unable to progress to additional nursing courses because the prerequisite for subsequent course enrollment was changed to a C− grade rather than a D− grade. They filed a suit asking for an injunction allowing them to continue in the nursing program. The students alleged that the change constituted a change in the curriculum *after* they had enrolled, and the change was therefore unfair. The trial court returned a verdict in favor of the students and granted the injunction. The college appealed.

The New York Appellate Division reversed the trial court, holding that the change that did occur was not a "curriculum change" but rather a "grading change." The court stated that even if it were a curriculum change, the faculty had an obligation to uphold academic standards, particularly when those standards involved clinical practice and the public's safety.[50] Furthermore, the court continued, the changes were communicated to the student body well in advance of the change's effective date.

Likewise, in *Crabtree v. California University of Pennsylvania*,[51] the Pennsylvania Commonwealth Court upheld the university's requirement of an additional 1,000-hour internship in a post-masters' certificate program for Mary Ann Crabtree. Ms. Crabtree had graduated from the school's psychology program in 1988 and then enrolled in the certificate program. The 1985–1987 catalog clearly stated that the certificate required 450 hours of an internship. The catalog also contained a statement that the university retained the right to alter statements or procedures in the catalog. In addition, the catalog stated that it was the student's responsibility to keep up with changes that might occur in requirements.

The student alleged that because she entered the university's program in 1986, the 1985–1987 catalog should control the number of hours she had to take to complete the certificate program.

The court, in supporting the university's decision, discussed the fact that the disclaimer in the catalog concerning changes in the requirements for the certificate allowed the university to make changes as it saw fit. Moreover, Ms. Crabtree was given adequate notice of the change by the university in announcements and a bulletin sent to all students enrolled in the program.[52]

Graduation

Academic institutions must also make careful decisions concerning the graduation of students, and the same principles discussed in the *Admission and Readmission* and *Advancement in the School or Program* sections apply to these decisions as well. Catalog and specific school or program documents must contain clear language and directives concerning graduation requirements, including any time limitations under which the student must operate, grade point average required for graduation, semester or quarter hours needed for graduation, any application process that the student must initiate *prior* to graduation, and any fees necessary. A student who feels aggrieved by an adverse decision concerning graduation can challenge it under the various legal mechanisms discussed earlier in this chapter; for example, breach of an express or implied contract term, violation of due process rights (if the school is public and the decision not to graduate the student rests upon some disciplinary action), or arbitrary or capricious decision by the school.

In *Eiland v. Wolf*,[53] for example, the Texas Court of Appeals for the First District (Houston) reviewed several allegations made by a medical student, Philip Wolf, concerning the decision of the University of Texas Medical Branch at Galveston not to graduate him from the medical school. At the trial level, the court granted declaratory relief and a permanent injunction against the school for Wolf's "wrongful dismissal" from the school after he failed his final course in the program. In essence, the trial court ordered that Wolf graduate and receive the degree of Doctor of Medicine. The school appealed the decision.

The appeals court, in reversing the trial court's holding, cited *Horowitz* in upholding the school's decision to dismiss Wolf and not graduate him. Characterizing the decision as an *academic* one, the court held no hearing was required (as Wolf alleged) and the process that did take place concerning the decision to dismiss the student was fair. Furthermore, the court continued, there was evidence in the trial record that the decision to dismiss Wolf was based on professional (faculty) judgment and therefore could not be overturned absent a void of academic decision making by faculty.[54]

Wolf's claim that the university, a public institution, violated his equal protection rights under the Fourteenth Amendment was also held invalid. Citing a U.S. Supreme Court case, *Regents of the University of Michigan v. Ewing*,[55] the court reiterated that generally academic decisions are not subject to rigorous judicial review. Therefore, absent evidence to support an allegation that the decision was "beyond the pale of reasoned academic decision-making," that decision must be upheld.[56]

Wolf's last count, a breach of contract claim, was based on the school catalog's language concerning graduation and its requirements. Distinguishing this case from the *Babb* case discussed in Table 20–1, the court held that in this case, the catalog contained a disclaimer reserving the right of the school to change its contents and negating the establishment of a contract with any student. In addition, the university's catalog expressly stated that the School of Medicine had the "authority" to drop any student from enrollment "if circumstances of a legal, moral, health, social or academic nature justify such a request."[57] Thus, no enforceable contract existed between Wolf and the university. Even if a contract did exist, the court concluded, the school and university adhered to the terms of the catalog (contract) without question.

Privacy

The student enrolled in a postsecondary academic institution has a right to privacy. That right has its basis in several legal arenas—state and federal constitutions and statutory law. The state and federal constitutional protections are firmly rooted in the Fourteenth Amendment to the U.S. Constitution. State protections of privacy are usually located in a parallel amendment, section, or article. The respective constitutions protect against violations of privacy by the state and federal government, and a student does not lose those protections when enrolled in primary, secondary, or postsecondary educational programs. Public entities have different obligations in maintaining the privacy of citizens, including students, than do private organizations, and educational institutions are no exception.

The student enrolled in a postsecondary academic institution has a right to privacy.

The academic institution may violate a student's constitutional right of privacy in several ways. One way in which it could be jeopardized is by intrusively seeking out private information from a student. "Overstepping" by academic faculty into unjustified areas may be challenged. Therefore, information sought by an academic institution or program must be germane to the reason for the initial inquiry.

A second way in which a student's right to privacy may be violated is a search of the student's room, locker, or person for whatever reason. When this occurs, the U.S. Constitution's Fourth Amendment protection against unreasonable searches and seizures and parallel state constitutional protections come into play. This student right will be discussed further in the section *Other Constitutional Rights*.

A student also has an interest in protecting the privacy of his or her student records. Although a state may protect releases of postsecondary student records by statute and/or case law, the federal Family Educational Rights and Privacy Act of 1974 was amended by the Buckley Amendment[58] and is the controlling law in this area.

The Buckley Amendment was passed to ensure a consistent approach to the release of a student's school record. Prior to its enactment, only a few states had any laws regulating the release of information in the student's school file. In addition, it was often difficult for the student or student's parents to obtain information contained in the school file for their own review. Thus, Congress tied access and release of student files to the receipt of federal funds from any applicable federal program administered by the Department of Education and applied the Act to both public and private "educational agencies."[59]

Briefly, the Buckley Amendment allows students 18 years of age and older the right of access to their records, the right to be informed of the school policy concerning that access, and the right to give consent for the release of information from their educational file, which includes "records, files, documents and other materials which contain information directly related to a student and are maintained by an educational agency or institution or a person acting for such agency or institution."[60] In addition, if there is anything in the educational record that the student objects to, procedures spelled out in the Act must be adopted by the educational agency to allow the student to challenge that information.

The Buckley Amendment was passed to ensure a consistent approach to the release of a student's school record.

Exceptions exist in the Act concerning the need for consent to be obtained prior to the release of information under certain circumstances and also for certain materials being exempt from access or review by the student. For example, consent need not be obtained from the student to release file information when the release is to other school officials, including teachers, within the school who have been determined by the institution to have a legitimate educational interest in that information; when the release is pursuant to a judicial order or lawful subpoena (although notification prior to release is required); when the release is to appropriate individuals who need the information in an emergency to protect the health or safety of the student or other persons; and in connection with a student's application for, or receipt of, financial aid.[61] Student "directory information," which includes name, address, major field of study, dates of attendance, and degree awarded may also be released without consent, unless a refusal is given by the student.[62] A student does not have access to teachers' and administrators' personal notes solely within the teachers' or administrators' possession; the student's parents do not have access to the student's medical, psychiatric, or other professional treatment records; and, if the student has signed a waiver of access, the student cannot review letters or statements of recommendation if used solely for the purpose for which they were intended. If the student requested notification of those individuals who gave such letters of recommendation, the school must notify the student when the letters are received.[63]

Academic institutions and their respective schools or departments must ensure adherence to the Buckley Amendment's mandates concerning the privacy and accessibility of student records. Not only may a student be harmed by unauthorized release of information or by not being able to review that which he or she is entitled to examine, but the academic institution may have funding terminated if noncompliance is proven. The development of policies and procedures consistent with those mandates by nursing programs can aid with conformity. In addition, the careful storing of student records, evaluations, and other materials concerning the student by the nursing program is also essential. Student information in faculty offices should also be carefully stored, with access to that information limited to the faculty member or his or her secretary.

Other Constitutional Rights

Searches and Seizures/Privacy

A student's interest in maintaining privacy also rests in federal and state constitutional protections against invasions of privacy under the prohibition against unreasonable searches and seizures by the government. The Fourth Amendment of the U.S. Constitution, and parallel state provisions, do not prohibit any and all searches and seizures. Rather, the ban extends only to unreasonable searches and, in some instances, to warrantless searches.[64]

Although it is clear that the constitutional protection against tyrannical governmental intrusion into privacy extends to students, how it applies has not always been clear. Initially, many of the cases concerning this right dealt with the student and his or her expectation of privacy in university- or college-sponsored student housing, whether in a residence hall or another type of dwelling. In those cases, courts have held that students do have an expectation of privacy in college- or university-sponsored housing, their possessions, and their person.[65] The expectation cannot be abrogated by the academic institution's reliance on the *in loco parentis* doctrine or its position as a "landlord" of the student. In other words, the institution cannot give consent to university or other police to conduct a search of the student's living quarters.[66]

There are exceptions to these limitations on an educational institution's ability to breach the privacy of students, however. One is when the student gives consent for a warrantless search under certain conditions. For example, the residence contract might contain a provision dealing with the ability of the university to enter and search a student's dwelling under very limited circumstances.[67] Or the student may orally consent to a search at the instant it is asked for by university or college officials. However, as with any provision in a housing contract, the search consented to would have to be clearly requested, narrowly drawn, and *not* include the personal belongings of a roommate.[68]

A second exception to the requirement of a warrant prior to a search is when an emergency exists and protection of the health and safety of other students is at issue, or when necessary to maintain "order and discipline." For this exception to apply, however, there must be a true emergency; that is, when the life or well-being of the students is of concern, such as a fire or when police are needed to provide assistance or help individuals in distress,[69] or when an incident is disrupting the functioning of the entity as an educational institution.[70] It is clear that if the university is simply conducting what has been termed an "administrative search," there is no emergency or disruption of the academic milieu. Moreover, when there is time to obtain a search warrant, the courts will usually require that one be obtained, unless consent for such searches has been obtained through the housing contract or from the student personally.[71]

A third exception concerning the need for a warrant before searching a student's residence is when an item is in the "plain view" of the school official. The plain-view doctrine has specific applicability to criminal law. It is also applied to student searches as well. Thus, when a school official or the police are lawfully in a student's room or home, and incriminating evidence is present in plain view of that officer or school official, it can be seized and used in a school disciplinary hearing, for example, or in a criminal trial. Of course, the question whether or not the evidence was seized pursuant to this doctrine is always subject to challenge and would occur under the "exclusionary rule" doctrine analyzed in Chapter 9. Generally speaking, however, because the rule has been interpreted by the U.S. Supreme Court as applying only in certain situations like criminal cases and administrative searches (e.g., Occupational Safety and Health Administration), its use in the academic setting is probably limited.

It is important to remember that the application of the rules covering unreasonable searches and seizures and student residences apply particularly to public academic institutions. Private institutions are less constrained by these constitutional protections. Yet, if local, state, or federal officials are involved in any search or seizure by a private academic agency, then the court would require adherence to those protections. In addition, the character of funding received by a private academic institution—from state or local taxes, for example—may color the institution more similar to a public rather than strictly private entity, and therefore necessitate adherence to privacy protections.

Drug and Alcohol Testing/Privacy

In recent years the character of the allegations of invasion of privacy actions of students has changed. Though privacy issues concerning a student's living quarters and belongings are still important, the issue of drugs, drug testing, and any subsequent actions taken by the academic institution against the student based on the test results has become the focus of this constitutionally based right.

It would be inaccurate to say that none of the early cases dealing with student privacy dealt with drugs, drug testing, or disciplinary actions against students. However, it has not been until recently that this focus has taken on monumental proportions.

The issue of a student's constitutional rights in relation to searches and drug testing had its birth in the public school arena. In the first U.S. Supreme Court case, *New Jersey v. T.L.O.*,[72] the search of a 14-year-old freshman's purse for cigarettes after the student was found smoking in violation of the school's rule was upheld by the Court, even when the search turned up marijuana and paraphernalia used to make and smoke the marijuana. In so holding, the Court said that although public school students do have an expectation of privacy when in school, the test for such a search is whether or not it was reasonable, taking into consideration all the circumstances surrounding the search. When there is a question of the student's conduct breaking the law or the rules of the school, that search will be justified under "ordinary circumstances," so long as the search is within reasonable parameters and scope to fulfill the objectives of the search and is not "excessively" intrusive given the student's age, sex, and nature of the alleged offense.[73]

In addition, the Court held that if the above criteria are met, there is no need for a search warrant *prior* to the search, so long as the student is under the school's authority. Even so, the Court also held that the Fourth Amendment's protection against unreasonable searches and seizures does apply to public school officials because they are representatives of the state and must therefore conduct themselves within the mandates also applicable to law enforcement officers.[74]

The issue of a student's constitutional rights in relation to searches and drug testing had its birth in the public school arena.

After the *T.L.O.* decision, cases shifted from searches of property to searches of individuals, mainly through drug testing programs, by using blood or urine analysis to determine whether drugs are present in the student's system at the time of the test. In 1995 the ability of high schools to test student athletes for drugs was supported by the U.S. Supreme Court in *Vernonia School District v. Acton.*[75] The Court upheld the Vernonia School District's initial testing (with the parents' consent) of all students when applying for any interscholastic sports team and then random testing thereafter. If consent was not obtained for the initial testing, the student could not be considered for the particular team. Likewise, if the student subsequently tested positive during random testing, several penalties were imposed, up to and including suspension from the team.[76]

James Acton did not feel it was fair to be tested for drugs, since he never had a drug problem and was an excellent student. His parents agreed and sued the school board, alleging that the policy violated the student's Fourth Amendment rights.

The U.S. Supreme Court held that no Fourth Amendment violation occurred because the school search was "reasonable under the circumstances," especially in view of the documented drug problem facing students and student athletes generally in Vernonia.[77] The policy was reasonable, the Court opined, because a student's legitimate expectation of privacy is lessened as a result of his or her constant supervision by school officials under the *in loco parentis* doctrine. Moreover, the Vernonia policy carefully fashioned an unobtrusive search (e.g., no direct observation of student giving specimen).[78] Last, the Court held that the policy was reasonable because there was a dire need for the testing to identify students who might be using drugs in order to help them overcome the problem and provide a safe interscholastic sports program.[79]

IMPLICATIONS FOR NURSING STUDENTS AND FACULTY

Nursing students who provide care to patients while under the influence of any drug that would impair their ability to provide safe care are problematic from a liability perspective for both the school and for the student. The school or program may have a clear interest, indeed may possess a clear duty, to evaluate those nursing students who are functioning in an impaired manner. How that interest or duty is carried out, however, will deter-mine whether or not any testing program passes judicial scrutiny if challenged. Therefore, nursing programs that consider testing nursing students for drug or alcohol use will need to do so very carefully.

To begin with, programs in public postsecondary institutions will need to conform strictly to constitutional protections as discussed so far. In addition, the utilization of a voluntary, as opposed to a mandatory, drug-testing program needs to be carefully evaluated. What standard will be applied when deciding to test a student must also be addressed. For example, in the *T.L.O.* case, one of the issues discussed was the fact that the "reasonable suspicion" of drug presence standard applicable to high school students would probably not apply to college students.[80] The appropriate standard for students in colleges or universities would probably be a "probable cause" one, thus eliminating any random testing under either approach.

Secondly, if a nursing school or program does decide to do any testing of student nurses, compliance with the *Drug-Free Schools and Communities Act of 1986* and its amendments[81] will be helpful. Although it has no specific discussion or requirements concerning drug testing, the Act does require that any institution of higher education receiving federal funds or any other form of financial assistance under any federal program adopt and implement a drug and alcohol abuse policy.[82] The Act requires several components to any adopted program, including standards of conduct prohibiting unlawful possession, use, or distribution of drugs and alcohol on campus; sanctions that will be imposed by the institution if the code of conduct is violated; and continual evaluation of the program once implemented.[83]

Schools of nursing have published articles concerning their established policies on drug and alcohol abuse and research findings covering substance abuse curriculum in nursing education programs.[84] Interestingly, as a way around the random testing issue, some policies require the nursing student to provide consent ("A Witness Contract") to be tested for drugs and alcohol and enter into treatment if any suspicious behavior is identified by faculty during their clinical or classroom experiences.[85]

Privacy must be maintained for the nursing student who is believed to be impaired while providing care to patients during clinical assignments—concerning the conduct in question, the testing itself, the procedure for gathering any blood or urine specimen, the test results, and any disciplinary actions taken as a consequence of a positive test result. Along this line, it is vital that clear due process protections are afforded the student who may be dismissed or otherwise disciplined by the program for a positive result.

Nursing school administrators and faculty must also be certain that they are not discriminating against the student who may have an alcohol or drug use problem in violation of state and federal antidiscrimination laws (e.g., ADA). For example, for a first offense, it may be wise to counsel the student to take a leave of absence to obtain treatment rather than suspend or dismiss the student. Then, after successful completion of treatment, the student may reapply pursuant to the school's leave of absence policy, and, if criteria are met, be able to resume active status in the program.

The policy and procedures concerning any testing of the nursing student must also carefully analyze the confirming test that is used and be cognizant of the fact that there are many viable criticisms of the accuracy of such tests. In addition, strict procedures must ensure that, from the collection of the specimen to its ultimate acceptance by the testing site, a "chain of custody" exists.[86] If there is any lapse in this chain, the student could successfully allege that a particular specimen does not belong to him or her.

Until the legal issues surrounding drug testing are resolved with more clarity, it may be prudent for nursing programs to develop other ways of dealing with the impaired student in the clinical area. Drug use that impairs a student's ability to safely provide patient care would be important to include in the school's and program's catalog as one of the grounds upon which disciplinary action may be taken against a student. Including information and research about chemical substance abuse in the school's curriculum would also be important in aiding students to increase their knowledge about chemical abuse. In addition, continuing education programs concerning drug use and treatment may also help the student identify the problem he or she is experiencing and therefore seek help voluntarily, thus eliminating further progression of the problem.

Open lines of communication between faculty and students may also be a valuable alternative for the student who needs treatment for chemical abuse. Faculty and administrators must be willing to confront students with evidence of impairment. In addition, suggesting ways the student can obtain the help he or she needs can be useful in aiding the student to complete educational and professional goals.

First Amendment Freedoms

First Amendment freedoms are important ones for any individual, and the student is no exception. The First Amendment guarantees freedom of peaceful assembly, speech, press, the establishment and exercise of religion, and petitioning the government to remedy grievances.[87] Early cases centering on student discharges violated these, and Fourteenth Amendment, rights when students were dismissed from postsecondary academic institutions for "conduct" that was not seen as conforming with a particular school's expectations of students. Unfortunately, allegations against academic institutions for breaching students' First Amendment protections still abound, and the judicial system continues to balance the academic entity's rights with those of the student body.

First Amendment freedoms are important ones for any individual, and the student is no exception.

The classic case setting forth students' free speech and assembly rights in an academic setting was *Tinker v. Des Moines Independent Community School District.*[88] Three public school students were suspended from school after protesting the government's involvement in the Vietnam War by wearing black armbands during school hours. The student's challenge was dismissed at the federal district court level and the dismissal was affirmed by the appeals court *en banc.* Because both court decisions were based on the principle that it was within the school board's power to dismiss the students, even without any evidence of disruption of school activities by the students, the U.S. Supreme Court reversed and remanded the case. In doing so, the Court held that the demonstration was peaceful and not disruptive and therefore was protected by the First and Fourteenth Amendments; that both students *and* teachers possess First Amendment rights, subject to the "special characteristics of the school environment"; and that the term *free speech* includes certain "symbolic acts" that express views.[89]

Tinker's holding was applied again by the U.S. Supreme Court in a case involving postsecondary students' First Amendment rights. In *Healy v. James*,[90] decided in 1972, a federal district court evaluated a situation that arose at Central Connecticut State College, where students' request for recognition of a local chapter of Students for a Democratic Society (SDS) was approved by the Student Affairs Committee. The college president denied the recognition on the basis that the organization's philosophy was contrary to the college's support of academic freedom and would be a disruptive force on campus. The denial had the effect of prohibiting the organization from utilizing school meeting rooms, bulletin boards, and newspapers.

The Supreme Court reversed and remanded the case to the trial court to determine if the organization would abide by campus rules and regulations applicable to any organization on campus. If so, then the college would be required to approve the SDS pursuant to those rules and regulations. Citing *Tinker,* the Court held that although First Amendment freedoms in the school setting must be balanced with the right of school officials to constitutionally "prescribe and control" conduct there, college classrooms are the "marketplace of ideas," and academic freedom must continue to be protected from unconstitutional infringement.[91]

The U.S. Supreme Court and respective federal courts have decided a plethora of First Amendment cases since these two important cases.[92] Generally, they uphold the exercise of a student's First Amendment rights in the academic milieu. However, the student's exercise of those rights may be limited if it materially and substantially disrupts others and the operation of the school, if damage or injury to property or person occurs, if it is for the purpose of producing lawless action, or if faculty or administrators are threatened.

Likewise, a student's freedom to exercise his or her religious beliefs has also generally been supported by the courts. This right, like those already discussed, may present itself in combination with the exercise of other First Amendment freedoms. For example, a nursing student who dresses a certain way because of religious beliefs may not feel that he or she can wear the nursing student uniform in clinical settings because it is against the dress requirements of his or her religion. Or a religious group may request recognition from college or nursing program officials to establish a chapter of that organization on campus.

Nursing faculty and administrators, whether in public or private institutions, would be wise to carefully study the latest case law in this area before developing any formal or informal policies concerning the handling of First Amendment freedoms. Certainly, consultation with legal counsel for the academic institution would be vital, not only in exploring the issues but also when a specific case or situation developed. In addition to developing a specific stance concerning First Amendment freedoms, school officials must ensure that any positions developed are applied in a just and equitable manner, that any restriction or limitation on First Amendment rights is factually based, and that the group is given the chance to comply with reasonable school requirements that may avoid the restriction or limitation. Last, but not least, faculty must keep up with any new case law developments concerning First Amendment rights.

Equal Protection of the Law

Equal protection of the law as a constitutional requirement means that no one person or persons shall be denied the protections of the law given other persons in like or similar circumstances.[93] Insofar as public postsecondary academic entities are concerned, it is important that faculty or administrative decisions not unduly support one student or a group of students to the exclusion or expense of another student or group.

Generally the cases alleging a denial of equal protection have been decided in favor of the college or university, mainly because the students involved in the cases were not in like or similar circumstances, or the alleged differences were permissible. However, some examples in which a violation of the equal protection clause was raised include not enforcing a cheating policy in the same manner against students and placing restrictions on the use of the student activity fund by a particular school organization.[94]

Sexual Harassment

Sexual harassment is a potential concern for all individuals, whether as an employee or as a student. Students are protected from sexual harassment (a form of sex/gender discrimination) under Title IX of the Education Amendments.[95] In *Gebser v. Lago Vista Independent School District*,[96] the U.S. Supreme Court established the parameters of liability for a school (in this case a high school) receiving Title IX funds. Briefly, the Court held that for an educational institution to be liable for the sexual harassment of a student *by a faculty member,* school officials would have to have "actual notice of . . . and . . . [be] deliberately indifferent to, the teacher's misconduct."[97]

In *Davis v. Monroe County Board of Education*,[98] the Court delineated an academic institution's liability for sexual harassment *by a student.* In *Davis,* the Court reemphasized the "deliberate indifference" standard articulated in *Gebser.* If school officials know about student-to-student sexual harassment and are knowingly indifferent to it when the harasser is "under the school's disciplinary authority," the educational institution might be liable.[99] Sexual harassment in this case was defined as "behavior . . . so severe, pervasive, and objectively offensive" that its victims are denied equal access to education that is protected under Title IX.[100]

Students should become familiar with any policies the academic institution has established concerning sexual harassment. If the student believes he or she is a victim of sexual harassment by either a student or a faculty member, the concerns should be brought to the immediate attention of the school official designated in the policy. Oftentimes, the resolution of such situations can be handled through specifically established dispute resolution mechanisms (e.g., mediation) or other resolution procedures (e.g., grievance policy).[101] If no dispute resolution mechanism exists in the academic institution specifically for sexual harassment, the student may be able to use the nursing program or institution's code of conduct or mission statement of the school as a basis for eliminating the harassment.

If, however, neither of these options is available and the student believes the behavior experienced is sexually harassing, he or she should seek advice from an attorney experienced in gender discrimination issues. Specific details concerning when the harassment occurred, who was notified in the institution, what interventions, if any, took place to rectify the problem, and any other details concerning the behavior will be important to share with the attorney. After a careful evaluation of the specific details, the attorney can then advise the student about the possibility of filing a suit to eliminate the conduct and often possibly other relief under Title IX (e.g., compensatory damages, attorney's fees).

ADDITIONAL STUDENT CONCERNS

Professional Negligence/Negligence

Students in postsecondary academic institutions may have additional concerns that accompany them as they progress through their academic careers. One such concern for the student is that of liability for alleged *negligent* care that is given by the student during the educational program. Professional negligence occurs when there is an allegation that a standard of care was breached, causing injury to a patient. The overall conduct standard for the professional nurse would be what ordinary, prudent, and reasonable professional nurses would have done in the same or similar circumstances. When professional negligence is alleged against a student nurse, the standard of the graduate professional nurse in the same or similar situation applies.[102] Thus the student must ensure that he or she is well prepared for any patient care assignments being undertaken, must ask for supervision or additional instruction when unsure of the care to be provided, and must ask for a change in assignment if not able to carry out the patient treatment in a safe manner. Furthermore, the nursing student should carry professional liability insurance to ensure some financial protection against the costs of legal representation. A professional liability policy would also provide a financial base from which a judgment can be paid should a verdict be entered against the student nurse.

When professional negligence is alleged against a student nurse, the standard of the graduate professional nurse in the same or similar situation applies.

Similarly, nursing students may be held responsible for their own nonnursing negligence, even when it takes place during school-related activities. For example, in *Central Security Mutual Insurance Company v. DePinto*,[103] a nursing student who was driving herself and other nursing students to a clinical placement in a college van was involved in an accident in which the driver of the other car was killed. At issue in the case was whether Ms. DePinto's father's automobile insurance excluded the van from being covered under the policy because the van was insured for "regular use." The court allowed the case to stand and held that the van was not being "used regularly," but was strictly limited to going to and returning from the clinical placement via a specified route. It is important to note here that the school was not sued directly in this case but was involved as an intervenor. Thus the case was allowed to go forward against the nursing student who was driving at the time of the accident.

Conformity with State Nurse Practice Act

Conformity with the state nurse practice act is another concern for the nursing student, both while progressing through the program and while awaiting licensure based upon successful passage of the state nursing boards. It is important for the student nurse to comply with all requirements concerning the provision of care while a student.

ETHICS CONNECTION 20–3

Faculty not only need to select what to teach and what to omit from ethics education; they also need to decide how and how not to teach ethics. A number of approaches are used. They range from the standard didactic method of introducing ethical theory, moral principles, and professional codes to clinical immersion experiences. One new approach, Narrative Pedagogy, is based on Diekelmann's[1] interpretive phenomenological research in nursing education. Narrative Pedagogy[2] offers new possibilities for ethics education in academic as well as clinical practice settings. Learning ethics and genetics is an appropriate exemplar for an innovative approach to schooling, learning, and teaching because

> the content for clinical practice is new and rapidly changing and the Human Genome Project[3] has led to ethical issues such as commercialization and profit seeking. . . . The commercialization, lack of governmental oversight and research outside of federally funded laboratories have contributed to ethical dilemmas of unimagined proportions. How can nurses in practice learn the as yet unthought, unanticipated ethical dilemmas related to genetic testing and gene therapy much less teach these to students or discuss them with other clinicians?[4]

Diekelmann and Diekelmann interpret the story of a teacher who shifts to a narrative pedagogical approach in two courses after current approaches to learning ethics and genetics have failed. The first course is an undergraduate maternity course and the second, a graduate women's health course. By doubling up on didactic content one week, the teacher and students have time for dialogue about the content-related issues the next week. On alternate weeks, the graduate and undergraduate students learn together. As the course unfolds, the teacher and students invite others in the community to participate in the biweekly dialogue. Undergraduate and graduate students, teachers, clinicians, and others in the community learn together on alternate weeks. The course becomes like "a Village Square" as word of the course spreads and more and more people ask to come to the gatherings. The teacher says, "We spend a lot of time thinking about the language of nursing practice . . . how we speak about ethical dilemmas we experience and . . . always, always we come back to language. How nurses control people with a technical language or . . . how by saying nothing we exonerate ourselves from participating in serious ethical dilemmas."[5] Throughout the courses, new questions emerge from the conversation. These are questions that often are central to practice but overlooked in the ethics literature. Diekelmann and Diekelmann conclude by reflecting that "new possibilities for ethics and genetics open up in the interpretive thinking of Narrative Pedagogy."[6] Narrative Pedagogy has merit as an approach to learning ethics because it is consistent with the emerging notion of communitarian ethics and the ethic of care.

---

[1]Nancy Diekelmann, "Creating a New Pedagogy for Nursing," 36(4) *Journal of Nursing Education* (1997), 147–148.
[2]Nancy Diekelmann and John Diekelmann. *Schooling Learning Teaching: Toward a Narrative Pedogogy.* (In press)
[3]See Chapters 3 and 11 for additional references to the Human Genome Project.
[4]Nancy Diekelmann and John Diekelmann. "Learning Ethics in Nursing and Genetics: Narrative Pedagogy and the Grounding of Values," 15(4) *Journal of Pediatric Nursing* (August 2000), 1–6. (In press)
[5]*Id.*
[6]*Id.*

For example, nurse practice acts require that patient care by students can be given only pursuant to a recognized nursing education program that meets faculty and clinical supervision requirements. The nursing student must also be aware of what restrictions are placed on his or her role when working as a nurse's aide or in other assistive roles. The student nurse must be careful not to perform responsibilities while in an assistive role that only a *licensed* nurse can perform pursuant to the nurse practice act. If that occurs, the student could be alleged to be practicing nursing without a license. Therefore, familiarity with the nursing practice act, and the rules and regulations to enforce it, is important, not only upon completion of the nursing program but during the time the student nurse is advancing toward graduation.

FACULTY RIGHTS AND CONCERNS

Although most of the chapter has thus far been devoted to student rights and concomitant faculty responsibilities, it is also important to highlight faculty rights and specific concerns that faculty may have when teaching. Faculty possess many rights when teaching in a postsecondary institution, including evaluation/grading rights and employment protections. New teaching/learning methodologies, like distance education and the use of computers and other technologies, raise new concerns for faculty. Likewise, liability concerns exist in relation to suits initiated by students alleging negligent teaching, defamation, and invasion of privacy, to name a few. Some of those concerns and rights will be briefly presented.

Liability Concerns

The potential liability a faculty member and the academic institution face for an alleged violation of a student's due process rights or failure to progress through a particular program has been presented earlier in this chapter. In fact, a study of 24 cases filed against nursing education programs between 1961 and September of 1989 indicated that, among other findings, nursing students, particularly in baccalaureate programs, are more prone to sue schools of nursing and nursing faculty than other students in postsecondary institutions.[104] Of the 24 cases included in the study, 10 of the 11 filed by nursing students involved allegations concerning

dismissals from, or denial of admissions to, nursing education programs.[105]

Educational Malpractice Suits

Admission and dismissal suits are not the only types of suits that faculty may be involved in. One additional allegation against faculty that may arise is that of educational malpractice. In this type of suit, the student alleges that the nursing faculty member breached his or her duty to teach effectively. As a direct and proximate result of this failure to teach properly, the student was not able to graduate or successfully pass state boards. The student may seek an injunction and ask the court to require the nursing program to graduate him or her, or the student may seek compensation for the failure to graduate and/or pass state boards.

Educational malpractice suits against any faculty, including nurse faculty, have not been successful to date. As early as 1979, courts have not supported this cause of action against *public* school teachers, reasoning that (1) identifying why a student did not learn would be difficult; (2) recognizing this type of cause of action would "open the floodgates" of litigation against teachers; and (3) allowing a suit for negligent teaching would also be a blatant interference by the judicial system in the administration of public schools.[106] Subsequent decisions involving faculty in postsecondary institutions have reached similar conclusions.[107]

Educational malpractice suits against . . . faculty, including nurse faculty, have not been successful to date.

Despite this protection, nurse faculty will want to continue to teach in a manner consistent with sound educational principles and in accordance with applicable standards. There is no question that nursing faculty have a basic duty to instruct students properly.[108] When, and if, a successful challenge alleging a breach of that duty will occur remains to be seen.

Being Named as a Defendant in a Suit

Nursing faculty may be named as a defendant in a suit filed by a student in one of two ways. Because the faculty member is an employee of the school or college, he or she may be sued as a named defendant, along with the school or college. So long as the student's allegations involve the faculty member's duties that are within the scope of his or her employment as a faculty member, then the faculty member can be named in the suit.

Nursing faculty may also be individually named in a suit by a student under the theory of personal liability. The student may sue the faculty member "individually" and as a faculty member if the student is unclear whether the conduct alleged against the faculty member was within the scope of the faculty's employment responsibilities, or if the conduct was "willful" or "intentional."[109]

Nursing faculty in public academic institutions may enjoy the benefit of sovereign or charitable immunity against tort actions given to the college or university where employed, depending on the particular state statute that affords the protection. If the immunity is absolute, the faculty member could not be sued successfully by a student when allegations concerning his or her employment duties were the basis of the suit. However, not all immunity protections are absolute, if they exist at all. Moreover, if the faculty member is sued individually, there may be no immunity protection. The faculty member will need to be knowledgeable about what protections, if any, are afforded to the institution and its faculty.

Grading and Evaluation of Students

Because of the emphasis on student rights in relation to evaluation and grading, faculty often think they do not possess any rights when making decisions about student competency in the clinical and academic area. However, nothing could be further from the truth. The *Horowitz* case presented earlier in this chapter provides support for faculty rights when professional judgments are made concerning the caliber of a student's abilities.

In its unanimous opinion, the U.S. Supreme Court relied on a long-standing precedent of lower court rulings holding that academic decisions (e.g., what is a passing grade, evaluations of students) are within the realm of the academic community alone.[110] Additionally, the Court stated that courts were not equipped with the expertise needed for such determinations.[111] Since the Supreme Court has not overruled its own opinion concerning this issue, the decision, and the principles it supports, can still be relied on.

Even so, faculty cannot make academic decisions arbitrarily, capriciously, or in a discriminatory manner. Rather, faculty judgments must be deliberate and careful, as the Court found existed in the *Horowitz* and *Clements* cases. In this regard, anecdotal notes specific to difficulties encountered by the student in both the classroom and clinical area are essential. Moreover, the faculty must inform the nursing student of the difficulties he or she is having in the program as well as the consequences if improvement does not occur (e.g., probation or dismissal). This will require the faculty to meet with the nursing student experiencing academic problems as required in the school of nursing policy. If faculty also use *Horowitz* and *Clements* as a guide, it appears that the more notice given the student, the better the faculty will comply with the student's due process obligations.

Any written materials given to nursing students during the time they are enrolled in the nursing school or program that govern their responsibilities, grading, and progression through the program should be carefully developed. School of nursing catalogs, syllabi, and descriptions of special projects need to include precise information informing the student of his or her responsibilities and how grading will occur. Objectives for each course and clinical rotation should be behaviorally defined.

Evaluation tools used by faculty must also be carefully developed. Because any evaluation is somewhat subjective, the tool should be as objective as possible and used in a consistent manner by the school of nursing faculty.

Nursing faculty in private and public academic institutions clearly *do not* need to provide a hearing for a student prior to dismissing the student from the program or school for academic reasons. However, if the faculty member is in doubt about the character of dismissal that is going to occur, it is best to provide the student with whatever protections are afforded students who are being dismissed for disciplinary reasons. A court will not fault a faculty member or institution for providing *more* protections to a student than was necessary, but a court may impose liability if required faculty and institution responsibilities were not met.

Employment

Nursing faculty teach at both private and public academic institutions. The faculty member may have a contract of employment for a definite period of time (e.g., 1 year) in either type of institution, or the faculty member may be tenured; that is, possess a property right to continued employment unless discharged "for cause."[112] A tenured position, although not a guarantee of lifetime employment,[113] is more secure for a number of reasons. First, it provides procedural protections for the faculty member when there is an allegation that "adequate cause" exists to terminate the faculty member's employment (e.g., incompetency, neglect of duties). Second, it limits the ability of the institution to terminate the faculty to for-cause situations, thus protecting the faculty member's academic freedom.[114] Even so, it affords no protection to the faculty member if the dismissal or termination is due to "noncausal" reasons such as the discontinuance of a program or financial exigency.

The faculty member may have a contract of employment for a definite period . . . or the faculty member may be tenured . . .

Although not as protective as tenure, a contract of employment with the institution means a faculty member may be dismissed only "for-cause" prior to the completion of the term of the contract. Moreover, if the nursing faculty member teaches at a public university or community college and is dismissed in violation of the contract of employment, he or she can sue, alleging an entitlement in continued employment pursuant to the contract and a violation of due process rights.[115] If, however, a contract of employment was not renewed at the end of its term (e.g., 1 year), absent a discriminatory motive or an intent to violate the faculty member's constitutional rights, the institution could do so without liability.[116]

There have been a large number of cases involving faculty terminations in academic institutions. The cases involving terminations "for cause" include insubordination (*Hillis v. Stephen F. Austin University*[117]), sexual harassment (*Lehman v. Board of Trustees of Whitman College*[118]), and neglecting one's duties (*White v. Board of Trustees of Western Wyoming Community College*[119]).

Faculty challenges to for-cause dismissals by public institutions include some of the same grounds public students have used to challenge decisions by faculty. They include violations of the faculty member's liberty rights under the Fourteenth Amendment's Due Process Clause (*Board of Regents v. Roth*[120]) and free speech under the First Amendment (*Connick v. Meyers*[121]).

Faculty challenges to for-cause dismissals by public institutions include some of the same grounds public students have used to challenge decisions by faculty.

Faculty members in private institutions have also mounted legal challenges to for-cause terminations that include breach of contract and discrimination. Both of these challenges have been used by faculty in public institutions as well.[122]

Faculty of nursing programs can avoid involvement in lawsuits surrounding employment termination by providing quality instruction to students. Adherence to the employment contract or requirements of tenured faculty is vital. Documented research and publication, as well as service on college or school committees, can help the nursing faculty member retain his or her current faculty status or, if desired, obtain a promotion or tenure.

If the faculty member believes that a termination has occurred unfairly or in violation of the employment contract or tenure, legal advice should be obtained as quickly as possible. At a minimum, the decision should be challenged through the established institutional procedures for dealing with decisions adverse to faculty. However, legal action may be necessary to obtain a fair resolution of the issue. However, reminiscent of the decision in the *Horowitz* case, courts generally defer to the decisions of institutions when terminations of tenured faculty occur. As one court opined:

> The management of the university is primarily the responsibility of those equipped with the special skills and sensitivities necessary for so delicate a task. One of the most sensitive func-

tions of the university administration is the appointment, promotion and retention of faculty. It is for this reason that the courts, and administrative agencies as well, should only rarely assume academic oversight, except with the greatest caution and restraint, in such areas as faculty appointment, promotion and tenure, especially in institutions of higher learning.[123]

Distance Learning

The use of computers in nursing education is growing at a rapid rate. On-line courses are available through many nursing education programs, including those at the State University of New York at Stony Brook, Lewis University in Romeoville, Illinois, and St. Joseph's College in Standish, Maine.[124] Advantages to students include flexibility in course scheduling, exposure to faculty expertise in many geographic locations, and eliminating travel time to and from the classroom. However, distance education raises legal and other concerns for faculty. Practical concerns include workload, class size, costs, skills and training, and competency in computer and other technological equipment.[125] The legal issues include copyright and ownership of the distance learning course or materials, standards for teaching and scholarship, and compensation for the "significant" greater time involved in the preparation and teaching of distance learning courses.[126] Ethical challenges include cheating by students (e.g., not doing the work personally) and accessing work done by others (e.g., purchasing papers or projects from other distance learning students).[127]

Nurse faculty considering the development of a distance learning course must work closely with other faculty and the educational institution as a whole to develop clear policies and practices concerning distance education. The proposed policies should be approved by the faculty or its representative, and the final, written procedures distributed to all faculty and administration.[128] Likewise, faculty need to establish rules and procedures for teaching-load credit in the preparation and delivery of the course or programs taught in this manner.[129] Moreover, the academic freedom of the faculty member offering distance learning courses should be well guarded in this teaching medium.

The ownership of materials developed and authored by faculty will need to be proactively determined *prior* to offering the course.[130] The ownership issues must include a determination of who exercises control over the future use and distribution of the materials.[131] Likewise, when the course should be revised or withdrawn due to changes in its content are necessary parameters to establish in order to avoid any possible suits from students and/or patients cared for by students alleging negligence by the faculty for using incorrect or outdated course materials.

SUMMARY OF PRINCIPLES AND APPLICATIONS

The world of academia is not an ivory tower insofar as legal issues go. Nursing students will continue to challenge faculty and institutional decisions. The study of suits filed against nursing education programs (discussed earlier in this chapter) indicated that of the 11 cases filed by students, 6 were decided in favor of the student.[132] Likewise, faculty will continue to challenge institutional decisions concerning their continued employment. As a result, student nurses and nursing faculty must remember that:

- Students do not leave their constitutional rights at the door of an academic institution

- Students in public postsecondary institutions have constitutional protections that are not available to students in private academic institutions. They include due process rights for disciplinary actions; freedom from undue restraints on First Amendment rights; and equal application of constitutional rights to all students similarly situated

- Students in private postsecondary institutions cannot be treated in an arbitrary, capricious, or discriminatory manner by school officials. Rather, notions of fair play, notice, and equality should be guidelines under which faculty operate vis-à-vis the student body

- Students in public or private institutions need not be given a hearing *prior* to dismissal from the school or program for academic reasons

- Students in private postsecondary institutions can utilize the contract theory when they allege that a violation of some written document—a school catalog—or implied contract provision has adversely affected them

- Any postsecondary institution receiving federal funds must conform to federal laws protecting handicap, age, religion, or sex

- Generally, faculty in schools of nursing have the ability and responsibility to evaluate students both academically and clinically. Those decisions will not be overturned by the courts unless they are found to be impulsive and without basis. Faculty are considered to be the "experts" in evaluating academic performance

- The Buckley Amendment protects the release of student records and information in both public and private postsecondary schools

- Drug testing of students in public and private postsecondary schools must be carefully evaluated

- Should nursing negligence be alleged against a student, the standard applied to the student will be what the ordinary, reasonable, and prudent graduate *professional* nurse would have done in the same or similar circumstances

- Student nurses must be familiar with their state nursing practice act throughout their career as nursing students as well as when they become licensed practitioners

- No suit against a faculty member for educational malpractice has yet been successful

- Nursing faculty may, in some instances, be sued as employees of an academic institution and individually as well

- An employment contract or tenure provides the nurse faculty member with more employment protection

- Nonrenewal of a teaching contract may be challenged if the reason for nonrenewal is discriminatory or intentionally violates a constitutionally protected right

- Distance learning requires faculty to be actively involved in the preparation, planning, and establishment of faculty protections for this nontraditional teaching methodology

TOPICS FOR FURTHER INQUIRY

1. Replicate the study of cases filed against school of nursing educational programs beginning with October 1989 until the present. Compare the findings with those of the first study. Identify differences, if any, and explain why they exist. Suggest additional areas of research for future studies in this area.

2. Evaluate a school of nursing's clinical evaluation tool for a particular clinical rotation. Analyze the tool in terms of clarity, behaviorally defined objectives, and consistency of use among faculty. Suggest areas of improvement.

3. Analyze a public nursing education program's catalog concerning due process rights of students in grading. Suggest where improvements might occur.

4. Draft a contract of employment for a nurse faculty member in either a public or private nursing education program. Include provisions for termination of the contract, renewal of the contract, and faculty responsibilities.

REFERENCES

1. See generally, William Kaplin and Barbara Lee. *The Law of Higher Education: A Comprehensive Guide to Legal Implications of Administrative Decision Making.* 3rd Edition. San Francisco, Cal.: Jossey-Bass, 1995, 1–75.
2. Henry Campbell Black. *Black's Law Dictionary.* 7th Edition. St. Paul, Minn.: West Publishing Group, 1999, 791.
3. Patricia Hollander, D. Parker Young, and Donald Gehring. *A Practical Guide to Legal Issues Affecting College Teachers.* Asheville, N.C.: College Administration Publications, 1995, 3 (The Higher Education Administration Series).
4. Ralph Chandler, Richard Enslen, and Peter Renstrom. *Constitutional Law Handbook.* 2nd Edition. Rochester, N.Y.: Lawyers Cooperative Publishing, 1993, 646 (with April 2000 cumulative supplement).
5. *Id.* at 697.
6. 294 F.2d 150 (5th Cir. 1961), *cert. denied,* 386 U.S. 930 (1961).
7. D. Parker Young and Donald Gehring. *The College Students and the Courts: Cases and Commentary.* Asheville, N.C.: College Administration Publications, 1986, 13-6.
8. *Dixon v. Alabama State Board of Education, supra* note 6, at 158–159.
9. *Id.*
10. 95 S. Ct. 729 (1975).
11. Young and Gehring, *supra* note 7, at 13-8.
12. *Id.* at 13-8 and 13-9.
13. *Id.*
14. *Goss v. Lopez, supra* note 10, at 732.
15. 435 U.S. 78, 98 S. Ct. 948 (1978).
16. Abigail Petersen, "*Board of Curators v. Horowitz,*" 6(4) *Hofstra Law Review* (Summer 1978), 1115.
17. *Id.* at 1116–1117.
18. *Id., citing Horowitz v. Board of Curators,* 74CV47-W-3 (W.D. Mo. November 14, 1975).
19. 538 F.2d 1317 (8th Cir. 1978).
20. Petersen, *supra* note 16, at 1120.
21. 435 U.S. at 85–90.
22. 435 U.S. at 92.
23. *Dixon v. Alabama State Board of Education, supra* note 8, at 157.
24. Chandler, Enslen, and Renstrom, *supra* note 4, at 1-1.
25. See, for example, *Hopwood v. Texas,* 78 F.3d 932 (5th Cir.), *cert. denied,* 116 S. Ct. 2580 (1996). In this case, the appeals court ruled that diversity does not provide a compelling interest for race-conscious decisions when considering students' admission into an educational program. The case is currently back in a federal appellate court for further consideration. John Alger, "Affirmative Action in Higher Education: A Current Legal Overview,"

(1999), 1. Available on the American Association of University Professors Web site at http://www.aaup.org. Accessed May 19, 2000.

26. *Id.* See also Jonathan Alger, "*Bakke—Still Breathing, But Barely,*" *ACADEME* (1998), located on the American Association of University Professors Web site, *supra* note 25. Accessed May 19, 2000.

27. 42 U.S.C. Section 12101 *et seq.* (1992).

28. Jason Searns, Jane Howard-Martin, and Diane Hopper. *Public Accommodations Under the Americans with Disabilities Act: Compliance and Litigation Manual.* St. Paul, Minn.: West Group, 2000, 77–110.

29. *Id.* at 9.

30. 42 U.S.C. Section 6101 *et seq.* (1975).

31. 835 F.2d 1000 (2nd Cir. 1987).

32. *Id.* at 1001–1003.

33. *Id.*

34. *Id.* at 1005.

35. 974 S.W.2d 351 (5th Cir. 1998).

36. Hollander, Young and Gehring, *supra* note 3, at 9–11.

37. 565 F.2d 2000 (1st Cir. 1977).

38. Young and Gehring, *supra* note 7, at 1–4 to 1–5.

39. *Id.* The federal trial court decision is located at 422 F. Supp. 1354 (1976).

40. 449 N.Y.S.2d 26 (1982).

41. 704 F.2d 713 (1983).

42. *Id.* at 715.

43. *Id.*

44. *Id.* at 716.

45. 514 F.2d 622 (10th Cir. 1975).

46. See also *Clayton v. Trustees of Princeton University,* 608 F. Supp. 413 (1985) (student suspension for cheating during a lab practicum exam); *Boehm v. University of Pennsylvania School of Veterinary Medicine,* 553 A.2d 575 (1990) (veterinary students accused by school of cheating; school decision upheld); *Abrahamiam v. City University,* 565 N.Y.S.2d 571 (1991) (student suspended for cheating on physics exam; decision upheld); *Gagne v. Trustees of Indiana University,* 692 N.E.2d 489 (1998) (law student expelled for making false statements on several applications concerning arrests or convictions for crimes; school decision upheld).

47. An excellent resource for decisions involving students with emotional problems is *The Dismissal of Students with Mental Disorders: Legal Issues, Policy Considerations and Alternative Responses* by Gary Pevala. Asheville, N.C.: College Administration Publications, 1985 (The Higher Education Administration Series). See also Sterns, Howard-Martin, and Hopper, *supra* note 28; Laura Rothstein. *Disabilities and the Law.* 2nd Edition. St. Paul, Minn.: West Group, 1997 (with regular updates).

48. See generally, Kaplin and Lee, *supra* note 1.

49. 359 N.Y.S.2d 120 (1974).

50. *Id.* at 121.

51. 606 A.2d 1239 (1992).

52. Chandler, Enslen, and Renstrom, *supra* note 4, at 1010.

53. 764 S.W.2d 827 (1989).

54. *Id.* at 833.

55. 474 U.S. 214 (1985).

56. *Supra* note 53, at 837.

57. *Id.* at 838.

58. Pub. L. No. 93-380, 20 U.S.C. Section 1232g *et seq.* (1974).

59. U.S.C. Section 1232g (a) (1) (A).

60. *Id.* at 1232g (4) (A).

61. *Id.* at 1232g (6) (b) (1) (A) through (I).

62. *Id.* at 1232g (5) (A) and (B).

63. *Id.* at 1232g (4) (A) and (B) and (5) (A) and (B). Proposed regulations amending the Buckley Amendment were published in the *Federal Register* on June 1, 1999. The proposed changes include (1) a provision to permit disclosure of educational records to authorized representatives of the U.S. Attorney General for law enforcement reasons without the student's consent; (2) the ability of the educational institution to release educational records without the prior written consent of the student or his or her parents when "legal action" is initiated by the student or parents; and (3) the ability of postsecondary institutions to disclose final results of any disciplinary proceeding against a student who is alleged to be a perpetrator of a crime of violence and the institution determines (in its proceedings) that the student did violate the institution's rules or policies governing that crime. 64, Fed. Reg. 29531–29535 (June 1, 1999). The proposed rules can be accessed on the World Wide Web at www.access.gpo.gov. Accessed May 19, 2000. The deadline for any comments concerning the rules was August 1, 1999. *Id.* at 29531. The reader will want to keep abreast of any developments regarding the proposed rules.

64. Chandler, Enslen, and Renstrom, *supra* note 4, at 221–297.

65. Gary Pavela, "Constitutional Issues in the Residence Halls," in *Administering College and University Housing.* Revised Edition. Gary Pavela, Editor. Asheville, N.C.: College Administration Publications, 1992, 25–30. (The Higher Education Administration Series).

66. *Id.*; see also entire text of *Administering College and University Housing.*

67. *Id.* at 25–30; see also Stephen T. Miller, "Contracts and Their Use in Housing," in *Administering College and University Housing, supra* note 65, at 61–76.

68. *Id.* The U.S. Supreme Court may be narrowing the protections afforded by the Fourth Amendment. Although the decisions have not involved searches in a college or university setting, the cases may have an impact upon a student's Fourth Amendment privacy rights. See, as examples, *Minnesota v. Carter,* 525 U.S. 83 (1998) (police look into an apartment window through "gap" in the closed venetian blinds and see people not living in the apartment bagging cocaine; Supreme Court holds that the search was not a violation of individuals' Fourth Amendment rights, as there is no expectation of privacy for someone "merely present" with the consent of the home owner/renter); *Ohio v. Robinette,* 117 S. Ct. 417 (1996) (man stopped in his car for speeding given verbal warning, then asked if anything illegal was in the car; Robinette answered no and consented to search of car. Marijuana and "a pill" were discovered and Robinette arrested for possession of a controlled substance. Supreme Court held that informing persons that they are "legally free to go" in a warning before search not necessary; all searches must be "measured in objective terms" and each case looked at by evaluating the totality of the circum-

stances that led to the search). Chandler, Enslen, and Renstrom, *supra* note 4.

69. Pavela, *supra* note 65, at 28.

70. See, for example, *People v. Lanthier,* 97 Cal. Rptr. at 297 (1971).

71. Pavela, *supra* note 65, at 26–28.

72. 469 U.S. 325 (1985).

73. *Id.* at 337–343.

74. *Id.*

75. 515 U.S. 646, 132 L. Ed. 2d 564 (1995).

76. *Id.* at 649–651.

77. *Id.* at 652–665.

78. *Id.*

79. *Id.*

80. *New Jersey v. T.L.O., supra* note 72.

81. 20 U.S.C.A. Section 111 *et seq.*; 20 U.S.C.A. Section 7101 *et seq.*; 34 C.F.R. Section 86.1 *et seq.*

82. *Id.*

83. *Id.*

84. See, for example, Marilyn Asteriadis, Virginia Davis, Joyce Masoodi, and Marcia Miller, "Chemical Impairment of Nursing Students: A Comprehensive Policy and Procedure," 20(2) *Nurse Educator* (March/April 1995), 19–22. See also, generally, D. Polk, K. Glendon, and C. DeVore, "The Chemically Dependent Student Nurse: Guidelines for Policy Development," 41 *Nursing Outlook* (1993), 166–170; E. Greenhill and K. Skinner, "Impaired Nursing Students: An Intervention Program," 30(8) *Journal of Nursing Education* (1991), 379–381; Gary Clark and Julie Stone, "Assessment of the Substance Abuse Curriculum in Schools of Nurse Anesthesia," 11(3) *Journal of Addictions Nursing* (1999), 123–135; Kathryn Kornegay, "Using Open Alcoholics Anonymous Meetings as a Teaching Strategy for Undergraduate Nursing Students," 11(1) *Journal of Addictions Nursing* (1999), 19–24.

85. Greenhill and Skinner, *supra* note 84.

86. Kevin Zeese, *Drug Testing Legal Manual and Practice Aids.* 2nd Edition. Deerfield, Ill.: Clark Boardman Callaghan, 1996 (with regular updates).

87. Chandler, Enslen, and Renstrom, *supra* note 4, at 75–219

88. 393 U.S. 503 (1969).

89. *Id.* at 506–514.

90. 92 S. Ct. 2338 (1972).

91. *Id.* at 2340.

92. See, generally, Chandler, Enslen, and Renstrom, *supra* note 4.

93. Chandler, Enslen, and Renstrom, *supra* note 4.

94. *Patterson v. Hunt,* 682 S.W.2d 508 (1984); *Rosenberger v. Rector and Visitors of University of Virginia,* 115 S. Ct. 2510 (1995).

95. 20 U.S.C. Section 1681 *et seq.* (1972).

96. 118 S. Ct. 1989 (1998).

97. *Id.*; William Kaplin, "Limited Liability for Sexual Harassment by Students," *Syntax Weekly Report* (1999), 1–3. Available on the College Administration Publications Web site at http://www.collegepubs.com. Accessed May 19, 2000.

98. 526 U.S. 629 (1999).

99. *Id.*; William Kaplin, *supra* note 97, at 1.

100. Kaplin, *supra* note 97, at 1, *citing Davis v. Monroe County Board of Education, supra* note 98.

101. *Id.* at 2. See also Kaplin and Lee, *supra* note 1, at 815–822.

102. Linda J. Shinn, "Yes, You Can Be Sued," in *Take Control: A Guide to Risk Management.* Linda Shinn, Editor. Chicago, Ill: Kirke-Van Orsdel, Inc. and Chicago Insurance Company, 1998, 6.

103. 681 P.2d 15 (Kan. 1984).

104. Lelia Helms and Kay Weiler, "Suing Programs of Nursing Education," 39(4) *Nursing Outlook,* 158–161.

105. *Id.*

106. *Donahue v. Copiague Union Free School District,* 418 N.Y.S.2d 375 (1979).

107. See *Tolman v. Cencor Career Colleges,* 851 P.2d 203 (1993).

108. Hollander, Young, and Gehring, *supra* note 3, at 27. See also *Alsider v. Brown Institute,* 592 N.W.2d 468 (Minn. 1999) wherein the appeals court again rejected an educational malpractice allegation against faculty but warned that "objectively measured failed promises" made by faculty to students *are* actionable.

109. *Id.*

110. Abigail Petersen, "*Board of Curators v. Horowitz,*" *supra* note 16, at 1123, *citing Gasper v. Burton,* 513 F.2d 843 (10th Cir. 1975); *Mustell v. Rose,* 211 So. 2d 489, 498, *cert. denied,* 393 U.S. (1968); *Barnard v. Inhabitants of Shelburne,* 102 N.E. 1095 (1913).

111. *Id.*

112. Joseph Beckman. *Faculty/Staff Nonrenewal and Dismissal for Cause in Institutions of Higher Education.* Asheville, N.C.: College Administration Publications, 1986, 4. See also Kaplin and Lee, *supra* note 1, at 150–370.

113. Hollander, Young, and Gehring, *supra* note 3, at 23.

114. *Id.*

115. *Id.* at 5.

116. *Id.* at 8.

117. 665 F.2d 547 (1982).

118. 576 P.2d 397 (1978).

119. 648 P.2d 421 (1982).

120. 408 U.S. 564 (1972).

121. 103 S. Ct. 1684 (1983).

122. See Beckman, *supra* note 112.

123. *New York Institute of Technology v. State Division of Human Rights,* 386 N.Y.S.2d 685, 688 (1976).

124. "Online Courses: The Forecast for Nursing Education," 1(1) *Excellence* (2000), 1.

125. *Id.* at 2.

126. American Association of University Professors. *Statement on Distance Learning,* 1–3. Available on the association's Web site at http://www.aaup.org. Accessed July 13, 1999.

127. See generally, Patricia Hollander. *Computers in Education: Legal Liabilities and Ethical Issues Concerning Their Use and Misuse.* Asheville, N.C.: College Administration Press, 1986.

128. AAUP, *supra* note 126, at 2–4.

129. *Id.*

130. American Association of University Professors. *Draft Statement on Copyright,* 1–4. Available on the association's Web site, *supra* note 126. Accessed July 13, 1999.

131. *Id.* at 3–4.

132. Lelia Helms and Kay Weiler, *supra* note 104.

The Nurse in Advanced Practice

21

Paula Henry, JD, NP-C, BSN, RN

The nursing profession has evolved to include several specialty practice areas in which the registered nurse has become a primary health care provider in the expanded role of advanced practice nurse (APN). An APN is a registered nurse who has successfully completed an additional course of study in a nursing specialty that provides specialized knowledge and skills to function in an expanded role. Figures from 1996 indicated that in the United States there were approximately 161,711 registered nurses academically prepared to function in the expanded role.[1] APNs generally fall into four categories: nurse anesthetist (CRNA), nurse-midwife (CNM), nurse practitioner (NP), and clinical nurse specialist (CNS). A 1990 Gallup poll conducted to determine the public's attitude toward health care and nursing showed that 86% of the public were receptive to having an APN as their primary care provider.[2] Recent consumer studies indicate continued satisfaction and acceptance of the APN as a primary care provider.[3] Research studies have established that APNs who provide basic primary care, when compared to physicians practicing in similar settings, are cost-effective, and APNs promote better patient compliance with health care treatment regimes, increased participation in prevention care, and improved access to care.[4] It is well documented that APNs are capable of and in fact provide high-quality care equal to, if not better than, the care provided by physicians in the primary care setting.[5]

Inherent in role expansion is the development of legal responsibilities that are unique to the advanced practice nurse. Understanding the important legal issues is necessary to fully comprehend the legal ramifications of an expanded role. The legal issues regarding role definition, scope of practice, standard of care, and overlapping functions will be discussed to provide a general framework for reference regarding advanced practice. Statutory authority and judicial recognition have addressed the definition of advanced practice and the nurse's ability to function fully in the expanded role.

DEFINITIONS OF ADVANCED PRACTICE NURSES

Of the four main categories of advanced practice that are recognized within the nursing profession, the common denominator in each category is the fact that the individual is a registered nurse. The hallmark of the expanded role is the advanced educational training in an area of specialization with the concurrent increase in responsibility, both professionally and legally. Role definition begins at the professional level with a review of the specific professional organizations' policy statements and the nursing literature. Regardless of the category of advanced practice, the APN's focus is on the provision of quality nursing care in the promotion of health and the prevention of illness. The APN's goal is to be able to legally practice to the fullest extent of the APN's education, skill, and training. To obtain autonomy, the APN must achieve professional independence in decision making and in defining the scope of practice.

Nurse Anesthetist

According to the American Association of Nurse Anesthetists, a nurse anesthetist is a professional registered nurse licensed to practice nursing who has become an anesthesia specialist by successfully completing an approved and accredited nurse anesthetist program.[6] In addition, to become certified, the nurse anesthetist must pass a national qualifying examination and then fulfill continuing education requirements every 2 years for recertification. Certified registered nurse anesthetists (CRNAs) provide anesthesia for dental, surgical, and obstetric procedures ranging from local to regional anesthesia.[7]

ETHICS CONNECTION 21–1

Nurse anesthetists have been providing quality anesthesia services in [the United States] for more than a century.[1] Early in the last century, their professional relationships were challenged when nurse anesthetists were accused of "practicing medicine without a license."[2] Although landmark decisions in Kentucky (1917) and California (1936) established that nurse anesthetists were practicing nursing, not medicine, their professional autonomy has been restricted by the federal requirement that nurse anesthetists be supervised by anesthesiologists. Therefore, 80% of certified registered nurse anesthetists (CRNAs) practice under the supervision of physicians, and 20% "function as sole anesthesia providers working and collaborating with surgeons and other licensed physicians."[3] Of these sole anesthesia providers, 70% practice in rural areas, "affording anesthesia and resuscitative services to these medical facilities for surgical, obstetrical, and trauma care."[4] This raises interesting ethical issues of distributive justice regarding differences of services between rural, urban, and suburban health care. If quality of anesthesia services is comparable between CRNAs and anesthesiologists for rural health care, how is that not the case in urban and suburban settings? CRNAs, regardless of practice location, are recertified every 2 years. As with all areas of nursing practice, professional autonomy must be balanced with competence and quality in the beneficent interest of patient safety and effectiveness.

In a spring 2000 move hotly contested by anesthesiologists, the Health Care Financing Administration (HCFA) announced that it would remove the requirement that nurse anesthetists must be supervised by anesthesiologists when administering anesthesia to Medicare patients. State statutes or hospital policy, then, would regulate supervision of nurse anesthetists. This HCFA change has important implications for CRNA practice, including the distributive justice issue of equity of compensation for professional services.

Enacted in 1965, Medicare (Title XVIII of the Social Security Act) reimbursed hospitals under Part A for "reasonable costs" of anesthesia services provided by hospital-employed certified nurse anesthetists (CRNAs). Anesthesiologists who employed and supervised CRNAs could bill under Part B as if they personally performed the care. Anesthesiologists who supervised CRNAs who were employed by a hospital could bill the same base units as if they did the care themselves, but their time units were halved.[5] This legislation supported the practice of anesthesiologists supervising as many as four or more nurse anesthetists at once and being reimbursed for anesthesia services for all the cases that were being supervised. Nurse anesthetists were being reimbursed for their services to the patient in one surgery suite, while anesthesiologists were receiving as much as or more than quadruple the fees of the CRNAs because they could supervise several cases simultaneously. The American Association of Nurse Anesthetists (AANA) has chipped away at that federal gift to anesthesiology practice for nearly 20 years, sometimes successfully, sometimes not. In an almost rhythmic patter of legislation, beginning with the Tax Equity and Fiscal Responsibility Act of 1982 (TEFRA),[6] equity issues of limiting the number of CRNAs an anesthesiologist can supervise at one time, reducing the conversion rate for anesthesiologists who supervise CRNAs, increasing the conversion rate for CRNAs, and direct reimbursement for CRNAs under Medicare, Part B have been statutorily gained, with occasional setbacks. Collaborative working relationships between CRNAs and anesthesiologists are an important focus of this specialty, despite the competing claims for reimbursement. These relationships are complicated further when the CRNAs are hospital employees, and the hospital costs of anesthesia services are part of the calculations.

Nurse anesthetists are at high risk for substance abuse because they have ready exposure and access to controlled substances. In response to this increased risk, the AANA has adopted a therapeutic approach to substance abuse and provides a variety of services to prevent substance abuse and educate CRNAs about substance abuse, prevention, recognition, and management. AANA also provides guidelines for the development of treatment programs for addicted nurse anesthetists. Guidelines include intervention, treatment, aftercare, and workplace reentry. In addition, the AANA maintains a hotline and provides peer assistance advisors for CRNAs.[7] These services protect privacy and confidentiality.

---

[1]American Association of Nurse Anesthetists. *Nurse Anesthetists—Providing Anesthesia into the Next Century Executive Summary.* (January 1997). Available at http://www.aana.com/library/execsummary.asp

[2]*Id.*

[3]American Association of Nurse Anesthetists. "Nurse Anesthetists and Anesthesiologists Practicing Together," in *Professional Practice Manual for Certified Registered Nurse Anesthetist. Position Statement No. 1.9.* Park Ridge, Ill.: Author, 1996. Available at http://www.aana.com/library/practice.asp

[4]*Supra* note 1.

[5]American Association of Nurse Anesthetists. *Nurse Anesthesia Reimbursement.* Retrieved on May 1, 2000, from http://www.aana.com/library/reimbursement.asp

[6]Tax Equity and Fiscal Responsibility Act of 1982 (Pub. L. No. 97-248).

[7]American Association of Nurse Anesthetists. *Peer Assistance.* Retrieved on May 1, 2000, from http://www.aana.com/peer/

The APN's goal is to be able to legally practice to the fullest extent of the APN's education, skill, and training.

Nurse anesthetists have been administering anesthesia for more than 100 years.[8] A certified nurse anesthetist administers 65% of all anesthesia in the United States, and the nurse anesthetist is the sole provider of anesthesia in more than 70% of rural hospitals in the United States.[9] Nurse anesthetists have the longest history of involvement with the legal profession, especially in the scope of practice arena.

Anesthesia is an example of the overlapping functions of physicians and nurses. When a certified nurse anesthetist (CRNA) provides anesthesia to a patient, that action is recognized as the practice of nursing.[10] When anesthesia is provided by a physician, it is the practice of medicine.[11] The recent furor over the Health Care Financing Administration's (HCFA) proposals to remove the federal requirement of physician supervision of the CRNA, and allow each state to decide the issue itself, has raised issues pertaining to the CRNA's autonomy and the economic issues which question the reimbursement for anesthesiologist supervision that is not required in 29 states.[12, 13] The bottom line in this turf battle is that for a hundred years, nurse anesthetists have been providing anesthesia in a safe, cost-effective, and highly competent manner.

Certified Nurse-Midwife

A certified nurse-midwife (CNM) is a registered nurse with additional education in the independent management of the aspect of women's health care that pertains to pregnancy, childbirth, postpartum, care of the newborn, and gynecology, including family planning.[14] This definition is consistent with the American College of Nurse-Midwives 1992 policy statement on nurse-midwifery practice.[15] Certified nurse-midwives provide maternal-fetal services in the traditional settings of clinics and hospitals, as well as in the nontraditional settings of birth centers and clients' homes.

The nurse-midwifery role has developed into an integral part of the health care team of attending physicians, residents in training, and nursing professionals which has improved access to care and significantly decreased the cost for maternity care.[16] Nurse-midwives have demonstrated that collaborative practice can exist in health care reform.

Nurse Practitioner

In the early 1970s, the American Nurses Association identified the role of nurse practitioner. A nurse practitioner (NP) is a registered nurse who with advanced educational preparation and advanced clinical competency is able to deliver primary health and medical care.[17]

The NP's functions include annual health screening, the diagnosis and management of common acute health problems, and the monitoring of chronic long-term health disorders. The NP's practice encompasses pediatrics, geriatrics, emergency medicine, family practice, obstetrics-gynecology, neonatology, adult medicine, and psychiatry, to name a few areas. Studies have shown that NPs provide safe, cost-efficient, and quality primary care.[18] A 1993 analysis of multiple studies done in the previous 10 years concluded that NPs provide care equivalent to or better than that of physicians.[19]

A 1993 analysis of multiple studies done in the previous 10 years concluded that NPs provide care equivalent to or better than that of physicians.

The total number of NPs in practice in the United States currently is close to 63,000.[20] Approximately 10% of the practicing NPs have established an independent practice.[21] NPs have expanded the role and are now practicing in the critical care settings of the NICU,[22] ICU,[23] and emergency department[24] as the primary provider for acutely ill patients. In 1996, an NP became the nurse manager of a primary care community health

---

ETHICS CONNECTION 21–2

Certified nurse-midwives are working toward being included in managed care plans. A report of the Pew Health Professions Commission and the University of California San Francisco Center for Health Professions Taskforce on Midwifery, *Charting a Course for the 21st Century: The Future of Midwifery,* acknowledges that the "U.S. is one of the few industrialized countries where midwives do not play a central role in the care of all or most pregnant women," and "urges reforms in the way midwives practice and are regulated, credentialed, and educated.[1] The report calls for the U.S. "health system to 'embrace' the midwifery model as an essential component of comprehensive care for women and their families." As with the clinical nurse specialists, the basic issue of distributive justice is the public's access to nurse-midwifery services. Gaining this access requires changes in public policy.

In addition to the goals of increased public understanding about the role of midwives and the intent to elevate the status of midwives within the health system, nurse-midwives are becoming more involved in political action. The taskforce chair commented, "midwives are underrepresented in policy and service development . . . having a place at the policy table and being recognized for their contributions toward the goals of managed care"[2] would be important accomplishments for nurse-mid-wifery.

Managed care may lead to policy changes that were not likely to occur under the fee-for-service system of health care. The percentage of births attended by midwives in 1996 was nearly double that of 1989. Nevertheless, this was only a small percentage (6.5%) of the total number of births. The medicalization of natural processes that has occurred during the age of science has become the norm and has helped to extinguish the practice of more natural birthing processes, such as those used by midwives. The taskforce report attributes this lack of recognition of midwifery to the different approaches to the birthing process used by midwives and to the need for shared authority between nurse-midwives and physicians.

Specifically, the taskforce recommends that certified nurse-midwives "be recognized as independent and collaborative practitioners, that laws and regulations permit full access to their services, that reimbursement rates be equitable and nondiscriminatory, that private credentialing entities avoid narrowing their scope of practice, and that education programs provide opportunities for inter-professional education and training experiences."[3] These policy initiatives in the interest of public access to certified nurse-midwifery services will take time. They represent an attempt to align moral issues of distributive justice, beneficence, and nurse and client autonomy with law and policy. Thus, certified nurse-midwifery legislation is "on the way" to being coextensive with ethics, but "not yet there."[4]

---

[1]Download and ordering information available at http://www.futurehealth.ucsf.edu/press_releases/midwifery.html

[2]*Id.*

[3]The Center for the Health Professions, University of California San Francisco. *Press Release: Taskforce Urges Inclusion of Midwifery in Managed Care Plans,* April 19, 1999. Available at http://www.futurehealth.ucsf.edu/press_releases/midwifery.html

[4]*Id.* See also National Council of State Boards of Nursing, Inc., "What Regulations of Advanced Nursing Practice Can Offer Health Care Reform," *Emerging Issues* (September 1993). Available at http://www.ncsbn.org/files/publications/positions/health/health2.asp This document identifies benefits that reportedly can accrue to various stakeholders as an outcome of advanced practice regulation.

---

center in Pennsylvania.[25] A year later, a group of nurse practitioners (Columbia Advanced Practice Nurses Association) opened an office practice in midtown Manhattan amidst an uproar from physicians and their organized groups in the area.[26] Two years later, the CAPNA group continued to grow and prosper.

The overlap of functions performed by NPs and physicians is well recognized within the medical-legal community. A recent study reported in the *Journal of the American Medical Association* showed that NPs who are functioning within their scope of practice provide care of equal quality to that of physicians in the same primary care practice.[27]

It is predicted that by the year 2005, the number of NPs will be equal to the number of practicing family practice physicians and the perception is that this growth will have a significant impact on access to care and the health care services workforce.[28]

ETHICS CONNECTION 21–3

For primary care NPs, some ethical issues are more similar to those of primary care physicians than they are to nursing ethics. The moral principles are the same; it is the situations that may vary. Sugarman,[1] a primary care physician, has identified common ethical problems that have relevance for primary care NPs. For example, NPs experience a tension between justice and beneficence when clients request inappropriate tests or treatments, such as antidepressant medications that are not medically indicated. They also are asked for inappropriate medical exemptions or privileges, such as being asked to certify that a client may not return to work, when the client is capable of working.

The just distribution of scarce resources is another ethical concern of NPs. Resources include not only the diagnostic and treatment costs but also the resource of time. As a consequence of managed care, NPs are experiencing pressure to limit time with patients. Many of the other ethical issues in NP practice are similar to the practice of other nurses, including confidentiality—particularly in the treatment of minors, informed consent, respecting client autonomy, and concern for just treatment of unserved and underserved populations.

In the early to mid-1990s, the number and variety of NPs increased dramatically, in part because of federal support for schools of nursing to develop master's level nurse practitioner programs. The number of programs proliferated. In some cases, the programs were soundly conceived and implemented. In other cases, particularly in schools where there were no other master's offerings in nursing, the quality of the programs was suspect.[2] The National Organization of Nurse Practitioner Faculty (NONPF) is a politically active organization that is concerned about quality of NP programs and is seeking separate accreditation for NP programs within schools of nursing. Although monitoring quality of NP programs is an important practice, the creation of yet another external accrediting body is costly for educational institutions and has the potential to drain resources from other programs of the school or university. Educational institutions are reconsidering specialty accreditation because of the high burden and questionable benefit of such accreditation, not only in nursing but also in other academic and professional disciplines. This is a distributive justice issue.

NPs experience autonomy issues similar to those of other APNs, such as certified nurse-midwives and certified registered nurse anesthetists. Many physicians work collaboratively with NPs. Others refer to NP practice with such phrases as "the dumbing down of medicine" and argue that NPs will not see the more complex possibilities in common health problems, such as sore throat. The Teachers' College, Columbia University pilot project that examined primary outcomes in patients who were treated by physicians or by nurse practitioners who were practicing autonomously found that NP quality of care is equal to that of physicians.[3] The ethical distributive justice issue of the public's access to choice in quality health care is a major concern of NPs. Prescriptive authority and other issues of NP practice are not solely issues of professional autonomy but also of distributive justice and—particularly in the case of pain management—beneficence. The American College of Nurse Practitioners (ACNP)[4] maintains an active electronic dialogue about legislative and other policy issues and initiatives regarding protection of the public, access to care, and other advanced practice issues.

[1] Jeremy Sugarman. *20 Common Problems—Ethics in Primary Care.* St. Louis: McGraw-Hill, 2000.

[2] American College of Nurse Practitioners. *Year 2000 National Nurse Practitioner Summit: Virginia Trotter Betts as Keynote Speaker Outlines NP Policy Role,* February 5–8, 2000. Available at http://www.nurse.org/acnp/summit/index.shtml

[3] M. O. Mundinger. "Primary Care Outcomes in Patients Treated by Nurse Practitioners or Physicians: A Randomized Trial," 283(1) *JAMA* (2000). Also available in full text at http://jama.ama-assn.org/issues/v283nl/full/joc90696.html

[4] See http://www.nurse.org/acnp/

Clinical Nurse Specialist

A lesser-known APN is the clinical nurse specialist (CNS). The American Nurses Association defines the clinical nurse specialist as a registered nurse who through graduate studies and supervised practice has become an expert in a defined area of knowledge and practice in a specific area of clinical nursing.[29] The CNS generally has a master's degree or a doctorate. Expert clinical practice is the *sine qua non* of the CNS, and includes various "subroles" such as clinical research, consultation, teaching, and leadership and administration.[30]

There are over 13,000 clinical nurse specialists providing care to patients in a variety of practice areas including cardiology, pulmonology, oncology, rheumatology, medical-surgical, pediatrics, and psychiatry, to name a few.[31] The number of practicing clinical nurse specialists by the year 2015 is expected to reach 31,000.[32] This predicted growth will be assisted by the passage of the 1997 Balanced Budget Act, which authorized the CNS to receive direct Medicare reimbursement.[33] Although role identification separate from nurse practitioners continues to evolve, clinical nurse specialists are clearly recognized as advanced practice nurses.

Of the four categories of advanced practice nurses, the CNS has had the least involvement with the legal system.

SCOPE OF PRACTICE OF ADVANCED PRACTICE NURSE

Scope of practice refers to the legal parameters in which the nurse is authorized to practice.[34] Each state, through its constitutional police powers, has the authority to enact licensing laws that govern health care professionals. Physicians have historically attempted to establish their exclusive right to practice medicine, which included the right to diagnose, treat, and prescribe medication, and made it illegal for any other professional to carry out these functions.

ETHICS CONNECTION 21–4

As is the case in other areas of advanced practice nursing, clinical nurse specialists (CNSs) are focusing on assuring the public's access to their services. Morally, access to health care goods and services often is cast as an issue of distributive justice. Indeed, justice is an issue for CNSs, as is securing professional autonomy through state statutes. The National Association of Clinical Nurse Specialists (NACNS) is using concerted, collective political action to secure such access to CNS services.[1] NACNS has developed model language for regulation of CNS practice at the state level. Rather than seek a second level of licensure, CNSs affirm that registration is adequate. CNSs are calling for statutes that include "a broad definition of Advanced Practice Nurses" (APNs) that would specify the types of APNs that are recognized in the state, including CNSs. They insist that the CNS title must be protected in statute. This title recognition is critically important for several reasons, including third-party reimbursement.

The CNS's scope of practice typically is broader than that of other APNs in that CNSs have direct as well as indirect patient care responsibilities. In a curious way that perhaps reflects federal and state roots in rugged individualism, direct patient care responsibilities are regulated; indirect responsibilities most often are not. Indirect responsibilities "are not the primary concern of the state in regulating health professionals."[2] Thus, the more narrow scope of practice is regulated and the broader scope that affects a broader range of patients is not safeguarded. NACNS describes the scope of CNS practice as having "three spheres of influence: patient, nursing personnel, and organization/system." Prescriptive authority is not necessarily required for all three spheres of practice. Thus, NACNS has taken the position that "prescriptive authority should be available to CNSs and should be optional." Prescriptive authority for CNSs should extend to "device prescription" so that CNSs may prescribe durable medical equipment to assist patients in self-care activities or to prescribe assistive devices to facilitate nursing care. A hydraulic lift, for example, is a device that would assist nursing care but not necessarily assist patient self-care. At present, many states grant device prescriptive authority to physical and/or occupational therapists or physical medicine physicians. When a rehabilitation nursing CNS, for example, determines that a patient requires an assistive device but not physical or occupational therapy, a therapist or physician still must be consulted. This practice both decreases the professional autonomy of the CNS and increases the cost to the patient and the health care system.

As with the other advanced practice nursing roles, CNSs are involved in influencing public policy that will improve clients' access to CNS services. As their practice expands and more technological tools of practice become available, issues related to crossing state boundaries and issues of electronic communication or "telehealth" are relevant to the ethics of CNS practice. Silva and Ludwick[3] have identified ethical issues relevant to interstate nursing practice from the perspective of autonomy, nonmaleficence, beneficence, justice and privacy/confidentiality.

---

[1]Clinical nurse specialist information available at http://www.nacns.org/updates/index.html
[2]*Id.*
[3]Mary Cipriano Silva and Ruth Ludwick, "Interstate Nursing Practice and Regulation: Ethical Issues for the 21st Century," *Online Journal of Issues in Nursing* (July 12, 1999). Available at http://www.nursingworld.org/ojin/ethicol/ethics_1.htm

The practice of medicine as a profession, however, does not possess a monopoly on who can legally provide health care services to a consumer. Certain functions traditionally performed by physicians are now legally recognized to be within the scope of practice of advanced practice nurses.[35]

APNs are held legally accountable for their own actions and are responsible for exercising independent and rational judgments based upon competent assessments of their patients when rendering nursing care.[36] Statutory law has established that the APN has the legal authority to practice under the individual nurse's license and that authority does not flow from a physician's or any other health care provider's license. There are several sources of law to determine the APN's scope of practice and the legal authorization to practice. These include each state's nurse practice act, specific statutory rules and regulations, professional standards, and case law.[37] Attorney general opinions, although not binding upon the court, are utilized to interpret scope-of-practice issues. It is imperative that the APN have knowledge of the laws that affect his or her individual practice and that address the legal parameters in which the APN may provide health care services.

APNs are held legally accountable for their own actions . . .

Unfortunately there is no uniformity among the sources of law governing the APN. As of 1998, only 26 states had a nurse practice act that authorized the advanced practice of nursing within that statutory framework.[38] Licensure regulations are the legal mechanism authorizing the practice of nursing, and they vary from state to state. Forty-seven states have enacted rules and regulations that govern the scope of practice of the APNs; however, eight states do not recognize a clinical nurse specialist as an APN.[39] Many states rely on the national standards developed by each specialty when defining the scope of practice.

State regulations are another source of law defining the scope of practice. Most nurse practice acts establish a board of nursing to regulate APNs, although some states establish separate boards (e.g., the nurse-midwifery board or the board of medicine that may regulate the APN).[40] There are

also separate regulations establishing prescriptive authority or reimbursement for services, which will impact the advanced practice of nursing and may place extensive restrictions on the scope of practice.[41] California has separate statutes that regulate the scope of practice of nurse-midwives, nurse practitioners, and nurse anesthetists. In 1998, California enacted separate statutes to recognize the role of the clinical nurse specialist and authorized regulations to be created to regulate the CNS's scope of practice.[42] Arizona and Arkansas also have separate statutes regulating nurse anesthetists.[43] By 1998 a total of 26 states authorized NPs to have a true independent scope of practice, defined as full independence without requiring physician supervision or collaboration.[44]

Independent practice is not defined by whether the APN functions "alone" or in collaboration with another or if the APN is reimbursed for the nursing services rendered. Independent practice is defined by the legal relationship of the APN within the health care arena. The Joint Commission on Accreditation of Healthcare Organizations defines a licensed independent practitioner as "an individual who is permitted by law and a health care institution to provide patient care services without direction or supervision within the scope of his/her license . . ."; this applies to APNs.[45] APNs have the educational preparation and clinical skills to function independently, because APNs are autonomous, responsible for their own judgment and actions, comply with national standards of practice, are licensed as professionals, and function within their scope of practice.

APNs have the educational preparation and clinical skills to function independently. . . .

Case law is an additional source of law that can define the APN's scope of practice. In recent years, courts were required to define the scope of practice of nurses in expanded roles and had to determine if the nurse was practicing medicine without a license. In fact, as early as the 1930s, a court was asked to address the legal issue of nurses administering general anesthesia.[46, 47] In 1983, the Missouri Supreme Court in *Sermchief v. Gonzales,*[48] discussed later in this chapter, interpreted the Missouri Nurse Practice Act to determine the NPs' scope of practice. The court held that the nurse practitioners' actions did not constitute the unlawful practice of medicine but rather constituted the practice of *nursing*.[49] The current approach of the courts is to recognize that nurses and physicians perform overlapping functions and procedures that were once the exclusive domain of medicine.

In certain instances, however, allegations have been brought that the APN is illegally engaged in the practice of medicine. In 1985, a Colorado court ruled that the services provided by a nurse practitioner in a rural clinic constituted the professional practice of nursing.[50] In 1986, an Illinois court ruled that a nurse practitioner who was hired by a competing practice group to provide gynecological services was not engaged in the practice of medicine but was within the practice of nursing[51]; and in 1990, the Supreme Court of New York upheld a jury verdict that a nurse practitioner was not engaged in the unauthorized practice of medicine when the NP performed the dermatological procedure of incision and drainage of the acne cysts of her patient.[52]

STANDARD OF CARE OF ADVANCED PRACTICE NURSE

Standard of care is the legal principle that underscores the premise that APNs must know the limits of their education, training, skills, and experience. The court in *Sermchief* stated that the hallmark of a professional is knowing the limits of one's professional knowledge.[53] The APN has the duty to render nursing services pursuant to the professional nursing standard of care. The APN's conduct is measured against that of a reasonably prudent professional nurse of similar knowledge and skill in similar or like circumstances.[54]

. . . the hallmark of a professional is knowing the limits of one's professional knowledge.

The APN's conduct is measured against that of a reasonably prudent

professional nurse of similar knowledge and skill in similar or like circumstances.

Case law has addressed the issue of the APN's standard of care, and some courts have held that the APN's standard of care may be the same as a physician's standard of care.[55] In *Fein v. Permanente Medical Group*,[56] for example (Key Case 21–6), the question of whether the standard of care of the nurse practitioner and that of the physician was the same was a major legal issue. In other cases, courts have held that the standard of care for the APN should be that of the APN and not that of a physician.[57] In those cases where the standard of care for the APN is held to be that of an APN in the same or similar circumstances, the standard is established by the testimony of an APN expert witness.[58] What these differing court opinions indicate is that the APN cannot rely on an APN standard of care being applied in *any* case involving an APN. Rather, it appears that the standard of care that is applied is very fact-specific to the case being litigated.

Perhaps the reliance on fact-specific analysis of the standard of care in a certain situation is why standard of care continues to be misunderstood and misapplied in certain situations. Each profession establishes its own standards of care; however, in certain circumstances the level of care, the procedure performed, and the service rendered may be the same within another profession. In actuality there is one standard which several different professions may have adopted as the standard of care within a specific profession.[59] For example, in the area of anesthesia, the necessary steps to obtain proper intubation of a patient, whether performed by an anesthesiologist (physician) or a nurse anesthetist, are exactly the same. Improperly placing an endotracheal tube is a negligent act regardless whether the anesthesiologist or the nurse anesthetist performed the intubation.[60] In performing the intubation, both professionals are expected to apply the same principles, follow the same recommended guidelines, perform the task with the same technique, and function within the same policy and procedures.[61] The minimum requirements to meet the standard of care within the respective professions may be the same, but the difference is the experience, training, and licensure of the different professions.

Unfortunately the courts, the lawyers, and the legal community fail to fully understand the scope of practice and standard of care of APNs. In 1997, in a bizarre ruling, the Texas Court of Appeals upheld the verdict of the jury which awarded $10 million dollars to a plaintiff against a Texas hospital even though the jury found the nurse anesthetist was not negligent.[62] The plaintiff suffered irreversible brain damage and is permanently disabled as the result of complications during her cesarean section. Expert testimony from a rival anesthesiologist that the hospital was negligent for failing to have the nurse anesthetist under the direct supervision of an anesthesiologist led to the inconsistent jury verdict.[63] The plaintiff's expert testified that the standard of care required physician supervision of the CRNA; however, as a matter of law in the state of Texas, the standard of care did not require physician supervision.[64]

There was no evidence presented that had an anesthesiologist been present to supervise the CRNA or had provided the anesthesia, the outcome would have been any different. In fact, the jury found the CRNA not to be negligent. The *La Croix* court failed to understand the CRNA's scope of practice and correct standard of care in this case. The case was appealed and the appellate court affirmed the lower court's findings, despite the fact that the decision inaccurately reflects the standard of care to be applied to a CRNA in Texas.[65]

To determine the standard of care of an APN a court may also consult professional organizations' policy statements which detail the levels of performance in a given specialty, such as the American Academy of Nurse Practitioners' *Standards of Practice*.[66] Written protocols or standardized procedures are guidelines that outline and authorize particular advanced practice functions and are generally developed in collaboration with a physician. The APN's written protocols are used to determine if the NP has met the standard of care.[67] Hospital policy and procedures[68] and collaborative practice agreements[69] can also be reviewed by the court to assist in identifying the standard of care of APNs.

Since each profession sets its own standard of care, the courts, in order to understand the standard of care to be applied, rely on expert testimony as to the specific standard of care. Expert testimony, however, will be required only if the opin-

ions being expressed are on an issue that is beyond the general knowledge of a layperson. For example, an allegation regarding the lack of informed consent may not require an expert's opinion as to the issue of whether a reasonable patient would have consented to the treatment. However, the issue regarding what needs to be disclosed by a provider in order to obtain informed consent would require expert testimony.

To establish that there was a breach of the standard of care by the APN, expert testimony must be presented. In the *Fein* case, for example, a physician who was head of a cardiology department provided expert testimony on behalf of the defendant NP regarding the NP's standard of care.[70] A primary care physician with experience in working with and supervising NPs was the plaintiff's expert witness regarding the standard of care of the NP in *Gugino v. Harvard Community Health Plan*.[71] In the *Jenkins* case, both parties had expert nurse practitioners to testify to the standard of care of the FNP in evaluating a patient with breast complaints.[72]

In an interesting situation, the Iowa Supreme Court overturned a jury verdict for the defense, ruling that the trial court erred when the judge did not permit a nurse anesthetist to testify as an expert regarding the negligence of an anesthesiologist.[73] In the *Carolan* case, the NA expert had over 27 years of experience in providing anesthesia to over 17,000 patients and thus was clearly qualified to testify to the standard of care required for proper position and padding of the patient's arm during the administration of anesthesia.[74] It remains crucial for the future development of the role of the APN that the standard of care be established by the testimony of a qualified APN expert, and APNs should strive to ensure that the legal community retains the appropriate expert on their behalf.

BARRIERS TO ADVANCED PRACTICE

In 1992, an economic study showed that an estimated $6.4 to $8.75 billion dollars could be saved annually if APNs were utilized to the full extent of their practice.[75] Practice barriers involving legal limitations on the scope of practice, prescriptive authority, and third-party reimbursement must be removed to permit consumers access to cost-effective and quality health care services. Organized medicine and restrictive legislation have created large obstacles preventing the APN from fully participating as a direct primary care provider in the health care arena. These practice barriers deny consumers their lawful right to choose their provider.

The legal authority to prescribe medications is the central barrier to the APN's legal and professional recognition as a primary care provider. The primary policy question is why there is failure to legally acknowledge the APN's ability and expertise to prescribe medications when APNs have been safely prescribing for the past 30 years.[76] APNs have, however, had to function in legal ambiguity and uncertainty to provide prescriptive services to their patients. The failure to have full legal prescriptive authority has caused delays in treatment and interruption in the continuity of care. Without clear legal authority, APNs have had to devise different mechanisms to implement their prescriptive treatment plan for their patients, which include (1) seeking out a physician to physically write the prescription; (2) utilizing presigned prescriptions; (3) phoning the prescription to the pharmacy under the physician's name; and (4) establishing written protocols delineating the drugs that can be furnished by the APN from a "laundry" list contained in a formulary. These prescriptive practices severely limit APNs' ability to practice to the full extent of their legally recognized expanded role.[77]

By 1998, 48 states had enacted statutes providing prescriptive authority for NPs and several states included other APNs.[78] Eighteen states have authorized NPs to independently prescribe medications.[79] A positive step toward prescriptive authority was taken when the Drug Enforcement Agency (DEA) licensed APNs as "mid-level practitioners" for the purpose of prescribing controlled substances. The APN must apply for and receive a DEA number. The APN can then prescribe controlled substances from Schedules II through V.[80] However, it is important to note that the APN can legally prescribe controlled substances with a DEA number only if allowed by the state in which the APN practices. As a result, state law determines which provider can legally obtain a DEA number and prescribe a controlled substance in that state. Despite the fact that APNs have proven their ability to safely prescribe medications, they continue to be barred from full legal recognition by short-sighted legislation backed by organized medicine and insurance companies fearful of losing economic control over the health care marketplace.

Consumers are being denied access to the primary care services of the APN when the insurance industry refuses to directly reimburse the APN for services rendered or when regulations are established to limit the reimbursement to the APN. Four main obstacles to direct reimbursement for APNs include (1) not covering services rendered, (2) not defining APNs as "qualified practitioners," (3) paying less to APNs than to other practitioners, and (4) paying the APN through a billing physician.[81] Federal and state statutes must be amended to remove the statutory barriers to the APN's practice. Providing direct reimbursement to the APN for services rendered will directly increase consumers' access to the health care provider of their choice.

Although some barriers are slowly being lowered (e.g., the direct Medicare reimbursement to NPs and CNSs), other barriers concerning "turf" and the degree of physician supervision are being raised.[82] Reform can be achieved only through federal and state legislative changes that will not only promote access to cost-efficient and quality health care but allow APNs to function fully within their scope of practice.

ETHICS CONNECTION 21–5

The *Code for Nurses with Interpretive Statements*[1] is relevant to both advanced and basic nursing practice. The anticipated *Code* revisions emphasize professional autonomy more strongly than in previous versions, and more clearly identify the patient or client as the entity to whom nurses are accountable. These changes and others are more consistent with advanced practice nursing than are earlier iterations. Issues of privacy and confidentiality, preventing harm, and acting fairly in the best interest of clients are moral practices of all nurses. "Ethics Connections" in this chapter have focused on ethical issues in advanced practice nursing that are different from or more extensive than those of basic nursing practice.

Ethics Connection continued on following page

Arguably, there are four advanced practice roles: certified nurse-midwives, clinical nurse specialists, nurse anesthetists, and nurse practitioners. Other highly educated and experienced nurses, such as nurse administrators, educators, and researchers, also consider themselves to be advanced practice nurses, although they generally are not acknowledged as such in state statutes. Although these latter groups may not need the same type of statutory regulation in advanced health assessment and prescriptive authority as advanced practice nurses who provide direct client care, they are engaged in an advanced level of nursing practice in its broadest sense.[2] Appropriate professional organizations must consider the fairness or justice of expanding the categories of "advanced practice nurses."

The variations in educational preparation for advanced practice roles raise ethical questions of distributive justice and beneficence. Currently, graduate level academic preparation is required for licensure or certification in most advanced practice roles. This was not always the case, however. For example, some associate degree programs prepared advanced practice nurses (APNs) who still practice in that role without having earned higher degrees. The fairness of requiring these nurses to earn graduate degrees must be balanced with public safety—a beneficence issue. Other equity or distributive issues are raised when APNs are compensated or reimbursed at the same level, regardless of educational level. Basic entry into practice issues are replicated in the early efforts to regulate and certify APNs.

Of the four categories of advanced practice nurses that are regulated in some states, there are formal and informal subdivisions. Clinical nurse specialists, for example, may be categorized according to client's chronological age or developmental status, function or physiological disorders, medical or surgical specialties, and the like. Thus, there may be clinical nurse specialists in gerontology, diabetes, orthopedics, rehabilitation nursing, and so on. Nurse practitioners generally, but not always, are primary care practitioners. According to the National Association of School Nurses (NASN),[3] both certified clinical nurse specialists and nurse practitioners may complete a formal course of study to become advanced practice school nurses. With all the possible categories of advanced practice nurses (APNs), there are common ethical concerns as well as unique ethical issues within each category.

Common ethical issues in advanced practice nursing include issues of clinical practice, social policy, certification and regulation, compensation or reimbursement, identity and professional autonomy, intra- and interdisciplinary communication, attaining and maintaining competence, and boundary issues with other disciplines and roles. Each of these sets of issues may be analyzed from the perspective of respect for autonomy, nonmaleficence, beneficence, and distributive justice as well as from the perspective of covenantal relationships.

All four advanced practice categories share a concern about increasing the public's access to APN services. This is a concern of distributive justice, autonomy, and beneficence. According to Betts,[4] advanced practice nurses are concerned about "access to care, patient-focused care, and delivery of health care by a variety of providers—to facilitate an ideal health care delivery system." Issues of universal access, delivery by a variety of providers, and facilitating the ideal health care delivery system lend themselves to ethical analysis from a moral principle perspective, focusing on distributive justice and beneficence. Patient-focused care and delivery of health care by a variety of providers involve the moral principle of respect for autonomy as well. Covenantal relationships or the ethic of care also is a useful way of exploring the ethical dimensions of these health policy issues (see Chapter 3).

Betts comments that the shift from a fee-for-service payment system to managed care has been the most rapid change in health care. When noting that managed care has held costs steady but has not improved access to care for the 44 million uninsured, Betts asks, "Is managed care making money for the providers by taking out inefficiencies or denying care?"[5] Betts asserts, "All the answers for what's wrong in health care today exist inherently within nursing. But nurses [and advanced practice nurses] have to be aware of current changes in health care and deficits within the . . . profession"[6] before they can implement a policy agenda. Despite its hyperbole, Betts's statement may contain an element of truth.

Denying care is maleficent. It places financial gain over human worth. The issue of managed care as a distributive justice issue is central to all of nursing practice, including advanced practice. Nurses are gaining more legitimate power in health care as managed care continues to emphasize aggregate health and cost containment—misguided though some of those cost-balancing efforts are. This is particularly the case for advanced practice nurses, whose professional autonomy had been constrained by lobbying efforts of wealthier, competing groups, such as physicians. These groups worked through their professional organizations to prevent or defeat legislation or deter private sector initiatives, such as health insurance corporations, from crafting legislation or policies that respected and expanded nursing's professional autonomous and collaborative practices. Professional prerogatives such as admitting privileges, prescriptive authority, and reimbursement for services are examples of issues of nursing autonomy that had been constrained under the guise of public beneficence. Nurses have been successful in negotiating some changes in these areas, but the overarching concern of distributive justice in acknowledging professional autonomy, and thus greater public access to health care, remains.

[1]American Nurses Association. *Code for Nurses with Interpretive Statements.* Kansas City, MO: Author, 1985.

[2]See also National Council of State Boards of Nursing, Inc. *National Council Position Paper: Advanced Clinical Nursing Practice,* 1986. Available at http://www.ncsbn.org/files/publications/positions/apcncor.asp

[3]National Association of School Nurses (NASN). *Position Statement on the Advanced Practice School Nurse,* October 1997. Available at http://www.nasn.org/issues/advan__prac.htm

[4]American College of Nurse Practitioners. *Year 2000 National Nurse Practitioner Summit: Virginia Trotter Betts as Keynote Speaker Outlines NP Policy Role,* February 5–8, 2000. Available at http://www.nurse.org/acnp/summit/index.shtml

[5]*Id.*

[6]*Id.*

LEGAL ISSUES IN ADVANCED PRACTICE

A comprehensive review of the reported cases involving advanced practice nurses reveals that relatively few have been filed, despite an increase of the expanded roles. Although some of the key cases presented contain more examples of one category of advanced practice than the others, this basically reflects the fact that certain APNs have a longer history of practice. As a result, that group has had earlier involvement with the legal system regarding role definition and scope-of-practice issues. The cases selected for analysis were chosen on the basis of the important legal principles that the case presented within a certain time frame.

> . . . *relatively few cases have been filed against APNs, despite an increase of the expanded roles.*

Nurse Anesthetist
Negligence, Negligence Per Se, and Respondeat Superior

The majority of reported cases filed against APNs involve an allegation of negligence; that is, that the APN breached the standard of care. Malpractice actions are filed when the professional's failure to meet the standard of care directly causes harm to the patient. Of the four categories of APNs, the nurse anesthetist has the longest history of practice and also has the greatest number of reported cases. The practice issues relating to the nurse anesthetist's negligence generally concern the selection, administration, and management of anesthesia and related procedures.

A 1985 Washington appellate case, *Brown v. Dahl,*[83] addressed the plaintiffs' allegations against

the nurse anesthetist for negligently administering the anesthetic; for failing to attempt corrective measures; and for failing to seek help in a timely manner. The plaintiffs also sued Dr. Dahl, the anesthesiologist, for lack of informed consent during the preanesthesia evaluation and negligence for allowing the nurse anesthetist to administer the anesthetic when he represented that he would personally administer it. The morning of surgery, the nurse anesthetist informed Mr. Brown that she would be administering the anesthesia during his procedure. The nurse anesthetist testified at trial that Mr. Brown did not voice any complaints regarding the fact that the nurse anesthetist would be administering the anesthesia instead of Dr. Dahl.

During the initial induction, Mr. Brown developed a partially obstructed airway and difficulties in breathing. The nurse anesthetist attempted to counteract the reaction, and when that was unsuccessful, finally requested assistance. After several attempts by Dr. Dahl, an airway was established; however, Mr. Brown had sustained cardiac arrest and suffered permanent physical and mental disabilities. The trial court ruled that there was enough evidence of the nurse anesthetist's negligence to proceed to trial. The jury, however, found the nurse anesthetist not negligent. Plaintiffs appealed, and the appellate court reversed the lower court because the court failed to give a jury instruction on *res ipsa loquitur*[84] and gave other improper instructions as well. The case was remanded to the lower court for a new trial.

The nurse anesthetist has the affirmative duty to monitor the effects of an anesthetic agent and the patient's condition. Failure to properly monitor that causes harm to the patient will result in the nurse anesthetist being held liable for negligence. Besides the *Brown* case, two other cases are illustrative of these legal principles.

The first is a 1985 North Carolina appellate case, *Ipock v. Gillmore,*[85] which upheld the jury's findings that the nurse anesthetist was negligent for failing to perform a proper preanesthetic evaluation and failing to properly monitor the patient during surgery. The patient underwent elective laparoscopy for sterilization, but because of medical complications, a total hysterectomy was performed. The patient suffered cardiac arrest during the procedure and suffered hypoxia and resultant brain damage caused by the nurse anesthetist's negligence during surgery.

The second case involves the failure of the anesthesiology team, which included an anesthesiologist, a nurse anesthetist, and a student nurse anesthetist, to properly monitor a patient's condition while she was undergoing a radiographic procedure under general anesthesia. In the Ohio case of *Lupton v. Torbey*,[86] the patient, at her request, underwent general anesthesia for a celiac axis radiographic study to confirm the diagnosis of arterial vascular constriction of the stomach, a condition that had caused her a long history of stomach pain. During the initial phase of the procedure, the anesthesiologist was supervising the nurse anesthetist; however, he left, leaving the nurse anesthetist and student to monitor the patient. Over the next 15 minutes, the nurse anesthetist failed to assess the patient's vital signs; however, he became concerned about how quickly the patient had responded to the anesthetic. The nurse anesthetist left to speak with the anesthesiologist, leaving the patient in the care of the student. Upon arrival, the radiologist discovered that the patient had no pulse, and emergency measures were instituted, but the patient suffered brain damage. Prior to completion of the trial, the anesthesiology team settled the case for $75,000.[87]

An illustration of a case involving the doctrine of *respondeat superior,* which resulted in a $1 million jury verdict, is the 1985 Michigan case *Theophelis v. Lansing General Hospital.*[88]

In *Theophelis,* the parents of a 7-year-old boy filed a wrongful death action against Lansing General Hospital alleging medical negligence in the administration of anesthesia during a tonsillectomy. Although the CRNA was not named as a defendant, the trial court held the hospital liable under the doctrine of *respondeat superior* for the negligence of the CRNA in failing to properly monitor the patient, and for the anesthesiologist's failure to properly supervise the CRNA.[89]

In Key Case 21–1, *Starcher v. Byrne,* the court found that the standard of care did not require the physical presence of the supervising physician while anesthesia was being administered by a CRNA.

In Key Case 21–2, the theory of negligence per se was used in a creative way.

KEY CASE 21–1 Starcher v. Byrne (1997)[90]

Patient has elective surgery and CRNA administers anesthesia

CRNA employed by an anesthesiologist

Surgeon is paged when CRNA begins anesthesia

Patient experiences bronchospasm resulting in irreversible brain damage

Suit is filed alleging the surgeon was negligent for not being physically present when CRNA administered anesthesia

FACTS: Mrs. Starcher was admitted to the hospital for an elective surgical procedure, repair of her ventral hernia. Anesthesia was to be administered by the CRNA, who was employed by an anesthesiologist.

As the CRNA began the induction, the surgeon received an emergency page and in compliance with hospital policy, remained in the operating suite but stepped outside of the operating room in order to answer the page while the CRNA was initiating anesthesia. While the surgeon was out of the operating room, the CRNA encountered problems with intubation. Upon the surgeon's return, the surgeon and CRNA determined that the patient was experiencing a bronchospasm and emergency treatment was instituted. Cardiopulmonary resuscitation was successful; however, due to the lack of oxygen to her brain, she suffered irreversible brain damage, resulting in a coma for several days and long-term physical and mental defects. Plaintiffs (the patient and her husband) brought a medical malpractice suit against the surgeon alleging the surgeon was negligent for not being physically present while the CRNA was administering anesthesia. The plaintiffs alleged that his failure to be present breached the standard of care.

KEY CASE 21-1	Starcher v. Byrne (1997)[90] *Continued*

The court returns verdict for surgeon

TRIAL COURT: At trial, the jury found in favor of the surgeon.

APPEALS COURT: The plaintiffs appealed, asserting that the weight of the evidence should have resulted in a plaintiff verdict. They also argued that the surgeon's absence meant that he failed to properly supervise the CRNA.

The Supreme Court of Mississippi upholds trial court verdict and dismisses the appeal

SUPREME COURT: The Supreme Court of Mississippi upheld the jury's verdict and dismissed the appeal. The Mississippi Supreme Court held that the standard of care of the supervising physician did not require that the supervising physician be physically present in the operating room while the CRNA administered anesthesia.

ANALYSIS: The *Starcher* case illustrates a case of attempting to apply the doctrine of *respondeat superior* to a supervising physician under a negligence per se theory of liability. In the *Starcher* case the CRNA's employer was an anesthesiologist who was not involved in the case. The only physician involved was the surgeon. Plaintiffs contended that the standard of practice required that CRNA administer anesthesia under the direction and physical presence of a licensed physician. Since the CRNA's employer was not involved in the case and not even at the hospital, plaintiffs contended that the surgeon was therefore in charge and supervising the CRNA. Plaintiffs asserted, under the theory of negligence per se, that there was a presumption that the standard of care had been breached because the surgeon was not physically present when the CRNA initiated the anesthesia.

In Mississippi, there is no separate statute that governs the CRNA's practice. The Mississippi Board of Nursing requires that nurse practitioners, including nurse anesthetists, must practice within a collaborative/consultative practice with a licensed physician. There is no requirement that the collaborative/ consulting physician be physically present at the time the APN is providing health care services.

Physician supervision is becoming an important issue for the APN in the medical-legal arena.[91]

KEY CASE 21-2	Mitchell v. Amarillo Hospital District (1993)[92]

FACTS: The plaintiff, Michael Mitchell, was admitted to a Texas hospital in February 1987 with the diagnosis of cardiac tamponade. Emergency cardiac surgery was scheduled, and a CRNA employed by the hospital administered the anesthesia. During the administration of the anesthesia, the patient suffered cardiac arrest. Although resuscitation efforts were successful, the patient suffered brain damage and died 3 years after the incident.

Civil rights suit filed against CRNA and others for death of patient

The family filed a civil rights claim against the CRNA, the surgeon, the hospital, and the medical director of the department of anesthesia.

Key Case continued on following page

KEY CASE 21–2   Mitchell v. Amarillo Hospital District (1993)[92] *Continued*

CRNA and surgeon settle case with plaintiffs

Trial court dismisses claims against remaining defendants

Plaintiffs appeal dismissal

Court of Appeals upholds trial court's decision

TRIAL COURT: The plaintiffs settled with the CRNA and the surgeon. However, they pursued their claim against the hospital and the head of the department of anesthesia. A summary judgment motion was filed by defendant and granted by the trial court.

Plaintiffs alleged that under the legal theory of negligence and negligence per se, the hospital deprived Mr. Mitchell of his civil rights by permitting a nurse anesthetist to illegally practice medicine, make independent decisions, and prescribe controlled drugs. Plaintiffs alleged numerous violations of state and federal statutes under the theory of negligence per se. The trial court dismissed the claims against the hospital and head of the anesthesiology department, which were based on a constitutional challenge that Mr. Mitchell's rights under the Fifth and Fourteenth Amendments of the U.S. Constitution had been violated. Plaintiffs filed an appeal.

APPEALS COURT: The Texas Court of Appeals upheld the trial court's decision and ruled that neither the acts of the CRNA nor the hospital's policy regarding nurse anesthetists constituted a deprivation of Mr. Mitchell's civil rights. It further upheld the finding that Texas law did not require a nurse anesthetist to be supervised by an anesthesiologist. Therefore, the actions of the CRNA did not violate any state statute.

ANALYSIS: *Mitchell* was a highly unusual case in which the action was based upon a denial of civil rights under a theory of negligence per se. It should be noted that nowhere did the plaintiffs allege that the CRNA negligently administered the anesthesia or that there was improper supervision. Plaintiffs' focus was on the advanced practice of the nurse anesthetist and the hospital's policy of permitting the nurse anesthetist to practice.

APNs should be aware that negligence and scope of practice allegations sometimes are clouded by unusual legal theories such as constitutional claims. It is equally significant that the *Mitchell* case was taken up on appeal from a summary judgment motion in which no evidence was introduced. It nonetheless procedurally resulted in the court determining the legality of the CRNA's practice and the hospital's policies regarding the expanded role of the CRNA.

It is also important to note that negligence per se claims are filed against APNs when an injury occurs and the APN's conduct that allegedly caused the injury is not included in a state statute or regulation that defines the APN's scope of practice. APNs must be cautious when providing care outside state-established scope-of-practice parameters. This may be particularly important for those APNs who are not specifically authorized to prescribe medications and treatments by state law or regulation. The potential for future negligence per se claims against APNs if an injury to a patient is alleged as a result of that prescribing is very real.

Res Ipsa Loquitur

This doctrine means "the thing speaks for itself." The essential elements that need to be proved in a *res ipsa loquitur* case are (1) that the plaintiff's injury would not have occurred under ordinary circumstances if someone had not been negligent;

(2) that the injury was the result of defendant's action while plaintiff was under the exclusive control of defendant; and (3) that the plaintiff did not contribute to or voluntarily act in a manner to cause the injury.[93]

This theory was asserted in *Morgan v. Children's Hospital*,[94] a 1985 case involving a nurse anesthetist's failure to adequately ventilate a patient undergoing a thymectomy procedure for the treatment of myasthenia gravis. The patient developed severe bradycardia, necessitating open cardiac massage, and although stabilized, he sustained global brain damage due to hypoxia as a result of the CRNA's negligence.[95] The trial court refused to give the *res ipsa loquitur* jury instruction, and a defense verdict was returned by the jury. The case was taken up on appeal, where the appellate court ruled that the lower court erred in failing to give the instruction, overturned the defense verdict, and remanded it for a new trial.[96]

Malpractice claims are frequently brought under the theory of *res ipsa loquitur* when the patient goes into surgery for a specific procedure and sustains an injury intraoperatively. CRNAs as part of the operating room team must be vigilant in their role in positioning and monitoring the patient.[97] Proper documentation of the procedures followed in positioning the patient and the padding utilized are essential if a *res ipsa loquitur* claim can be successfully defeated.[98]

Vicarious Liability and Borrowed Servant

Vicarious liability is the legal doctrine that holds one person legally accountable for the acts of another person. Generally a principal/agent relationship must exist in which the principal has control over or directs the actions of the agent in order for the doctrine to apply. The borrowed servant rule may apply when an employee is temporarily under the control of another with regard not only to the work to be performed but also the manner in which the work should be performed. This theory is illustrated in the case of *Harris v. Miller*.

KEY CASE 21-3   Harris v. Miller (1991)[99]

Nurse anesthetist administers anesthesia improperly and delays administering needed blood to patient

FACTS: In June 1981, Etta Harris underwent back surgery for treatment of a ruptured disc. Dr. Miller, an orthopedic surgeon, performed the surgery, and the anesthesia was administered by CRNA William Hawks, who was employed by Beaufort County Hospital. The hospital did not have an anesthesiologist on staff, and its policy was that the nurse anesthetist would administer anesthesia under the responsibility and supervision of the surgeon performing the surgery. Dr. Miller was a private practitioner and not on the hospital staff. A preanesthetic evaluation was performed by the CRNA, but the CRNA failed to interpret the patient's chest X-ray properly and did not identify the enlarged heart that could lead to decreased heart function under certain anesthetics employed during surgery.

At the beginning of the surgical procedures, the patient's blood pressure dropped and her heart rate was elevated to an abnormally high rate. The CRNA testified that he thought these changes resulted from the fact that the patient was not responding to the anesthetic and increased the anesthesia.

Approximately 1 hour later, while the operation was continuing, the patient's blood pressure remained low, and the surgeon noticed that the patient had lost 300 to 400 cc of blood, an amount twice the normal expected loss. The surgeon ordered the CRNA to administer blood; however, the CRNA delayed carrying out this order for approximately 40 minutes.

Key Case continued on following page

KEY CASE 21–3   Harris v. Miller (1991)[99] *Continued*

Meanwhile, the patient's blood pressure continued to remain at an extremely low level, and the CRNA failed to notify the surgeon of the patient's critical condition for approximately another 1½ hours. Resuscitative efforts were instituted, and a vascular surgeon performed an exploratory laparotomy and found the aorta flaccid. The vascular surgeon clamped the patient's aorta so that blood flow would not enter the legs and the patient's blood pressure would return.

Patient's injuries include vocal cord paralysis, a permanent tracheostomy, and brain damage

The patient was admitted to the ICU, where she remained comatose for an extended period of time. When the patient regained consciousness, her vocal cords were paralyzed, and she had a permanent tracheostomy and residual disabilities as a result of the brain damage suffered because of improper ventilation during the procedure. A postoperative X-ray revealed that the endotracheal tube was improperly positioned in the right lung, leaving the left lung unventilated. Further evidence indicated that, during the procedure, the CRNA failed to listen for bilateral breath sounds after intubation.

Patient files a medical malpractice claim against the CRNA, doctor, and hospital

The patient spent 8 months in a rehabilitation center before being discharged home to be cared for by her husband. Mrs. Harris filed a medical malpractice claim against the CRNA, medical doctor, and hospital in 1983. She died 6 years later as a result of her injuries. The family was substituted as the plaintiffs in Mrs. Harris's medical malpractice claim and it was amended to include a wrongful death claim against the doctor. In 1987 the plaintiffs settled their claim against the CRNA and the hospital.

Trial court grants surgeon's motion for directed verdict

TRIAL COURT: A jury trial was held. At the conclusion of the evidence, the defendant surgeon moved for a directed verdict. The trial court granted the surgeon's motion on the grounds that the undisputed evidence showed that the CRNA's negligence caused the injury and that the surgeon was not vicariously liable for the actions of the CRNA. The trial court's decision was based on the fact that plaintiffs failed to establish that the surgeon had a master-servant relationship under the doctrine known as the borrowed servant rule. Although the CRNA was employed by the hospital, plaintiffs argued that the CRNA was loaned to the surgeon and according to hospital policy was under the surgeon's control and responsibility.

Plaintiffs appeal trial court decision

Plaintiffs appealed by a writ of certiorari requesting the court of appeals to review the trial court's decision in granting the directed verdict.

Appellate court affirms trial court decision

COURT OF APPEALS: The Court of Appeals for North Carolina granted a hearing on the issue of whether the trial court erred in granting the directed verdict on the basis that the surgeon was not vicariously liable for the acts of the CRNA. It affirmed the trial court's decision.

The appellate court dealt with whether the evidence showed that the surgeon had sufficient control of the CRNA's acts and therefore he should be liable under the borrowed servant rule.

| **KEY CASE 21–3** | Harris v. Miller (1991)[99] *Continued* |

Plaintiff appeals court of appeals decision to Supreme Court of North Carolina

Although the appellate court interpreted the hospital's manual as evidence that the surgeon had the right of supervision, the court made a distinction between the power to supervise and the power to control. In addition, it rejected plaintiff's argument that the surgeon's testimony was evidence that he was ultimately responsible for the quality of care given to a patient and held that the surgeon did not have the right to control the CRNA's actions.

APPEAL TO SUPREME COURT OF NORTH CAROLINA: The plaintiff appealed the decision of the court of appeals to the Supreme Court of North Carolina. The supreme court on review held that there was sufficient evidence for the case to be heard by the jury under the doctrine of vicarious liability of the surgeon. The North Carolina Supreme Court disagreed with the court of appeals' interpretation of the language of the hospital manual and interpreted the manual in the light most favorable to plaintiff, holding that the language could be interpreted that the surgeon was responsible for the selection and proper administration of the anesthetic agent.

The supreme court believed that the surgeon, on the basis of the hospital policy manual and the doctor's testimony, held the right to control the CRNA's actions and in fact at one point in time ordered the CRNA to stop administering all anesthesia and give the patient 100% oxygen as a remedial measure.[100]

The supreme court reversed the court of appeals' decision and granted the plaintiff a new trial against the surgeon[101] on the theory of vicarious liability and negligent supervision of the CRNA. Plaintiffs could not retry their negligence claim against the surgeon for the bleeding problem.

ANALYSIS: The *Harris* case is illustrative of the legal principle that other health care providers may be liable for an APN's negligent actions if the supervising provider has control over the APN's acts. The right of control may be determined through an analysis of a facility's policy manuals. Whether an individual will be viewed as an employer and be held vicariously liable will depend on the facts of each case. Under the doctrine of vicarious liability, the right of control is two pronged—the right to control the result of an individual's action and the right to control the means to reach that result. In the *Harris* case, the policy manual established the surgeon's right to control the result of the anesthesia actions, and in fact the surgeon may have assumed that right when he ordered the CRNA to perform certain tasks.

The primary lesson contained in the *Harris* case is that when APNs develop their practice, they should not allow policies and procedures or hospital standards to create a legal relationship with other health care providers beyond that established by statutes or case law.

Nurse-Midwives

A review of the legal literature reveals only a few reported civil cases involving nurse-midwives[102] and even fewer for nurse practitioners and clinical nurse specialists. However, APNs have been involved in criminal allegations for the illegal practice of medicine[103] and in antitrust cases.[104, 105]

RNs who function in an expanded role but lack required certification have been charged and convicted of the illegal practice of medicine.[106] In the *Bowland* case, an RN who held herself out as a midwife was criminally convicted for failing to meet the California statutory requirement of certification. The *Bowland* case is illustrative of the legal premise that an APN who fails to comply with statutory certification requirements may be criminally prosecuted.

> *. . . an APN who fails to comply with statutory certification requirements may be criminally prosecuted.*

A negligence per se theory was asserted against a nurse-midwife in *Lustig v. The Birthplace*[107] and was the basis for a $725,000 settlement for the wrongful death of a mother and child due to a nurse-midwife's breach of the statutory duty to consult a physician when there was a significant change in either the mother's or child's condition.[108] The nurse-midwife, who followed the mother throughout her pregnancy and labor, failed to recognize changes in the mother's condition that were consistent with preeclampsia and resulted in the stillbirth of the child and the death of the mother 2 days later.[109]

In 1999, there were two significant settlements of medical malpractice claims involving CNMs.[110]

In the first case, just before trial, a CNM and her supervising obstetrician settled the malpractice claim against them as individuals for $1 million. The allegations against the supervising physician were for his failure to timely respond and not for negligent supervision.[111] After a trial against the hospital, the jury found that the CNM was an agent of the hospital and thus the hospital was vicariously liable for failing to obtain timely medical intervention when the baby showed fetal distress. After trial, the case was settled for a confidential amount.[112] In the second case, the CNM was again alleged to have failed to timely obtain a medical consult and to have assumed too much responsibility. The case settled for $3.5 million and again an obstetrician participated in the settlement as the result of his delay in providing care.[113]

In another 1999 case, a CNM successfully argued that she had the right to rely on the medical judgment of the obstetricians who worked with her and received a verdict in her favor. However, the jury awarded $2.8 million against the remaining defendants.[114]

The most important legal principle that the APN should understand is that each and every APN is responsible for his or her wrongful actions or omissions that cause harm to another.[115]

Vicarious liability is based upon one party having the right of control over another.[116] The APN has the responsibility to define the legal relationship with any other health care provider and must understand that vicarious liability will not be presumed, nor does it take the place of the APN's own liability.

In a 1990 malpractice case involving a nurse-midwife's failure to monitor and treat a mother's hypertension and preeclampsia, a federal district court found the nurse-midwife negligent. That case is presented in Key Case 21–4.

KEY CASE 21–4   Anderson v. United States (1990)[117]

Mother followed during pregnancy by nurse-midwife employed by Indian Health Service

FACTS: On September 12, 1984, the minor plaintiff, Casey Anderson, was born to Marie Anderson, an 18-year-old primipara, at the Fort Yates Indian Health Services Hospital in North Dakota. During plaintiff's pregnancy, labor, and delivery, she was followed by a nurse-midwife, Dorothy Meyer, who was an employee of the Indian Health Services and was qualified to deliver babies in low-risk pregnancies. Plaintiff saw an obstetrician on one of her prenatal visits who informed her that she was progressing well.

Mother develops preeclamptic state, but staff does not intervene medically

During plaintiff's labor, the staff recorded elevations of her blood pressure, which were the presenting signs of pregnancy-induced hypertension. Although fetal monitoring was done on two separate occasions, the staff failed to recognize plaintiff's preeclamptic medical problem. Meconium staining was also present at the time plaintiff's membranes were ruptured, and there was evidence at the time of delivery that meconium aspiration had occurred. The baby was lethargic and required resuscitation at the time of his birth.

He is now 5 years old and is severely disabled. He is unable to walk, crawl, talk, see, or control his bowel movements, and he must be fed through a jejunostomy tube.

Mother files a malpractice suit alleging negligent failure to timely diagnose and treat pregnancy-induced hypertension and preeclampsia

Plaintiff filed a medical malpractice claim, alleging negligence in the failure to timely diagnose and treat plaintiff's pregnancy-induced hypertension and preeclampsia resulting in the minor plaintiff suffering from intrapartum asphyxia and being born with severe and permanent brain injuries and cerebral palsy.

U.S. FEDERAL DISTRICT COURT DECISION: This case was filed in the U.S. District Court, as the Fort Yates Indian Health Services Hospital in North Dakota is a medical facility operated by the United States in the Standing Rock Indian Reservation. The suit was filed pursuant to the Federal Tort Claims Act.[118]

Court rules the hospital, including nurse-midwife, negligent, and their negligence caused birth injuries

A bench trial was held, and the trier of fact ruled that the staff at the Fort Yates Hospital, including the nurse-midwife, was negligent in failing to timely diagnose and treat plaintiff's pregnancy-induced hypertension and preeclampsia, which proximately caused the minor plaintiff to suffer intrapartum asphyxia and severe permanent brain injuries.

The defendant, the United States, was held liable for approximately $3.4 million economic damages, and an additional $525,000 was awarded to the maternal grandmother on her loss of consortium claim under the doctrine of *in loco parentis* as she had assumed financial and physical responsibility of caring for the baby since his birth. A trust was established to handle the minor plaintiff's financial needs.

APPEALS COURT: No appeal was made by either party.

ANALYSIS: The significance of the *Anderson* case is that it was one of the very few reported cases that dealt with the expanded role of the nurse-midwife. It is also representative of the fact that APNs whose practice setting is a federal or government entity are not immune from allegations of negligence.

APNs who are employees of government are not immune from negligence suits

The *Anderson* case also reflects the deep-pocket theory and the doctrine of *respondeat superior*, as the action was brought against the United States as the principal for the actions of its agents who were acting within their scope of employment at the federally operated medical facility.

Nurse Practitioner

Failure to inform a patient of known risks and a delay in the proper treatment of an infection were two of the allegations against the nurse practitioner (NP) in *Gugino v. Harvard Community Health Plan.*[119] On the basis of medical expert testimony, the NP was held liable for the failure to inform the patient in 1975 of the known risk of infection associated with an IUD, the Dalkon shield, which the patient had had inserted in 1972. In addition, the NP was liable for the 48-hour delay in instituting the proper treatment, thereby necessitating the patient to undergo a total hysterectomy for multiple abscesses.[120] The courts have held that the APN must keep abreast of the medical research regarding implanted devices. The APN has a continuing duty to inform his or her patients of any known risk associated with a course of treatment or a device, whether past or present. It should be noted, however, that the APN will be held accountable only if the APN knew or should have known about the treatment or device.

Another example of the NP's failure to warn of known risks is the wrongful death claim filed against the county and the manufacturer of a polio vaccine for the actions of a pediatric NP in the case of *Sheenan v. Pima County.*[121] The allegations claimed that the pediatric NP was negligent for failing to inform the parent of the danger of contracting polio after receiving the vaccine. The appellate court upheld the defense verdict on the grounds that the mother (the plaintiff), even if informed of the risk, would still have permitted her child to receive the vaccine. However, the court found that the pediatric NP, as a learned intermediary and the one most knowledgeable regarding the risks, had the duty to disclose to the mother the

1 in 5 million risk of contracting the disease. The legal premise that the APN has constructive knowledge of the risks of treatment and drugs was established when the court acknowledged the advanced practice of professional nurses.[122]

The APN has a continuing duty to inform his or her patients of any known risk associated with a course of treatment or a device, whether past or present.

There is a recognized affirmative duty to refer the patient to another health care provider or specialist if the patient's condition is beyond the APN's skill or knowledge.

In *Sermchief v. Gonzales* the court recognized that NPs who function in an advanced role must be aware of the limits of their knowledge and the limits contained in the written standing orders and protocols. There is a recognized affirmative duty to refer the patient to another health care provider or specialist if the patient's condition is beyond the APN's skill or knowledge.

Allegations of the APN's failure to institute proper treatment can be asserted against the APN, as illustrated in the well-known *Fein v. Permanente* case.

KEY CASE 21–5   Sermchief v. Gonzales (1983)[123]

Two NPs provide obstetrical, gynecological, and family planning care to patients via standing orders and written protocols developed by physicians

FACTS: Two NPs and five physicians were employed by the East Missouri Action Agency to provide obstetrical, gynecological, and family planning services to low-income patients. NPs Janice Burgess, a family planning practitioner, and Suzanne Solari, an obstetric-gynecologic practitioner, provided competent health care services pursuant to written standing orders and protocols developed by the physicians. In fact, there were no allegations that the NPs' actions had caused harm to any client.

Complaint against nurses and physicians about services filed with licensing agency

Board of agency decides to seek criminal charges against NPs for practicing medicine without a license and against physicians for aiding and abetting that unauthorized practice

Nurses and physicians file suit asking for injunctive and declaratory relief

Court rules against NPs and physicians

The Missouri Supreme Court reverses the lower court, holding that the NPs were practicing nursing as defined in the Missouri Nurse Practice Act

In 1980, a confidential complaint was filed with the Missouri State Board of Registration for the Healing Arts alleging that the NPs were practicing medicine without a license and that the physicians, by developing written standing orders and protocols, were aiding and abetting unauthorized practice of medicine.

Upon investigation of the complaint, the Board decided to seek criminal charges against the NPs and hold a hearing to decide if the physicians' licenses should be revoked or suspended. Upon learning of the board's actions, the NPs and physicians, through their attorneys, obtained a temporary restraining order against the board, prohibiting the board from acting further. An action for declaratory and injunctive relief was filed with the court, seeking a court order to permanently prohibit the board from interfering with their practice, challenging the constitutionality of Missouri's Medical Practice Act, and asking for a determination that the NPs' actions constituted professional nursing.

TRIAL COURT DECISION: The trial court heard expert testimony from both sides and ruled on behalf of the board. The court held that the NPs' actions constituted the unlawful practice of medicine and enjoined them from performing any activities pursuant to their protocols unless a physician was on site at the time. The court further upheld the constitutionality of the Medical Practice Act, and thus the NPs had adequate notice that their actions were unlawful.

Regarding the physicians, the court ruled they were not immune from the board's actions and would need to respond to the allegations of aiding and abetting the unauthorized practice of medicine.

The lower court's decision was appealed to the Missouri Supreme Court.

MISSOURI SUPREME COURT DECISION: The Missouri Supreme Court reversed the lower court's decision and ordered that judgment be entered for the NPs and physicians. The supreme court held that the NPs' acts were authorized under Missouri's State Nurse Practice Act, and therefore their acts did not constitute the unlawful practice of medicine.

The supreme court recognized that the legislature's intent was to authorize the expanding scope of nurse practice when the nurse practice act was revised, by having an open-ended definition of professional nursing and by eliminating the requirement that a physician directly supervise nursing functions. The court did not address the NPs' level of training or degree of skill, as the board's challenge was directed only toward the NPs' legal right to act pursuant to the standing orders and protocols.

At the time of the appeal, the only basis of the court's review was the comparison of the medical practice act and the nurse practice act and the evidence presented at the time of trial, despite the fact that amicus briefs by advocates for the nursing profession were filed urging the court to rule in favor of defendants.

ANALYSIS: The *Sermchief* case is important, as it was the first legal challenge to address the legality of the APN's scope of practice. The

Key Case continued on following page

| KEY CASE 21–5 | Sermchief v. Gonzales (1983)[123] *Continued* |

Supreme Court of Missouri acknowledged that the state had recognized the expanded role of nurses when the nurse practice act was revised in 1975. The court applied the rule of statutory interpretation in comparing the medical practice act and the nurse practice act to determine the NP's scope of practice.

This case is also significant as the court, by recognizing the expanded role of nursing practice, articulated the legal premise that APNs also have the responsibility to act in a professional manner and know the limits of their professional knowledge. This would include the duty to act within the limits of standing orders and protocols and the duty to refer when a patient's needs exceed the APN's scope of practice.

| KEY CASE 21–6 | Fein v. Permanente Medical Group (1985)[124] |

Patient experiences chest pain and calls Kaiser Health Plan physician, who could not see him

Patient sees NP, who, in consultation with physician-supervisor, determines chest pain due to muscle spasm

Chest pain persists, so patient returns and sees a physician in Plan; diagnosis of muscle spasm also made by this physician

Pain persists and ECG obtained on third visit

Myocardial infarction diagnosed and patient admitted to CCU

FACTS: In February 1976, a 34-year-old attorney, Lawrence Fein, experienced, over a 5-day period, brief intermittent episodes of chest pain while exercising and while working. As a Kaiser Health Plan member, he contacted his primary care physician on February 26, 1976, for an appointment, but his physician did not have an open appointment available, and he was given an appointment that afternoon with Family NP Cheryl Welch, who was working under the supervision of physician-consultant Dr. Winthrop Frantz. Mr. Fein was aware that Ms. Welch was an NP and did not request to be seen by a doctor. After examining Mr. Fein, Ms. Welch consulted Dr. Frantz, who wrote a prescription for Valium, and Ms. Welch informed Mr. Fein that they believed his pain was due to muscle spasms.

At about 1 o'clock the next morning, the patient awoke with severe chest pains and was taken to the Kaiser Emergency Room where he was treated by Dr. Redding. After obtaining a chest X-ray and examining him, Dr. Redding concluded the patient was suffering from muscle spasms and ordered pain medication. The patient also continued to suffer from intermittent chest pain, which became more severe the next afternoon. He was again seen in Kaiser Emergency Room, where, after an ECG was obtained, an acute myocardial infarction was diagnosed, and he was admitted to the Cardiac Care Unit. The patient was able to return to part-time work within 8 months of the incident and full-time within 1 to 2 years. At the time of trial, he was able to engage in all of his prior recreational activities.

Suit filed by patient alleging failure to timely diagnose and treat heart attack

In February 1977, Mr. Fein filed a medical malpractice claim alleging failure to timely diagnose and treat his heart attack.

TRIAL COURT DECISION: A jury trial was held and expert testimony was presented. Plaintiff's cardiology expert testified that plaintiff's presenting signs and symptoms were consistent with an imminent heart attack, and at the time plaintiff saw the NP an ECG should have been ordered. Plaintiff's expert also testified that Dr. Redding should have ordered an ECG, and if an ECG had been obtained, the plaintiff's impending myocardial infarction could have been identified and medical intervention instituted to prevent or minimize the attack.

Jury returns negligence verdict against the health plan due to conduct of NP and physicians

Despite testimony by the NP and the emergency room physician and the defense experts, the jury ruled in favor of the plaintiff, and judgment was entered against the Permanente Medical Group for the negligent conduct of the NP and the two physicians (Frantz and Redding). The jury awarded approximately $1.2 million dollars for noneconomic and economic damages, which were reduced under statutory law.

Both parties appealed the lower court's decision.

APPEALS COURT DECISION: The plaintiff appealed the lower court's decision on the grounds that the judgment in his favor should not be reduced under the California statutes limiting noneconomic damages to $250,000, nor should receipt of any disability benefits reduce the amount of economic damages. The appellate court upheld the California statutes as being constitutional and affirmed the trial court's ruling to reduce the award.

Plaintiff loses appeal to fight reduction of noneconomic damages

Health plan appeals several issues, including the jury instructions regarding the NP standard of care

The defendant medical group appealed the lower court's decision on several grounds pertaining to voir dire jury selection, causation and damage issues, denial of periodic payment, and the jury instruction regarding the standard of care of the NP.

The lower court had instructed the jury that the standard of care required of an NP when the NP examines a patient or makes a diagnosis is the standard of care of a physician and surgeon duly licensed to practice medicine in the state of California. The appellate court, based upon its review of California's Nurse Practice Act and the legislature's intent to recognize the existence of overlapping functions between physicians and RNs, held that the lower court erred in the NP's standard of care instruction to the jury.

Appeals court rules the lower court's applications of a physician standard of care to an NP in error

Appeals court upholds decision of lower court, as the use of the wrong standard of care did not affect judgment

However, although the trial court erred in its jury instruction, the appellate court upheld the plaintiff's verdict on the grounds that the lower court's error did not affect the judgment and would not warrant a reversal. In fact, the appellate court ruled that although there were errors by the trial court, none warranted a reversal, and therefore the judgment remained as entered.

It should be noted that the appellate decision was not unanimous, and several appellate justices dissented.

SECOND APPEAL REQUEST: The petition for rehearing filed by the plaintiff/appellant was denied on April 4, 1985.

ANALYSIS: The *Fein* case is the landmark case that addresses the standard of care of NPs and therefore is the precedent in California that

Key Case continued on following page

KEY CASE 21–6   Fein v. Permanente Medical Group (1985)[124] *Continued*

identifies the professional standard that the APN's conduct will be measured against in a negligence action.

An important issue in the legal recognition of the APN is the fact that in *Fein* a physician who was not an NP expert testified to the standard of care of the NP. To ensure that the appropriate professional standard is being applied, APNs should challenge any physician's expert qualifications in an action brought against them.

The *Fein* case is also significant for the principle that the NP standard of care will be applied only as long as the NP is functioning within the scope of the NP's practice. Because Ms. Welch consulted her physician-consultant and was acting within her scope of practice as a Family NP (even though her actions were found to be negligent), the standard her conduct would be measured against would be the NP standard. Functioning outside the scope of practice would expose the NP to a nonnurse standard of care.

In 1993 in the case of *Adams v. Krueger,* a nurse practitioner was held liable for the misdiagnosis of a patient's condition.[125] During the trial, the jury found the NP was 41% negligent, the physician who prescribed the ointment for the patient's misdiagnosed condition was held 10% negligent, and the patient was 49% negligent.[126] The district court, however, imputed the NP's negligence to her employer the physician, reasoning that he was responsible for the actions of his employee, the nurse practitioner.[127] The court of appeals affirmed the district court reasoning.[128]

In the 1996 case *Jenkins v. Payne,* a medical malpractice claim was brought against a nurse practitioner and five physicians for failing to timely diagnose Paget's disease in a patient that they had been continuously treating over a 2-year period of time. The trial court's judgment of $1 million against the family practice physician and the nurse practitioner was affirmed by the Virginia Supreme Court. This case is discussed in more detail in Key Case 21–7.

KEY CASE 21–7   Jenkins v. Payne (1996)[129]

Patient sees NP for nipple discharge and scabbing of left breast

Pain and discharge in left breast nipple continues

NP refers the patient to a dermatologist for the left breast nipple irritation

FACTS: In January 1991, the patient, Veronica Payne, was initially seen by a nurse practitioner, who was supervised by a family practice physician, for complaints of a discharge and scabbing of her left breast nipple. The NP ordered a mammogram, which was reported as negative. The NP prescribed antibiotics for the problem.

Six months later the patient returned to see the NP with complaints of continuing pain and discharge from her left breast nipple. The NP refered the patient to a dermatologist for treatment of the persistent left breast irritation. The NP did not document the fact that she had any discussions with the patient regarding the possibility of breast cancer or the need for a biopsy.

Treatment continues with gynecologist and NP but with no relief from left breast nipple irritation

The patient was seen by a gynecologist on October 21, 1991 and on November 8, 1991 for her breast complaints. The gynecologist prescribed antibiotics and a topical steroid cream and diagnosed her as having eczema. The gynecologist documented a past history that the patient had an inflamed and bleeding left nipple for 1½ years. Ms. Payne maintained that the gynecologist reassured her that she did not have breast cancer. During 1992, the patient was seen several times by the NP and the gynecologist. Neither of these health care providers documented that they had reexamined the patient's breasts or inquired whether the problem still persisted.

Patient diagnosed in terminal stage of Paget's disease with lymph node metastasis

On September 23, 1992 the NP performed a breast exam on Ms. Payne and discovered multiple masses in the patient's left breast. In December 1992, Ms. Payne was diagnosed with Paget's disease in the terminal stage with lymph node metastasis. Ms. Payne died in April 1994.

Patient dies in 1994 after filing malpractice claim against the NP and five physicians

Prior to her death, Ms. Payne filed a medical malpractice claim against the NP and five physicians, alleging the failure to diagnose and treat her breast cancer and for the misdiagnosis.

TRIAL COURT: Evidence was presented by experts that Paget's disease is a cancer of the nipple and milk ducts and classic symptoms of this disease are discharge, skin lesions, nipple inflammation, and irritation. In the early stages, the cancer is noninvasive, and there is a 90% survival rate if treatment is instituted before the cancer becomes invasive. Ms. Payne's surgical oncologist testified that Ms. Payne had a 10-year survival probability of nearly 90% had her cancer been diagnosed when it was noninvasive. The plaintiff's expert surgical oncologist testified that Ms. Payne's cancer became invasive 3 to 6 months prior to the December 1992 diagnosis.

The NP's supervising physician testified that he was responsible for the care of all patients treated by the NP and held daily discussions with the NP regarding her treatment of any seriously ill patients. He acknowledged that he knew a biopsy was necessary in order to differentiate Paget's disease from a benign problem. He testified that he was aware of Ms. Payne's breast problem and in January 1992, he recognized that there was a chance Ms. Payne had Paget's disease but did not discuss this possibility with the NP or the patient.

Expert testimony was given at the trial that the supervising physician and the NP breached the standard of care by failing to recognize the symptoms of breast cancer, by failing to refer the patient for a biopsy, and for misdiagnosing the problem as an infection.

Both the plaintiff and defense presented expert nurse practitioners to testify on the standard of care.

After Ms. Payne's death during trial, suit is amended to include a wrongful death claim

While the action was pending Ms. Payne died as a result of her disease, and the claim was amended to allege a cause of action for wrongful death.

Jury awards $1.1 million to family of patient

TRIAL COURT DECISION: The jury awarded a $1.1 million verdict against the defendants. The gynecologist settled his claim for $450,000 prior to trial.

Key Case continued on following page

KEY CASE 21–7	Jenkins v. Payne (1996)[129] *Continued*

Appellate court confirms jury's verdict

An appeal was filed by the defendants alleging that the gynecologist was the sole proximate cause of Ms. Payne's death.

APPEAL COURT DECISION: The appellate court affirmed the trial court's jury verdict.

ANALYSIS: The NP was held liable for misdiagnosing Ms. Payne's condition and failing to recognize the symptoms of breast cancer. The NP also breached the standard of care for failing to follow up with the patient as to whether the treatment she had prescribed was effective. The lack of documentation about any discussion regarding a biopsy and the possibility of breast cancer was also significant.

The supervising physician, although not directly involved in seeing the patient, through his discussions with the NP suspected that Ms. Payne may have had Paget's disease but did not tell the NP or the patient, nor did he refer her for a biopsy.

Tragic events can occur when the NP fails to timely diagnose and follow up on a patient's problem.

Clinical Nurse Specialist

The title clinical nurse specialist (CNS) has been recognized by the nursing profession since the 1930s, and historically, the role developed in the psychiatric nursing area. The role of the CNS has expanded into most facets of patient care, including case management, consultation, research, and education. However, there is some confusion regarding the role of the CNS. In 1998, legislation in California was enacted which recognized the role of the certified nurse specialist as an APN.[130] In 1994, one article discussed the CNS role as a cardiovascular nurse interventionist.[131] In the legal arena, however, a review of the reported case law does not reveal any cases specifically involving the CNS.

Even so, the CNS is faced with similar practice hurdles and liability issues that other APNs have had to confront. The legal issues pertaining to informed consent, especially in the research setting, and the duty to appropriately monitor and inform a patient of any known risks or dangers are applicable to the CNS's practice.

Inability to receive third-party reimbursement has previously prevented the CNS from being hired instead of another professional whose services are reimbursed.[132]

Since recent changes in the federal Medicare regulations allows the CNS to receive direct reimbursement, the role of the CNS will become more recognized and in turn be under increased legal scrutiny.[133] Regardless of the practice setting, the CNS, along with the other APNs, is a provider of direct patient care and is capable of functioning independently or interdependently in a highly competent and cost-effective manner.

SUMMARY OF PRINCIPLES AND APPLICATIONS

The APN's role in health care reform is slowly progressing. There are serious legal barriers preventing APNs from functioning to the fullest extent of their education, training, and skills. After more than 30 years, the APN continues to face legal obstacles regarding prescriptive authority, direct reimbursement, and scope-of-practice issues.

Recent advances in prescriptive authority, reimbursement,[134] and the growth of the number of APNs actively practicing has led to increased concerns and renewed turf battles within physicians' organizations. Scope of practice and physician supervision issues are being raised in an attempt to limit the APN's practice. APNs must be constantly vigilant to any erosion of the gains already achieved and be proactive in establishing their role within the health care workforce.

Legal recognition must catch up to the realities of the APN's practice to allow patients full access to quality and cost-efficient health care by highly competent health care providers. The time has come for APNs to take their rightful and legal place in the promotion of health and reduction of health costs. It is imperative that to continue to provide competent and high-quality health care and to achieve a truly independent and autonomous practice, the APN must understand the legal principles pertaining to scope of practice, the standard of care, and the current legal theories. Therefore, the APN should:

- Be able to identify the practice issues that may expose him or her to allegations of malpractice

- Keep abreast of the changes in the laws that govern advanced practice

- Be familiar with the legal theories of *respondeat superior* and vicarious liability when the APN is acting in the role of employer or principal

- Adhere to the standards of care pertaining to the APN's area of specialty

- Develop written protocols and standardized procedures when required by state law in order to comply with those state statutes and regulations

- Identify the legal authority to perform overlapping functions

- Form collaborative practices with other health care professionals

- Identify the barriers to practice and the mechanism to achieve full prescriptive authority and reimbursement

TOPICS FOR FURTHER INQUIRY

1. Design a study to evaluate the consumer's knowledge and recognition of the APN's role in health care.

2. Help develop an APN national database regarding unreported legal cases that involve an APN's practice but may not name the APN as a defendant.

3. Compare and contrast the effectiveness of collaborative practice agreements and employment agreements for the APN.

4. Write a paper analyzing APN educational programs in at least two states to determine the existence and amount of time spent regarding the legal and ethical aspects of advanced practice.

5. Design a study to evaluate insurance companies' recognition of the APN role. Identify how the recognition

occurs (e.g., direct reimbursement, amount reimbursed) and where changes in each system should occur.

6. Develop a marketing plan to improve the visibility of the APN's role in health care in your state.

7. Draft a realistic proposal to educate legislators regarding the necessity for full prescriptive authority for APNs.

8. Design a study to evaluate NP and CNS cost-effectiveness within the Medicare system.

9. Compare and contrast prescribing procedures of NPs with those of physicians. Identify why differences exist and how the differences can be minimized.

REFERENCES

1. Anthony Kovner and Steven Jonas, Editors. *Health Care Delivery in the United States.* 6th Edition. New York: Springer Publishing Company, 1999, 82–83, *citing* Division of Nursing, Bureau of Health Professions, Health Resources and Service Administration. *Advance Notes from the National Survey of Registered Nurses.* Rockville, Md.: Author, 1997.

2. K. O'Connor, "Advanced Practice Nurses in an Environment of Health Care Reform," 19 *MCN* (March/April 1994), 68, *citing* "Omnibus Poll," Lincoln, Nebraska, Gallup Organization, 1993.

3. American Nurses Association. *Nurse Practitioner and Certified Midwives: A Meta-Analysis of Process of Care, Clinical Outcomes and Cost-Effectiveness of Nurses in Primary Care Roles.* Washington D.C.: American Nurses Publishing, 1993.

4. A. Catlin and M. McAuliffe, "Proliferation of Non-Physician Providers as Reported in the Journal of the American Medical Association (JAMA), 1998," 31 *Image: Journal of Nursing Scholarship* (1999), 175–177.

5. A. L. Andersen, C. L. Gilliss, and L. Yoder. "Practice Environment for Nurse Practitioners in California: Identifying Barriers," 165 *Western Journal of Medicine* (1996), 109–214. See also, Mary Mundinger, Robert Kane, Elizabeth Lenz, Annette Totten, and others, "Primary Care Outcomes in Patients Treated by Nurse Practitioners or Physicians," 283(1) *JAMA* (2000), accessed January 28, 2000, at http://jama.ama-assn.org/issues/v283nl/full/joc90696.html

6. American Association of Nurse Anesthetists. *Legal Issues in Nurse Anesthesia Practice.* Park Ridge, Ill.: Author, Anesthetists, accessed on January 29, 2000, at the association's home page, http://www.aana.com

7. A. Inglis and D. Kjervik, "Empowerment of Advanced Practice Nurses: Regulation Reform Needed to Increase Access to Care," 21(2) *Journal of Law, Medicine, & Ethics* (1993), 194. See also, American Association of Nurse Anesthetists. *Scope and Standards for Nurse Anesthesia Practice.* Park Ridge, Ill.: Author, 1998.

8. American Association of Nurse Anesthetists. *Nurse Anesthesia . . . No Longer the Best Kept Secret in Health Care.*

Park Ridge, Ill.: Author, accessed on January 31, 2000, at the association's home page, *supra* note 6.

9. *Id.*

10. Gene Blumenreich, "Legal Briefs: Anesthesia—It's Finally the Practice of Medicine," 67 *Journal of the American Association of Nurse Anesthetists (JAANA)* (April, 1999), 109–112.

11. *Id.*

12. A. Federwisch, "CRNA Autonomy—Nurse Anesthetists Fight Latest Skirmish," *Nurseweek* (Dec. 14, 1998), 23.

13. "Medical Gloves Come Off in Fight Over Anesthesia," Associated Press, *Chicago Tribune,* Tuesday, Dec. 29, 1998, Section 1, 11.

14. D. Williams, "Credentialing Certified Nurse Midwives," 39 *Journal of Nurse-Midwifery* (July/Aug. 1994), 258.

15. *Id.* at 259.

16. L. Ament and L. Hanson, "Model for the Future," *Nursing and Health Care Perspectives* (1999), 26–33. See also, Laura Mackler, "The Doctor's Still In But New Study Funds Midwives on the Increase," Associated Press, December 2, 1999, accessed January 29, 2000 at http://abcnews.go.com/sections/living/dailynews/midwives991202.html

17. American Academy of Nurse Practitioners. *Standards of Practice,* accessed July 9, 1998, at the academy's home page at http://www.aanp.org

18. J. Schultz, G. Liptak, and J. Fioravanti, "Nurse Practitioners' Effectiveness in NICU," 25(1) *Nursing Management* (Oct. 1994), 50.

19. American Nurses Association, *supra* note 3.

20. M. Ventura and D. Grandinetti, "NP Progress Report: A Survey," 62(7) *RN* (1999), 33–35.

21. *Id.*

22. J. Beal, D. Maguire, and R. Carr, "Neonatal Nurse Practitioners: Identity as Advanced Practice Nurses," 25 *JOGNN* (1996), 401–406.

23. V. Knaus, S. Felton, S. Burton, P. Fobes, and K. Davis, "The Use of Nurse Practitioners in the Acute Care Setting," 27 *JONA* (1997), 20–27.

24. E. Nelson, S. Van Cleve, M. Swartz, W. Kessen, and P. McCarthy, "Improving the Use of Early Followup Care After Emergency Department Visits," 145 *AJDC* (1991), 440–444.

25. J. Kerekes, M. Jenkins, and D. Torrise, "Nurse-Managed Primary Care," 27 *Nursing Management* (1996), 44–47.

26. D. Grandinetti, "NP Progress Report: How Is This Practice Doing?" 62(7) *RN* (1999), 36–38.

27. Mary Mundinger and others, *supra* note 5.

28. R. Cooper, P. Laud, and C. Dietrich, "Current and Projected Workforce of Non-Physician Clinicians," 280(9) *JAMA* (1998), 788–794. See also, R. Cooper, T. Henderson, and C. Dietrich, "Roles of Nonphysician Clinicians as Autonomous Providers of Patient Care," 280(9) *JAMA* (1998), 795–801.

29. D. Askin, K. Bennett, and C. Shapiro, "The Clinical Nurse Specialist and the Research Process," 23(4) *JOGNN* (May 1994), 336.

30. A. Henrick and J. Appleyard, "Clinical Nurse Specialists and Nurse Practitioners: Who Are They, What Do They Do, and What Challenges Do They Face?" in *Current Issues in Nursing.* Joanne McCloskey and Helen Grace, Editors. 5th Edition. St. Louis, Mo.: Mosby, 1997, 18–24.

31. S. Wong, "Reimbursement to Advanced Practice Nurses (APNs) Through Medicare," 31 *Image: Journal of Nursing Scholarship* (1999), 167–169.

32. R. Cooper, P. Laud, and C. Dietrich, *supra* note 28.

33. S. Wong, *supra* note 31.

34. A. Inglis and D. Kjervik, *supra* note 7 at 197.

35. G. Blumenreich, "The Overlap Between the Practice of Medicine and the Practice of Nursing," 66 *JAANA* (1998), 11–15.

36. K. O'Connor, *supra* note 2, at 66.

37. See generally, Carolyn Buppert. *Nurse Practitioner's Business Practice & Legal Guide.* Gaithersburg, Md.: Aspen Publishers, 1999.

38. L. Pearson, "Annual Update of How Each State Stands on Legislative Issues Affecting Advanced Nursing Practice," *Nurse Practitioner* (1998), 14–66.

39. *Id.* at 22–53.

40. D. Williams, *supra* note 14, at 259.

41. G. Birkholz and D. Walker, "Strategies for State Statutory Language Changes Granting Fully Independent Nurse Practitioner Practice," *Nurse Practitioner* (1994), 54.

42. L. Pearson, *supra* note 38, at 16.

43. G. Burkholz and D. Walker, *supra* note 41, at 54.

44. L. Pearson, *supra* note 38, at 26.

45. D. Williams, *supra* note 14, at 260.

46. *Chalmers-Francis v. Nelson,* 6 Cal.2d 402, 57 P.2d 1312 (1936).

47. *State v. Borah,* 51 Ariz. 318, 76 P.2d 757 (1938).

48. 660 S.W.2d 683 (Mo. enbanc 1983).

49. *Id.*

50. *Professional Health Care Inc. v. Bigsby,* 709 P.2d 86 (Colo. 1995).

51. *Prentice Medical Corporation v. Todd,* 145 Ill. App. 3d 692, 495 N.E.2d 1044, 99 Ill. Dec. 309 (1986).

52. *Hoffson v. Orentreic,* 168 A.D.2d 243 (1990).

53. 660 S.W.2d 683, 690.

54. Buppert, *supra* note 37, at 217–221.

55. *Id.* at 220.

56. 38 Cal. 3d 137, 695 P.2d 665; 211 Cal. Rptr. 368 (1985).

57. 300 N.W.2d 380, 382 (Mich. App. 1980).

58. Buppert, *supra* note 37, at 220.

59. G. Blumenreich, "Standard of Care," 65 *JAANA* (1997), 523–526.

60. *Id.* at 525.

61. G. Blumenreich, "Expert Testimony," 64 *JAANA* (1996), 517–520.

62. *Denton Regional Medical Center v. La Croix,* 947 S.W.2d 941 (1997).

63. G. Blumenreich, "La Croix Case," 65 *JAANA* (1997), 419–422.

64. *Denton v. La Croix, supra* note 62.

65. Blumenreich, *supra* note 63.

66. American Academy of Nurse Practitioners, *supra* note 17.

67. *Fein v. Permanente Medical Group, supra* note 56.

68. See, for example, *Czubinsky v. Doctors Hospital,* 139 Cal. App. 3d 361, 188 Cal. Rptr. 685 (1983).

69. M. Sebas, "Developing a Collaborative Practice Agreement for the Primary Care Setting," 19 *Nurse Practitioner* (March 1993), 49.

70. 38 Cal.3d 137, 695 P.2d 665, 211 Cal. Rptr. 368 (1985).

71. 380 Mass. 464, 403 N.E.2d 1166 (1980).

72. *Jenkins v. Payne,* 465 S.E.2d 795 (Va. 1996).

73. *Carolan v. Hill,* 553 N.W.2d 882 (Iowa 1996).
74. *Id.*
75. A. Inglis and D. Kjervik, *supra* note 7, at 193.
76. *Id.* at 198.
77. *Id.*
78. L. Pearson, *supra* note 38, at 17.
79. *Id.* at 19.
80. Buppert, *supra* note 37, at 131–132, 173.
81. Bonnie Faherty, "Advanced Practice Nursing: What's All the Fuss?" 2(3) *Journal of Nursing Law* (1995), 12.
82. See, as examples, Cooper, Henderson, and Dietrich, *supra* note 28; C. Pierson, "APNs in Home Care," 99(10) *AJN* (1999), 22–23; K. Grumbach and J. Coffman, "Physicians and Nonphysician Clinicians: Complements or Competitors?" 280(9) *JAMA* (1998), 825–826 (editorial); H. P. Leblanc, B. Simon, D. Garard, R. Nawrot, and others, "Attitudes Toward the Utilization of Certified Nurse Midwives Among Physicians and Midwives in Illinois and Indiana," 3(3) *Center Research Briefs* (1997), accessed January 29, 2000, at Southern Illinois University at Carbondale's home page at http://www.siu.edu (Center for Rural Health and Social Service Development).
83. 705 P.2d 781 (Wash. App. 1985).
84. *Res ipsa loquitur* is discussed at length in Chapters 4 and 5.
85. 326 S.E.2d 271 (N.C. App. 1985).
86. 480 N.E.2d 464 (Ohio 1985).
87. *Id.* at 464.
88. 366 N.W.2d 249 (1985).
89. *Id.*
90. 687 So. 2d 737 (Miss.) 1992.
91. See, for example, *Glassman v. Castello,* 986 P.2d 1050 (Kan. 1999). The Kansas Supreme Court reversed a lower court decision holding a CRNA 99% liable and the obstetrician 1% liable for the death of the mother during a cesarean section that resulted in the delivery of a healthy baby. The Kansas Supreme Court cited Kansas law, which stated that "the duties and functions of a registered nurse anesthetist" are performed "in an interdependent role as a member of a physician . . . directed team." The nature and extent of the obstetrician's duty to direct and supervise the CRNA was, according to the court, a factual issue for the jury. A. David Tammello, "Are Doctors Responsible for Negligence of CRNAs?" 40(8) *Nursing Law's Regan Report* (January 2000), 2.
92. 855 S.W.2d 857 (1993).
93. *Res ipsa loquitur* is discussed in depth in Chapters 4 and 5.
94. 480 N.E.2d 464 (1985).
95. *Id.* at 465.
96. *Id.* at 476.
97. See, for example, *Pommier v. Savoy Memorial Hospital,* 1998 WL 391121 (La. App. 3d Cir.) 1998.
98. See, for example, *Shahires v. Louisiana State University,* 680 So. 2d 1352 (La. App. 2d Cir.) 1996.
99. 407 S.E.2d 556 (1991).
100. G. Blumenreich, "*Harris v. Miller*" 62 *Journal of American Association of Nurse Anesthetists* (June 1994), 210.
101. 438 S.E. 2d 731 (1994).
102. S. Jenkins, "The Myth of Vicarious Liability," 39 *Journal of Nurse-Midwifery* (March/April 1994), 106.
103. See *Sermchief v. Gonzalez, supra* note 48.
104. *Bahn v. NME Hosp. Inc.,* 772 F.2d 1467 (9th Cir. 1985).
105. *Nurse Midwifery Assoc. v. Hibbett,* 577 F. Supp. 1273 (D. Tenn., 1983).
106. *Bowland v. Municipal Court for Santa Cruz County,* 18 Cal.3d 479, 556 P.2d 1081, 134 Cal. Rptr. 630 (1976).
107. No. 83-2-07528-9, Wash. King's County Superior Crt., decided Sept. 9, 1983 as reported in 27 ATLA Law Rptr. 87 (March 1984).
108. *Id.*
109. *Id.*
110. D. Rubsamen, "Multimillion Dollar Damage Award for Perinatal Brain Damage," 29 *Professional Liability Newsletter* (October 1999).
111. *Id.*
112. *Id.*
113. *Id.*
114. *Id.*
115. *Id.*
116. See *Harris v. Miller,* 335 N.C. 379, 438 S.E.2d 731 (1994).
117. 731 F. Supp. 391 (1990).
118. 28 U.S.C. 2671 *et seq.*
119. 403 N.E.2d 1166 (1980).
120. *Id.*
121. 660 P.2d 486 (1983).
122. See, for example, Buppert, *supra* note 37, at 238–244.
123. 660 S.W.2d 683, 690 (Mo. enbanc 1983).
124. 38 Cal.3d 137, 696 P.2d 665, 211 Cal. Rptr. 368 (1985).
125. 856 P.2d 864 (1993).
126. *Id.*
127. *Id.*
128. *Id.*
129. 465 S.E.2d 795 (1996).
130. L. Pearson, *supra* note 38.
131. Mary Engles and Marguerite Engles, "Cardiovascular Nurse Interventionist: An Emerging New Role," 15(5) *Nursing and Health Care* (April 1994).
132. See, generally, Buppert, *supra* note 37 and Henrick and Appleyard, *supra* note 30.
133. A. Catlin and M. McAuliffe, *supra* note 4.
134. The Health Care Financing Administration (HCFA) has published its final rule establishing Medicare payments for advanced practice nurses. The rule can be accessed on the *Federal Register* home page at www.access.gpo.gov.

The Nurse as Entrepreneur

22

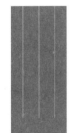

KEY PRINCIPLES

- Sole Proprietorship
- Partnership
- Corporation
- Professional Service Corporation
- Professional Association
- Antitrust Laws
- Insurance

Perhaps one of the clearest examples of advanced practice for any nurse is owning and operating his or her own business. Whether that business be involved in the delivery of health care (e.g., a nurse staffing agency) or the selling of health care products such as operating room equipment designed by the nurse, important legal issues must be analyzed and decided upon *before* the business is even initiated. Furthermore, there are many legal concerns that continue to be important long after the business is "up and running." This chapter will explore those issues within a general framework applicable to any business in which the nurse functions.

PRELIMINARY CONSIDERATIONS

Review of Professional Guidelines

An entrepreneur is defined as one who initiates and assumes the financial risks of a new enterprise and usually manages the enterprise as well.[1] A nurse entrepreneur is a nurse who performs those functions, not only to establish and maintain a successful business but also to make quality nursing care and nursing more available to the public.[2] This dual role requires nurse entrepreneurs to be accountable and responsible not only to themselves, the profession, and employees but also to consumers of health care. This accountability requires the nurse entrepreneur to be clear about adhering to professional guidelines, standards, and ethical principles. Therefore, one of the initial steps that must be undertaken by the future nurse entrepreneur is a thorough review of professional guidelines, standards, and ethical principles to ensure both philosophical and practical compliance with them.

> *One of the initial steps that must be undertaken by the future nurse entrepreneur is a thorough review of professional guidelines, standards, and ethical principles to ensure both philosophical and practical compliance with them.*

Although the review may vary somewhat based on the nature of the nurse entrepreneur's business, the documents to be examined would include professional association standards, such as the American Nurses Association's Code for Nurses with Interpretive Statements,[3] its Scope and Standards of Advanced Practice Registered Nursing,[4] as well as scope of practice guidelines for particular specialties.

Community Analysis

Once the nurse thoroughly understands the professional underpinnings of the prospective business, the next stage in the preliminary phase is to consider carefully the prospective business idea. This includes evaluating the need for the future business and should therefore involve a clear "needs assessment" in the geographic location where the business is to be. This can be done on a formal or informal basis. Formally, for example, the nurse could obtain statistics from the appropriate state department that compiles information concerning the business being considered. If the nurse is considering a temporary staffing agency, for example, but discovers that the community is flooded with such agencies, it may not be in the best interest of the nurse or consumer to establish another there. Informally the nurse can review local telephone books to determine locations and numbers of current businesses identical or similar to the one being considered and can canvass them to obtain information concerning the services they provide.

In addition to evaluating competition, the nurse entrepreneur will also need to analyze such factors as available workforce (if employees will be needed), location of the business (proximity to a hospital or clinic, if that need is present), cost of office space and whether renting or purchasing the space is best, and what options are available for marketing the business once it is established.

Initial Review of State and Federal Laws Affecting Business

The nurse also needs to evaluate what laws will pertain to the business. Although this step should also take place later in the formation of the enterprise, it is essential initially to ensure that the business can, in fact, be legally operated in the state. For example, if the nurse entrepreneur is contemplating establishing a home health care agency, a review of state licensing laws and respective rules and regulations, nurse practice and other professional practice acts, and reimbursement laws would be necessary to aid the nurse in determining if such a business can be legally and successfully established.

Financial Constraints

Because establishing a business takes an enormous amount of capital at the onset, the nurse entrepreneur will need to do an analysis of his or her financial status, not only for this initial outlay

but also for the time needed for the business to show a profit. Many experts in the field of consulting to entrepreneurs suggest that it may take as long as 3 years before a business begins to show a profit. Therefore, nurse entrepreneurs will need to evaluate how they will financially support the business and themselves during the time necessary for the business to grow. It may be, for example, that the nurse will have to work full- or part-time in a salaried position in addition to putting time into the business venture.

Many experts in the field of consulting to entrepreneurs suggest that it may take as long as 3 years before a business begins to show a profit.

Self-Analysis

The preliminary step of analyzing oneself is perhaps one of the most important. Traditionally, nurses have worked for others, either in a health care delivery setting, such as a hospital, or in a physician's office or clinic. Furthermore, until recently, professional nursing education has focused little attention on business concepts or principles. The nurse entrepreneur must carefully evaluate the personal and professional strengths and weaknesses that will help or inhibit business success. Strengths include:

- Resourcefulness
- Creativity
- Ability to withstand uncertainty
- Some experience in business
- Completion of a course or courses in business organizations, management, and/or finance
- Established social supports, including family
- A mentor or consultant who can be looked to for advice
- Flexibility

CONSULTING WITH EXPERTS

Once the preliminary steps have been completed, the nurse entrepreneur should put the business idea in writing, clearly outlining its nature, purpose, proposed general location, and other information decided upon during the preliminary phase. Then it is essential that the nurse consult with experts who can offer guidance through the maze of establishing and running the business.

It is essential that the nurse consult with experts who can offer guidance through the maze of establishing and running the business.

Consultation with an Attorney

The nurse entrepreneur will need to obtain accurate and up-to-date information concerning establishing the business consistent with the laws of the state where the business will be located. Many times, identifying an attorney well versed about a particular subject can be difficult, but not impossible. Information of this kind can be obtained from the state nurses' association, from local bar associations with lawyer referral services, from the national or local nurse attorney association, or from friends or colleagues who have established their own business.

It is important that the attorney selected is familiar with licensing laws, practice acts, business structures, and employment laws (if employees will be utilized). Equally important, however, is the nurse entrepreneur's comfort level with the attorney selected. The attorney should not only be viewed as an expert who will legally establish the business in the correct manner, but also as a resource the nurse entrepreneur can consult as the business changes. It is vital, then, that the attorney–nurse entrepreneur relationship be a solid one that can continue over time.

Business Structure

One of the first issues that will need to be determined when legal advice concerning the business is obtained is what organizational form the business will take. Generally there are three fairly universal organizational structures for businesses: the sole proprietorship, the partnership, and the corporation. These structures are governed by state law and may therefore vary slightly from state to state. Furthermore, some states have developed a fourth business structure option, the professional association. Variations on these four arrangements also exist, including the joint venture and the syndicate, but this chapter will focus on the four most common business models.

SOLE PROPRIETORSHIP. This business model is the least complicated of all of the business structures and is excellent for the nurse entrepreneur who wants to establish a solo nursing practice, such as a private psychotherapy practice or a consulting service. The sole proprietor is, in effect, the business, and therefore any assets or liabilities belong to the owner. The nurse would declare income and expenses from the business as his or her own, and any profit would be taxed to him or her. In addition, the nurse would be required to pay estimated self-employment taxes, health insurance, and other costs normally paid by the business if it had been established under a different organizational structure.[5]

If the nurse entrepreneur decides to utilize this form for the business, help such as secretarial services or additional nurses to provide client services may still be necessary. Usually those individuals are not considered employees, but are viewed as contractors who contract with the sole proprietor for the services. If they are independent contractors—that is, individuals working for themselves—they would be responsible for any and all taxes on income paid to them by the nurse entrepreneur. If, however, the nurse contracted with a secretarial agency, for example, for typing services, then the agency would be responsible for paying the agency employee and reporting that income to the Internal Revenue Service.

In considering the sole proprietorship, the nurse entrepreneur will also want to obtain advice from an attorney concerning the need to register the business with the state, city, or county office established to handle any business with an assumed or fictitious name. For example, if the nurse has decided to call the consulting business NURSE CONSULTANTS, then the nurse will need to register the business in the assumed or fictitious name index so that, if need be, the nurse can be readily identified as the owner of the business, and any additional information about the business, such as its starting date, can be obtained. If, however, the nurse decides to use his or her name as the business name, then there is usually no need to register the business with the assumed name office.

PARTNERSHIP. A partnership is a voluntary arrangement whereby two or more individuals co-own and carry on a business for profit.[6] A formal partnership arrangement is created by a document called a partnership agreement, and the nurse entrepreneur's attorney must represent the nurse's interests in developing and finalizing that agreement. If the partners decide not to formalize their business relationship in a written agreement, most states have a statute (e.g., the Uniform Partnership Act) that formalizes the relationship by governing the rights and responsibilities of individuals in the partnership to ensure that the owners fulfill obligations to themselves and the public. The nurse entrepreneur will want to seek a specific opinion from his or her attorney as to which approach is best to take for the proposed business.

Regardless of which option is selected, a partnership has legal implications that must be carefully evaluated by the nurse. To begin with, each partner can bind the other(s) in relation to the operation of the business, and each is personally responsible for the business debts incurred by the other(s). Moreover, the partnership arrangement is not a flexible one. If, for example, two nurses have established a nurse-managed center as a partnership, and one of them decides to leave the practice, then the partnership must be dissolved and a *new* one formed. Each partner is responsible for his or her share of the business expenses and taxes according to the partnership agreement or partnership statute.

In addition to the general partnership arrangement, the nurse entrepreneur will want to explore with his or her attorney any advantages of establishing a *limited partnership.* Unlike the general partner, a limited partner supplies money to the business but has no say in its operation, delivery of services, or any other aspect of the business. Moreover, the limited partner's share of liability is restricted to that which he or she has contributed to the business. This may be a valuable option for the nurse entrepreneur needing financial resources to begin the venture.

Again, as with the sole proprietorship, if an assumed name is utilized, it must be registered with the assumed name index, regardless of the type of partnership formed.

CORPORATION. A corporation is a very formalized business structure. Controlled by state, county, or national law, it is an entity established by incorporators to conduct business. The incorporators fill out and file articles of incorporation with the state, county, or national office empowered with granting corporation status. In a state, that office is the secretary of state, and information required includes the name of the corporation, its purpose (e.g., to provide nursing care to the public), and the amount of financial backing initially available at incorporation.

The name of the corporation is an important piece of the filing process. It cannot be identical to any other business name in the state, so the attorney will need to search the corporation list to determine if the selected name is available and, if it has not been used already, to reserve it for the nurse's use. In addition, if the name of the business will be an assumed one, it must also be registered as such with the secretary of state.

When the appropriate office determines that the potential business has complied with all of its requirements, it will send the incorporators a certificate of incorporation and an incorporation number. In addition, the corporation is listed on the state's domestic corporation list, and to remain "in good standing" on that list, the corporation must file renewal papers and pay a filing fee on an annual basis.

Unlike the sole proprietorship and the partnership, the corporation must be managed by a board of directors who are elected by the owner/incorporators and the stockholders, if stock is issued. The board members manage the business through established guidelines, called bylaws, and are accountable to the owners and stockholders for the decisions they make.

Unlike the sole proprietorship and the partnership, the corporation must be managed by a board of directors who are elected by the owner/ incorporators and the stockholders, if stock is issued. The board members manage the business through established guidelines, called bylaws, and are accountable to the owners and stockholders for the decisions they make.

The corporation as a formal entity has interesting legal characteristics. To begin with, it has a "perpetual existence." In other words, once established, it survives any changes in ownership or purpose, although those changes must be communicated to the registration office and be consistent with its bylaws. In addition, the corporate structure protects the personal civil liability of the owners/incorporators and board of directors because it is a legal creature that can be sued and can accept financial responsibility for judgments entered against it.

PROFESSIONAL CORPORATION. The corporation the nurse entrepreneur will be establishing is usually not a general business corporation but rather a professional service corporation. Also governed by state, county, or national law, the professional corporate structure is also very formalized but is specific to professionals (e.g., nurses, dentists, and lawyers) establishing and rendering specific *professional* services to the public. Because the corporation is rendering a specific service, most state laws require the owners and shareholders of the corporation to be licensed in the same profession as the services provided by it. Also, a professional service corporation does not insulate its owners and shareholders from personal civil liability for malpractice, nor does it alter the professionals' ethical obligations and responsibilities to the clients.[7]

The opportunity to start a professional service corporation may not be readily available to the nurse entrepreneur, for its existence varies from state to state. The attorney consulted can advise the nurse on the availability of this form of business. For example, it may be that the statutory language of the professional corporation act does not expressly exclude nurses from incorporating, or it may clearly include nurses by referring to the state nurse practice act. Also important for the nurse and the attorney to evaluate is whether or not the corporation can render only one professional service, such as nursing, or can provide more than one, such as nursing and medical care.

Because of the traditional professional service corporation principle that all owners/incorporators must be licensed in the same profession, it has been only recently that multidisciplinary professional service corporations have been readily available to professionals. As a group, however, nurses have not been included in many of the updated state professional service corporation statutes. Therefore, if the nurse entrepreneur is contemplating a business that requires multidisciplinary services, and the option of incorporating such a business structure is not available, then the nurse will have to abandon the idea of a professional service corporation and utilize another organizational model.

PROFESSIONAL ASSOCIATION. The professional association option may be available to the nurse entrepreneur in his or her state and, depending on the state statute, may provide an alternative to the prohibition against a multidisciplinary business entity. The attorney consulted by the nurse will need to review the state law to determine if this possibility exists, and if so, what if any restrictions are present. Generally, however, the alternative allows the formation of a professional *association,* as opposed to a corporation or partnership, by identified professional groups such as nursing and medicine; requires the establishment of a written association agreement that governs the business entity; and requires that the name of the business utilize the term *associates, associated,* or similar title.[8]

Insurance

The nurse entrepreneur will need to explore the various insurance needs he or she will have when initiating a business, and discussing this with the attorney is important. Moreover, the attorney can review policies of insurance being considered or purchased by the nurse and suggest areas of concern that may need to be further explored in consultation with the insurance company and its agent. At a minimum, premises liability insurance and professional liability insurance will be required. Additional insurance concerns depend on whether or not the nurse entrepreneur will hire employees; for example, under state law, employers are mandated to contribute to workers' compensation and unemployment insurance for their employees. Also important to consider, whether or not employees are utilized, is the need for health insurance.

The nurse entrepreneur will need to explore the various insurance needs he or she will have when initiating a business . . .

PREMISES LIABILITY INSURANCE. This type of insurance contract protects the physical plant of the business from loss that might occur from fire, water damage, flooding or other natural disasters, and theft. Also important to insure against loss will be the contents of the business office; that is, furniture, equipment, including computers and typewriters, and products, if any, sold or developed by the business. Many premises liability policies offer the replacement of business contents on a current market value basis, while others do not. It is important that the nurse be clear about what type of premises liability policy needs to be purchased.

In addition to protecting the business itself, a premises liability policy also covers injuries to clients that occur at the place of business. For example, if a nurse-midwife provides services at a clinic site, and a client should slip on the clinic floor, any injuries that are found to result from that slip could be covered under the liability policy.

Other situations covered by these policies may include suits against the business owner for other injuries to clients, such as defamation and false imprisonment. Further, coverage may be available for injuries sustained while driving a motor vehicle if in connection with the operation of the business.

Specific exclusions vary from policy to policy, but most often the exclusions include professional liability coverage.

PROFESSIONAL LIABILITY INSURANCE. Whenever the nurse is providing a *professional* nursing service, such as client counseling, client teaching, or direct nursing care, professional liability insurance is essential. As with premises liability policies, professional liability policies vary, and the nurse will need to be certain that the insurance purchased will adequately cover the nurse's role in the business venture. This will require a thorough review of the policy terms, not only with legal counsel but with the insurance company and agent as well.

Specific points on which to seek clarification include the type of nursing service(s) covered by the policy; what types of nursing services, if any, are excluded; whether the policy is a claims-made or an occurrence policy (the latter being the better one to purchase if possible); what deductibles, if any, are applicable; and the coverage limits of the policy. Moreover, if the nurse entrepreneur utilizes employees who will provide nursing or other services, the nurse will need to consider providing professional liability insurance coverage for them

as well. Conversely, if the business will be contracting with other professionals to provide such services, those professionals will need to be informed that they must carry their own liability insurance and show proof of coverage to the nurse entrepreneur.

PRODUCT LIABILITY INSURANCE. If the nurse entrepreneur will be designing and/or marketing a product to be utilized in health care, such as an operating room instrument or an intravenous device, the state and federal product liability law will need to be carefully reviewed with counsel. An insurance plan also needs to be purchased to insure the nurse entrepreneur against lawsuits based on product liability law. Liability principles in product liability are based in "strict liability" or negligence theories. Because of the uniqueness of this area of law and the potential for culpability due to various roles the nurse entrepreneur may undertake, including a designer or supplier of health care delivery products, adequate and appropriate product liability insurance is a must.

Other Areas

Additional areas that need to be discussed with legal counsel by the nurse entrepreneur will depend on the nature of the business. For example, if employees will be utilized, the nurse must develop an employee handbook, job descriptions, and a policy and procedure manual to aid in establishing the working relationship between those employees and the nurse employer. In addition, mandatory compliance with any employee benefit packages, including contributions to workers' compensation funds, will need to be explored.[9] Furthermore, the nurse will want to consult with legal counsel on a regular basis to comply with changes in the law that might occur in relation to employee rights.

Consultation with an Accountant

Retaining an accountant is important to any entrepreneur or business executive, because the financial considerations in running a business are just as important as the legal considerations. As with the attorney consultant, the nurse entrepreneur should select an accountant with whom the many concerns of establishing and maintaining a business can be comfortably discussed and clarified. The accountant-client relationship will continue over time, and therefore it is essential that the accountant selected be accessible, responsive, and informed about the needs and concerns of the nurse entrepreneur. Identifying that type of accountant may be initially difficult if the nurse has not consulted with an accountant in the past, but referral sources to assist the nurse include the attorney consultant, professional associations for accountants, and colleagues or friends utilizing accountant services.

Although the exact topics to be discussed with the accountant will vary based on the nature of the nurse entrepreneur's business, there are several areas that should be explored regardless of the type of business. Those areas include tax implications of the business structure, implications of various financing options for the business, and establishing a bookkeeping system for the enterprise.

Tax Implications

Regardless of what form the organization of the business takes, there is no doubt that any and all income derived from the business must be declared to the Internal Revenue Service and state tax offices pursuant to federal and state tax laws. How these laws affect the business structures varies, however. For example, if the business is organized as a sole proprietorship, income is reported through the owner's Social Security number, and any income that remains after legitimate expenses are deducted becomes profit assessed to the sole owner. When operating a business as a sole proprietor, estimated income tax payments may need to be paid to ensure that adequate tax payments are being made throughout the taxable year.

> *Regardless of what form the organization of the business takes, there is no doubt that any and all income derived from the business must be declared . . . pursuant to federal and state tax laws.*

If the nurse entrepreneur decides to establish the business as a corporation, different tax rules apply. For example, any and all dividends paid to shareholders must be declared as income, in addition to any profit the corporation possesses.

Of course, profit exists only after legitimate expenses are deducted, but federal tax laws have greatly decreased the ability of the corporation to fully deduct expenses.

The nurse entrepreneur will want to carefully evaluate the best business structure in light of the current tax laws to enable the business to receive maximum benefit from the applicable law.

Financing the Business

Whatever form the business takes, financing it adequately is one of the most important aspects of establishing an enterprise. If the business is "undercapitalized," it may not be given the chance to prove itself in the long run. Therefore the nurse entrepreneur will need to carefully determine how much will be needed to get the business "up and running"; how income will be generated and where the income will come from; how much to pay in employees' salaries, if they are to be used; and how long, if at all, the nurse can exist without personal income from the business. The accountant can help the nurse estimate those costs and suggest the best way to deal with financing, especially as it relates to obtaining the maximum benefits in terms of tax liability. For example, it may be best for the nurse entrepreneur to combine a number of financing possibilities—a small bank loan and personal finances—rather than borrow all of the money from a bank. Or, it may be best to explore financing from government agencies, such as the Small Business Administration. If any type of loan is received, the nurse entrepreneur will want the accountant and attorney to review the document for guidance as to how it will affect tax and other liabilities.

Bookkeeping

The nurse entrepreneur will save much time and anguish if a good system of bookkeeping is established from the start of the business and carried out faithfully as the business develops and grows. The accountant's advice can be invaluable. Documentation of income received, expenses paid, equipment purchased, and salaries of employees and the business owners or officers are just a few areas that must be explored. Detailed receipts of equipment purchased and expenses paid are vital. Documents supporting compliance with state laws requiring employer contributions to unemployment compensation and workers' compensation funds will also be necessary. Once established, the bookkeeping system stands as a ready defense should state or federal agencies request documentation of the business operation. It also provides a quick source of information needed by the accountant when preparing the business income tax returns.

Other Consultants

In addition to conferring with the consultants already discussed, additional support and information can be obtained through consultants specific to the nurse entrepreneur's needs. Additional ones to consider, either initially or at some future time in the business's growth, would include an employee benefits counselor; a marketing and/or advertising agent, if appropriate; an attorney specializing in patent, trademark, and copyright law; a financial planner; and a personal banker.

ANTITRUST CONCERNS

Assuming that the nurse entrepreneur is able to successfully master the maze of setting up a business, another obstacle will loom on the horizon—competition, or the resistance of other health care providers to allowing that business to flourish. Although professional groups other than nurses have begun to provide health care services in nontraditional roles and settings, this resistance is keenly felt by nurse entrepreneurs because of what has been termed their dependent role—that is, the delivery of health care under the direct or indirect supervision of a physician, regardless of the health care delivery setting.[10] This "dependent" status, coupled with the economic climate of health care delivery today *and* the positive impact that nurses functioning in nontraditional roles and settings have had on providing quality patient care at reasonable rates, has set the stage for attempts to limit, restrict, and/or boycott nurse-owned businesses.

Types of Barriers for Nurse Entrepreneurs

Many types of trade restraints on a nurse entrepreneur's practice have been identified. Four will be discussed: licensing constraints; limitations on, or nonexistence of, third-party reimbursement; inability to obtain admitting privileges to health care facilities; and inability to obtain physician supervisors or collaborators.[11]

Licensing Restrictions

Licensing restrictions effectively limit any nurse's practice. If the state nurse practice act does not provide for more "independent" practice, this restriction can quite literally sound the "death knell" for the nurse-entrepreneur contemplating a nontraditional role inconsistent with the state statute. A complaint filed by the state attorney's office alleging the unauthorized practice of medicine, for example, may simply be too much for many nurses to risk, even if the judgment ultimately favors the nurse, as was the case in *Sermchief v. Gonzales*, discussed in Chapter 21.

Many types of trade restraints on a nurse entrepreneur's practice have been identified: licensing constraints; limitations on, or nonexistence of, third-party reimbursement; inability to obtain admitting privileges; and inability to obtain physician supervisors or collaborators.

Reimbursement Concerns

Similarly, the inability of the nurse entrepreneur to count on payment of fees for nursing care from third-party payers, whether the services occur in a home, hospital, or clinic, effectively destroys the financial viability of the enterprise. Figures indicate that, for example, in 1995, 32% of the $988 billion dollars spent for health purposes was paid through insurance companies.[12] The types of health insurance plans include Medicare and Medicaid, employer-sponsored programs, and many managed care plans. Clearly, if a patient cannot utilize health insurance benefits to cover the cost of being seen by a nurse, the patient may not consider seeking out those services regardless of the quality of care provided.

Inability to Obtain Admitting Privileges

To the nurse entrepreneur providing care to clients in an outpatient clinic, or to a nurse-midwife needing to utilize a hospital's services to deliver a patient's child, lack of admitting privileges effectively renders the nurse entrepreneur's services worthless. Although some institutions have granted admitting privileges to certain groups of nurse entrepreneurs, such as nurse-midwives, such privileges are clearly under the control of the medical staff, who continue to see *any* nontraditional health care provider of similar services as a potential threat to their own practice. As a result, those nurses who have obtained staff/admitting privileges are in the minority.

Lack of Physician Supervisors or Collaborators

Regardless of what state statutory framework exists in relation to expanded nurse roles, few, if any, allow the nurse to function totally independent of the physician. Thus, physician backup is essential to ensure that the nurse entrepreneur is practicing "nursing" as opposed to "medicine." This backup may take the form of a joint practice or a corporation. Or it may take the form of a "collaborative" arrangement with a physician for supervision, standing orders, and utilization of the physician for admissions to the appropriate health care facility. In either case, if no such physician collaboration or supervision exists, the nurse entrepreneur cannot deliver nursing services without risking liability for the unauthorized practice of medicine. Furthermore, many patients will not consider a nurse for the provision of nursing services unless they can clearly obtain access to whatever health care delivery system may be needed.

ANTITRUST LAWS AND THEIR IMPACT ON TRADE RESTRICTIONS

Antitrust laws, on both the federal and state level, prohibit anticompetitive measures, such as contracts, monopolies, boycotts, or other conduct that effectively constrains commerce or trade. The main federal antitrust laws are the Sherman Antitrust Act, the Clayton Act, and the Federal Trade Commission Act, all of which prohibit anticompetitive measures among states—that is, affecting interstate commerce—and among foreign nations. A proven violation of the federal laws may be enforced by one or both agencies empowered to administer and enforce the federal antitrust laws: the Department of Justice (Antitrust Division) and the Federal Trade Commission. Criminal and/or civil liability is possible for proven violations. Like-

wise, state antitrust laws ban anticompetitive measures within the respective state and, if proven, also result in civil and/or criminal sanctions.

Antitrust laws . . . prohibit anticompetitive measures, such as contracts, monopolies, boycotts, or other conduct that effectively constrains commerce or trade.

The Sherman Act

The Sherman Act basically forbids any measure that effectively limits competition in interstate commerce and trade among foreign nations. Composed of Sections 1 and 2, it prohibits contractual relationships, "combinations and conspiracies" that restrain trade, and monopolies, "attempted monopolies and conspiracies to monopolize."[13]

The Clayton Act

The Clayton Act, and its amendment known as the Robinson-Patman Act, bans price fixing and exclusive dealings involving contracts and tying arrangements that substantially lessen competition. Furthermore, it outlaws any merger, acquisition, or joint venture by corporate entities that may result in a monopoly anywhere in the country by any line of commerce.[14]

The Federal Trade Commission Act

This federal law, enforced by the Federal Trade Commission and empowered only to bring civil actions against alleged offenders, bans any and all unfair methods of competition and unfair deceptive practices or acts, which include false or misleading advertising or misrepresentations to the public.[15]

Specific Applications of Federal Antitrust Laws

In addition to the above-described measures, other key factors must exist before one or more of the acts will apply. Under the Sherman Act, for example, an "agreement" or "conspiracy" must exist between distinct individuals, groups of individuals, or entities that negatively affects competition. Once such an agreement or conspiracy has been found to exist, then the court must determine if the agreement is a *per se* violation of the act; that is, if it is so potentially harmful to competition that nothing will justify its existence.[16] The courts have found *per se* violations in price fixing, tying arrangements (one party sells a product—e.g., durable medical equipment—only on the condition the buyer purchase another product from the seller—e.g., home care intravenous equipment), and boycotts (attempting to refuse to deal with certain health care providers or provider groups to prevent their presence in the marketplace).[17]

If no *per se* violation exists, the court hears evidence concerning the intent of the agreement and its effect on competition and the marketplace. This has been called the "rule-of-reason" test, meaning that if the agreement does not "unreasonably" restrain trade, there is no violation of Section 1 of the Act.[18]

In the health care arena, the courts have critically analyzed whether conduct alleged to be anticompetitive really is so or whether it is motivated by "legitimate" objectives such as concern for quality patient care or safety, and whether there is an adverse effect on quality, price, or availability of services.[19] When the conduct can clearly be supported by a legitimate basis and does not adversely affect the marketplace, courts usually do not rule against the conduct.

In addition to the above analysis, the court also evaluates other factors, including the pertinent market for the product or service, the applicable geographic market for the product or service, and whether or not the alleged violator has "monopoly power" (the power to control prices or exclude competition) in the relevant market.

State Laws

If an agreement between two or more separate persons or organizations does not negatively affect interstate commerce, but does affect competition within a state, then a state's antitrust law may apply to that alleged limitation on competition and the marketplace. For example, Illinois' Antitrust Act was passed to promote the unhampered growth of commerce and industry within Illinois by banning restraints of trade, such as monopolies,

price fixing, and allocating or dividing customers or supplies.[20] In addition to criminal sanctions, the Act provides for civil remedies against any person, corporation, or group, including injunctions, divestiture of property, and dissolution of domestic corporations or associations.[21]

Exceptions to Antitrust Laws

The federal and respective state antitrust laws both contain exemptions or exceptions to the general prohibition on restraining trade. General exemptions and exceptions include (1) activities of labor organizations or their members; (2) the purchase of stock for investment purposes not intended to lessen competition; and (3) religious and charitable activities of not-for-profit organizations that are exclusively religious or charitable. Additionally, under the McCarren-Ferguson Act the "business of insurance," when regulated by state law and the state's regulation is not coercive, intimidating, or a boycott, is also exempt from the antitrust laws.[22]

The federal antitrust laws also provide an exception for peer review activities required under the Health Care Quality Improvement Act. However, it is important to note that the Health Care Quality Improvement Act's protection is narrowly defined in terms of its requirements for protection and the type of conduct it covers (called "safe harbor" provisions).[23] For example, a court would probably not grant immunity for alleged anticompetitive behavior by any professional association, such as the American Medical Association, that did not allow a physician membership in its organization because the physician had established a joint practice with an advanced practice nurse.

IMPLICATIONS FOR NURSE ENTREPRENEURS

At least one antitrust case involving nurses in independent practice has been decided that illustrates the concepts, principles, and theories discussed thus far. It is interesting that of all the antitrust methods possible to use against nurse entrepreneurs, two that seem to occur most often are the tying arrangement and the boycott. One well-known case that illustrates the illegality of a boycott against a nurse anesthetist is presented in Key Case 22–1.

The decision in the *Oltz* case is an exception to the general lack of success experienced by entrepreneurs challenging practice arrangements, in-

FACTS: The nurse anesthetist plaintiff, Tafford Oltz, was providing anesthesia services to St. Peter's Hospital in Helena, Montana, the only hospital of two in the city that provided services to the general public and was able to offer surgery services. The arrangement Mr. Oltz had with the hospital was an independent contractor arrangement; that is, he provided services, submitted his fee to the hospital—not the patient—and the contractual arrangement was on a month-by-month basis. When Mr. Oltz began his arrangement with the hospital, there were three anesthesiologists also working for the hospital, but that number increased to four shortly after Mr. Oltz began working with the hospital. It became clear that the plaintiff's services were in direct competition with the anesthesiologists' services because of Oltz's popularity with the surgical staff and his lower fees for the anesthesia services he rendered. During this period of discontent among the anesthesiologists, they decided to organize the anesthesia services into a department of anesthesia. With the hospital administrator and board apprised of the actions of the anesthesiologists, Oltz was taken off the anesthesia call schedule, and policies were adopted requiring supervision of anesthesia services solely by anesthesiologists (prior to the policy, they could be supervised by the surgeon or obstetrician). The hospital eventually cancelled his contract with the hospital.

Oltz's contract was reinstated, however, after Mr. Oltz's attorney and the state's attorney general's office wrote the hospital, threatening to sue if the contract cancellation were not rescinded. Although the contract was going to be reinstated, three of the four anesthesiologists threatened to leave, and the board then entered into an exclusive anesthesia contract with the anesthesiologists in Helena. Mr. Oltz was offered a salaried position at $40,000 a year, but he refused the offer and filed suit against the hospital and the four anesthesiologists, alleging a violation of Section 1 of the Sherman Act in that the defendants had conspired to boycott his services and to exclude his services from the marketplace.

Hospital found to conspire to boycott nurse anesthetist's services

TRIAL COURT: The federal trial court for the District of Montana, after the four doctors settled with Mr. Oltz and paid him damages, found for the plaintiff. Because the verdict also involved awarding damages to Mr. Oltz that were contested by both parties, both sought an appeal of the trial court's decision.

APPEALS COURT: The Ninth Circuit Court of Appeals affirmed the trial court's decision and remanded the case to that court on certain issues. Specifically, the appeals court held that competition for anesthesia services was severely restricted as a result of the actions of the hospital, as evidenced by increased prices for such services and by excluding Mr. Oltz's services from the marketplace; that the anesthesiologists' and the hospital's interests were different enough to allow the application of the Sherman Act to the hospital; that the relevant market for anesthesia services was from the area around the hospital; that a conspiracy existed to exclude Mr. Oltz's services; and that a new trial on the damages awarded to Mr. Oltz should take place.

Anesthesia services severely restricted because of exclusive arrangement with anesthesiologists

Key Case continued on following page

KEY CASE 22–1	Oltz v. St. Peter's Community Hospital (1988)[24] *Continued*

A conspiracy to boycott services did exist

At the trial for damages, Oltz was awarded a significant monetary award of three times his actual losses because of the defendants' conduct ("treble damages").

ANALYSIS: The *Oltz* case is an important one because it illustrates the successful application of the Sherman Act to a situation in which quality services were being offered at a lower price to the public, and it was that economic competition that affected two significant areas of anesthesia services in the marketplace—the anesthesia services provided by the nurse anesthetist and the anesthesiologists and the resulting contest for staff privileges. It is also important in that the case deals with a rural hospital, and it may be that in rural areas, competition must be more carefully safeguarded, especially when such competition is limited initially simply because the choices of services in the marketplace are fewer than in urban areas.[25]

cluding exclusive contracts with a group of providers, as an illegal boycott. Even so, the nurse entrepreneur who believes that such illegal action may be occurring must obtain a legal opinion as to his or her possibility of success if a suit is contemplated under Section 1 of the Sherman Act.

> *It is interesting that of all the antitrust methods possible to use against nurse entrepreneurs, two that seem to occur most often are the tying arrangement and the boycott.*

The nurse entrepreneur must also keep in mind that litigation under the antitrust laws is difficult because of its highly technical and complex nature. For example, in a U.S. Supreme Court case, *Jefferson Parish Hospital v. Hyde*,[26] an anesthesiologist claimed that the hospital's exclusive agreement for anesthesia services with a group of which he was not a member excluded him from the provision of those services and, in effect, established a tying arrangement.

The Court, in ruling against Hyde, held that no *per se* violation of the Sherman Act had occurred because patients could be admitted to another hospi-

tal in the area if they wanted to. Because the exclusive arrangement was not a *per se* violation, the Court then applied the rule-of-reason test. The Court opined that because patients could seek hospitalization elsewhere, no reasonable restraint on competition existed, and no tying arrangement was proven.

For the nurse entrepreneur, the *Hyde* decision clearly indicates that in order to challenge a consumer's inability to select the nurse as a health care provider because the nurse is not included in a group of providers the health care delivery system uses, he or she must show that (1) the market for the services provided is the same for both providers; (2) market power is under the control of the target facility or group; and (3) there is a clear, documented demand for the nurse's services.[27]

> *The nurse entrepreneur will need to stand ready to challenge conduct and arrangements that interfere with the nurse's right to provide quality, low-cost care to consumers and to practice in a manner consistent with the nurse's education, scope of practice, and experience.*

ETHICS CONNECTION 22–1

Nurses in entrepreneurial roles may benefit from the increased competition for provision of health care goods and services that accompanies managed care. In a sense, the "playing field" is being leveled by managed care. Traditional providers must compete in the marketplace for continuing contracts and other arrangements with those who purchase their goods and services. Nurse entrepreneurs, thus, may be competing in a fairer marketplace. Attempts to restrain trade and squelch new businesses still will occur, of course. However, health care delivery is in transition, and those who can provide the best quality services for the least cost are more likely to be successful than they would have been in the recent past. From an ethical perspective, perhaps the marketplace for nurse entrepreneurs is becoming more just than it had been.

Nurse entrepreneurs not only need to be aware of nursing ethics but also should be well informed about business ethics. As businesspeople, they have more professional autonomy than do most other nurses. The benefits of increased autonomy may be accompanied by burdens. One burden is the possibility of professional isolation. This isolation can be minimized or avoided when entrepreneurs are part of a moral community of other nurses and business colleagues. Through such a community, nurse entrepreneurs can stay current in their entrepreneurial practice area and engage in dialogue about common ethical issues. They may realize that what they had thought were individual issues in their own business may, in fact, be social policy issues of access or reimbursement.

Another potential burden is the danger of becoming so absorbed in learning how to manage a business that their competency in the nursing practice or health care service they are delivering becomes outdated. Again, immersion in a moral community may help to safeguard the entrepreneur's continuing competency. Finally, there is a danger in losing one's identity as a nurse. Entrepreneurship is vitally important for nursing's collective autonomy, and it is compromised by nurses who no longer refer to themselves as nurses but only by the business title. This is not only the case for individuals who own their own businesses or share in the ownership. It is especially disturbing when nurse politicians, who have opportunities to support nursing's social justice agenda, do not identify themselves as nurses. Whenever individual nurses succeed in independent or collaborative roles, all of nursing benefits. So, too, will the public as they become more aware of the scope and quality of nursing services that are available to them through nurse entrepreneurship and advanced and basic practice roles.

What impact the antitrust laws will ultimately have on managed care and the many health care delivery organizational arrangements that are developing remains to be seen. The nurse contemplating the establishment of a business within this ever-changing health care delivery environment will need to watch carefully for developments in this area. The nurse entrepreneur must be able to provide care with or within current—and future—organizational structures in order to be successful in a business established to provide health care services. Will exclusive arrangements with certain providers continue to be upheld by the court? Will mergers of major hospitals eliminate competition in the selection of health care and health care providers by consumers? Will provider networks illegally set fees in violation of the Federal Trade Commission mandates and the antitrust laws?

Although the answers to these and other questions involving antitrust law cannot be easily answered, the nurse entrepreneur will need to stand ready to challenge conduct and arrangements that interfere with the nurse's right to provide quality, low-cost care to consumers and to practice in a manner consistent with the nurse's education, scope of practice, and experience.

SUMMARY OF PRINCIPLES AND APPLICATIONS

There are many concerns and obstacles in setting up and running a business. Other concerns not covered in this chapter, such as insurance fraud and abuse when receiving third-party reimbursement from insurance plans, must also be considered by the nurse entrepreneur. In addition, preparation, hard work, and continued updating of information vital to the business's operation will be required. The following principles are essential:

- A thorough assessment of self, the business structure, and the service to be provided is vital

- Consultation with experts in business, law, accounting, and other identified areas is mandatory *before* one sets out to establish a business venture

- Ongoing relationships with experts are necessary to ensure compliance with current and future laws when maintaining a business

- The organizational structure of the business—whether it be a sole proprietorship, partnership, professional association, or corporation—must be carefully decided after fully exploring the tax, accounting, and legal ramifications of that structure

- The potential for antitrust concerns—whether through the establishment of a monopoly, a tying arrangement, or a conspiracy—must be kept in mind when establishing a business that may compete with other businesses or health care providers in the marketplace

- The major federal antitrust laws include the Sherman Act, the Clayton Act, and the Federal Trade Commission Act. Generally all three prohibit any restriction of competition in the marketplace; exceptions to that rule are activities that do not include interstate commerce, state actions, and labor organizations' activities

- In addition to federal antitrust laws, state statutes to preserve competition in the marketplace must also be reviewed

- Nurse entrepreneurs must be ready to challenge obstacles to the establishment of their businesses not only in court but through legislative and other processes that deter the expansion and growth of autonomous practice

TOPICS FOR FURTHER INQUIRY

1. Develop an interview guide for use in interviewing at least three nurse entrepreneurs currently in business in your state. Evaluate areas of difficulty for the nurse entrepreneur and how those areas of difficulty were resolved. Identify and analyze how each nurse entrepreneur obtained information to establish and run his or her business. Identify any anticompetitive experiences the nurses had to resolve, and how they did so.

2. Write a paper on the types of business structures available to a nurse in your state. Compare and contrast each type of structure and analyze how any limitations on a nurse's business may affect antitrust or other laws (e.g., state nurse practice act).

3. Develop a proposal to amend one of the federal antitrust laws in view of the changes in health care delivery. Include such areas as who would be affected by the proposal, how changes in initiating a case alleging a

violation of the proposal would be handled, and the purpose of the proposed changes.

4. Conduct a confidential survey in your community to identify those health care delivery systems that allow advanced practice nurses to obtain admitting privileges in their facility. Analyze how that process is different, if at all, for other health care providers with admitting privileges. Also evaluate the nurse's ability to obtain admitting privileges in more than one facility. Suggest changes in current processes or propose procedures to initiate admitting privileges in the facilities surveyed.

REFERENCES

1. Henry Campbell Black. *Black's Law Dictionary*. 7th Edition. St. Paul, Minn.: West Group, 1999, 554.
2. See generally, Mary Mundinger, Robert Kane, Elizabeth Lenz, Annette Totten, and others, "Primary Care Outcomes in Patients Treated by Nurse Practitioners or Physicians: A Randomized Trial," 283(1) *JAMA* (2000), 59–68; Center for Rural Health and Social Service Development, Southern Illinois University at Carbondale, "Attitudes Toward the Utilization of Certified Nurse Midwives Among Physicians and Midwives in Illinois and Indiana," 3(3) *Center Research Briefs* (1997). Available at Southern Illinois University's Web site at http://www.siu.edu. Accessed January 29, 2000; also see Chapter 21.
3. American Nurses Association, Kansas City, Mo., 1985.
4. American Nurses Association, Washington, D.C., 1996.
5. Carolyn Buppert. *Nurse Practitioner's Business Practice & Legal Guide*. Gaithersburg, Md.: Aspen Publishers, 1999, 321.
6. Black, *supra* note 1, at 1142.
7. Buppert, *supra* note 5, at 323.
8. See, for example, 805 ILCS 305/0.01 *et seq.* (1992) (*Professional Association Act*—Illinois).
9. See generally, Chapter 16 (The Nurse as Employee).
10. Bonnie Faherty, "Advanced Practice Nursing: What's All the Fuss?" 2(3) *Journal of Nursing Law* (1995), 9–17; see also Chapter 21 for a more detailed discussion of the issue; Marlene Wilken, "Policy Implementation," in *Health Policy & Politics: A Nurse's Guide*. Gaithersburg, Md.: Aspen Publishers, 1999, 210–211.
11. *Id.*
12. Anthony Kovner and Steven Jones. *Health Care Delivery in the United States*. 6th Edition. New York: Springer Publishing Company, 1999, 36–37.
13. 15 U.S.C. Sections 1 and 2 (1914).
14. 15 U.S.C. Sections 13, 14, 15, and 18 (1914).
15. 15 U.S.C. Section 45 (1914).
16. Robert Miller. *Problems in Hospital Law*. 7th Edition. Gaithersburg, Md.: Aspen Publishers, 1996, 128.
17. *Id.*
18. Christopher Kerns, Carol Gerner, and Ciara Ryan, Editors. *Health Care Liability Deskbook*. 4th Edition. St. Paul, Minn.: West Group, 1998, 17-3 (with regular updates).
19. See generally, *Id.*
20. 740 ILCS 10/3 (1982).

21. *Id.* at 10/7.
22. See, for example, U.S.C.A. Chapter 15 Section 17 (1914); 740 ILCS 10/5 (1987); 15 U.S.C.A. Section 10/2(b).
23. Kerns, Gerner, and Ryan, *supra* note 18, at 17–16.
24. 861 F.2d 1440 (9th Cir. 1988).
25. See, for example, *BCB Anesthesia Care v. Passavant Area Memorial Hospital Association,* 36 F.3d 664 (7th Cir. 1994). Certified registered nurse anesthetists (CRNAs) appealed a federal district court decision dismissing their suit that alleged the hospital's termination of their contract and replacing them with anesthesiologists was a tying arrangement to boycott their services and to fix prices under the Sherman Act. The Seventh Circuit Court of Appeals affirmed the trial court's dismissal of the case, opining that *one* hospital's decision concerning staffing did not unreasonably impact upon competition. Kerns, Gerner, and Ryan, *supra* note 18, at 17-32.
26. 466 U.S. 2 (1984).
27. See, generally, Miller, *supra* note 16; Kerns, Gerner, and Ryan, *supra* note 18.

Interview Guidelines and Assessment Criteria for Choosing an Attorney

As this book illustrates, a nurse may be involved in various types of lawsuits. Whether a defendant in a professional malpractice suit or a suit involving another type of tort, or a plaintiff whose constitutional right of due process has been violated by a public academic institution, one needs legal services to properly defend or initiate a suit.

A lawsuit, however, is not the only reason a nurse may need legal services. A nurse entrepreneur needs advice to establish and run a business. A nurse may need a contract developed or interpreted before signing, or a staff nurse may seek an opinion about practice concerns and liabilities.

Despite the many situations that require an attorney, nurses and the general public know little about the law, attorneys, or how to obtain legal advice or representation. When a clear legal problem exists, or when seeking advice and counsel before a problem arises, identifying an attorney who can provide early competent counsel and advice is essential. In addition, competent representation is imperative if the nurse is involved in a specific court case.

This appendix provides general guidelines for the nurse in seeking legal counsel, regardless of the situation within which that need arises.

SOME INFORMATION ABOUT LAWYERS

A lawyer (also called an attorney, counselor, attorney at law, barrister, or solicitor) is an individual who has a minimum of a bachelor's degree *and* a law degree (J.D. or L.L.B.). Some attorneys, however, have additional degrees. Master's degrees in law (L.L.M.) are possible in tax, patent, and health care law, for example. Those attorneys who practiced another profession prior to law may have graduate degrees in that particular field. For example, lawyers who practiced nursing prior to law may have a master's degree in nursing. Doctoral

degrees also exist in law. For example, a Doctor of Juridical Science (S.J.D.) in Health Law and Policy is offered by Loyola University of Chicago School of Law through its Institute for Health Law.

The basic law degree is granted after completion of law school, which generally takes 3 years if one attends full time. Master's programs in law are usually 1 to 2 years in length.

To practice law, the law school graduate must apply to sit for the state bar examination. The examination is given twice yearly (February and July) throughout the country. The application process to sit for the bar is detailed, and the applicant must provide information concerning education, jobs held, all prior addresses, involvement in any lawsuits as a defendant or plaintiff, and character references.

Once completed, the application and the information contained in it are reviewed by the state supreme court (or its committee). Essentially, the character and fitness of the applicant to sit for the bar, and ultimately to practice law in that state, are evaluated.

If the applicant is approved to sit for the bar examination and passes, the individual is issued a license to practice law in the state. At swearing-in ceremonies the attorney takes an oath to, among other things, defend the federal and state constitutions. The lawyer is then licensed to practice law in the state and must comply with state requirements concerning that practice, including types of practice, advertising, license renewal mandates, and professional ethics.

The lawyer who is licensed to practice in a particular state may also want to practice in the federal court system. In some states, such as Illinois, a specific application to the federal court system is necessary to do trial work in the federal courts located in that state. A lawyer may also choose to apply for admission to practice before the U.S. Supreme Court.

IDENTIFYING THE LEGAL PROBLEM

The first task for the nurse is to identify the legal problem that exists. This is important because it helps identify the type of attorney needed and also facilitates early intervention. For example, if a nurse is served with a summons and complaint naming him or her as a defendant in a professional negligence lawsuit, an attorney who concentrates his or her practice (or specializes) in the defense of malpractice suits is necessary. If, in contrast, the nurse employee is concerned about being disciplined by the employer for something that occurred at work, consultation with an attorney with experience in employment law is wise.

HOW TO FIND AN ATTORNEY

Once the legal problem is identified, the next step for the nurse is to find an attorney for the specific purpose of determining whether or not his or her services will be utilized. This is perhaps the most difficult step for the nurse. The local yellow pages, radio and television ads, and the Internet are several sources for identifying attorneys who practice in a particular state. Although readily available, these sources may not be the most efficient ways to locate an attorney.

Other sources that may be helpful, used in conjunction with the above or alone, include:

- Referral from a friend or colleague who has utilized an attorney for the same or similar problem
- Referral from another attorney whose services have been used for other legal advice or services
- Local or state bar associations (many operate lawyer referral services to the public)
- Other professional associations such as The American Association of Nurse Attorneys, and state nurses' associations or organizations
- An attorney who has presented a seminar or presented a paper at a professional meeting
- Information services (directories, special yellow pages) about attorneys available in public libraries or law libraries (located at the local or state courthouse)
- A prepaid legal service plan, if a member
- Legal clinics or legal aid organizations, if low-cost legal services are needed and one is eligible

If the nurse is covered under a professional liability insurance policy and is named in a suit, contacting the insurance carrier is necessary, as discussed in Chapter 5. An attorney will be assigned to the case. Although the nurse may not have control over the attorney who is assigned to the case, he or she can evaluate the attorney with the guidelines below. If the nurse is not comfortable with the attorney, the nurse should discuss this discomfort with the attorney and the insurance company. If the difficulties identified by the nurse cannot be resolved, another attorney can be assigned to the case.

HOW TO SELECT AN ATTORNEY

Once the nurse has identified a potential source for an attorney, determination of *which* attorney will be utilized or retained is next. The selection process can occur either during a face-to-face meeting with the attorney or an initial telephone consultation, although a meeting is preferable. In either case, the attorney may or may not charge a fee for the consultation. This should be clarified by the nurse at the onset of the consultation.

The decision to select a particular attorney is best achieved by formulating certain questions concerning the attorney, the practice, the particular case or situation, the legal work required, and the nurse's role in the case. In addition, the nurse's impressions of the attorney and the ability to work with him or her are also important areas to explore.

These areas are important because the nurse will be paying the attorney to represent him or her in all dealings concerning the legal matter in question. Therefore, selecting an attorney whom the nurse trusts and is comfortable with is just as important as evaluating the attorney's skill and expertise.

The following are sample questions for the nurse to consider.

The Attorney

- How long has the attorney been practicing law?
- How many similar cases has the attorney handled?
- Does the attorney represent individuals? Businesses and organizations? Both?
- If the attorney cannot or will not take the case, can a referral be made?

- When is the best time to contact the attorney during office hours?
- If the case is taken, how does the attorney handle keeping clients abreast of developments (e.g., phone calls, letters)?

The Attorney's Law Practice

- How much will the case and services cost? There are several fee arrangement possibilities listed in Table A–1.
- Will the agreement be placed in writing and signed by both the attorney and the client?
- Will a monthly bill (invoice) be sent indicating the time spent on the case or situation?
- Will the attorney be the only lawyer working on the case or situation? If not, who else will be? What will be the additional cost to the nurse, if any?
- What are the chances of success with the case or situation?
- What strategies will the attorney utilize in the case or situation?
- How long will a resolution of the particular problem take?
- If an appeal is necessary, what additional costs will there be? What additional time frames can be expected? What are the chances of success on appeal?

- If the situation involves criminal law or concerns, will the attorney (or firm) represent the nurse in that case? What additional costs/fees will there be?
- When can the nurse expect the attorney to respond to calls or letters (e.g., within 24 hours, by phone, or by written correspondence)?

The Nurse Client's Role

The nurse plays an important part in the overall success of any legal matter, whether during the initial consultation or during the progression of the case or legal matter. The attorney can do his or her job only if apprised accurately, completely, and honestly about the legal matter. Therefore, the following are questions for the nurse client to explore with the attorney concerning his or her role:

- What information or additional documents does the attorney need, both at the initial meeting and afterward?
- When should the nurse contact the attorney (e.g., when a new development arises, when documents are received)?
- What should the nurse do when anyone in the case or situation contacts the nurse per-

---

TABLE A–1

Legal Fee Arrangements

NAME OF ARRANGEMENT	EXPLANATION
Contingent fee	Used for civil cases in which the nurse is a plaintiff (e.g., when nurse sues employer for defamation); a percentage of money received for client goes to attorney; nurse must clarify if contingent amount to attorney is from gross amount awarded or deducted after expenses (e.g., court costs, subpoena fees); usual amount is $33\frac{1}{3}\%$, but some states regulate this arrangement in certain cases (e.g., professional negligence)
Hourly fee	Based on attorney's fixed hourly rate for any and all legal work, including court appearances, drafting of documents, conferences; out-of-pocket expenses (e.g., court costs, delivery fees) are also billed to client; nurse should clarify if any legal work is billed at a higher rate (e.g., court appearances)
Retainer fee	Utilized alone or in conjunction with hourly fee; nurse pays certain amount to attorney as initial payment on case or to have attorney available for legal work needed (e.g., establishing a patient care clinic); initial retainer will most probably be supplemented by additional retainers
Flat fee/fee for service	Amount is agreed to for services regardless of amount of legal work needed; used in "simple" or uncomplicated matters (e.g., review of documents or basic advance directive); out-of-pocket expenses billed to client

Data from Henry Campbell Black. *Black's Law Dictionary.* 7th Edition. St. Paul, Minn.: West Group, 1999; Barbara Youngberg. *The Risk Manager's Desk Reference.* 2nd Edition. Gaithersburg, Md.: Aspen Publishers, 1998; Lawrence Baum. *American Courts: Process and Policy.* 4th Edition. Boston: Houghton Mifflin, 1998.

sonally (e.g., the attorney for another party, the employer)?

- How can the nurse help the attorney with the legal work needed (e.g., gathering information, supplying addresses)?

If the nurse is unclear about what to do in a particular situation after a case has been instituted or an attorney retained, the best approach is to contact the attorney before anything is done. Something that the nurse sees as unrelated to the case or legal situation at the time may turn out to be intertwined in it. Therefore, seeking preventive advice from the nurse's attorney is always judicious.

The Nurse's Impressions/Ability to Work with the Attorney

This aspect of the selection process is very important, as discussed earlier. During the initial meeting or telephone conversation, the nurse should rely on what he or she thinks and feels about the attorney. For example:

- Is the attorney clear in his or her explanation of the legal issues involved in the case or situation?
- Is the attorney's full attention given to the nurse during that time or does the attorney allow other clients or staff to interrupt for nonemergent matters?
- Does the attorney make the nurse feel at ease and appear interested in the case or legal situation?
- Does the attorney "pressure" the nurse into making a decision about utilizing the attorney or provide time for the nurse to think about the choice?
- Does the attorney interact with the nurse in a respectful manner?

If the nurse client decides to choose the attorney to represent him or her, then that agreement can be formalized and finalized. If, however, the nurse is not comfortable with the attorney, or wishes to explore other attorneys, the nurse should inform the attorney of that decision. The nurse can simply state that some time is needed to think about the information received before deciding whether to retain the attorney's services. A call to the attorney concerning a decision not to retain his or her services is helpful to the attorney so that the consultation file can be closed.

PROFESSIONAL RESPONSIBILITIES OF THE ATTORNEY

An attorney, like any other professional, must conform his or her conduct to ethical rules that govern the practice of law and the representation of clients. The rules are included in a model Code of Professional Responsibility adopted by the American Bar Association (ABA). Each state has adopted its own code of ethics. Those codes either adopt the entire ABA model code or are based on it. In either case, the state code is enforced by the state supreme court's disciplinary committee or commission.

The code of ethics establishes standards of conduct and lists prohibited conduct. If a violation of the code allegedly occurs, a complaint can be made to the committee or commission. The committee or commission investigates the complaint and, if appropriate, determines sanctions against the lawyer after a disciplinary proceeding or other procedures are completed.

Areas included in the code of interest to the nurse client include the requirements of:

- Maintaining confidentiality between the attorney and client with exceptions clearly delineated
- Representing the client fully, independently, zealously, and within the bounds of the law
- Avoiding conflicts of interest between a client and others, including the attorney himself or herself
- Withdrawing from representation of a client only in identified situations, with protections afforded the client

The last provision of a state code of ethics is important. Although the nurse client is able to terminate the attorney-client relationship at any time, the attorney is not able to do so. Rather, the attorney can end the representation only when, as examples, the client asks the attorney to do something illegal (e.g., destroy evidence) or utilize the judicial system inappropriately (e.g., to harass someone or obstruct justice). If a case is pending in court or other legal proceeding (e.g., administrative action), withdrawal can occur only with permission of the court or hearing officer.

Regardless of the reasons for the withdrawal and when it takes place, the attorney must make every effort to avoid "unduly prejudicing" the client. This includes, of course, providing adequate notice to the client and the court or other tribunal and providing the client with his or her file, along with any original documents.

When Difficulties Arise between Attorney and Client

If the nurse client experiences problems with the selected attorney, a frank discussion with him or her should be initiated by the nurse. It is hoped that identifying the problems will aid in their resolution. If not, the nurse should terminate the relationship and obtain the services of another attorney if the legal case/situation has not been resolved.

If the nurse believes the attorney may have violated any of the ethical rules, the attorney should be reported to the state disciplinary committee or commission. In addition, if the nurse believes the attorney handled the case or situation negligently, then consultation with an attorney who handles professional liability suits against attorneys is advised. Moreover, if the attorney's conduct violates any criminal laws (e.g., personal use of the client's money, forging a signature on a settlement check), then contacting the police or state's attorney or state's attorney general's office is advisable.

Guidelines for Legal Research

The nurse who takes a course in law and nursing or who seeks out legal information for any other reason needs to have a basic understanding of legal research so that a particular law, regulation, or case can be easily located. Law libraries are organized differently than other libraries with which the nurse is familiar. In addition, legal research is also unique in comparison with the research the nurse does when preparing a paper or obtaining information for his or her clinical research project.

Although the most comprehensive source of legal information can be found in a law library (e.g., at a law school or court building), some legal references may also be found in local public libraries (e.g., state statute books, texts). Regardless of location, certain basic information is necessary.

LEGAL REFERENCES

Many types of legal references are helpful when one is doing legal research. Similar to nursing research, the sources can be described as *primary* and *secondary*. Obviously the use of primary sources is preferred and more scholarly than the use of secondary sources. In fact, in the law, relying on secondary sources can be disastrous because laws and case decisions can and do change on a regular basis.

Some of the more common primary sources are listed in Table B–1.

Secondary sources are those that enhance the primary sources. Some of the more common ones are listed in Table B–2.

UNDERSTANDING LEGAL CITATIONS

In Table B–1, examples of statute and case citations are listed. Citations must also be understood to find the specific case or statute of interest to the nurse. Samples of statute citations are listed

in Table B–3, and examples of case citations in Table B–4.

It should be noted that the researcher may see both the "official" and "unofficial" reporting citations for a case in the citation. If so, the researcher can find the same case using either reporting system available. The following case citation gives both the state (official) and the regional (unofficial) citation:

> *Prairie v. University of Chicago Hospitals,* 298 Ill. App. 3d 316, 698 N.E.2d 611 (1998).

Also, the history of a case is seen in the case citation. The following citation tells the researcher the path the case has taken in the various courts of the judicial system:

> *Kevorkian v. Arnett,* 939 F. Supp. 725 (C.D. Cal.), *cert. denied sub nom. Lundgren v. Doe,* 117 S. Ct. 413 (1996), *vacated & appeal dismissed,* 136 F.3d 1360 (9th Cir. 1998).

ANALYZING STATUTES AND CASE DECISIONS

Statutes

When you analyze a statute, it is important to read the act in its entirety to get an overview of its intent and purpose. Most statutes contain the following sections: Title, Legislative Purpose, Definitions, Exceptions, and Penalties for Violations of the act. In addition, most statutes have cross-references, additional references, and cases decided under the act that can help with a more in-depth understanding of the act.

Because laws can change frequently, the nurse must also check the back of each volume of the statute book being used for the "pocket part." The pocket part is published in a thin, tissue-paper supplement that fits into the back cover of each volume. If many changes have occurred, a paperback supplement might be used in place of the

TABLE B–1

Selected Primary Legal References

NAME	STATE/ FEDERAL	INFORMATION INCLUDED	SAMPLE CITATION
United States Code (U.S.C.)	F	Laws of federal gov't	42 U.S.C. § 1983
Code of Federal Regulations (C.F.R.)	F	Regulations promulgated by rulemaking to enforce federal laws	40 C.F.R. § 405.53 (1980)
Illinois Compiled Statutes (ILCS)	S	Laws of the state of Illinois	401 ILCS 50/4 (1989 & supplement)
Illinois Administrative Code (IL. Adm. Code)	S	Regulations promulgated by rulemaking to enforce state laws	68 IL. Adm. Code 1220.110 et seq.
United States Supreme Court Decisions (U.S.)	F	Supreme Court opinions	Roe v. Wade, 410 U.S. 113 (1973)
Federal Reporter (F.2d)	F	U.S. District Courts of Appeals Decisions, Second Series	Kranson v. Valley Crest Nursing Home, 755 F.2d 46 (3rd Cir. 1985)
Northwestern Reporter (N.W.2d)	S	Unofficial reporting system for most state appellate decisions in region covered (North and South Dakota, Nebraska, Iowa, Minnesota, Wisconsin, and Michigan), Second Series	In re Kowakski, 382 N.W.2d 862 (Minn. Ct. App. 1986)

Data from *The Bluebook: A Uniform System of Citation.* 16th Edition. Cambridge, Mass.: Harvard Law Review Association, 1996.

TABLE B–2

Selected Secondary Legal Resources

NAME AND PUBLISHER	INFORMATION INCLUDED	SAMPLE CITATION
Disabilities and the Law— West Group	Textbook on disabilities law	Laura Rothstein, Disabilities and the Law (2d ed. 1997)
Annals of Heart Law—Loyola University Chicago School of Law, Institute for Health Law and National Health Lawyers Association	Articles on health law	Kathleen Vyborny, *Legal and Political Issues Facing Telemedicine,* 5 Annals of Health Law 61–119 (1996)
Personnel Law—Prentice-Hall	Textbook on personnel law	Kenneth Sovereign, Personnel Law (4th ed. 1998)
Medicare and Medicaid Guide—Commerce Clearing House (CCH)	Unofficial compilation of materials from Medicare and Medicaid (also called a "service")	Medicare & Medicaid Guide (CCH) § 1401

Data from *The Bluebook: A Uniform System of Citation.* 16th Edition. Cambridge, Mass.: Harvard Law Review Association, 1996.

TABLE B–3

Sample Statute Citations

NAME	VOL. NO.	TITLE OF SET	SECTION NO.	YEAR
Administrative Procedure Act (F)	5	U.S.C.	552 et seq.	(1946, as amended)
Illinois Nursing and Advanced Practice Nursing Act (S)	225	ILCS	65/5-1	(1998)

TABLE B–4				
Sample Case Citations				
NAME	VOL.	REPORTING SET/PAGE	COURT INFO.	COMMENTS
Miller v. Spicer	822	F. Supp. 158	(D. Del. 1993)	Miller is the plaintiff, Spicer the defendant
In re Custody of a Minor	434	N.E.2d 601	(Mass., 1982)	"In re" means "in the matter of," when court decides a matter without formally including adversarial parties
People v. Wassil	658	A.2d 548	(Conn., 1995)	In criminal cases, the plaintiff is always the people of the state, as represented by the state's attorney or attorney general

"pocket part." The pocket part or supplement contains any recent changes in the laws contained in the volume (including new court decisions interpreting the particular statute) and must be consulted before research is considered complete.

Cases

Most case decisions are reported in a standard format. The arrangement of the information may vary somewhat, but most often includes:

- The case name
- Case citation information (e.g., the docket number, date of decision, name of court rendering decision)
- A brief case summary, which informs the reader of the facts of the case, lower court decision(s), and how the case came before the deciding court (judicial history)
- "Headnote" designations, which inform the reader of the specific points of law discussed in the case
- The names of the attorneys for each party in the case, the judge(s) who heard and decided the case, and the names of any judge(s) who did not take part in the decision
- The text of the opinion, which includes the facts, identification of the issue(s), the reasoning utilized, the court's decision/holding on each issue, and the disposition of the case (e.g., reversal of the lower court decision, remand to the lower court with specific instructions)
- The text of any concurring and dissenting opinion(s) of the other judges (e.g., at appellate or state or federal supreme court level)

No case decision can be relied on until it is checked to determine if it is still "good law." Changes in court decisions can occur when, for example, an appellate court (or other higher court) reverses a lower court decision, or an administrative agency decision is judicially reviewed by the appropriate state or federal court.

At one time, the process of checking case decisions was done by hand and was the only method for ensuring the status of a case. The process was called "shepardizing" after the publisher of the soft-cover books that were consulted (*Shepard's Case Citations*). With this method, still used today when computer-assisted legal research is not available, the researcher must use the current case citation and check it in all of the *Shepard's* volumes *after* the date of the decision for guidance as to the case's current status.

COMPUTER-BASED LEGAL RESEARCH

The use of computers and computer software has revolutionized legal research. The Internet provides a myriad of free information about, for example, U.S. Supreme Court decisions, federal and state court decisions, legislation and administrative rules passed by respective state legislatures and Congress, and legal journal articles. Some of the addresses for various sites providing this information appear in Appendix C.

It is important for the reader to note, however, that not all Internet sites can be relied upon as accurate and up-to-date. Regardless of how legal research is conducted on the Internet, the same principles that apply to more "traditional" legal research (e.g., making sure the case or statute under consideration has not been amended or over-turned, using current secondary sources) also apply to computer-based research.

Accurate and up-to-date information can be obtained through subscribed-to legal databases of-fered by legal publishing houses such as Lexis Publishing and West Group, to name a few. In addition, texts and self-help books on computer-based legal research can help guide the researcher to appropriate Internet Web sites.

Annotated List of Selected Useful Internet Sites

The following World Wide Web sites are just a few of the many available sites containing valuable information for the reader in the areas of law, ethics, and nursing practice. Every attempt has been made to ensure the accuracy of the web addresses. However, as the reader knows, the web is changing every day. As a result, the reader may need to use additional searches to locate these addresses.

In the interest of saving space, the following addresses do not include an essential part of a web address: http://www. Please be certain to add this part of the address to those listed before searching for them.

NAME OF ORGANIZATION	WORLD WIDE WEB ADDRESS	COMMENTS
American Nurses Association	nursingworld.org/	Updates on national issues affecting nursing; cases; ANA position statements; articles; links to other web sites
American Society of Healthcare Risk Management	ashrm.org/	Useful information on risk management principles; cases
Centers for Disease Control and Prevention	cdc.gov/	Statistics; articles; prevention guidelines; searches
Department of Health and Human Services	os.dhhs.gov/	Statistics; research reports; specific disease information; searches; links to other web sites
Government Printing Office (GPO)	access.gpo.gov/	Link to GPO; access connects to Federal Register, Congressional bills, Congressional records; lists documents of federal government and how to obtain
Joint Commission on Accreditation of Health Care Organizations (JCAHO)	jcaho.org/	Information about JCAHO; can register complaints; publications; articles
Journal of the American Medical Association	jama.ama-assn.org/	Articles in JAMA
National Association of School Nurses	nasn.org/	Information about NASA; searches; association statements on practice issues
National Council of State Boards of Nursing	ncsbn.org/	Information about council; searches for nurse practice acts; articles; updates on national issues in nursing
National Institute for Occupational Health and Safety (NIOSH)	cdc.gov/niosh/	Occupational safety and health information; NIOSH ALERTS; case studies; links to other web sites
National Institutes of Health	nih.gov/	Health information; special reports; links to other web sites
National League for Nursing (NLN)	nln.org/	Information on nursing practice, education, and research
Occupational Safety and Health Administration (OSHA)	osha.gov/	Compliance directives; OSHA standards; press releases; searches
Sigma Theta Tau National Honor Society Of Nursing	stti-web.iupui.edu/	Virginia Henderson Library (searches); journal service; links to other web sites
U.S. House of Representatives	house.gov/	Information about House and members; text and status of bills; searches; links to other web sites with text of laws
U.S. Senate	senate.gov/	Information about Senate and members; text and status of bills; searches; links to other web sites
U.S. Supreme Court	law.cornell.edu/supct.table.html	Supreme Court decisions by topic or party name; searches

Index

Note: Page numbers in *italics* refer to illustrations, page numbers followed by a t refer to tables.